T0219413

At a Glance

Pocket Atlas of Human Anatomy

Founded by Heinz Feneis

Wolfgang Dauber, MD
Institute of Anatomy
University of Tuebingen
Tuebingen, Germany

5th revised edition

907 illustrations

Thieme
Stuttgart · New York

Translator: Stephanie Kramer, BA, Dipl Trans, IoL, Berlin, Germany

Illustrator: Professor Gerhard Spitzer

1st German edition 1967, published under the title *Anatomische Bildnomenklatur*

2nd German edition 1970	7th German edition 1993
1st Italian edition 1970	2nd Dutch edition 1993
3rd German edition 1972	2nd Greek edition 1994
1st Polish edition 1973	3rd English edition 1994
4th German edition 1974	3rd Spanish edition 1994
1st Spanish edition 1974	3rd Danish edition 1995
1st Japanese edition 1974	1st Russian edition 1996
1st Portuguese edition	2nd Czech edition 1996
1976	3rd Swedish edition 1996
1st English edition 1976	2nd Turkish edition 1997
1st Danish edition 1977	8th German edition 1998
1st Swedish edition 1979	1st Indonesian edition
1st Czech edition 1981	1998
5th German edition 1982	1st Basque edition 1998
2nd Danish edition 1983	3rd Danish edition 1999
2nd Japanese edition 1983	4th Spanish edition 2000
1st Dutch edition 1984	4th English edition 2000
2nd Swedish edition 1984	2nd Chinese edition 2001
2nd English edition 1985	3rd Turkish edition 2001
1st French edition 1986	4th Swedish edition 2001
2nd Polish edition 1986	2nd Portuguese edition
6th German edition 1988	2002
2nd Italian edition 1989	4th Polish edition 2003
2nd Spanish edition 1989	2nd Russian edition 2005
1st Turkish edition 1990	3rd Greek edition 2005
1st Greek edition 1991	5th Spanish edition 2006
1st Chinese edition 1991	4th Dutch edition 2006
1st Icelandic edition 1992	5th Swedish edition 2006
3rd Polish edition 1992	1st Korean edition 2006

Library of Congress Cataloging-in-Publication Data is available from the publisher.

This book is an authorized and revised translation of the 9th German edition published and copyrighted 2005 by Georg Thieme Verlag, Stuttgart, Germany. Title of the German edition: Feneis' Bild-Lexikon der Anatomie.

Important note: Medicine is an ever-changing science undergoing continual development. Research and clinical experience are continually expanding our knowledge, in particular our knowledge of proper treatment and drug therapy. Insofar as this book mentions any dosage or application, readers may rest assured that the authors, editors, and publishers have made every effort to ensure that such references are in accordance with **the state of knowledge at the time of production of the book.**

Nevertheless, this does not involve, imply, or express any guarantee or responsibility on the part of the publishers in respect to any dosage instructions and forms of applications stated in the book. **Every user is requested to examine carefully** the manufacturers' leaflets accompanying each drug and to check, if necessary in consultation with a physician or specialist, whether the dosage schedules mentioned therein or the contraindications stated by the manufacturers differ from the statements made in the present book. Such examination is particularly important with drugs that are either rarely used or have been newly released on the market. Every dosage schedule or every form of application used is entirely at the user's own risk and responsibility. The authors and publishers request every user to report to the publishers any discrepancies or inaccuracies noticed. If errors in this work are found after publication, errata will be posted at www.thieme.com on the product description page.

© 1976, 2007 Georg Thieme Verlag
Rüdigerstrasse 14, 70469 Stuttgart, Germany
http://www.thieme.de
Thieme New York, 333 Seventh Avenue,
New York, NY 10001, USA
http://www.thieme.com

Typesetting by Hagedorn Kommunikation, Viernheim
Printed in Germany by Appl, Wemding
ISBN-10: 3-13-511205-5 (GTV)
ISBN-13: 978-3-13-511205-3 (GTV)
ISBN-10: 1-58890-558-6 (TNY)
ISBN-13: 978-1-58890-558-1 (TNY)
1 2 3 4 5 6

Preface

The adoption of new official nomenclature by the "Federative Committee on Anatomical Terminology" (FCAT) has made a complete revision of the *Pocket Atlas of Human Anatomy* necessary. In its latest edition, the *Terminologia Anatomica* has incorporated results from more recent studies, mostly from research on the urogenital and central nervous systems. This has greatly expanded the total number of terms.

A number of these findings are derived from experiments on animals. The FCAT has added such findings to the *Terminologia Anatomica* without noting their origins in animal experimentation.

Experience has shown, however, that such findings and their interpretation can initially be applied to human beings only with the greatest caution. Relevant text passages thus alert the reader again to the uncertainty of such terms.

As we had already observed while writing earlier editions of this work, newly added terms have not been annotated by the FCAT. Attempts at obtaining more information from the committee were fruitless, with the result that certain terms remain without further explanation. These are listed in the "Notes" on page 474.

In a welcome revision, the commission has now added an official terminology to the Latin terminology. This simplifies communication between speakers of various languages and makes it more precise. Efforts by the FCAT to establish official definitions of terms that until now have been controversial (e.g., fascia) are equally welcome.

The customary Anglophone numbering of cranial nerves with roman numerals and of spinal nerves, vertebrae, and spinal segments with arabic numerals has been adopted. Otherwise, numbering schemes follow *Terminologia Anatomica.*

As in previous editions, colleagues and students offered comments and suggestions, which for the most part have been incorporated. I would like to thank all of them for their efforts, in particular Dr. C. Walther, for his dedication and perseverance in making informed and knowledgeable suggestions. Because of the wish expressed by students to have the "General Terminology" at the front of the book, I have placed that section at the beginning.

Professor Gerhard Spitzer was responsible once again, as in all previous editions, for designing the illustrations. With characteristic mastery he revised existing drawings, added new ones, and ensured their seamless incorporation into the sequence of illustrations. I owe him my deepest gratitude for his exacting collaborative efforts.

I would like to thank Georg Thieme Verlag and its employees, especially, Ms. Profittlich, Ms. Mauch, and Mr. Zepf, for their patience and understanding and for the harmonious collaboration that went into creating this edition.

Translation of the present edition into English was performed by Stephanie Kramer, who did so with perseverance and skill. My sincere thanks to her and to Gabriele Kuhn for her careful assistance during the completion of this edition.

Wolfgang Dauber

1

1 *GENERAL ANATOMY.*
2 *PARTS OF HUMAN BODY.*
3 **Head.**
4 *Forehead.* Front half of the head; frons. A
5 *Occiput.* Back of the head. B
6 *Temple.* A
7 *Ear.*
8 *Face.* A
9 *Eye.*
10 *Cheek.* C
11 *Nose.*
12 *Mouth.*
13 *Chin.*
14 **Neck.** The superior border of the neck runs along an imaginary line that extends from the inferior margin of the mandible to the mastoid process and continues along the superior nuchal line to the external occipital protuberance. Its inferior border extends from the upper border of the manubrium of the sternum, along the clavicle, over the acromion and the spine of the scapula to the spinous process of C 7. A B
15 **Trunk.** Torso. A B C
16 *Thorax.* The part of the trunk between the neck and the abdomen. It is supported by the skeletal framework of the thoracic cage. The inferior boundary of the thorax is formed by the inferior thoracic aperture and the diaphragm. A
17 *Front of chest.* C
18 *Abdomen.* The part of the trunk bounded by the thorax, the superior border of the wing of the ilium, the inguinal ligament, and the pubic symphysis. A, C
19 *Pelvis.* The part of the trunk bounded by the abdomen and the pelvic diaphragm. The greater and lesser pelvis are divided by the linea terminalis.
20 *Back.* Posterior aspect of the trunk. B
21 **Upper limb.** It consists of the shoulder girdle and the free appendage.
22 *Pectoral girdle; Shoulder girdle.* Its skeletal framework consists of the scapulae and the clavicles. A B
23 *Axilla.* Connective tissue space between the arm and the lateral wall of the thorax. C
24 *Arm.* A
25 *Elbow.*
26 *Forearm.* A
27 *Hand.*
28 *Wrist.* A
29 *Metacarpus.* A
30 *Palm.* A
31 *Dorsum of hand.*
32 *Fingers including thumb.*

33 **Lower limb.** It consists of the pelvic girdle and the free appendage.
34 *Pelvic girdle.* Its supporting skeletal framework consists of the hip bones. C
35 *Buttocks.* B
36 *Hip.* Region of articulation between the pelvis and the free lower limbs. C
37 *Thigh.* A B
38 *Knee.* C
39 *Posterior part of knee.* C
40 *Leg.* A
41 *Calf.* B C
42 *Foot.*
43 *Ankle.* A
44 *Heel.* B
45 *Metatarsus.* A
46 *Sole.* B
47 *Dorsum of foot.* C
48 *Toes.*
49 **Cavities.**
50 *Cranial cavity.*
51 *Thoracic cavity.*
52 *Abdominopelvic cavity.*
53 *Abdominal cavity.*
54 *Pelvic cavity.*

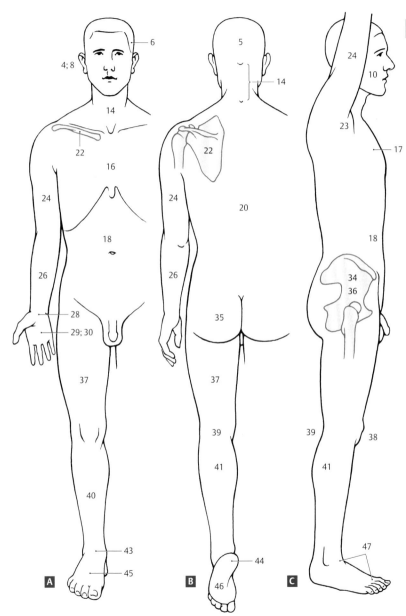

1 *GENERAL TERMS*

2 **Vertical.**

3 **Horizontal.** A

4 **Median.** Located in the median plane.

5 **Coronal.** Located parallel to the coronal suture. A

6 **Sagittal.** Located in parallel anteroposterior planes. A

7 **Right.**

8 **Left.**

9 **Intermediate.** Situated in between two structures or extremes.

10 **Medial.** Located near the midline.

11 **Lateral.** Located away from the median plane.

12 **Anterior.** Located at or near the front.

13 **Posterior.** Located at or near the back.

14 **Ventral.** Located near the front of the body.

15 **Dorsal.** Located near the back of the body.

16 **Frontal.** Pertaining to the forehead; parallel to the forehead.

17 **Occipital.** At or near the back of the head. A

18 **Superior.** Upper; closer to the head.

19 **Inferior.** Lower; closer to the base of the spine.

20 **Cranial.** Situated at or closer to the cranium.

21 **Caudal.** Situated closer to the tail.

22 **Rostral.** Situated toward the beak.

23 **Apical.** Pertaining to the apex; facing the apex.

24 **Basal.** Pertaining to the base, facing the base.

25 **Basilar.** Pertaining to the cranial base; near the cranial base.

26 **Middle.** Located in the middle.

27 **Transverse.** Crosswise; horizontal.

28 **Transverse.** Positioned horizontally.

29 **Longitudinal.** Positioned longitudinally.

30 **Axial.** Located near an axis. Pertaining to the axis, i.e., the second cervical vertebra.

31 **External.** Located on the outer surface.

32 **Internal.** Located on the inner surface.

33 **Luminal.** Pertaining to or located near the lumen.

34 **Superficial.** Located near the surface.

35 **Deep.** Lying further below the surface.

36 **Proximal.** Located near the trunk. B

37 **Distal.** Located away from the trunk. B

38 **Central.** Located in the midpoint.

39 **Peripheral.** Situated away from the center.

40 **Radial.** Pertaining to or located near the radius. B

41 **Ulnar.** Pertaining to or located near the ulna. B

42 **Fibular; Peroneal.** Pertaining or situated near the fibula. B

43 **Tibial.** Pertaining to or situated near the tibia. B

44 **Palmar; Volar.** Pertaining to or situated near the palm of the hand. B

45 **Plantar.** Pertaining to or situated near the sole of the foot. B

46 **Flexor.**

47 **Extensor.**

48 *PLANES, LINES, AND REGIONS.*

49 **Anterior median line.** Vertical midline through the anterior of the trunk. C

50 **Sternal line.** An imaginary line that passes through the lateral border of the sternum. C

51 **Parasternal line.** An imaginary vertical line that runs through a point midway between the sternal and midclavicular lines. C

52 **Midclavicular line.** An imaginary vertical line that passes through the midpoint of the clavicle. C

53 **Mammillary line; Nipple line.** An imaginary line that is sometimes identical to the midclavicular line. C

54 **Anterior axillary line.** An imaginary line that passes through the anterior axillary fold. C

55 **Midaxillary line.** An imaginary line that passes through a point midway between the anterior and posterior axillary lines. C

56 **Posterior axillary line.** An imaginary line that passes through the posterior axillary fold. B C

57 **Scapular line.** An imaginary vertical line that runs through the inferior angle of the scapula. B

58 **Paravertebral line.** An imaginary vertical line that is visible only on radiographs, passing through the ends of the transverse processes. B

59 **Posterior median line.** Vertical midline through the posterior of the trunk.

60 **Frontal planes; Coronal planes.** Planes that are parallel to the surface of the forehead and at right angles to the median plane and a horizontal plane. A

61 **Horizontal planes.** Planes that are at right angles to the median planes and a frontal plane. A

62 **Sagittal planes.** Planes at right angles to the frontal and horizontal planes. A

63 *Median plane; Median sagittal plane.* Plane of symmetry that divides the body into two equal halves. A

64 *Paramedian planes.* Planes that are parallel to, to the immediate right and left of, the median plane. A

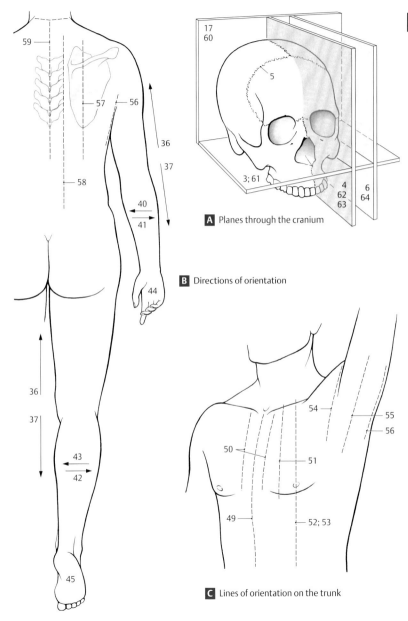

A Planes through the cranium

B Directions of orientation

C Lines of orientation on the trunk

1

1 **Transverse planes.** These include the following specific horizontal planes. A

2 *Transpyloric plane.* Horizontal plane that passes through the midpoint between the upper margin of the pubic symphysis and upper border of the manubrium of the sternum. A

3 *Subcostal plane.* Horizontal plane through the inferior margin of the tenth costal cartilage. A

4 *Supracristal plane.* Horizontal plane through the uppermost point of the iliac crest. It transects the vertebral column at the level of the fourth lumbar spinous process. A

5 *Intertubercular plane.* Horizontal plane that transects the tubercula of the iliac crest. A

6 *Interspinous plane.* Horizontal plane that passes through the anterior superior iliac spines. A

7 **Regions of head.**

8 **Frontal region.** Forehead region. B

9 **Parietal region.** Region overlying the parietal bone. B C

10 **Occipital region.** Region overlying the occipital bone. B C

11 **Temporal region.** Region overlying the squamous part of the temporal bone. B C

12 **Auricular region.** Region around the ear. A

13 **Mastoid region.** Region overlying the mastoid process. B C

14 **Facial region.** Anatomical regions of the face.

15 *Suprapalpebral sulcus.* Groove located above the upper eyelid. B

16 *Orbital region.* Area involving the orbit. B

17 *Infrapalpebral sulcus.* Groove located below the lower eyelid. B

18 *Buccal region.* Cheek area. B

20 *Parotid region.* Region overlying the parotid gland and the masseter muscle. B

21 *[[Retromandibular fossa]].* Fossa extending medially along the ramus of the mandible to behind the temporomandibular joint. It contains the parotid gland and veins.

22 *Zygomatic region.* Region about the zygomatic bone. B

23 *Nasal region.* Region about the nose. B

24 *Nasolabial sulcus.* Groove that extends from the ala of the nose to the labial commissure. B

25 *Oral region.* Area around the oral fissure. B

26 *Mentolabial sulcus.* Mentolabial furrow. B

27 *Mental region.* Chin area. B

28 **Regions of neck.** B

29 **Anterior cervical region; Anterior triangle.** Triangular region bounded by the midline of the neck, the anterior border of the sternocleidomastoid muscle, and the inferior margin of the mandible.

30 *Submandibular triangle.* Triangular region bounded by the mandible and the two bellies of the digastric muscle. B

31 *Carotid triangle.* Triangular region bounded by the sternocleidomastoid muscle, the posterior belly of the digastric muscle, and the superior belly of the omohyoid muscle. B

32 *Muscular triangle; Omotracheal triangle.* Triangular region bounded by the midline, the anterior border of the sternocleidomastoid muscle, and the superior belly of the omohyoid muscle. B

33 *Submental triangle.* Triangular region below the chin between the hyoid bone and the two anterior bellies of the digastric muscle. B

34 **Sternocleidomastoid region.** Region overlying the sternocleidomastoid muscle. B

35 *Lesser supraclavicular fossa.* Small hollow between the origins on the sternum and the clavicle of the sternocleidomastoid muscle. B

36 **Lateral cervical region; Posterior triangle.** Triangular region bounded by the clavicle, the anterior border of the trapezius muscle, and the posterior border of the sternocleidomastoid muscle. B

37 *Omoclavicular triangle, Subclavian triangle.* Triangular region limited by the clavicle and the sternocleidomastoid and omohyoid muscles. B

38 *Greater supraclavicular fossa.* Depression in the skin overlying the omoclavicular triangle. B

39 **Posterior cervical region.** C

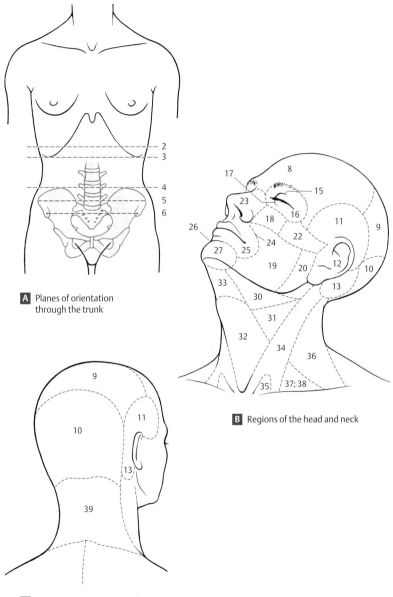

A Planes of orientation through the trunk

B Regions of the head and neck

C Head and posterior cervical regions

1

1 **Anterior and lateral thoracic regions.**

2 **Presternal region.** Region in front of the sternum. C

3 **Infraclavicular fossa (Mohrenheim's fossa).** Depression in the skin overlying the clavipectoral triangle. C

4 **Clavipectoral triangle; Deltopectoral triangle.** Triangular region bounded by the deltoid muscle, the pectoralis major muscle, and the clavicle. C

5 **Pectoral region.** The area overlying the pectoralis major muscle. C

6 *Lateral pectoral region.* Region lateral to the mammary and inframammary regions. C

7 *Mammary region.* The area pertaining to the breast. C

8 *Inframammary region.* The area below the mammary region. C

9 **Axillary region.** Region between both axillary folds. A

10 **Axillary fossa.** A

11 **Abdominal regions.**

12 **Hypochondrium.** Region lateral to the midclavicular line and between the pectoral region and the subcostal plane. C

13 **Epigastric region; Epigastric fossa.** Area below the pectoral region and between the two midclavicular lines and the subcostal plane. C

14 **Flank; Lateral region.** Region lateral to the midclavicular line between the subcostal plane and the supracristal plane. C

15 **Umbilical region.** Region bounded by the two midclavicular lines, the subcostal plane, and the supracristal plane. C

16 **Groin; Inguinal region.** Region lateral to the midclavicular line between the supracristal plane and the inguinal ligament. C

17 **Pubic region.** Region bounded by the two midclavicular lines, the supracristal plane, and the inguinal ligament. C

18 **Regions of back.**

19 **Vertebral region.** Strip overlying the vertebral column. B

20 **Sacral region.** Region overlying the sacrum. B

21 *Coccygeal foveola.* Small depression overlying the coccyx.

22 **Scapular region.** Region overlying the scapula. B

23 **Infrascapular region.** Area between the scapular region and the lumbar region. B

24 **Lumbar region.** Area between the iliac crest and the infrascapular region. B

25 **Perineal region.**

26 **Anal triangle.** Region around the anus that is bordered anteriorly by an imaginary line connecting the two ischial tuberosities. D

27 **Urogenital region.** Region around the perineum that is located anterior to an imaginary line connecting the two ischial tuberosities. D

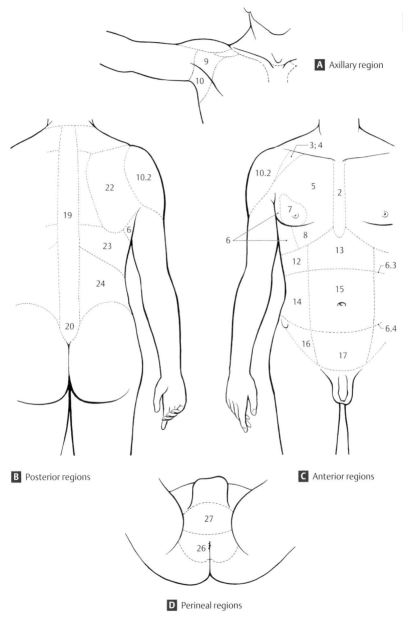

A Axillary region

B Posterior regions

C Anterior regions

D Perineal regions

1

1   **Regions of upper limb.**

2   **Deltoid region.** Region overlying the deltoid muscle. A B

3   **Brachial region.** Arm region.

4   *Anterior region of arm.* B

5   Lateral bicipital groove. B

6   Medial bicipital groove. B

7   *Posterior region of arm.* A

8   **Cubital region.** Elbow region.

9   *Anterior region of elbow.* B

10   *Cubital fossa.* A

11   *Posterior region of elbow.* A

12   **Antebrachial region.** Forearm region.

13   *Anterior region of forearm.* B

14   *Posterior region of forearm.* A

15   *Radial border; Lateral border.*

16   *Ulnar border; Medial border.*

17   **Hand region.**

18   *Carpal region.* Region about the wrist.

19   *Anterior region of wrist.* Anterior (flexor) surface of the wrist. A

20   *Posterior region of wrist.* Posterior (extensor) surface of the wrist. B

21   *Dorsum of hand.* B

22   *Palm; Palmar region.* A

23   *Thenar eminence.* Ball of the thumb.

24   *Hypothenar eminence.* Ball of the little finger.

25   *Metacarpal region.*

26   *Digits of hand;* Fingers including thumb.

27   *Thumb.*

28   *Index finger.*

29   *Middle finger.*

30   *Ring finger.*

31   *Little finger.*

32   *Palmar surfaces of fingers.* Flexor surfaces of the fingers.

33   *Dorsal surfaces of fingers.* Extensor surfaces of the fingers.

34   **Regions of lower limb.**

35   **Gluteal region.** Region overlying the gluteal muscles. A

36   *Intergluteal cleft; Natal cleft.* Anal cleft. Indentation between the buttocks.

37   *Gluteal fold.* Fold passing over the gluteus maximus muscle that forms the inferior boundary of the buttocks when the hip joint is extended. A

38   **Hip region.**

39   **Femoral region.** Thigh region.

40   *Anterior region of thigh.* B

41   *Femoral triangle.* Triangular region bounded by the inguinal ligament, the sartorius muscle, and the gracilis muscle. B

42   *Posterior region of thigh.* A

43   **Knee region.**

44   *Anterior region of knee.* B

45   *Posterior region of knee.* A

46   *Popliteal fossa.* A

47   **Leg region.**

48   *Anterior region of leg.* B

49   *Posterior region of leg.* A

50   *Sural region.* Calf region. A

51   *Anterior talocrural region; Anterior ankle region.* Region anterior to the talocrural joint. B

52   *Posterior talocrural region; Posterior ankle region.* Region posterior to the talocrural joint. A

53   *Lateral retromalleolar region.* Region posterior to the lateral malleolus. A

54   *Medial retromalleolar region.* Region anterior to the medial malleolus.

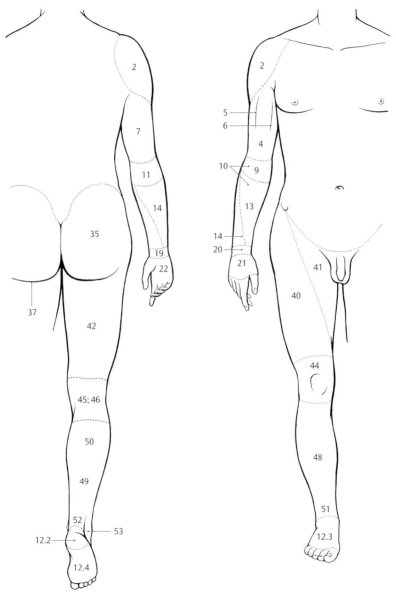

A Posterior regions

B Anterior regions

1

1 **Foot region.**

2 *Heel region.*

3 *Dorsum of foot; Dorsal region of foot.*

4 *Sole; Plantar region.*

5 *Lateral border of foot; Fibular border of foot; Peroneal border of foot.*

6 *Medial border of foot; Tibial border of foot.*

7 *Longitudinal arch of foot.* The longitudinal arch consists of two parts.

8 *Lateral part.* It extends from the calcaneal tuberosity over the cuboid to the heads of the fourth and fifth metatarsals. C

9 *Medial part.* It extends from the calcaneal tuberosity over the talus, navicular, and three cuneiform bones to the heads of the first three metatarsals. C

10 *Proximal transverse arch of foot.* Transverse arch of the midfoot, which is composed of the navicular, cuneiform, and cuboid. It reaches its highest point below the cuneiform bones. I, II, and III. A

11 *Distal transverse arch of foot.* Transverse arch of the forefoot, which is composed of the first five metatarsals. B

12 *Ankle region.* Anatomically: the region about the tarsus. Clinically: hindfoot, consisting of the talus and calcaneus; midfoot, consisting of the remaining tarsal bones and corresponding soft tissues.

13 *Metatarsal region.* Anatomically: the region about the metatarsus. Clinically: forefoot, consisting of the metatarsals, phalanges, and the soft tissues. C

14 *Digits of foot; Toes.* C

15 *Great toe (I).*

16 *Second toe (II), Third toe (III), Fourth toe (IV).*

17 *Little toe; Fifth toe (V).*

18 *Plantar surfaces of toes.*

19 *Dorsal surfaces of toes.*

20 SYSTEMIC ANATOMY.

21 BONES; SKELETAL SYSTEM.

22 **Bony part.**

23 *Cortical bone.* Superficial layer formed by the outer circumferential lamellae.

24 *Compact bone.* Dense bony substance formed by osteons.

25 *Spongy bone; Trabecular bone.* Loosely organized bone substance with interstices filled with bone marrow.

26 **Cartilaginous part (of the skeleton).**

27 **Membranous part (of the skeleton).**

28 *Periosteum.* Outer sheath consisting of two layers that invests the bone tissue, gives attachment to tendons and ligaments, and nourishes the outer vessels of the bone.

29 *Perichondrium.* It transitions into cartilage without a clear border between the two.

30 **Axial skeleton.** Vertebral column, ribs, and sternum.

31 **Appendicular skeleton.** Bones of the limbs.

32 **Long bone.** Long bone, e.g., the fibula.

33 **Short bone.** Short bone, e.g., the carpal bones.

34 **Flat bone.** Flat bone, e.g., the parietal bone.

35 **Irregular bone.** Irregular bone, e.g., the sphenoid.

36 **Pneumatized bone.** Bone that contains pneumatized cells, e.g., the ethmoid.

37 **Sesamoid bone.** Bone embedded in tendons or ligaments that acts as a shock absorber.

38 **Diaphysis.** Shaft of a bone.

39 **Epiphysis.** End of a long bone involved in growth during development stages.

40 *Epiphysial cartilage.*

41 *Epiphysial plate; Growth plate.* Zone of cartilage between the diaphysis and the epiphysis that is responsible for longitudinal bone growth.

42 *Epiphysial line.* Line visible on radiographs and in sections of bone that marks the former site of the epiphysial plate.

43 **Metaphysis.** Zone of growth of the diaphysis toward the epiphysis.

44 **Apophysis.** Part of an epiphysis that arises from its own ossification center, e.g., the greater trochanter.

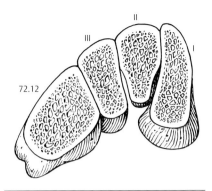

A Proximal transverse arch of the foot, anterior view

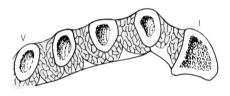

B Distal transverse arch of the foot, anterior view

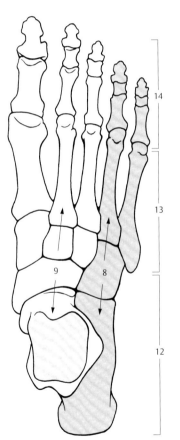

C Bones of the foot, superior view

1

1 **Tuber; Tuberosity.** Roundish, bony protuberance, e.g., the ischial tuberosity.

2 **Tubercle.** Small bony protuberance, e.g., the lesser tubercle.

3 **Tuberosity.** Roughened area on the external surface of a bone, e.g., the masseteric tuberosity.

4 **Eminence.** Elongated protuberance, e.g., the cruciform eminence.

5 **Process.** Bony process, e.g., the transverse process of a vertebra.

6 **Condyle.** Articular eminence, e.g., the condyle of the humerus.

7 **Epicondyle.** Bony projection on a condyle, e.g., the medial epicondyle of the humerus.

8 **Crest; Ridge.** Bony ridge or crest, e.g., the iliac crest.

9 **Line.** Bony line or ridge, e.g., the linea aspera.

10 **Notch.** Indentation or recess, e.g., the acetabular notch.

11 **Fossa.** Depression, e.g., the cubital fossa.

12 **Groove.** Trench, furrow, e.g., the carotid groove.

13 **Articular surface.** Surface of a joint.

14 **Medullary cavity; Marrow cavity.**

15 **Endosteum.** Medullary cavity lining that is similar to periosteum.

16 **Yellow bone marrow.** Yellow, fatty bone marrow.

17 **Red bone marrow.** Red, hematopoietic bone marrow.

18 **Nutrient foramen.** Opening of the nutrient canal at the surface of the bone.

19 **Nutrient canal.** Canal for the passage of vessels nourishing the bone.

20 **Ossification center.** Site during bone development for the onset of ossification of bones preformed in cartilage.

21 *Primary ossification center.* Onset of ossification in a cartilaginous part of a bone, e.g., the diaphysis in long bones. The epiphyses initially remain cartilaginous.

22 *Secondary ossification center.* Center that appears later than the primary ossification center, e.g., the epiphyses of long bones.

23 *JOINTS; ARTICULAR SYSTEM.*

24 **Bony joints.**

25 *Synarthrosis.* Articulation in which the bones are connected by fibrous connective tissue or cartilage.

26 *Fibrous joint.* Articulation in which two bones are joined by tough connective tissue consisting of collagen fibers or occasionally elastic fibers.

27 Syndesmosis. Ligamentous articulation in which two bones are joined by connective tissue usually consisting of parallel collagen or elastic fibers.

28 Gomphosis; Socket. Joint at the insertion of a tooth in the dental alveoli.

29 Interosseous membrane. Sheet of connective tissue consisting of tough collagen fibers that joins two bones.

30 Suture. Special type of syndesmosis.

31 Plane suture. Connection between bones in a plane, e.g., between the zygomatic bone and the maxilla.

32 Squamous suture. Platelike suture, e.g., at the temporal bone.

33 Limbous suture. Special type of squamous suture with interlocking, overlapping borders.

34 Serrate suture. Dentate suture, e.g., the sagittal suture.

35 Denticulate suture. Jagged suture, e.g., the lambdoid suture.

36 Schindylesis. Articulation between a ridge and a groove, e.g., between the vomer and the sphenoid.

37 *Cartilaginous joint.*

38 Synchondrosis. Articulation in which the bones are joined by hyaline cartilage, e.g., epiphysial plates.

39 Symphysis; Secondary cartilaginous joint. Articulation in which the hyaline cartilage at the ends of bones is connected by fibrocartilage, e.g., the pubic symphysis.

40 Epiphysial cartilage; Primary cartilaginous joint. Hyaline cartilage located at the ends of long bones.

41 *Bony union*; *Synostosis.* Union of adjacent bones, e.g., the hip bones.

42 *Synovial joint*; *Diarthrosis.* Joint that has an articular cavity with an inner lining.

43 *Articular surface.*

44 *Articular cavity.*

45 *Articular fossa.*

46 *Articular head.*

47 *Labrum.* Lip of fibrocartilage around the margin of an articular fossa.

48 *Joint capsule*; *Articular capsule.*

1   Fibrous layer; Fibrous membrane. Connective tissue layer of the joint capsule that is often reinforced by ligaments.

2   Synovial membrane; Synovial layer. Inner layer of the joint capsule that is composed of epithelioid cells of mainly two types (lacking a basement membrane) overlying loose connective tissue containing vessels, nerves, and adipose cells.

3   Synovial folds. The synovial folds project into the articular cavity.

4   Synovial villi.

5   Synovial fluid. Lubricant secreted by the synovial membrane that lines the joint capsule.

6   *Articular disc.* Disc that divides the articular cavity into two separate spaces.

7   *Meniscus.* Ringlike articular disc, e.g., in the knee joint.

8   *Ligaments.*

9   Intracapsular ligaments. Ligaments located within the joint capsule, e.g., the cruciate ligaments of the knee joint.

10 Capsular ligaments. Reinforcing ligaments extending from external to within the joint capsule, e.g., the collateral ligaments of the interphalangeal joints of the hand.

11 Extracapsular ligaments. Ligaments located outside of the joint capsule, e.g., the fibular collateral ligament of the knee joint.

12 *Articular recess.* Convexity in the joint capsule, e.g., the subpopliteal recess.

13 *Simple joint.* Articulation formed by only two bones, e.g., the hip joint.

14 *Complex joint.* Joint that consists of more than two bones, e.g., the wrist joint.

15 *Plane joint.* Joint in which the articular surfaces are nearly level, e.g., the zygapophysial joints.

16 *Cylindrical joint.* Collective term for the following uniaxial joints.

17 Pivot joint. Joints such as the proximal and distal radioulnar joints.

18 Hinge joint. Joint such as the humeroulnar joint.

19 *Bicondylar joint.* Joint that has a transverse main axis and an axis parallel to the longitudinal axis of the skeleton, e.g., the knee joint.

20 *Saddle joint.* Joint with two axes, e.g., the metacarpophalangeal joint of the thumb.

21 *Condylar joint*; *Ellipsoid joint.* Joint with two axes such as the wrist joint.

22 *Ball and socket joint*; *Spheroidal joint.* Multiaxial joint such as the shoulder joint.

23 Cotyloid joint; enarthrosis. Spheroidal joint such as the hip joint.

24 *Amphiarthrosis.* Inflexible joint. Joint in which motion is limited by a tight joint capsule and ligaments, e.g., the sacroiliac joint.

25 **Abduction.** Movement to lateral, away from the body.

26 **Adduction.** Movement toward the body.

27 **Lateral rotation; External rotation.** Outward rotation around a longitudinal axis.

28 **Medial rotation; Internal rotation.** Inward rotation around a longitudinal axis.

29 **Circumduction.** Circular movement, e.g., the motion of the arm in the shoulder joint.

30 **Flexion.** Bending the trunk or limbs.

31 **Extension.** Straightening the trunk or limbs.

32 **Pronation.** Rotational movement of the forearm so that the dorsum of the hand is facing upward. Raising the lateral margin of the foot.

33 **Supination.** Rotation of the forearm so that the palm of the hand is facing upward Raising the medial margin of the foot.

34 **Opposition.** Placing the thumb in opposition to the fingers; the little finger can also be slightly opposed.

35 **Reposition.** Returning to the original position or site.

36 ***MUSCLES; MUSCULAR SYSTEM.***

37 **Head.** Head of a muscle.

38 **Belly.** Belly of a muscle.

39 **Attachment.**

40 **[[Origin]]**

41 **Fixed end.** Part of the skeleton that remains fixed.

42 **Mobile end.** Part of the skeleton being moved.

43 **Fusiform muscle.** Spindle-shaped **muscle.**

44 **Flat muscle.**

45 **Straight muscle.**

46 **Triangular muscle.**

47 **Quadrate muscle.**

48 **Two-bellied muscle.**

49 **Two-headed muscle.**

50 **Three-headed muscle.**

51 **Four-headed muscle.**

1

1 **Semipennate muscle; Unipennate muscle.** Muscle that is penniform on one side.

2 **Pennate muscle; Bipennate muscle.** Muscle that is penniform on two sides.

3 **Multipennate muscle.** Muscle with multiple penniform fiber arrangements.

4 **Orbicular muscle.** Circular muscle.

5 **Cutaneous muscle.** Skin muscle.

6 **Abductor muscle.** Muscle that is used in abduction.

7 **Adductor muscle.** Muscle that is used in adduction.

8 **Rotator muscle.** Muscle that causes rotation.

9 **Flexor muscle.**

10 **Extensor muscle.**

11 **Pronator muscle.** Muscle that causes pronation.

12 **Supinator muscle.** Muscle that causes supination.

13 **Opponens muscle.** Muscle that causes opposition.

14 **Sphincter muscle.**

15 **Dilator muscle.** Muscle that causes dilation.

16 **Compartment.** Enclosure of muscle tissue in fascia. A compartment usually envelops a muscle group and is limited by bone and fascia.

17 **Fascia.** Inclusive term for all divisible connective tissue aggregations that can form sheaths and coverings.

18 *Fascia of head and neck.*

19 *Fascia of trunk.* It comprises the following five types of fascia.

20 *Parietal fascia.* Generic term for fascia lining the wall of a body cavity deep to the parietal layer of the serosa. It can occur as an independent structure, e.g., endothoracic fascia.

21 *Extraserosal fascia.* Generic term for all connective tissue structures found between the parietal fascia and the visceral fascia. It usually occurs as ligaments in the pelvis, e.g., the cardinal ligament.

22 *Visceral fascia.* Generic term for fascia that is immediately deep to the visceral layer of the serosa. It can also occur as a separate part of the subserous layer, e.g., with abundant adipose tissue.

23 *Fascia of limbs.*

24 *Fascia of muscles.*

25 Investing layer. Sheath of fascia surrounding a muscle or muscle group. The term also is used for epimysium.

26 Fascia of individual muscle; Muscle sheath. Connective tissue sheath surrounding one muscle.

27 **Epimysium.** External sheath of connective tissue surrounding a muscle.

28 **Perimysium.** Sheath of connective tissue investing bundles of muscle fibers.

29 **Endomysium.** Sheath of connective tissue surrounding a single muscle fiber enclosed in sarcolemma.

30 **Tendon.**

31 *Intermediate tendon.*

32 *Tendinous intersection.* Intermediate tendons of the rectus abdominis muscle.

33 **Aponeurosis.** Flattened tendon.

34 **Tendinous arch.** Thickened arch of fascia that gives origin to muscle fibers.

35 **Muscular trochlea.** Pulleylike structure that changes the direction of pull of a tendon, e.g., the sustentaculum tali, around which the tendon of the flexor hallucis longus muscle passes.

36 **Synovial bursa.** Sac of synovial fluid that reduces friction between muscle and bone.

37 *TENDON SHEATHS AND BURSAE.*

38 **Subcutaneous bursa.** Bursa that is located just beneath the skin.

39 **Submuscular bursa.** Bursa situated deep to a muscle.

40 **Subfascial bursa.** Bursa situated deep to a fascia.

41 **Subtendinous bursa.** Bursa situated deep to a tendon.

42 **Tendon sheath.** It reduces the frictional resistance of a tendon.

43 *Fibrous sheath.* The part of the tendon sheath that is composed of fibrous tissue.

44 *Synovial sheath.* Inner layer of the tendon sheath, which secretes a lubricant.

45 *Mesotendon.* Connection between a tendon and a tendon sheath that resembles a mesentery and contains vessels.

1 *CARDIOVASCULAR SYSTEM.*

2 **Blood vessel.**

3 **Arteriolovenular anastomosis; Arteriovenous anastomosis.** Intercommunication between an artery and a vein.

4 **Artery.**

5 **Nutrient artery.** Artery that supplies tissues with nutrients.

6 **Arteriole.** Small artery immediately preceding a capillary.

7 **Arterial circle.** Ring of anastomosing arteries.

8 **Vascular circle.** Ring of anastomosing veins.

9 **Cistern.** Dilatation of a lymphatic vessel.

10 **Blood.**

11 **Vascular plexus.**

12 **Venous plexus.**

13 **Arterial plexus.**

14 **Rete mirabile.** Two consecutive capillary networks; e.g., in the kidney.

15 **Articular vascular plexus.** Network of vessels around a joint; e.g., genicular anastomosis.

16 **Venous plexus.**

17 **Sinus venosus.** Venous channel that lacks a typical venous wall, e.g., the sagittal sinus.

18 **Tunica externa.** Outer layer of a blood vessel wall.

19 **Tunica intima.** Inner layer of a blood vessel wall.

20 **Tunica media.** Middle layer of a blood vessel wall.

21 **Valve.** Valvular structure, e.g., the mitral valve.

22 *Cusp.* Small valve. Often crescent-shaped part of a valve system, e.g., the semilunar cusps.

23 *Cusp.* Scalloped leaflets in a valve system, e.g., the anterior cusps of the right and left atrioventricular valves.

24 **Venous valve.**

25 **Anastomotic vessel.**

26 **Capillary.**

27 **Collateral vessel.** Vessel that forms a shunt.

28 **Sinusoid.** Specially formed segment of a vessel with thin walls and a larger lumen.

29 **Vasa vasorum.** Blood vessels that supply the vessel walls.

30 **Vessels of nerves.** Vessels that supply nerves.

31 **Vein.**

32 **Vena comitans.** Accompanying vein. It travels with an artery that supports its functioning.

33 **Cutaneous vein.**

34 **Emissary vein.** Vein that passes through the cranial bones to external.

35 **Nutrient vein.** Vessel that nourishes tissues.

36 **Deep vein.** Vein that lies deep to the fascia.

37 **Superficial vein.** Cutaneous vein. It lies on the fascia of the limbs.

38 **Venule.** Small vein that immediately follows a capillary.

39 **Lymphatic vessel.**

40 *Superficial lymph vessel.* Vessel that lies on the fascia of the limbs.

41 *Deep lymph vessel.* Vessel that lies deep to the fascia of the limbs and often accompanies blood vessels.

42 *Lymphatic plexus.* Plexus that is located deeper than the lymphatic capillary plexus, e.g., in the corium of the skin or just beneath it.

43 *Lymphatic valvule.*

44 **Lymph.**

45 **Lymphatic capillary.** Vessel with a blind beginning and permeable walls.

46 **Lymphatic rete.** Network of lymphatic capillaries close to their beginning.

47 *NERVOUS SYSTEM.*

48 **Nerve fiber.**

49 **Neuron.**

50 **Perikaryon.** Cell body of a neuron.

51 **Synapse.** Point of contact between neurons or between a neuron and other cells.

52 **Neuroglia.** Interstitial tissue of the nervous system.

53 *CENTRAL NERVOUS SYSTEM.*

54 **Gray matter; Gray substance.** Mass of neural cell bodies.

55 *Nucleus.* Cluster of neurons outside of the cortex.

56 *Nucleus of cranial nerve.*

57 Nucleus of origin.

58 Terminal nucleus.

59 *Column.* Column-shaped collection of neurons, e.g., in the spinal cord.

60 *Lamina.* Platelike layer of tissue, e.g., neuronal layers in the neocortex.

1

1 **White matter; White substance.** Mass of myelinated nerve fibers.

2 *Funiculus.* Cordlike tissue structure; bundle of nerve fibers.

3 *Tract.* Collection of nerve fibers with a common origin and termination. It can also contain other fibers.

4 *Fasciculus; Fascicle.* Clearly bordered bundle of nerve fibers that can contain more than one tract.

5 *Commissure.* Fiber tract that connects areas in one hemisphere to the corresponding areas in the other.

6 *Lemniscus.* Specific term for ascending sensory nerve fibers in the brainstem.

7 *Fiber.*

8 *Association fiber.* Fiber that connects cortical regions within one hemisphere.

9 *Commissural fiber.* Fiber that connects regions in each of the two hemispheres with each other.

10 *Projection fiber.* Fiber that connects the cerebral cortex with subcortical regions. Corticipetal and corticifugal fibers.

11 *Decussation.* Intersection of fibers in the midline.

12 *Stria.* Striped appearance produced as more rapidly growing neurons force apart existing cell areas during development of the hemispheres.

13 **Reticular formation.** Loosely organized cells and nerve fibers with only a small number of nuclei that influence movement, circulation, respiration, and the sleep–wake cycle.

14 **Ependyma.** Cellular lining of the ventricles in the central nervous system.

15 **CEREBELLUM.**

16 **Cerebellar fissures.** Deep furrows between the folds of the cerebellum that branch off into smaller fissures deep within the furrows.

17 **Folia of cerebellum.** Folds in the cerebellum that are separated by fissures.

18 **Hemisphere of cerebellum (H II–H X).**

19 **Vallecula of cerebellum.** Deep median furrow on the inferior aspect of the cerebellar hemispheres that is occupied by the medulla oblongata.

20 **Vermis of cerebellum (I–X).** Unpaired region of the cerebellum, part of which is phylogenetically older.

21 **TELENCEPHALON; CEREBRUM.** Endbrain. It arises from the prosencephalon.

22 CEREBRAL HEMISPHERE.

23 **Cerebral cortex.** Pallium. Mantle that covers most of the brainstem in each hemisphere.

24 **Cerebral gyri.** Cerebral convolutions, around 1 cm wide.

25 **Cerebral lobes.** The four cerebral lobes: frontal, parietal, temporal, and occipital.

26 **Cerebral sulci.** Grooves between the cerebral convolutions.

27 **Longitudinal cerebral fissure.** Deep longitudinal cleft that divides the cerebral hemispheres and houses the falx cerebri.

28 **Transverse cerebral fissure.** Fissure between the corpus callosum and the fornix above the thalamus and the roof of the third ventricle below.

29 **Lateral cerebral fossa.** Space deep in the lateral sulcus.

30 **Superior margin.** Upper border between the superolateral face and the medial surface of a hemisphere.

31 **Inferomedial margin.** Lower medial border between the medial and inferior surfaces of a hemisphere.

32 **Inferolateral margin.** Lower lateral border between the superolateral and inferior surfaces of a hemisphere.

33 *PERIPHERAL NERVOUS SYSTEM.* It begins at the surface of the brain and the spinal cord.

34 **Ganglion.** Cluster of neuron cell bodies that appears as a visible thickening of the nerve.

35 *Capsule of ganglion.* Connective tissue capsule of a ganglion.

36 *Stroma of ganglion.* Inner connective tissue of a ganglion.

37 **Craniospinal sensory ganglion.** Collective term for the following two ganglia.

38 *Spinal ganglion; Dorsal root ganglion.* The ganglion belonging to the dorsal root.

39 *Cranial sensory ganglion.* The spinal ganglion equivalent of a cranial nerve.

1 **Autonomic ganglion.** Ganglion belonging to the autonomic nervous system.

2 *Preganglionic nerve fibers.* Myelinated nerve fibers traveling to the ganglia of the visceral nerves.

3 *Postganglionic nerve fibers.* Unmyelinated nerve fibers traveling from the visceral ganglia to the visceral organs.

4 *Sympathetic ganglion.* Ganglia which are mainly present in the sympathetic trunk.

5 *Parasympathetic ganglion.* Ganglion of the parasympathetic system, e.g., ciliary ganglion.

6 **Nerve.**

7 *Endoneurium.* Loose connective tissue spread between the basal membranes of individual nerve fibers.

8 *Perineurium.* Connective-tissue sheath surrounding a bundle of nerve fibers. It consists of concentric lamellae of epithelioid connective-tissue cells interspersed with collagen fibers. Diffusion barrier.

9 *Epineurium.* Outer connective-tissue sheath surrounding a nerve.

10 *Afferent nerve fibers.* Nerve fibers that conduct impulses into the central nervous system.

11 *Efferent nerve fibers.* Nerve fibers that conduct impulses away from the central nervous system.

12 *Somatic nerve fibers.* Somatic or animal nerve fibers. Counterpart to the autonomic nerves (visceral nerves).

13 *Autonomic nerve fibers.* Nerve fibers that supply the viscera.

14 **Motor nerve.** Nerve that contains only fibers for innervating muscle. Afferent fibers, e.g., from muscle spindles, are not included this definition.

15 **Sensory nerve.** Nerve that contains afferent fibers that convey impulses from a nerve ending into the central nervous system. *Terminologia Anatomica* does not distinguish between the two definitions of sensory nerve, a distinction commonly made in European languages, which use two different terms. A sensory nerve can describe either any afferent nerve that transmits impulses toward the central nervous system or, more specifically, an afferent nerve that conveys impulses from specific sensory receiving areas such as the nose, eye, petrous part of temporal bone, and gustatory regions.

16 **Mixed nerve.** Nerve that contains both motor and sensory fibers. By definition, it can refer to a nerve that contains both somatic and visceral fibers.

17 *Cutaneous branch.* Cutaneous nerve or branch that innervates the skin.

18 *Articular branch.* Nerve or branch that innervates a joint.

19 *Muscular branch.* Nerve or branch that innervates muscle.

20 **Spinal nerve.** It is formed by the union of an anterior and posterior root.

21 *Rootlets.* Fine root fibers that exit from the spinal cord and attach to the anterior and posterior roots of the individual spinal nerves.

22 *Anterior root; Motor root; Ventral root.*

23 *Posterior root; Sensory root; Dorsal root.*

24 *Trunk of spinal nerve.* The part of the spinal nerve located between the union of the anterior and posterior roots and the departure of the first branch.

25 *Meningeal branch, Recurrent branch.* Branch that passes anterior to the spinal nerve through the intervertebral foramen to the meninges, where it forms a plexus with other meningeal branches. It contains sensory and sympathetic fibers.

26 *Ramus communicans.* Communicating branch between the spinal nerve and the sympathetic trunk.

27 *Anterior ramus.* Larger anterior branch of a spinal nerve, which can form a plexus with adjacent fibers. In the thoracic region it supplies branches to the intercostal nerves.

28 *Posterior ramus.* Smaller branch that supplies the skin of the back and the autochthonous back musculature.

29 **Cauda equina.** Mass of nerves that is formed by all spinal nerve roots from L1 or L2 downward and the terminal filum.

30 *Spinal nerve plexus.* Nerve plexuses in the cervical, lumbar, and sacral regions that distribute nerves to the limbs.

31 **Cranial nerve.**

32 **Autonomic nerve.** Nerve that supplies the viscera.

33 **Autonomic branch.** Nerve branch that supplies the viscera.

34 **Autonomic plexus.** Any plexus belonging to the autonomic part of the peripheral nervous system.

35 **Visceral plexus.**

36 *Vascular plexus.* Nerve plexus containing sensory and autonomic nerve fibers for the innervation of blood vessels.

37 *Periarterial plexus.* Nerve plexuses situated in the adventitia of the arteries.

38 *Vascular nerves.*

2

1 *SYSTEMIC ANATOMY.*

2 *BONES; SKELETAL SYSTEM.*

3 *CRANIUM.*

4 **Neurocranium; Brain box.**

5 **Viscerocranium.** Its border with the neurocranium extends from the root of the nose over the supraorbital margin to the lateral external acoustic meatus.

6 **Chondrocranium.** Cartilaginous part of the cranium present during embryonic stages that later forms a part of the cranial base.

7 **Desmocranium.** Structure arising from cranial bones formed by direct ossification.

8 **Pericranium.** Periosteum of the external surface of the cranium.

9 **Facial aspect; Frontal aspect.** View of the cranium from anterior. A

10 **Forehead.** A F

11 **Nasion.** Midpoint in the suture between the frontal and nasal bones. A F

12 **Superior aspect; Vertical aspect.** View of the cranium from superior. C

13 **Occiput.** Posterior aspect of the head. C F

14 **Vertex.** Highest point of the central part of the cranial vault. F

15 **Bregma.** Meeting point of the sagittal and coronal sutures. C

16 **Occipital aspect.** View of the cranium from posterior. B

17 **Lambda.** Point where the sagittal and lambdoid sutures meet. B

18 **Inion.** Outermost point on the external occipital protuberance. Point used in anthropological measurements. B F

19 **Lateral aspect.** Lateral view of the cranium. F

20 **Pterion.** Area in which frontal, parietal, temporal, and sphenoidal bones meet. F

21 **Asterion.** Point where the lambdoid suture and the occipitomastoid suture meet. F

22 **Gonion.** Most inferior, posterior, and lateral point on the angle of the mandible.

23 **Temporal fossa.** Shallow depression on the lateral wall of the cranium. It extends from the temporal lines to the level of the infratemporal crest of the greater wing of the sphenoid and laterally to the inferior border of the zygomatic arch. F

24 **Zygomatic arch.** Arch formed by the zygomatic process of the temporal bone and the temporal process of the zygomatic bone. F

25 **Infratemporal fossa.** Prolongation of the temporal fossa to inferior, which extends medially to the pterygoid process of the temporal bone. It contains the inferior part of the temporal muscle, the lateral pterygoid muscle, vessels, and nerves. F

26 **Pterygopalatine fossa.** Continuation of the infratemporal fossa to medial between the maxillary tuberosity, the perpendicular plate of the palatine bone, and the pterygoid process. It narrows inferiorly to continue as the greater palatine canal. F G H

27 **Pterygomaxillary fissure.** Opening that is occasionally found connecting the infratemporal fossa with the pterygopalatine fossa. It is bounded by the maxillary tuberosity and the lateral plate of the pterygoid process. G H

28 **Fontanelles.** Membrane-filled gaps between the cranial bones in children. J K

29 *Anterior fontanelle.* Quadrilateral gap located in the anterior part of the sagittal suture between the parietal and frontal bones. It closes by the second or third year of life. J K

30 *Posterior fontanelle.* Triangular gap located at the junction of the sagittal and lambdoid sutures, i.e., between the parietal and occipital bones. It closes within three months after birth. J K

31 *Sphenoidal fontanelle.* Space on the lateral side of the cranium between the frontal, parietal, temporal, and sphenoidal bones. J

32 *Mastoid fontanelle.* Space on the lateral side of the cranium between the parietal, occipital, and temporal bones. J

33 **Calvaria.** Skull cap, which is curved longitudinally and transversely. It is formed by the squamous parts of the frontal and parietal bones together with the upper portion of the squamous part of the occipital bone. D

34 *External table.* Outer layer of compact bone of the calvaria. D E

35 *Diploe.* Special layer of spongy bone between the external and internal tables of the calvaria. D E

36 *Diploic canals.* Wide canals located in the diploe for the passage of veins. E

37 *Internal table.* Inner layer of compact bone of the calvaria. E

38 *Groove for superior sagittal sinus.* Shallow depression for the superior sagittal sinus. D E

39 *Granular foveolae (Pacchionian granulations).* Small pits for the arachnoid granulations. D E

40 *Venous grooves.* Occasional grooves on the internal wall of the parietal bone that give passage to veins.

41 *Arterial grooves.* Grooves on the internal wall of the cranium that mainly give passage to the middle meningeal artery and its branches. D

42 *[Sutural bone].* Bones that are occasionally found interposed in cranial sutures.

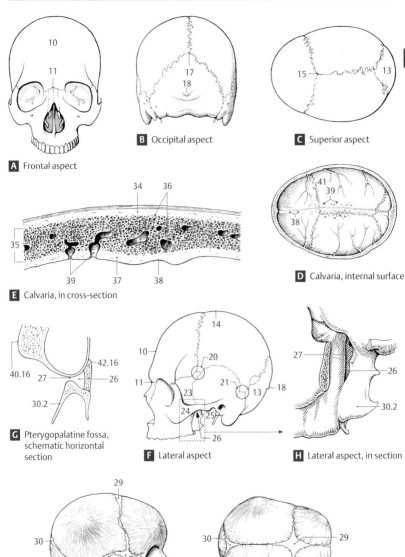

A Frontal aspect

B Occipital aspect

C Superior aspect

E Calvaria, in cross-section

D Calvaria, internal surface

G Pterygopalatine fossa, schematic horizontal section

F Lateral aspect

H Lateral aspect, in section

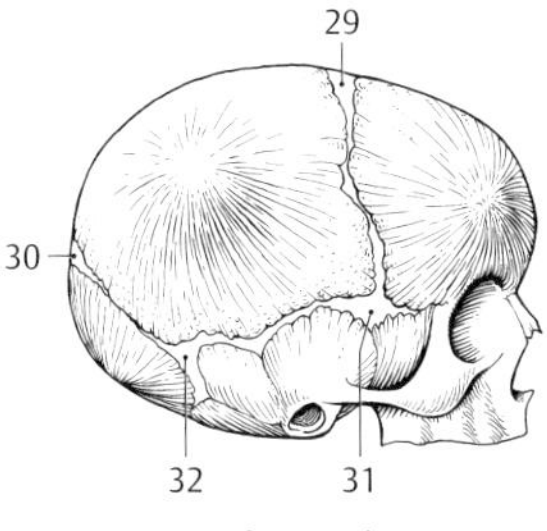

J Neonate cranium from right

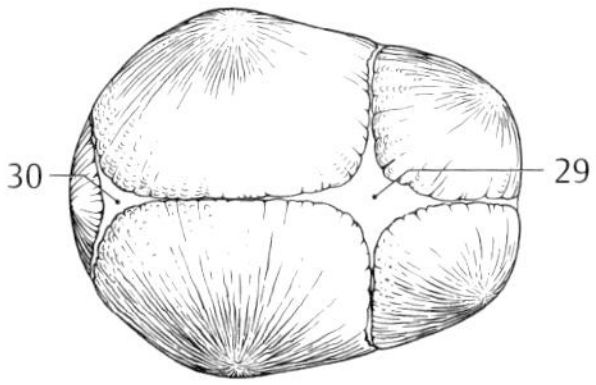

K Neonate cranium, superior view

2

1 **Cranial base; Basicranium.** A B

2 *Internal surface of cranial base.* A

3 *Anterior cranial fossa.* Fossa that extends from the wall of the frontal bone to the lesser wing of the sphenoid. A

4 *Impressions of cerebral gyri.* Shallow depressions that correspond the cerebral gyri. A

5 *Middle cranial fossa.* Fossa that is bounded by the lesser wing of the sphenoid and by the superior border of the petrous part of the temporal bone. A

6 *Posterior cranial fossa.* Fossa that is bounded by the superior border of the petrous part of the temporal bone and the posterior cranial wall. A

7 Clivus. Bony structure that slopes downward from the dorsum sellae to the foramen magnum. It is formed by the occipital bone and the sphenoid. A B

8 *Sphenopetrosal fissure.* Prolongation of the petrosquamous fissure to medial that is continuous with the foramen lacerum. Passage of the lesser petrosal nerve and exit of the chorda tympani from the cranium. A B

9 *Petro-occipital fissure.* Medial continuation of the jugular foramen that extends from the temporal bone to the occipital bone. A B

10 *External surface of cranial base.* B

11 *Jugular foramen.* Opening between the occipital bone and the petrous part of the temporal bone that is subdivided by connective tissue. Union of the sigmoid sinus and inferior petrosal sinus. It transmits the internal jugular vein and cranial nerves IX, X, XI. A B

12 *Foramen lacerum.* Irregularly bordered aperture that is closed with fibrocartilage. It is located between the apex of the petrous part of the temporal bone and the sphenoid in the middle cranial fossa and gives passage to the deep petrosal nerve and the greater petrosal nerve. A B

13 *Bony palate.* B C

14 *Greater palatine canal.* Canal formed by the palatine bone and the maxilla for transmission of the descending palatine artery and the greater palatine nerve. B C

15 *Greater palatine foramen.* Opening near the posterior border of the bony palate between the palatine bone and the maxilla. The greater palatine canal ends here. B C

16 *Lesser palatine foramina.* Openings to the lesser palatine canals. C

17 *Incisive fossa.* Match-head-sized depression covered with epithelium into which the incisive canals open by the incisive foramina. C

18 *Incisive canals.* Canals that extend from the floor of the nasal cavity on both sides of the nasal septum to the palate, where they unite as the incisive fossa. C

19 *Incisive foramina.* Between two and four openings of the incisive canals. C

20 *[Palatine torus].* Long protuberance that is occasionally found extending toward the oral cavity in the midline of the bony palate. C

21 *Palatovaginal canal.* Narrow canal between the vaginal process of the sphenoid and the sphenoidal process of the palatine bone that transmits a branch of the maxillary artery and the pharyngeal branch of the pterygopalatine ganglion. p. 30.8.

22 *Vomerovaginal canal.* Small canal between the vaginal process of the sphenoid and the vomer for the passage of a branch of the sphenopalatine artery. p. 30.9

23 *Vomerorostral canal.* Tiny canal between the vomer and the sphenoidal rostrum.

24 **Orbit.** Orbital cavity that contains the eyeball and its appendages.

25 *Orbital cavity.* D

26 *Orbital opening.* Anterior opening of the orbital cavity. D

27 *Orbital margin.* D

28 Supra-orbital margin. Upper border of the orbital opening. D

29 Infra-orbital margin. Lower border of the orbital opening. D

30 Lateral margin. Lateral border of the orbital opening. D

31 Medial margin. Medial border of the orbital opening. D

2

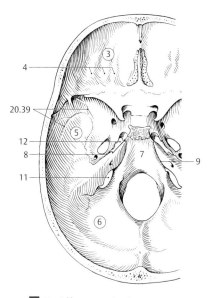

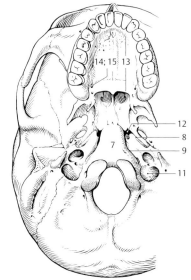

A Cranial base, superior view

B Cranial base, inferior view

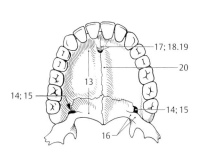

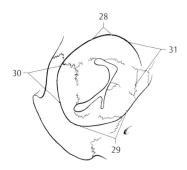

C Hard palate, inferior view

D Outline of right orbit

2

1 *Roof of orbit.* A

2 *Floor of orbit.* A

3 *Lateral wall of orbit.* A

4 *Medial wall of orbit.* A

5 *Anterior ethmoidal foramen.* Anterior opening in the medial wall of the orbit between the frontal bone and the ethmoid. It transmits the anterior ethmoidal nerve and the anterior ethmoidal vessels from the anterior cranial fossa. A

6 *Posterior ethmoidal foramen.* Posterior opening in the medial wall of the orbit between the frontal bone and the ethmoid for the passage of the posterior ethmoidal vessels and the posterior ethmoidal nerve. A

7 *Lacrimal groove.* Groovelike beginning of the nasolacrimal canal. A

8 *Fossa for lacrimal sac.* Widened depression at the beginning of the nasolacrimal canal for the lacrimal sac. A

9 *Superior orbital fissure.* Opening in the upper part of the orbit between the greater and lesser wings of the sphenoid that connects the cranial and orbital cavities. It transmits the ophthalmic, oculomotor, trochlear, and abducens nerves and the superior ophthalmic vein. A

10 *Inferior orbital fissure.* Opening between the greater wing of the sphenoid and the orbital surface of the maxilla. It transmits the zygomatic nerve, infraorbital nerve, and accompanying vessels. A

11 **Nasolacrimal canal.** Opening below the inferior nasal concha. A

12 **Bony nasal cavity.** A B

13 *Bony nasal septum.* Partition formed by the vomer and the perpendicular plate of the ethmoid. A

14 *Piriform aperture.* Pear-shaped anterior nasal opening in the bony cranium. A B

15 *Superior nasal meatus.* Nasal passage located above the middle nasal conchae. B

16 *Middle nasal meatus.* Nasal passage located between the inferior and middle nasal conchae. B

17 *Inferior nasal meatus.* Nasal passage located below the inferior nasal concha. B

18 *Opening of nasolacrimal canal.* Opening located below the inferior nasal concha. A

19 *Common nasal meatus.* Cavity between the nasal conchae and the nasal septum.

20 *Spheno-ethmoidal recess.* Cleft above the superior nasal concha. B

21 *Nasopharyngeal meatus.* The part of the nasal cavity extending from the posterior margin of the nasal conchae to the choana. B

22 *Choana; Posterior nasal aperture.* Either of two openings located between the nasal cavity and the nasopharyngeal meatus. B

23 *Sphenopalatine foramen.* Opening in the superior part of the pterygopalatine fossa that connects it with the nasal cavity. The palatine bone contributes the greater portion and the sphenoid the lesser portion. B

2

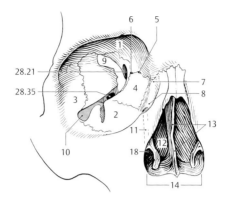

A Right bony orbital cavity

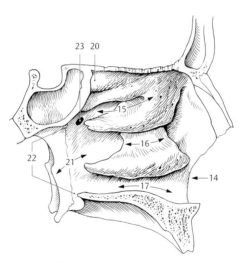

B Lateral wall of the nose with frontal and sphenoidal sinuses

2

1   *BONES OF CRANIUM.*

2   **Occipital bone.** Bone located between the sphenoidal, temporal, and parietal bones. A B C

3   **Foramen magnum.** Large opening in the occipital bone for the medulla oblongata, vessels, and nerves. A B C

4   *Basion.* Midpoint on the anterior margin of the foramen magnum. B

5   *Opisthion.* Midpoint on the posterior margin of the foramen magnum. A B

6   **Basilar part of occipital bone.** The part that ascends from the foramen magnum to the spheno-occipital synchondrosis. A B C

7   *Pharyngeal tubercle.* Small protuberance on the inferior aspect of the basilar part of the occipital bone that provides attachment to the pharyngeal raphe. A C

8   **Lateral part of occipital bone.** The part that is lateral to the foramen magnum. A B

9   **Squamous part of occipital bone.** The part that is posterior to the foramen magnum. A B C

10   *Mastoid border.* Margin of the occipital bone that articulates with the temporal bone. A

11   *Lambdoid border.* Articulates with the parietal bone. A

12   *[Interparietal bone].* Anatomical variant in which a transverse suture nearly separates the upper half of the squamous part of the occipital bone: Inca bone.

13   **Occipital condyle.** Spherical eminence for articulation with the atlas. A B C

14   **Condylar canal.** Passageway for transmission of a vein that begins at the sigmoid sinus and ends posterior to the occipital condyle. A B C

15   **Hypoglossal canal.** Passageway that begins superolateral to the foramen magnum and ends anterolateral to the occipital condyle. It transmits CN XII and a venous plexus. A B C

16   **Condylar fossa.** Depression located posterior to the occipital condyle into which the condylar canal opens. B

17   **Jugular tubercle.** Small protuberance above the hypoglossal canal. A B C

18   **Jugular notch.** Recess that, together with the petrous part of temporal bone, forms the jugular foramen. A C

19   **Jugular process.** Projection located lateral to the jugular foramen that is visible internally and externally. It corresponds to the transverse process of a vertebra. A B C

20   **Intrajugular process.** Process that occasionally divides the jugular foramen into a lateral compartment for the passage of the internal jugular vein and a medial compartment for the transmission of nerves. C

21   **External occipital protuberance.** Easily palpable bony projection at the border between the occipital and nuchal planes. B

22   **[External occipital crest].** Bony ridge that is occasionally present between the external occipital protuberance and the foramen magnum. B

23   **Highest nuchal line.** Curved line that extends laterally from the superior margin of the external occipital protuberance. It gives origin to the occipital belly of the epicranius muscle. B

24   **Superior nuchal line.** Transverse ridge at the level of the external occipital protuberance. The area between it and the highest nuchal line gives origin to the trapezius muscle. B

25   **Inferior nuchal line.** Transverse ridge that extends from the superior nuchal line to the foramen magnum. The area between the inferior and superior nuchal lines gives attachment to the semispinalis capitis muscle. B

26   **[[Nuchal plane]].** Surface below the external occipital protuberance. Attachment site for muscles of the neck. B

27   **Occipital plane.** Surface above the external occipital protuberance. B C

28   **Cruciform eminence.** Bony projection in the shape of a cross with the internal occipital protuberance at its center. A

29   **Internal occipital protuberance.** Projection on the internal surface opposite the external occipital protuberance. It forms the midpoint of the cruciform eminence. A

30   **[Internal occipital crest].** Inconstant thickened bony ridge that extends from the internal occipital protuberance to the foramen magnum. A

31   **Groove for superior sagittal sinus.** A

32   **Groove for transverse sinus.** A

33   **Groove for sigmoid sinus.** Groove that transmits the sigmoid sinus before it enters the jugular foramen. A C

34   **Groove for occipital sinus.** A

35   **Groove for marginal sinus.** Groove that is occasionally present along the inferior margin of the foramen magnum for the passage of the marginal sinus. A

36   **[Paramastoid process].** Projection that is occasionally found on the jugular process. It is directed toward the transverse process of the atlas. C

37   **Cerebral fossa.** Depression that lodges the occipital lobes. A

38   **Cerebellar fossa.** Depression that lodges the cerebellum. A

2

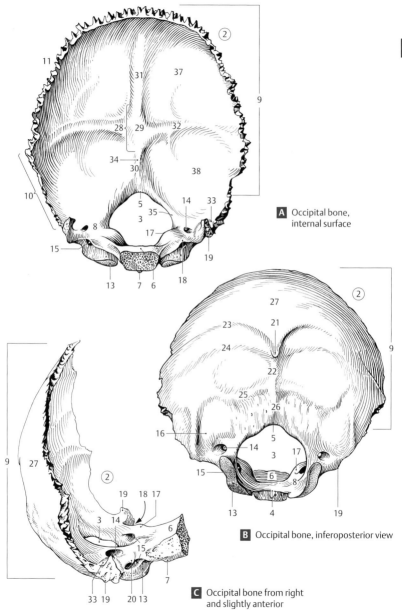

A Occipital bone, internal surface

B Occipital bone, inferoposterior view

C Occipital bone from right and slightly anterior

1 **Sphenoid; Sphenoidal bone.** Bone located between the frontal, occipital, and temporal bones. A B C

2 **Body of sphenoid.** The part of the sphenoid between the wings of the sphenoid and their processes. A B

3 *Jugum sphenoidale; Sphenoidal yoke.* The part of the body of the sphenoid that connects the lesser wings of the sphenoid. A

4 *Limbus of sphenoid.* Posterior border of the jugum sphenoidale. It is continuous with the anterior clinoid process.

5 *Prechiasmatic sulcus.* Groove between the right and left optic canals. A

6 *Sella turcica.* It is located above the sphenoidal sinus and houses the pituitary gland. A

7 *Tuberculum sellae.* Small protuberance in front of the sella turcica. A

8 *[Middle clinoid process].* Small protuberance that is occasionally present on both sides of the tuberculum sellae. A

9 *Hypophysial fossa.* Hollow for reception of the pituitary gland. A

10 *Dorsum sellae.* Posterior wall of the sella turcica. A C

11 *Posterior clinoid process.* Protuberance on both sides of the dorsum sellae. A C

12 *Carotid sulcus.* Rather S-shaped groove on the lateral surface of the sphenoid for the passage of the internal carotid artery. A

13 *Sphenoidal lingula.* Pointed process that is located lateral to the entrance of the internal carotid artery into the cranial cavity. A

14 *Sphenoidal crest.* Median bony ridge on the anterior surface of the body of the sphenoid that articulates with the perpendicular plate of the ethmoid. C

15 *Sphenoidal rostrum.* Prolongation of the sphenoidal crest to inferior that articulates with the vomer. C

16 *Sphenoidal sinus.* Paired sphenoidal sinuses. C

17 *Septum of sphenoidal sinuses.* Septum that divides the right and left sphenoidal sinuses. C

18 *Opening of sphenoidal sinus.* Anterior opening of the sphenoidal sinus into the spheno-ethmoidal recess. C

19 *Sphenoidal concha.* Originally a pair of separate, hollow bones. It is united with the body of the sphenoid to form part of the anterior and inferior wall of the sphenoidal sinus. C

20 **Lesser wing of sphenoid.** A B C

21 *Optic canal.* Canal for transmission of the optic nerves and the ophthalmic artery. A, p. 25 A

22 *Anterior clinoid process.* Projection from the lesser wing of the sphenoid bone that is directed posteriorly toward the middle and posterior clinoid processes. A

23 *Superior orbital fissure.* Cleft between the greater and lesser wings of the sphenoid for the passage of nerves and the superior ophthalmic vein. A B C

24 **Greater wing of sphenoid.** A B C

25 *Cerebral surface.* Surface of the greater wing of the sphenoid facing the brain. A

26 *Temporal surface.* Lateral facing surface of the greater wing of the sphenoid. B C

27 *Infratemporal surface.* Horizontal, inferior surface of the greater wing of the sphenoid.

28 *Infratemporal crest.* Bony ridge between the (vertical) temporal surface and the (horizontal) infratemporal surface of the greater wing of the sphenoid. B C

29 *Maxillary surface.* Surface of the greater wing of the sphenoid facing the maxilla. The foramen rotundum opens here. C

30 *Orbital surface.* Surface of the greater wing of the sphenoid facing the orbit. C

31 *Zygomatic margin.* Border of the greater wing of the sphenoid for articulation with the zygomatic bone. C

32 *Frontal margin.* Border of the greater wing of the sphenoid that is united with the frontal bone. A

33 *Parietal margin.* Border of the greater wing of the sphenoid that is united with the parietal bone. C

34 *Squamosal margin.* Squamous part of the greater wing of the sphenoid that articulates with the temporal bone. A

35 *Foramen rotundum.* Foramen that opens anteriorly into the pterygopalatine fossa. It transmits the maxillary nerve. A B C, p. 25 A

36 *Foramen ovale.* Opening for the passage of the mandibular nerve anteromedial to the foramen spinosum. A B

37 *[Sphenoidal emissary foramen].* Foramen that is occasionally present medial to the foramen ovale for the passage of an emissary vein from the cavernous sinus. A B

38 *Foramen spinosum.* Opening posterolateral to the foramen ovale for the passage of the middle meningeal artery. A B

39 *[Foramen petrosum].* Opening that is occasionally present between the foramen ovale and the foramen spinosum for the passage of the lesser petrosal nerve. A B

40 *Spine of sphenoid bone.* Inferiorly projecting tip of the greater wing of the sphenoid. A B

41 *Sulcus of auditory tube.* Shallow groove on the inferior surface of the greater wing of the sphenoid lateral to the root of the pterygoid process that lodges the auditory tube. B

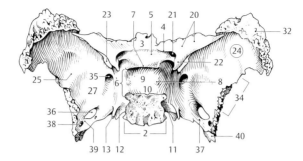

A Sphenoid, superior view

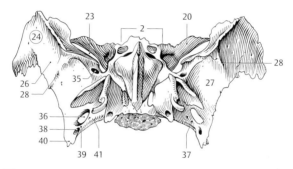

B Sphenoid, anteroinferior view

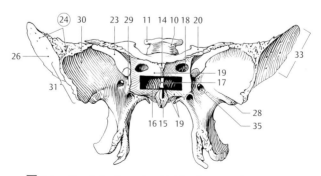

C Sphenoid, anterior view, sphenoidal sinus fenestrated

2

1 **Pterygoid process of the sphenoid.** A B

2 *Lateral plate of the pterygoid process.* A B

3 *Medial plate of the pterygoid process.* A B

4 **Pterygoid notch.** Notch located between the lateral and medial plates of the pterygoid process. It is open inferiorly and lodges the pyramidal process of the palatine bone. A

5 **Pterygoid fossa.** Depression between the lateral and medial plates of the pterygoid process for the medial pterygoid muscle. A B

6 **Scaphoid fossa.** Elongated depression on the root of the medial plate of the pterygoid process that lodges the thickened cartilaginous part of the auditory tube. The tensor veli palatini muscle takes origin at its lateral margin. A

7 **Vaginal process.** Small bony ridge medial to the root of the medial plate of the pterygoid process. It is bounded on its lateral side by a small depression. A B

8 *Palatovaginal groove.* Groove that joins the palatine bone to form the palatovaginal canal. A B

9 *Vomerovaginal groove.* Groove that unites with the vomer to form the vomerovaginal canal. A B

10 **Pterygoid hamulus.** Hooked process on the end of the medial plate of the pterygoid process. A B

11 *Groove of pterygoid hamulus.* Groove that forms a pulley for the tensor veli palatini muscle. B

12 **Pterygoid canal (vidian canal).** Canal that runs anteriorly in the base of the pterygoid process. It transmits the greater and deep petrosal nerves to the pterygopalatine ganglion in the pterygopalatine fossa. A

13 **Pterygospinous process.** Pointed spinous projection on the posterior border of the lateral plate of the pterygoid process. A

14 **Temporal bone.** Bone located between the occipital, sphenoidal, and parietal bones. It consists of petrous, tympanic, and squamous parts. C D E

15 **Petrous part of temporal bone.** The part of the temporal bone that contains the internal ear. D

16 *Occipital margin.* Border of the petrous part of the temporal bone that articulates with the occipital bone. C D

17 *Mastoid process.* Projection behind the external acoustic meatus that contains the mastoid cells. C E

18 *Mastoid notch.* Notch on the inferior surface of the petrous part of the temporal bone, medial to the mastoid process. Origin of the posterior belly of the digastric muscle. C

19 *Groove for sigmoid sinus.* Groove in the posterior cranial fossa that lodges the sigmoid sinus. D

20 *Occipital groove.* Groove for transmission of the occipital artery. It is situated medial to the mastoid notch, close to the occipital margin. C

21 *Mastoid foramen.* Opening behind the mastoid process for transmission of the mastoid emissary vein. C D

22 *Facial canal.* Canal for transmission of the facial nerve. It begins at the internal acoustic opening and ends at the stylomastoid foramen. C D E

23 *Geniculum of facial canal.* Sharp bend in the facial canal just below the anterior surface of the petrous part of temporal bone, near the hiatus for the greater petrosal nerve. D

24 *Canaliculus for chorda tympani.* Narrow passageway for the chorda tympani that begins at the facial canal and opens into the tympanic cavity. D E

25 *Apex of petrous part of temporal bone.* Anteromedially directed tip of the petrous part of the temporal bone. C D

26 *Carotid canal.* Canal for the passage of the internal carotid artery. C

27 External opening of carotid canal. Opening in the external cranial base between the jugular foramen and the musculotubal canal. C, p. 33 B

28 Internal opening of the carotid canal. Internal opening of the carotid canal at the apex of the petrous part of the temporal bone. C, p. 33 B

29 *Caroticotympanic canaliculi.* Tiny canals at the beginning of the carotid canal that transmit small branches of the internal carotid artery and the carotid plexus to the tympanic cavity. C

30 *Musculotubal canal.* Pair of canals located anterior to the carotid canal that extend into the tympanic cavity, one for the auditory tube and the other for the tensor tympani muscle. C E

31 Canal for tensor tympani. Upper canal for the tensor tympani muscle. E

32 Canal for auditory tube. Lower canal for the auditory tube. E

33 Septum of musculotubal canal. Bony septum that divides the canals for the tensor tympani and the auditory tube. E

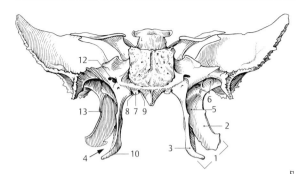

A Sphenoid, posterior view

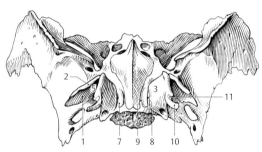

B Sphenoid, inferior view

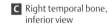

C Right temporal bone, inferior view

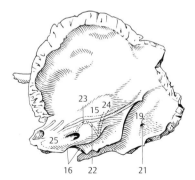

D Right temporal bone, internal surface

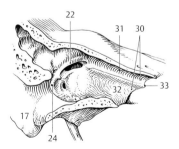

E Right temporal bone, anterolateral view in cross-section

2

1 *Anterior surface of petrous part of temporal bone.* A C

2 *Tegmen tympani.* Roof of the tympanic cavity located lateral to the arcuate eminence. C

3 *Arcuate eminence.* Prominence in the anterior surface of the petrous part of the temporal bone caused by the anterior semicircular canal. A C

4 *Hiatus for greater petrosal nerve.* Opening in the anterior surface of the petrous part of the temporal bone for the passage of the greater petrosal nerve, which arises from the facial nerve. A C

5 *Hiatus for lesser petrosal nerve.* Opening in the anterior surface of the petrous part of the temporal bone below the greater petrosal nerve. A C

6 *Groove for greater petrosal nerve.* Groove for transmission of the greater petrosal nerve, extending anteromedially from the hiatus for the greater petrosal nerve to the foramen lacerum. C

7 *Groove for lesser petrosal nerve.* Groove for transmission of the lesser petrosal nerve, extending from the hiatus for the lesser petrosal nerve to the foramen lacerum. C

8 *Trigeminal impression.* Shallow depression on the anterior surface of the apex of the petrous part of the temporal bone that lodges the trigeminal ganglion. C

9 *Superior border of petrous part of temporal bone.* A C

10 *Groove for superior petrosal sinus.* Depression on the superior border of the petrous part of the temporal bone that lodges the petrosal sinus. A C

11 *Posterior surface of petrous part of temporal bone.* A

12 *Internal acoustic opening.* Opening of the internal acoustic meatus in the posterior surface of the petrous part of the temporal bone. A

13 *Internal acoustic meatus.* Passageway that transmits CN VII, CN VIII, and vessels. A

14 *Subarcuate fossa.* Depression located posterosuperior to the internal acoustic meatus for the fetal flocculus. A

15 *Vestibular canaliculus.* Narrow canal that extends from the endolymphatic space of the internal ear to the posterior surface of the petrous part of the temporal bone.

16 *Opening of vestibular canaliculus.* A

17 *Posterior border of petrous part of temporal bone.* A B

18 *Groove for inferior petrosal sinus.* A

19 *Jugular notch.* Notch that forms the anterior margin of the jugular foramen. A B

20 *Inferior surface of petrous part of temporal bone.* B

21 *Jugular fossa.* Widening of the jugular foramen that contains the superior bulb of the jugular vein. B

22 Cochlear canaliculus. Bony canal that lodges the cochlear aqueduct.

23 Opening of cochlear canaliculus. Opening of the cochlear canaliculus located anteromedial to the jugular fossa. B

24 Mastoid canaliculus. Tiny canal that begins at the jugular fossa for the passage of the auricular branch of the vagus nerve. B

25 *Intrajugular process.* Projection that divides the jugular foramen into a posterolateral part for the passage of the jugular vein and an anteromedial part for transmission of CN IX, X, and XI. A B

26 *Styloid process.* Long bony process in front of the stylomastoid foramen. It is a relic of the hyoid arch. A B D

27 *Stylomastoid foramen.* External opening of the facial canal behind the styloid process and between the mastoid process and the jugular fossa. B

28 *Tympanic canaliculus.* Tiny canal in the petrosal fossula for the passage of the tympanic nerve and the inferior tympanic artery. B

29 *Petrosal fossula.* Small depression on the ridge between the carotid canal and the jugular fossa for the tympanic ganglion of glossopharyngeal nerve. B

30 *Tympanic cavity.* Cleftlike pneumatized space between the bony labyrinth and the tympanic membrane.

31 *Petrotympanic fissure.* (glaserian fissure). Fissure located posteromedial to the mandibular fossa between the tympanic part and the visible strip of the petrous part of the temporal bone. Its medial part can lodge the chorda tympani. B D

32 *Petrosquamous fissure.* Fissure located on the cranial base in front of the glaserian fissure and between the visible strip of the petrous part and the squamous part of the temporal bone. B C

33 *Tympanosquamous fissure.* Lateral continuation of the petrotympanic and petrosquamous fissures after they unite. B D

34 *Tympanomastoid fissure.* Suture between the tympanic part of the temporal bone and the mastoid process. The auricular branch of the vagus nerve exits here. B D

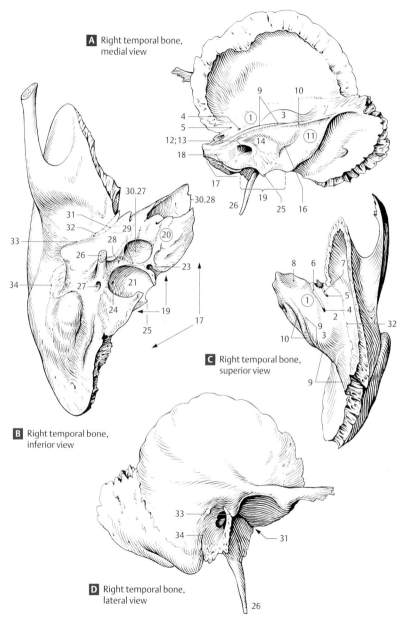

A Right temporal bone, medial view

B Right temporal bone, inferior view

C Right temporal bone, superior view

D Right temporal bone, lateral view

2

1 **Tympanic part of temporal bone.** The part of the temporal bone that forms most of the wall of the bony acoustic meatus except for the posterior, superior portion. B

2 *Tympanic ring.* Bony ring, the upper part of which is still open in newborns. A

3 *External acoustic opening.* Opening to the external acoustic meatus. B

4 *External acoustic meatus.* B

5 *Greater tympanic spine.* Anterior border of the tympanic ring formed by the tympanic part of the temporal bone. A

6 *Lesser tympanic spine.* Posterior border of the tympanic ring formed by the tympanic part of the temporal bone. A

7 *Tympanic sulcus.* Groove that provides attachment to the tympanic membrane. A

8 *Tympanic notch.* Convexity between the greater and lesser tympanic spines. In newborns it is the gap between the upper ends of the incomplete tympanic ring. It is later filled by the squamous part of the temporal bone. A

9 *Sheath of styloid process.* Sheath-like ridge formed by the tympanic part of the temporal bone that encloses the root of the styloid process. A

10 **Squamous part of temporal bone.** The part of the temporal bone that is inserted between the sphenoidal, parietal, and occipital bones. B

11 *Parietal border.* Upper margin that articulates with the parietal bone. B

12 *Parietal notch.* Notch between the posterior border of the squamous part of the temporal bone and the superior border of the mastoid process. B

13 *Sphenoidal margin.* Anterior border articulating with the sphenoid. B

14 *Temporal surface.* Outer surface that is largely covered by the temporal muscle. B

15 *Groove for middle temporal artery.* Groove that transmits the middle temporal artery. B

16 *Zygomatic process.* Projection from the temporal bone that contributes to the zygomatic arch. B

17 *Supramastoid crest.* Prolongation of the border of the zygomatic arch as the inferior temporal line of the parietal bone. B

18 *Suprameatal triangle.* Small depression located above the suprameatal spine and lateral to the mastoid antrum. B

19 *[Suprameatal spine].* Projection that gives attachment to the cartilaginous external acoustic meatus. B

20 **Mandibular fossa.** Articular fossa of the temporomandibular joint. B

21 *Articular surface.* Articular surface for the head of mandible. B

22 **Articular tubercle.** Rounded projection anterior to the mandibular fossa. B

23 **Cerebral surface.** Internal surface of the squamous part of the temporal bone that faces the brain.

24 **Parietal bone.** Bone located between the occipital, frontal, sphenoidal, and temporal bones. C D

25 **Internal surface.** Surface of the parietal bone facing the brain. C

26 *Groove for sigmoid sinus.* Groove near the mastoid angle of the parietal bone for the passage of the sigmoid sinus. C

27 *Groove for superior sagittal sinus.* C

28 *Grooves for arteries.*

29 *Groove for middle meningeal artery.* C

30 *External surface.* Surface of the parietal bone facing the scalp. D

31 *Superior temporal line.* Curved line for attachment of the temporal fascia. It forms the superior border of the temporal plane. D

32 *Inferior temporal line.* Curved line giving origin to the temporal muscle. D

33 *Parietal tuber; Parietal eminence.* Projection located near the center of the external surface of the parietal bone. D

34 **Occipital border.** Border of the parietal bone that faces the occipital bone. C D

35 **Squamosal border.** Inferior margin of the parietal bone that is directed toward the temporal bone. C D

36 **Sagittal border.** Superior margin of the parietal bone located in the sagittal suture. C D

37 **Frontal border.** Anterior border of the parietal bone that articulates with the frontal bone. C D

38 **Frontal angle.** Anterosuperior angle of the parietal bone. C D

39 **Occipital angle.** Posterosuperior angle of the parietal bone. C D

40 **Sphenoidal angle.** Anteroinferior angle of the parietal bone. C D

41 **Mastoid angle.** Posteroinferior angle of the parietal bone. C D

42 **Parietal foramen.** Opening that is usually located in the posterosuperior part of the parietal bone for the passage of the parietal emissary vein. C D

2

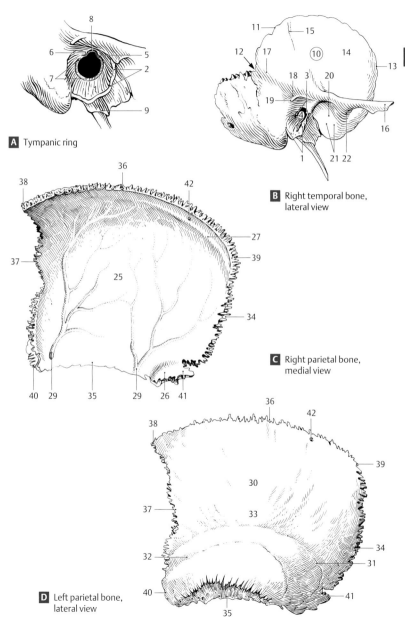

A Tympanic ring

B Right temporal bone, lateral view

C Right parietal bone, medial view

D Left parietal bone, lateral view

2

1 **Frontal bone.** A B C

2 **Squamous part of frontal bone.** A C

3 *External surface of frontal bone.* A

4 *Frontal tuber; Frontal eminence.* A

5 *Superciliary arch.* Bony protuberance above the supra-orbital margin. A B

6 *Glabella.* Area between the eyebrows. A

7 *[Frontal suture; Metopic suture].* Suture that normally fuses by the second or third year of life. Persists in 7–8% of people of European descent. A

8 *Supra-orbital margin.* A B

9 Supra-orbital notch/foramen. Notch or opening in the supra-orbital margin for the passage of the supra-orbital artery and the lateral branch of the supra-orbital nerve. Pressure point for the first division of the trigeminal nerve. A B

10 Frontal notch/foramen. Notch or opening medial to the supra-orbital foramen for the passage of the supratrochlear artery and the medial branch of the supra-orbital nerve. A B

11 *Temporal surface.* External, lateral surface of the frontal bone. A B

12 *Parietal margin.* Posterior border articulating with the parietal bone. A C

13 *Temporal line of frontal bone.* Continuation of the united superior and inferior temporal lines of the parietal bone. A

14 *Zygomatic process of frontal bone.* Process situated lateral to the orbit for articulation with the zygomatic bone. A B C

15 *Internal surface.* Surface of the frontal bone that faces the brain. C

16 *Frontal crest.* Anteromedial bony ridge that serves as attachment for the falx cerebri. C

17 *Groove for superior sagittal sinus.* Prolongation of the frontal crest for the passage of the superior sagittal sinus. C

18 *Foramen cecum.* Canal behind the frontal crest that usually has a blind end. If it is patent, it transmits an emissary vein. C

19 *Nasal part.* Bony segment located between the two orbital parts of the frontal bone. A B

20 *Nasal spine.* Medially situated sharp process of the nasal part of the frontal bone. A B C

21 *Nasal margin.* Serrated inferior border of the nasal part of the frontal bone that articulates on either side with the nasal bone and the frontal process of the maxilla. A B C

22 **Orbital part.** The part that forms the roof of the orbit. A B C

23 *Orbital surface.* Surface of the frontal bone that faces the orbit. B

24 *[Trochlear spine].* Small bony spicule that is occasionally present in the anterosuperior part of the medial angle of the eye. It gives attachment to the superior oblique muscle. A

25 *Trochlear fovea.* Small concavity that gives attachment to a fibrous pulley of the superior oblique muscle. A B

26 *Fossa for lacrimal gland; Lacrimal fossa.* Depression for the lacrimal gland in the lateral angle of the eye. B

27 **Sphenoidal margin.** Border between the orbital part of the frontal bone and the greater wing of the sphenoid. B

28 **Ethmoidal notch.** Notch between the right and left orbital parts of the frontal bone into which the ethmoid is inserted. B

29 **Frontal sinus.** It is an average of 3 cm high, 2.5 cm wide, and often extends 1.8 cm posteriorly, forming part of the roof of the orbit. A

30 *Opening of frontal sinus.* Medial opening in the floor of the frontal sinus for the drainage of discharge into the ethmoidal infundibulum located below the middle nasal concha. B C

31 *Septum of frontal sinuses.* Partition that divides the right and left frontal sinuses. A

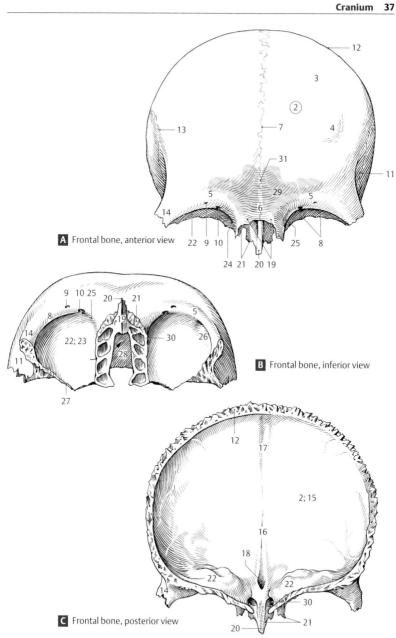

A Frontal bone, anterior view

B Frontal bone, inferior view

C Frontal bone, posterior view

2

1 **Ethmoid; Ethmoidal bone.** Unpaired bone inserted in the ethmoidal notch of the frontal bone. A B C D

2 **Cribriform plate.** Horizontal, elongated bony plate located in the median plane that forms the boundary between the nasal cavity and the anterior cranial fossa. B

3 **Cribriform foramina.** Openings in the cribriform plate for the passage of the olfactory nerves. B

4 **Crista galli.** Small bony projection in the cranial cavity to which the falx cerebri is firmly attached. A B C D

5 *Ala of crista galli.* Winglike pair of processes for attachment of the crista galli to the frontal crest. A B C D

6 **Perpendicular plate.** Vertical bony plate that is located inferior to the cribriform plate and forms the posterosuperior part of the nasal septum. A B C

7 **Ethmoidal labyrinth.** Collective term for the ethmoidal cells located between the orbital and nasal cavities.

8 *Anterior ethmoidal cells.* Cells that open between the middle and inferior nasal conchae. A C

9 *Middle ethmoidal cells.* These cells have the same opening as the anterior ethmoidal cells. C

10 *Posterior ethmoidal cells.* Cells that open above the middle nasal concha. C

11 *Orbital plate.* Especially thin plate of bone that forms part of the medial wall of the orbit. C

12 *Supreme nasal concha.* Uppermost rudimentary nasal concha. D

13 *Superior nasal concha.* A D

14 *Middle nasal concha.* A C D

15 *Ethmoidal bulla.* Especially large and protruding anterior ethmoidal cell that narrows the wide opening of the maxillary sinus. A

16 *Uncinate process.* Hooked process directed posteroinferiorly. It is almost completely concealed by the middle nasal concha. It projects across the wide opening to the maxillary sinus. A C

17 *Ethmoidal infundibulum.* Passageway below the middle nasal concha for the drainage of mucinous material. The frontal sinus, maxillary sinus, and anterior ethmoidal cells open here. A C

18 *Hiatus semilunaris.* Opening of the ethmoidal infundibulum between ethmoidal bulla and the uncinate process. C

19 **Inferior nasal concha.** The independent lower nasal concha, which is attached to the lateral nasal wall. E

20 **Lacrimal process.** Process that projects anterosuperiorly from the inferior nasal concha toward the lacrimal bone. E

21 **Maxillary process.** Lateral process that forms part of the medial wall of the maxillary sinus. E

22 **Ethmoidal process.** Process that is united with the uncinate process of the ethmoid. E

23 **Lacrimal bone.** Bone located in the orbit in front of the orbital plate of the ethmoid. F

24 **Posterior lacrimal crest.** Vertical posterior bounding bone at the entrance to the nasolacrimal canal. F

25 **Lacrimal groove.** Groovelike beginning of the nasolacrimal canal. F

26 **Lacrimal hamulus.** Hooked process projecting anterolaterally at the entrance to the nasolacrimal canal. F

27 **Fossa for lacrimal sac.** Widened beginning of the nasolacrimal canal for the lacrimal sac. F

28 **Nasal bone.** Bone located between the right and left frontal processes of the maxilla. Its superior end articulates with the frontal bone. G

29 **Ethmoidal groove.** Longitudinal groove on the inferior surface of the nasal bone for the passage of the external nasal branch of the anterior ethmoidal nerve. G

30 **Nasal foramina.** Inconstant opening for the passage of external nasal branches of the anterior ethmoidal nerve and small branches of the ophthalmic artery and vein.

31 **Vomer.** Unpaired bone of the cranial base. It forms the lower part of the nasal septum and is situated between the sphenoid, maxilla, palatine bone, and perpendicular plate of the ethmoid. H

32 **Ala of vomer.** Winglike process that articulates with the sphenoidal rostrum and, laterally, with the palatine bone. H

33 **Vomerine groove.** Oblique groove for transmission of the nasopalatine nerve and its accompanying vessels. H

34 **Vomerine crest of choana.** Posterior border of the vomer. H

35 **Cuneiform part of vomer.** Wedge-shaped part of the vomer. H

2

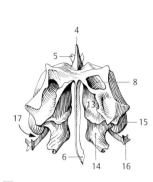

A Ethmoid, posterior view

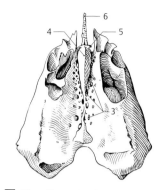

B Ethmoid, superior view

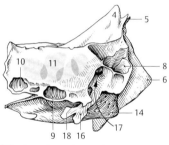

C Ethmoid, view from right

D Left half of ethmoid without perpendicular plate, medial view

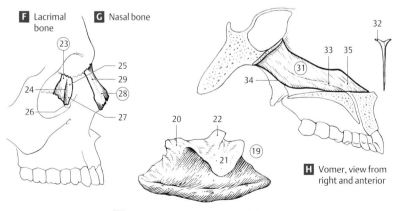

F Lacrimal bone **G** Nasal bone

H Vomer, view from right and anterior

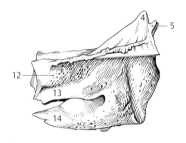

E Left inferior nasal concha, lateral view

1 **Maxilla.** A B

2 **Body of maxilla.** Central part of the maxilla enclosing the maxillary sinus. A

3 *Orbital surface.* The part of the body that forms the largest surface of the floor of the orbit. A

4 *Infra-orbital canal.* Canal for the passage of the infra-orbital nerve and artery between the orbit and the roof of the maxillary sinus. A

5 *Infra-orbital groove.* Groove at the beginning of the infra-orbital canal, beginning at the inferior orbital fissure. A

6 *Infra-orbital margin.* Lower margin of the orbit that is partly formed by the maxilla. A

7 *Anterior surface of maxilla.* A

8 *Infra-orbital foramen.* Opening of the infra-orbital canal from which the infra-orbital nerve and accompanying vessel emerge. Pressure point for the second division of the trigeminal nerve. A

9 *Canine fossa.* Depression below the infra-orbital foramen that gives origin to the levator anguli oris muscle. A

10 *Nasal notch.* Curved margin of the bony piriform aperture. A

11 *Anterior nasal spine.* Spinous projection situated in the middle of the inferior border of the piriform aperture for attachment of the cartilaginous nasal septum. A B

12 *Zygomaticomaxillary suture.* Suture that is occasionally still present in the orbit extending along the infra-orbital canal to the infra-orbital foramen. A

13 *Infratemporal surface.* Surface of the maxilla posterior to the zygomatic process. A

14 *Alveolar foramina.* Small openings on the infratemporal surface for the passage of nerves and vessels to the molars teeth. A

15 *Alveolar canals.* Canals beginning at the alveolar foramina for the passage of nerves and vessels that supply the molar teeth. A

16 *Maxillary tuberosity.* Thin-walled protuberance on the posterior wall of the maxillary sinus. A

17 *Nasal surface.* Medial surface of the maxilla that forms the lateral wall of the nasal cavity. B

18 *Lacrimal groove.* Depression for the nasolacrimal canal. B

19 Conchal crest. Nearly horizontal ridge providing attachment for the inferior nasal concha. B

20 Lacrimal margin. Border of the maxilla that articulates with the lacrimal bone. A B

21 Maxillary hiatus. Large opening in the maxillary sinus. It is narrowed by the uncinate process, the inferior nasal concha, and the palatine bone. B

22 *Greater palatine groove.* Groove along the posterior border of the maxilla, which forms part of the greater palatine canal for transmission of the greater palatine nerve and the descending palatine artery. B

23 *Maxillary sinus.* It measures over 3 cm vertically and sagittally and 2.5 cm in the frontal plane. Its floor is usually at least 1 cm below the floor of the nose and its lowest point is usually at the level of the first molar. B

24 **Frontal process of maxilla.** A B

25 *Anterior lacrimal crest.* Bony ridge of the frontal process at the entrance to the nasolacrimal canal. A

26 *Lacrimal notch.* Notch for the lacrimal hamulus at the entrance to the nasolacrimal canal. B

27 *Ethmoidal crest.* Oblique ridge on the medial surface providing attachment for the anterior end of the middle nasal conchae. B

28 **Zygomatic process of maxilla.** Lateral process of the maxilla for articulation with the zygomatic bone. A

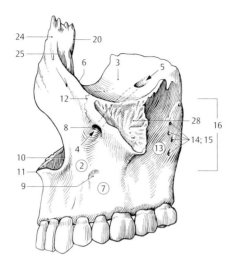

A Left maxilla, lateral view

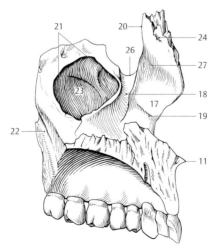

B Left maxilla, medial view

1 **Palatine process of maxilla.** Horizontal bony plate. The two processes form the anterior two-thirds of the hard palate. A B C

2 *Nasal crest.* Bony ridge formed by the union of the two processes in the midline. Site of attachment for the nasal septum. B

3 *[Incisive bone*; *premaxilla].* Embryonic bone that develops into part of the maxilla. A

4 *Incisive canals.* They begin as a pair of canals on the floor of the nasal cavity and unite on the palate in a single incisive fossa. A B

5 *[Incisive suture].* Suture only visible during development between the palatine process of the maxilla and the incisive bone. It normally extends from the incisive foramen to the space between the canine tooth and the second incisor tooth. A

6 *Palatine spines.* Bony ridges along the palatine grooves. A

7 *Palatine grooves.* Grooves running from posterior to anterior on the inferior surface of the palate transmitting nerves and vessels from the greater palatine foramen. A

8 **Alveolar process.** Ridged process bearing the teeth. A

9 *Alveolar arch.* Curved, free border of the alveolar process. A

10 *Dental alveoli.* Sockets in the alveolar process for reception of the roots of the teeth. A

11 *Interalveolar septa.* Bony ridges between adjacent dental alveoli. A

12 *Interradicular septa.* Bony partitions in the alveoli of multirooted teeth. A

13 *Alveolar yokes.* Eminences on the external surface of maxilla produced by the dental alveoli. A B

14 *Incisive foramina.* Openings of the incisive canals into the incisive fossa. A

15 **Palatine bone.** Bone that extends from the posterior border of the maxilla to the sphenoid. A B D E

16 **Perpendicular plate of palatine bone.** Vertical bony plate contributing to the walls of the nasal and maxillary sinuses. B C D E

17 *Nasal surface.* Surface of the perpendicular plate of the palatine bone facing the nose. E

18 *Maxillary surface.* External surface of the perpendicular plate of the palatine bone. Its posterior part borders with the pterygopalatine fossa from medial, and its anterior part with the maxillary sinus from posterior. D

19 *Sphenopalatine notch.* Semi-oval notch between the orbital process and the sphenoidal process of the perpendicular plate of the palatine bone. D E

20 *Greater palatine groove.* Channel that unites with the greater palatine groove of the maxilla to form the greater palatine canal, which lodges the greater palatine nerve and the descending palatine artery. D E

21 *Pyramidal process.* The inferoposterior end of the perpendicular plate of the palatine bone, which is inserted in the pterygoid notch. A C D E

22 *Lesser palatine canals.* Canals in the pyramidal process for passage of the lesser palatine nerves and arteries. A

23 *Conchal crest.* Ridge providing attachment for the posterior end of the inferior nasal concha. D E

24 *Ethmoidal crest.* Ridge providing attachment for the posterior end of the middle nasal concha. D E

25 *Orbital process.* Anterosuperiorly projecting process located between the maxilla, ethmoid, and sphenoid. D E

26 *Sphenoidal process.* Process behind the sphenopalatine notch that borders with the body and the vaginal process of the sphenoid. D E

27 **Horizontal plate of palatine bone.** It forms the posterior third of the hard palate and thus the floor of the nasal cavity. A B D E

28 *Nasal surface.* Surface of the horizontal plate that faces the nose. A

29 *Palatine surface.* Surface of the horizontal plate that faces the oral cavity. A D

30 *Lesser palatine foramina.* Openings of the lesser palatine canals. A

31 *Posterior nasal spine.* Posteromedian tip of the nasal crest. A B E

32 *Nasal crest.* Median bony ridge along the union with the opposing palatine bone. B D E

33 *Palatine crest.* Transverse ridge that is frequently present on the inferior surface of the horizontal plate near its posterior margin. A

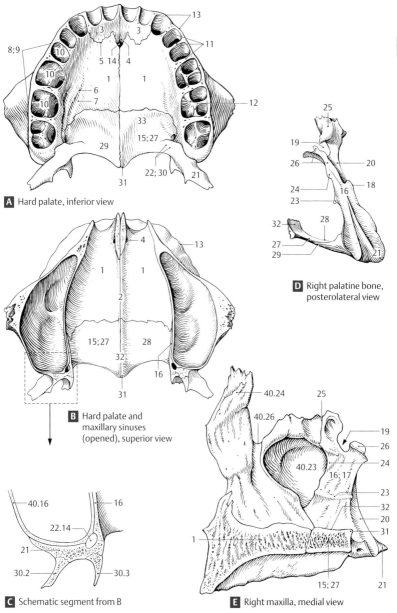

A Hard palate, inferior view

B Hard palate and maxillary sinuses (opened), superior view

C Schematic segment from B

D Right palatine bone, posterolateral view

E Right maxilla, medial view

2

1 **Zygomatic bone.** The zygomatic bone is inserted between the temporal bone, frontal bone, and maxilla. It forms a large part of the lateral wall of the orbit and part of the zygomatic arch. A B

2 **Lateral surface of zygomatic bone.** A

3 **Temporal surface.** Surface of the zygomatic bone facing the temporal fossa. B

4 **Orbital surface.** Surface of the zygomatic bone facing the orbit. A B

5 **Temporal process.** Posteriorly directed process that unites with the zygomatic process of the temporal bone to form the zygomatic arch. A B

6 **Frontal process.** Projection that articulates with the zygomatic process of the frontal bone and with the greater wing of the sphenoid. A B

7 **Orbital tubercle.** Small protuberance on the internal surface of the lateral orbital margin that gives attachment to the lateral palpebral ligament and other structures. A B

8 **[Marginal tubercle].** Small tubercle that is occasionally present on the posterior margin of the frontal process for attachment of the temporal fascia. A B

9 **Zygomatico-orbital foramen.** Foramen on the orbital surface of the zygomatic bone for the entrance of the zygomatic nerve. A B

10 **Zygomaticofacial foramen.** Opening on the lateral surface of the zygomatic bone through which the zygomaticofacial branch of the zygomatic nerve emerges. A

11 **Zygomaticotemporal foramen.** Opening on the temporal surface of the zygomatic bone through which the zygomaticotemporal branch of the zygomatic nerve emerges. B

12 **Mandible.** C D E F

13 **Body of mandible.** Horizontal part of the mandible to which the rami of the mandible are attached. C

14 *Base of mandible.* Lower part of the body of the mandible, excluding the alveolar part. C

15 *[Mandibular symphysis].* Fibrous tissue bridge at the junction of the right and left halves of the mandible in the midline. It ossifies by the first year of life.

16 *Mental protuberance.* C

17 *Mental tubercle.* Prominence on either side of the mental protuberance. C

18 *[[Gnathion]].* Point used for measurements, located in the midline on the inferior margin of the mandible. C D

19 *Mental foramen.* Opening below the first or second premolar tooth for passage of the mental nerve. Pressure point for the third division of the trigeminal nerve. C

20 *Oblique line.* Oblique ridge that extends from the ramus of the mandible to the external surface of the body of mandible. C F

21 *Digastric fossa.* Paired pea-sized or bean-sized depressions near the mental protuberance just above the inferior margin of the mandible for attachment of the anterior belly of the digastric muscle. D

22 *Superior mental spine*; *Superior genial spine.* Upper process projecting lingually that gives origin to the genioglossus muscle. D

23 *Inferior mental spine*; *Inferior genial spine.* Lower process projecting lingually that gives origin to the geniohyoid muscle. D

24 *Mylohyoid line.* Oblique ridge extending on the body of the mandible from posterosuperior to anteroinferior, giving origin to the mylohyoid muscle. At its posterior end the mylopharyngeal part of the superior constrictor muscle of the pharynx takes origin. The lingual nerve enters the oral cavity between the two muscles. D

25 *[Mandibular torus].* Bony outgrowth above the mylohyoid line at the level of the premolars. Possible hindrance to dental prostheses. D

26 *Sublingual fossa.* Concavity that lodges the sublingual gland on the anterior part of the body of the mandible above the mylohyoid line. D

27 *Submandibular fossa.* Depression below the mylohyoid line on the posterior half of the body of mandible. D

28 *Alveolar part.* Pectinate process on the base of mandible that houses the roots of the teeth. C

29 *Alveolar arch.* Parabolic free margin of the alveolar part. E

30 *Dental alveoli.* Sockets for reception and fixation of the roots of the teeth. E

31 *Interalveolar septa.* Bony partitions between the dental alveoli. E

32 *Interradicular septa.* Bony partitions between the roots of a single tooth. E

33 *Alveolar yokes.* Eminences on the external surface of the mandible produced by the dental alveoli. C E

34 *Retromolar triangle.* Bony triangle behind the last molar teeth of the mandible. Site of attachment for the pterygomandibular raphe. F

35 *Retromolar fossa.* Depression in the retromolar triangle. F

36 *[[Crista buccinatoria]].* Rounded bony ridge extending from the coronoid process to the medial, distal side of the third molar tooth. It forms the medial boundary of the retromolar triangle. F, p. 47 A

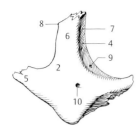

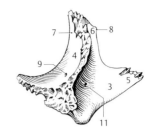

A Zygomatic bone, lateral view

B Zygomatic bone, medial view

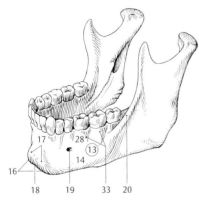

C Mandible

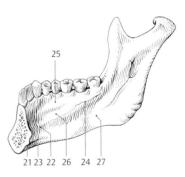

D Mandible, medial view

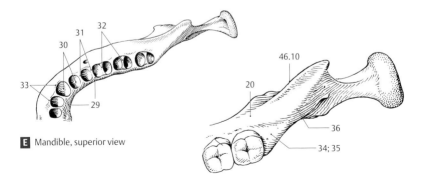

E Mandible, superior view

F Mandible segment,
superior view

1 **Ramus of mandible.** Projection that forms the ascending ramus of the mandible. A

2 *Angle of mandible.* Angle formed between the body and the ramus of the mandible. It is sharpest in adults and wider in newborns and elderly, edentulous individuals (ca. 140°). A

3 *[Masseteric tuberosity].* Roughened area that is occasionally present on the external surface of the angle of the mandible that gives attachment to the masseter muscle. A

4 *[Pterygoid tuberosity].* Roughened area that is occasionally present on the internal surface of the mandible near the angle of the mandible. Attachment site for the medial pterygoid muscle. A

5 *Mandibular foramen.* Opening on the internal aspect of the ramus of the mandible. Beginning of the mandibular canal which lies about 1 cm above the occlusal plane. A

6 *Lingula.* Thin bony projection in front of the mandibular foramen that gives attachment to the sphenomandibular ligament. A

7 *Mandibular canal.* Bony canal within the mandible that transmits the inferior alveolar artery and nerve. It begins at the mandibular foramen and passes beneath the roots of the teeth to the mental foramen. A

8 *Mylohyoid groove.* Groove that begins at the mandibular foramen and extends anteroinferiorly, transmitting the mylohyoid nerve and the mylohyoid branch of the inferior alveolar artery. A

9 *Coronoid process.* Muscular process that is separated by the mandibular notch from the condylar process to posterior. Attachment site of the temporal muscle. A

10 *Temporal crest.* Bony ridge that extends from the coronoid process to the oblique line. It gives attachment of the temporal muscle. A, p. 45 F

11 *Mandibular notch.* Notch between the condylar and coronoid processes. The masseteric nerve and vessels pass over it to supply the masseter muscle. A

12 *Condylar process.* Articular process. A

13 *Head of mandible.* Articular head of the mandible. A

14 *Neck of mandible.* Narrowed part of the mandible below the head of the mandible. A

15 *Pterygoid fovea.* Anteromedial depression below the head of the mandible for attachment of the lateral pterygoid muscle. A

16 **Hyoid bone.** Bone that already begins to ossify before birth. B

17 **Body of hyoid bone.** Anterior segment between the right and left lesser horns. B

18 *Lesser horn of hyoid bone.* Small horn on the hyoid bone. B

19 *Greater horn of hyoid bone.* Larger horn on the hyoid bone. B

20 ***VERTEBRAL COLUMN.*** C D

21 **Primary curvature.** Primary curvature occurring during embryological development as a result of anterior embryonic flexion. It persists as the two kyphoses. D

22 *Thoracic kyphosis.* C D

23 *Sacral kyphosis.* C D

24 **Secondary curvatures.** Curvatures that arise from fetal muscular movements. They are more functional in origin and persist as lordoses. D

25 *Cervical lordosis.* C D

26 *Lumbar lordosis.* C D

27 **Scoliosis.** Pathological lateral bending deformity of the spine.

2

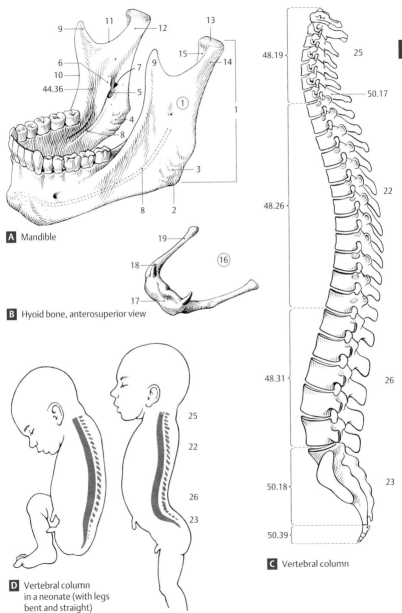

A Mandible

B Hyoid bone, anterosuperior view

C Vertebral column

D Vertebral column in a neonate (with legs bent and straight)

2

1   **Vertebra.**

2   **Vertebral body.** A B C D

3   *Intervertebral surface.* Surface of a vertebral body facing the adjacent vertebra. B D

4   *Anular epiphysis.* Epiphyseal ring around the surfaces of the vertebral bodies. Peripheral bony ridge. B

5   **Vertebral arch.** It forms the posterior and lateral boundaries of the vertebral foramen. C D

6   *Pedicle.* The part of the vertebral arch located on the vertebral body between the superior and inferior vertebral notches. B D

7   *Lamina.* Flattened posterior part of the vertebral arch. C

8   **Intervertebral foramen.** Opening between two adjacent vertebrae for the passage of a spinal nerve and small vessels. It is bounded by two adjacent vertebral notches (above and below), the vertebral bodies, and the intervertebral disc. B

9   **Superior vertebral notch.** Notch on the upper surface of the pedicle. B

10 **Inferior vertebral notch.** Notch on the lower surface of the pedicle. B

11 **Vertebral foramen.** Opening in the vertebra that is bounded by the vertebral arch and the vertebral body. The combined vertebral foramina form the vertebral canal. C D

12 **Vertebral canal.** Passageway formed by all of the vertebral foramina together. It extends from the foramen magnum to the sacral hiatus and contains the spinal cord. A B

13 **Spinous process.** The spinous processes of C1–C6 are bifid. B C D

14 **Transverse process.** A B C

15 **Superior articular process.** Superiorly projecting articular process on the vertebral arch. B C D

16 *Superior articular facet.* Surface of the superior articular process covered with cartilage for articulation with the inferior articular facet. C

17 **Inferior articular process.** Inferiorly projecting articular process on the vertebral arch that projects inferiorly. B C

18 *Inferior articular facet.* Surface of the inferior articular process covered with cartilage for articulation with the superior articular facet.

19 CERVICAL VERTEBRAE (C1–C7). The seven cervical vertebrae. A, p. 47 C

20 **Uncus of body; Uncinate process.** Upward projection from the lateral margin of the body of a cervical vertebra. Bone spurs can occasionally form here and impinge on the spinal nerves. A C

21 **Foramen transversarium.** Opening in the transverse processes of the cervical vertebrae for the passage of the vertebral artery and vein. A C

22 **Anterior tubercle.** Anterior protuberance found on the second to seventh cervical vertebrae for muscle attachment. A C

23 **Posterior tubercle.** Posterior protuberance on the second to seventh cervical vertebrae for muscle attachment. A C

24 **Carotid tubercle.** Prominent anterior tubercle on the sixth cervical vertebra. Possible compression of the common carotid artery from anterior. A

25 **Groove for spinal nerve.** Groove on the transverse processes of the third through seventh cervical vertebrae that transmits the spinal nerves emerging from the intervertebral foramen. A C

26 THORACIC VERTEBRAE (T1–T12). The twelve thoracic vertebrae. p. 47 C

27 **Superior costal facet.** Articular fossa for the head of the rib located on the superior margin of the vertebral body at the root of the vertebral arch. B

28 **Inferior costal facet.** Articular fossa for the head of the rib located on the inferior margin of the vertebral body below the root of vertebral arch. B

29 **Transverse costal facet.** Fossa for articulation with the tubercle of the rib. B

30 **Uncus of body of first thoracic vertebra; Uncinate process of first thoracic vertebra.** Body of the first thoracic vertebra, which strongly resembles that of a cervical vertebra. The uncinate process projects mainly to dorsal.

31 LUMBAR VERTEBRAE (L1–L5). The five lumbar vertebrae. p. 47 C

32 **Accessory process.** Rudiment of the original transverse process of the lumbar vertebrae projecting posteriorly from the base of the costal process. D

33 **Costal process.** A single transverse process formed by a rudimentary rib. D

34 **Mamillary process.** Small protuberance on the lateral surface of the superior articular process of the lumbar vertebrae. D

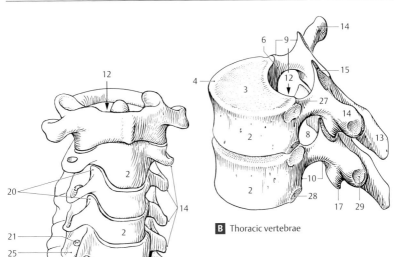

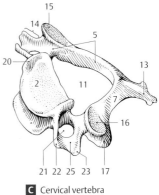

B Thoracic vertebrae

A Cervical vertebrae, anterolateral view

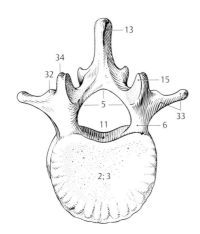

C Cervical vertebra

D Lumbar vertebra, superior view

1 **Atlas (C1).** First cervical vertebra. It does not have a body. A

2 **Lateral mass.** Thickened part of the atlas in place of the lacking vertebral body, which supports the cranium. A

3 *Superior articular surface.* Elliptical and concave articular surface of the atlas. A

4 *Inferior articular surface.* Roundish, slightly convex surface with a cartilage lining. A

5 **Anterior arch of the atlas.** A

6 *Facet for dens.* Articular fossa on the inner surface of the anterior arch for articulation with the dens of the axis. A

7 *Anterior tubercle of atlas.* A

8 **Posterior arch of atlas.** A

9 *Groove for vertebral artery.* Groove on the arch of the atlas behind the lateral mass that transmits the vertebral artery. A

10 *[Canal for vertebral artery].* The groove for the vertebral artery is sometimes converted into a canal.

11 *Posterior tubercle.* Rudiment of the spinous process. A

12 **Axis (C2).** Second cervical vertebra. B

13 **Dens of axis.** B

14 *Apex of dens.* Attachment site of the apical ligament of the dens. B

15 **Anterior articular facet of dens.** B

16 *Posterior articular facet of dens.* B

17 **Vertebra prominens (C7).** Seventh cervical vertebra. Its name originates from its prominent spinous process (in 70%). p. 47 C

18 SACRUM [SACRAL VERTEBRAE 1–5]. The sacrum consists of five fused vertebrae. C D F, p. 47 C

19 **Base of sacrum.** Broad superior surface of the sacrum, which comprises the first sacral vertebra. F

20 *Promontory of sacrum.* Upper margin of the base of the sacrum, which projects especially far into the pelvic girdle. F

21 *Ala of sacrum*; *Wing of sacrum.* Bone mass lateral to the first sacral vertebra. Upper part of the lateral part of the sacrum. F

22 *Superior articular process.* C F

23 **Lateral part of sacrum.** Lateral bone mass of the sacrum formed by the transverse processes and remnants of ribs. C F

24 *Auricular surface.* Ear-shaped surface at the level of the upper 2–3 sacral vertebrae for articulation with the ilium. C

25 *Sacral tuberosity.* Roughened area behind the auricular surface, giving attachment to the sacroiliac ligaments. C

26 *Pelvic surface.* Concave surface on the anterior aspect of sacrum that faces the pelvis. F

27 *Transverse ridges.* Four ridges on the anterior surface of the sacrum that mark where the five vertebral bodies are united. F

28 *Intervertebral foramina.* Openings at the sites of the original superior and inferior notches. D

29 *Anterior sacral foramina.* Openings in the anterior surface of the sacrum for the exit of the sacral nerves. They were formed by the fusion of vertebrae, rudimentary ribs, and ossified ligaments. D F

30 **Dorsal surface.** Posterior convex surface of the sacrum. C

31 *Median sacral crest.* Median ridge formed by the union of rudiments of the spinous processes of the sacral vertebrae. C

32 *Posterior sacral foramina.* Posterior counterparts of the anterior sacral foramina. C

33 *Intermediate sacral crest.* Remnants of articular processes located on both sides of the median sacral crest. C

34 *Lateral sacral crest.* Lateral series of rudimentary transverse processes on the right and left sides of the dorsal surface of the sacrum. C

35 *Sacral cornu*; *Sacral horn.* Inferiorly projecting process located to the right and left of the sacral hiatus. C

36 *Sacral canal.* Inferior end of the vertebral canal. C D

37 *Sacral hiatus.* Opening in the posterior wall of the sacral canal that is usually found in both lower sacral vertebrae, giving passage to the terminal filum. Injection site for epidural anesthesia. C

38 **Apex of sacrum.** Inferiorly directed tip of the sacrum, which articulates with the coccyx. C F

39 COCCYX (COCCYGEALVERTEBRAE 1–4). The coccyx usually consists of four rudimentary vertebrae. E, p. 47 C

40 **Coccygeal cornu.** Remnant of the superior articular process. E

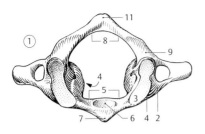

A Atlas, superior view

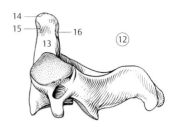

B Axis, from left

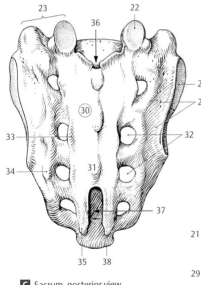

C Sacrum, posterior view

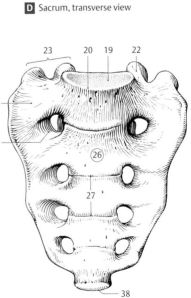

D Sacrum, transverse view

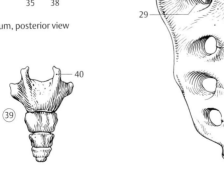

E Coccyx, posterior view

F Sacrum, anterior view

2

1 *THORACIC SKELEON.*

2 **Ribs (I–XII).** D

3 **True ribs (I–VII).** The first seven ribs, which are joined directly to the sternum by cartilage. This distinguishes them from the last five ribs. D

4 **False ribs (VIII–XII).** The last five ribs, which are not directly connected to the sternum by cartilage. D

5 *Floating ribs (XI-XII).* The eleventh and twelfth ribs are not connected to the costal arch. D

6 **Costal cartilage.** Cartilage at the anterior end of the ribs. D

7 **Rib.** D

8 **Head of rib.** The part of the rib that articulates with the vertebral column. A

9 *Articular facet of head of rib.* A B

10 **Crest of head of rib.** Small ridge that divides the articular facet into two surfaces. B

11 **Neck of rib.** The part of the rib located lateral to the head of the rib. A B

12 *Crest of neck of rib.* Sharp ridge on the superior border of the neck of the rib. A

13 **Body of rib; Shaft of rib.** The part of the rib that is continuous with the neck. A B

14 *Tubercle of rib.* Protuberance on the posterior surface between the neck and the body of the rib. A B

15 *Articular facet of tubercle of rib.* Surface for articulation with the transverse process of the thoracic vertebra. A B

16 *Angle of rib.* Site where the rib changes direction from dorsolateral to ventral. A B

17 *Costal groove.* Groove on the inferior border of the rib for the passage of the intercostal artery, vein, and nerve. B

18 *Crest of rib.* Sharp inferior border of a rib.

19 **First rib (I).** The only rib that is only bent around the edge. A D

20 *Scalene tubercle.* Small tubercle on the first rib for attachment of the anterior scalene muscle. A

21 *Groove for subclavian artery.* Groove on the first rib posterior to the scalene tubercle for the passage of the subclavian artery. A

22 *Groove for subclavian vein.* Groove on the first rib anterior to the scalene tubercle for the passage of the subclavian vein. A

23 **Second rib (II).** Rib that begins at the level of the sternal angle. It is easily palpated. A D

24 *Tuberosity for serratus anterior.* Roughened area on the second rib from which the anterior serratus muscle takes origin. A D

25 **[Cervical rib].** Accessory rib at C7 that can irritate the brachial plexus.

26 **[Lumbar rib].**

27 **Sternum.** C D

28 **Manubrium of sternum.** The part of the sternum above the sternal angle. C D

29 *Clavicular notch.* Notch for the sternoclavicular joint. C D

30 *Jugular notch; Suprasternal notch.* Notch at the superior border of the manubrium of the sternum. D

31 **Sternal angle.** (Angle of Ludovicus). Angle between the body and the manubrium of the sternum, which is palpable through the skin. C D

32 **Body of sternum.** The part of the sternum between the manubrium and the xiphoid process. C D

33 **Xiphoid process.** Cartilaginous end of the sternum. C D

34 **Costal notches.** Notches for the costal cartilages. C D

35 **[Suprasternal bones].** Ossicles that are occasionally found in the ligaments of the sternoclavicular joint. Remnants of the earlier episternum.

36 **Thoracic cage.**

37 **Thoracic cavity.**

38 **Superior thoracic aperture; Thoracic inlet.** Upper opening of the thoracic cavity. D

39 **Inferior thoracic aperture; Thoracic outlet.** Lower opening of the thoracic cavity. D

40 **Pulmonary groove of thorax.** One groove each to the right and left of the vertebral column for the dorsal part of the lungs. D

41 **Costal margin; Costal arch.** Arch formed by the cartilages of the seventh to tenth ribs. D

42 **Intercostal space.** Space between adjacent ribs.

43 **Infrasternal angle; Subcostal angle.** Angle between right and left costal arches. D

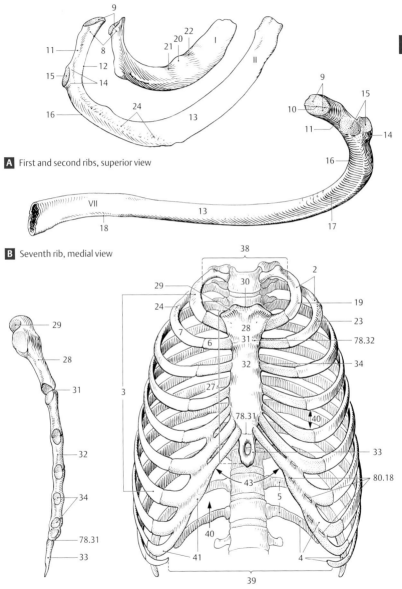

A First and second ribs, superior view

B Seventh rib, medial view

C Sternum, view from right

D Thoracic cage, anterior view

2

1 *BONES OF UPPER LIMB.*

2 **PECTORAL GIRDLE; SHOULDER GIRDLE.** A

3 **Scapula.** Shoulder blade. B C

4 **Costal surface.** Scapular surface facing the ribs. C

5 *Subscapular fossa.* Concavity on the costal surface of the scapula. C

6 **Posterior surface.** Scapular surface facing the skin of the back. B

7 *Spine of scapula.* Rather long bony ridge on the posterior surface of the scapula that is continuous with the acromion. B C

8 *Deltoid tubercle.* Tubercle at the root of the spine of the scapula that affords attachment to the overlapping tendons of the trapezius and deltoid muscles. B

9 *Supraspinous fossa.* Fossa that extends from above the spine to the superior border of the scapula. A B

10 *Infraspinous fossa.* Fossa that extends from below the spine to the inferior angle of the scapula. A B

11 **Acromion.** Free end of the spine of the scapula that projects over the head of the humerus. A B C

12 *Clavicular facet.* Articular facet for the clavicle. C

13 *Acromial angle.* Sharp bend where the spine of the scapula passes into the lateral margin of the acromion. B

14 **Medial border.** Border of the scapula facing the vertebral column. B C

15 **Lateral border.** Border of the scapula facing the humerus. B C

16 **Superior border.** Upper border of the scapula. B C

17 *Suprascapular notch.* Notch in the superior border of the scapula medial to the coracoid process for the passage of the suprascapular nerve. B C

18 **Inferior angle.** Lower angle of the scapula. B C

19 **Lateral angle.** Lateral angle of the scapula that bears the glenoid cavity. B C

20 **Superior angle.** Superomedial angle of the scapula. B C

21 **Glenoid cavity.** Articular fossa forming part of the shoulder joint. C

22 **Infraglenoid tubercle.** Small tubercle below the glenoid cavity for the origin of the long head of the triceps brachii muscle. B C

23 **Supraglenoid tubercle.** Small tubercle above the margin of the glenoid cavity for the origin of the long head of the biceps brachii muscle. C

24 **Neck of scapula.** The part of the scapula medial to the margin of the glenoid cavity. B C

25 **Coracoid process.** Hooked process that projects anteriorly from the superior border of the scapula just lateral to the suprascapular notch. Attachment site of the pectoralis minor muscle and origin of the short head of the biceps brachii and coracobrachialis muscles. A B C

26 **Clavicle.** A D

27 **Sternal end.** Thickened end of the clavicle (triangular in cross-section) facing the sternum. D

28 *Sternal facet.* Articular surface facing the sternum. D

29 *Impression for costoclavicular ligament.* Roughened area and depression on the inferior surface near the sternal end of the clavicle that gives attachment to the costoclavicular ligament. D

30 **Shaft of clavicle; Body of clavicle.** Middle portion of the clavicle. D

31 *Subclavian groove; Groove for subclavius.* Deep, elongated groove for attachment of the subclavian muscle. D

32 **Acromial end.** Prolate end of the clavicle facing the acromion. D

33 *Acromial facet.* Articular facet of the clavicle facing posterolaterally. D

34 *Tuberosity for coracoclavicular ligament.* Roughened area on the inferior surface of the acromial end of the clavicle for attachment of the coracoclavicular ligament. D

35 *Conoid tubercle.* Small eminence on the tuberosity that gives attachment to the conoid portion of the coracoclavicular ligament. D

36 *Trapezoid line.* Ridge on the tuberosity that gives attachment to the trapezoid portion of the coracoclavicular ligament. D

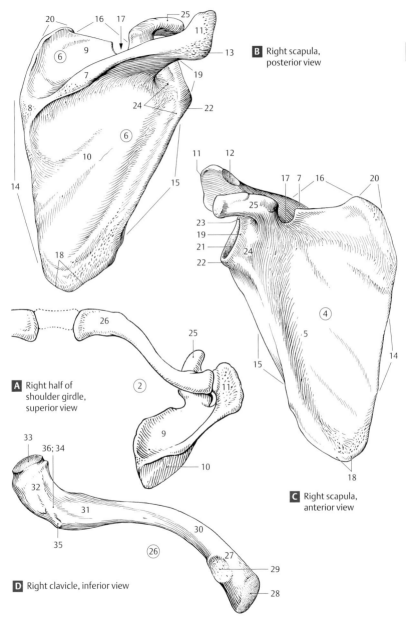

B Right scapula, posterior view

A Right half of shoulder girdle, superior view

C Right scapula, anterior view

D Right clavicle, inferior view

2

1 **FREE PART OF UPPER LIMB.**

2 **Humerus.** The bone of the upper arm. A B

3 **Head of humerus.** A B

4 **Anatomical neck.** Area bounded by the head of the humerus at one end and the greater and lesser tubercles at the other. A B

5 **Surgical neck.** Area distal to the greater and lesser tubercles. A B

6 **Greater tubercle of humerus.** Large protuberance on the lateral surface of the humerus for muscle attachment. A B

7 **Lesser tubercle of humerus.** Small protuberance on the anterior surface of the humerus for muscle attachment. A

8 *Intertubercular sulcus*; *Bicipital groove.* Groove between the two tubercles for passage of the tendon of the long head of the biceps brachii muscle. A

9 *Crest of greater tubercle*; *Lateral lip.* Bony ridge extending distalward from the greater tubercle that gives attachment to the pectoralis major muscle. A

10 *Crest of lesser tubercle*; *Medial lip.* Bony ridge extending distalward from the lesser tubercle that gives attachment to the teres major and latissimus dorsi muscles. A

11 **Shaft of humerus; Body of humerus.** Area between the two ends of the humerus. A B

12 *Anteromedial surface.* Area medial to the prolongation of the crest of the greater tubercle. A

13 *Anterolateral surface.* Area lateral to the prolongation of the crest of the greater tubercle. A

14 *Posterior surface.* B

15 *Radial groove*; *Groove for radial nerve.* Spiral groove for the radial nerve that passes from the posterior surface of the humerus around the lateral border to reach the anterolateral surface. B

16 *Medial border.* Its distal end is continuous with the medial supracondylar ridge. A B

17 *Medial supraepicondylar ridge*; *Medial supracondylar ridge.* Sharp, inferior end of the medial border of the humerus. It is continuous with the medial epicondyle. A B

18 *[Supracondylar process].* Bone spur of phylogenetic origin that is occasionally found (1%) at the medial border of the distal humerus. A

19 *Lateral border.* Its distal end is continuous with the lateral supracondylar ridge. A B

20 *Lateral supraepicondylar ridge*; *Lateral supracondylar ridge.* Sharp, inferior end of the lateral border of the humerus that is continuous with the lateral epicondyle. A B

21 *Deltoid tuberosity.* Roughened area on the anterolateral surface of the humerus near the middle of the shaft for attachment of the deltoid muscle. A B

22 **Condyle of humerus.** Distal end of the humerus between the epicondyles comprising the olecranon fossa, radial fossa, and articular surfaces. A B

23 *Capitulum of humerus.* Rounded eminence on the condyle for articulation with the radius. A

24 *Trochlea of humerus.* Cylindrical projection on the condyle for articulation with the ulna. A B

25 *Olecranon fossa.* Deep concavity above the trochlea on the posterior aspect of the humerus that receives the olecranon during elbow extension. B

26 *Coronoid fossa.* Depression on the anterior aspect of the humerus proximal to the trochlea that receives the coronoid process of the ulna during elbow flexion. A

27 *Radial fossa.* Anterior depression above the head of the humerus for reception of the head of the radius when the elbow joint is strongly flexed. A

28 **Medial epicondyle.** Protuberance that gives origin to the flexor muscles of the forearm. A B

29 *Groove for ulnar nerve.* Groove on the posterior surface of the medial epicondyle that transmits the ulnar nerve. B

30 **Lateral epicondyle.** Protuberance located lateral to the head of the humerus that gives origin to the extensor muscles of the forearm. A B

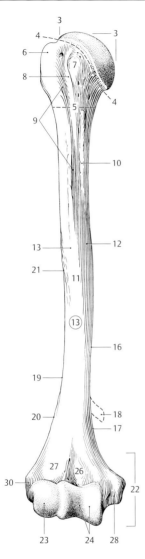

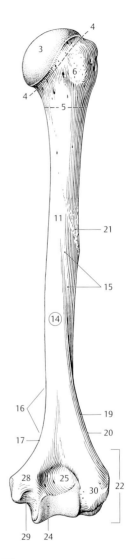

A Right humerus,
anterior view

B Right humerus,
posterior view

1 **Radius.** One of the two bones of the forearm. It is lateral to the ulna. A B C

2 **Head of radius.** Part of the radius that articulates with the capitulum of the humerus. A B

3 *Articular facet.* Concavity that receives the capitulum of the humerus. B

4 *Articular circumference of head of radius.* Rimlike surface around the head of the radius for articulation with the radial notch of the ulna. A B

5 **Neck of radius.** Slender region at the proximal end of the radius between the head of the radius and the radial tuberosity. A B

6 **Shaft of radius; Body of radius.** A B

7 *Radial tuberosity.* Roughened prominence on the medial aspect of the radius about 2 cm distal to its proximal end for attachment of the biceps brachii muscle. p. 115 A B

8 *Posterior surface.* B C

9 *Anterior surface.* A C

10 *Lateral surface.* A C

11 *Pronator tuberosity.* Attachment site of the pronator teres muscle. B

12 *Interosseous border.* Margin facing the ulna and giving attachment to the interosseous membrane. A B C

13 *Posterior border.* B C

14 *Anterior border.* Border of the radius that faces anterolaterally. A C

15 **Radial styloid process.** Projection from the lateral surface of the distal end of the radius. A B

16 **Suprastyloid crest.** Ridge above the styloid process giving attachment to the brachioradialis muscle. A

17 **Dorsal tubercle.** Bony ridge that is often palpable through the skin between the grooves for the extensor pollicis longus and the extensor carpi radialis brevis muscles. B

18 **Groove for extensor muscle tendons.** B

19 **Ulnar notch.** Roundish cavity on the distal end of the radius for articulation with the ulna. A B

20 **Carpal articular surface.** Surface facing distalward for articulation with the wrist. A

21 **Ulna.** Medial forearm bone. A B C

22 **Olecranon.** Proximal, posterior end of the ulna. Attachment site of the triceps brachii muscle. B

23 **Coronoid process.** Projection at the anterior end of the trochlear notch. A

24 *Tuberosity of ulna.* Roughened area distal to the coronoid process for attachment of the brachialis muscle. A

25 *Radial notch.* Superolateral surface for articulation with the articular circumference of the radius. A

26 **Trochlear notch.** Articular surface on the proximal end of the ulna for articulation with the trochlea of the humerus. A

27 **Shaft of ulna; Body of ulna.** A B

28 *Posterior surface.* B C

29 *Anterior surface.* A C

30 *Medial surface.* Surface facing the trunk. B C

31 *Interosseous border.* Attachment site of the interosseous membrane. A B C

32 *Posterior border.* B C

33 *Anterior border.* Margin facing anteromedially. A C

34 *Supinator crest.* Bony ridge extending distalward from the radial notch on the posterior surface of the shaft that gives origin to the supinator muscle. A B

35 **Head of ulna.** The head of the ulna located at its distal end. A B

36 *Articular circumference.* Anterolateral articular surface for articulation with the ulnar notch of the radius. A

37 *Ulnar styloid process.* Peglike process on the distal end of the ulna. Site of attachment for the articular disc of the distal radioulnar joint and the ulnar collateral ligament. A B

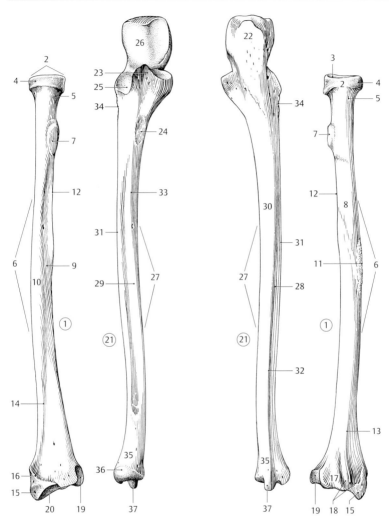

A Right radius and ulna, anterior view

B Right radius and ulna, posterior view

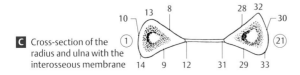

C Cross-section of the radius and ulna with the interosseous membrane

2

1 BONES OF HAND.

2 **Carpal bones.** The eight wrist bones. A B C

3 **[Os centrale].** Accessory wrist bone that is occasionally present between the capitate, scaphoid, and trapezoid. It normally fuses with the scaphoid. C

4 **Scaphoid.** Bone situated between the lunate and trapezium. A B

5 *Tubercle of scaphoid.* Prominence on the anterior surface of the scaphoid. It protrudes visibly with radial abduction of the hand. A

6 **Lunate.** Bone situated between the scaphoid and triquetrum. A B

7 **Triquetrum.** Bone dorsal to the pisiform between the hamate and lunate. A B

8 **Pisiform.** Bone located on the palmar side of the triquetrum. It is actually a sesamoid bone embedded in the tendon of the flexor carpi ulnaris muscle. A B

9 **Trapezium.** Bone situated between the first metacarpal and the scaphoid. A B

10 *Tubercle of trapezium.* Tubercle situated distal to the tubercle of the scaphoid and radial to the groove for the flexor carpi radialis muscle. A

11 **Trapezoid.** Bone located between the second metacarpal, scaphoid, trapezium, and capitate. A B

12 **Capitate.** Centrally located bone between the third metacarpal and the lunate. A B

13 **Hamate.** Bone located between the fourth and fifth metacarpals, the capitate, and the triquetrum. A B

14 *Hook of hamate.* Hooked process distal to the pisiform on the palmar aspect of the hamate. A

15 **Carpal groove.** Palmar groove between the tubercles of the scaphoid and trapezium on the radial side and the hook of hamate and pisiform on the ulnar side. It is converted by a transverse ligament into a closed canal for the flexor tendons of the fingers. A

16 **Metacarpals (I–V).** Metacarpal bones of the hand. A B

17 **Base of metacarpal bone.** Broad proximal end. A B

18 **Shaft of metacarpal bone; Body of metacarpal bone.** A B

19 **Head of metacarpal bone.** Distal articular head. A B

20 **Styloid process of third metacarpal (III).** Dorsal process at the base of the third metacarpal radial to the capitate. B

21 **Phalanges.** Bones of the fingers; digital bones. A B

22 **Proximal phalanx.** Proximal bone of a finger. A B

23 **Middle phalanx.** Middle bone of a finger. A B

24 **Distal phalanx.** Distal bone of a finger; ungual phalanx. A B

25 *Tuberosity of distal phalanx.* Roughened area on the distal flexor surface of the distal phalanx giving attachment to the tactile elevation. A

26 **Base of phalanx.** Thicker proximal end that bears the articular surface. A B

27 **Shaft of phalanx; Body of phalanx.** Shaft of a finger bone. A B

28 **Head of phalanx.** Distal head of a finger bone. A B

29 *Trochlea of phalanx.* The pulleylike head of the proximal and middle phalanges. A B

30 **Sesamoid bones.** Bones embedded in tendons or ligaments. A

2

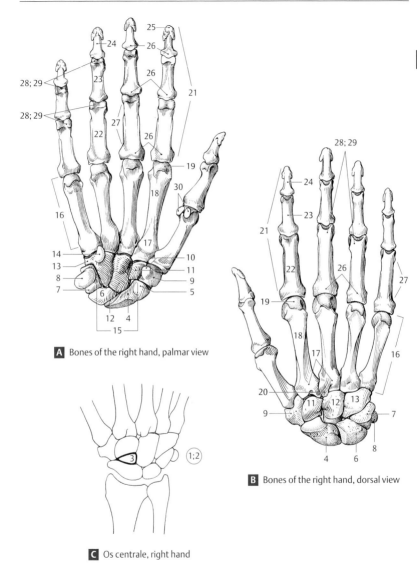

A Bones of the right hand, palmar view

B Bones of the right hand, dorsal view

C Os centrale, right hand

2

1 *BONES OF LOWER LIMB.*

2 **PELVIC GIRDLE.** The pelvic girdle consists of the two hip bones. The hip bones are connected at the pubic symphysis and, along with the sacrum, comprise the bony pelvis (pelvic girdle). D

3 HIP BONE; COXAL BONE; PELVIC BONE. Bony structure comprising the ilium, ischium, and pubis. A B C D

4 **Acetabulum.** Articular fossa of the hip joint formed by the ilium, pubis, and ischium. A

5 *Acetabular margin.* Prominent border that is interrupted by the acetabular notch. A

6 *Acetabular fossa.* Depression in the acetabulum that is surrounded by the lunate surface of the acetabulum. A

7 *Acetabular notch.* Notch in the lunate surface facing the obturator foramen. It is continuous with the acetabular fossa. A

8 *Lunate surface.* Articular surface of the acetabulum which is crescent-shaped and lined with cartilage. A

9 **Ischiopubic ramus.** Semicircumferential inferior border of the obturator foramen, formed by the ramus of the ischium and the inferior pubic ramus. A C

10 **Obturator foramen.** Round opening in the pelvis in which the obturator membrane replaces the bone. A B C

11 **Greater sciatic notch.** Notch between the posterior inferior iliac spine and the ischial spine. A C

12 **Ilium.** A C

13 **Body of ilium.** Main bony part of the ilium. Its inferior end is involved in formation of the acetabulum. A C

14 *Supra-acetabular groove.* Groove between the acetabular margin and the body of the ilium. A

15 **Ala of ilium; Wing of ilium.** A C

16 **Arcuate line.** Bony line at the boundary between the lesser and greater pelvis. C

17 **Iliac crest.** A C

18 *Outer lip.* Outer border of the iliac crest that gives attachment to the external oblique muscle of the abdomen. A

19 *Tuberculum of iliac crest.* Palpable projection on the outer lip about 5 cm posterior to the anterior superior iliac spine at the junction of the anterior gluteal line and the iliac crest. A

20 *Intermediate zone.* Rough bony area between the outer and inner lips of the iliac crest that gives origin to the internal oblique muscle of the abdomen. A

21 *Inner lip.* Bony ridge on the inner margin of the iliac crest that gives origin to the transverse abdominal muscle. A C

22 *Anterior superior iliac spine.* Bony projection at the anterior border of the iliac crest giving origin to the sartorius muscle. A C

23 *Anterior inferior iliac spine.* Bony projection at the anterior border of the ilium giving origin to the rectus femoris muscle. A C

24 *Posterior superior iliac spine.* Bony projection at the posterior border of the iliac crest. A C

25 *Posterior inferior iliac spine.* Bony projection at the superior border of the greater sciatic notch. A C

26 *Iliac fossa.* Depression on the inner aspect of the wing of the ilium. C

27 **Gluteal surface.** External surface of the wing of the ilium. A

28 *Anterior gluteal line.* Flat ridge near the center of the wing of the ilium, between the origins of the gluteus minimus and gluteus maximus muscles. A

29 *Posterior gluteal line.* Bony ridge between the origins of the gluteus medius and gluteus maximus muscles. A

30 *Inferior gluteal line.* Bony ridge above the acetabulum running between the origins of the gluteus minimus and rectus femoris muscles. A

31 **Sacropelvic surface.** Surface of the dorsal ilium facing the sacrum and consisting of the following two parts. C

32 *Auricular surface.* Ear-shaped surface for articulation with the sacrum. It is lined with fibrocartilage. C

33 *Iliac tuberosity.* Roughened area posterosuperior to the auricular surface for attachment of the sacroiliac ligaments. C

34 **Ischium.** Bone involved in formation of the acetabulum. It surrounds the obturator foramen from inferoposterior. A B C

35 **Body of ischium.** The part of the ischium above the obturator foramen. A B

36 **Ramus of ischium.** The part of the ischium below the obturator foramen. Its anterior end articulates with the inferior pubic ramus. A B

37 *Ischial tuberosity.* Bony prominence at the inferior border of the lesser sciatic notch. A C

38 **Ischial spine.** Bony process between the greater and lesser sciatic notches. A C

39 **Lesser sciatic notch.** Notch between the ischial spine and the ischial tuberosity. A C

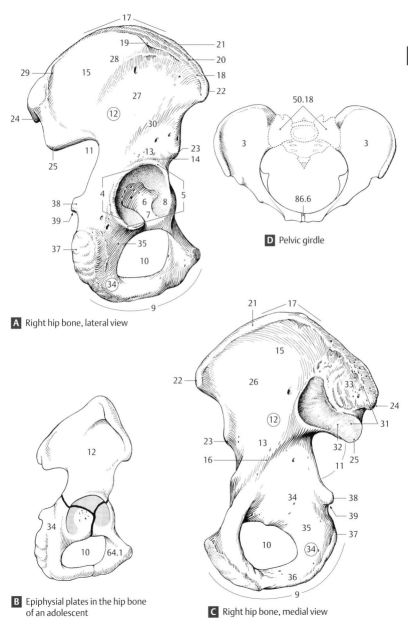

A Right hip bone, lateral view

D Pelvic girdle

B Epiphysial plates in the hip bone of an adolescent

C Right hip bone, medial view

1 **Pubis.** Bone involved in formation of the acetabulum and the anterior and inferior borders of the obturator foramen. A B

2 **Body of pubis.** A B

3 *Pubic tubercle.* Tubercle situated anterolateral to the pubic symphysis. A B

4 *Symphysial surface.* Medial surface of the body of the pubis facing its counterpart. B

5 *Pubic crest.* Ridge that extends medially from the pubic tubercle to the symphysis, giving attachment to the rectus abdominis muscle. A B

6 **Superior pubic ramus.** The part of the pubis above the obturator foramen. A B

7 *Iliopubic ramus.* Flat eminence near the proximal part of the pubis. A B

8 *Pecten pubis*; *Pectineal line.* Sharp, bony continuation of the arcuate line extending to the pubic tubercle. Origin of the pectineus muscle. A B

9 *Obturator crest.* Inferior border of the superior pubic ramus that gives origin to the pubofemoral ligament. A

10 *Obturator groove.* Groove on the obturator crest along the obturator foramen. A B

11 *Anterior obturator tubercle.* Small protuberance anterior to the obturator groove. A B

12 *[Posterior obturator tubercle].* Small protuberance that is occasionally present at the end of the obturator groove. A B

13 **Inferior pubic ramus.** The part of the pubis that is anteroinferior to the obturator foramen, between the pubic symphysis and the suture line with the ischium. A B

14 PELVIS.

15 **Pelvic cavity.**

16 **Pubic arch.** Arch below the pubic symphysis that is formed by the right and left pubic rami. C

17 **Subpubic angle.** The angle between the right and left inferior pubic rami (average of 75° in men and 90–100° in women). C

18 **Greater pelvis; False pelvis.** Region of the pelvis above the linea terminalis between the two wings of the ilium.

19 **Lesser pelvis; True pelvis.** Region of the pelvis below the linea terminalis.

20 **Linea terminalis.** Line extending from the promontory of the sacrum along the arcuate line, the pecten pubis, to the superior border of the pubic symphysis. It marks the boundary between the greater and lesser pelvis as well as the plane of the pelvic inlet. C E

21 **Pelvic inlet.** Upper opening of the lesser pelvis along the linea terminalis. C

22 **Pelvic outlet.** Lower opening of the lesser pelvis between the coccyx, the ischial tuberosities, and the inferior pubic rami. D

23 **Axis of pelvis.** Imaginary line passing through the midpoints of all diameters from the pubic symphysis to the anterior surface of the sacrum. The fetal head follows its course during birth. F

24 **Transverse diameter.** The transverse diameter of the pelvis is about 13 cm. E

25 **Oblique diameter.** It passes obliquely forward from the sacroiliac joint to the iliopubic ramus on the opposite side of the pelvis and is about 12.5 cm long. E

26 **Anatomical conjugate.** Distance between the anterosuperior border of the pubic symphysis and the promontory of the sacrum. D

27 **True conjugate.** Distance between the posterosuperior border of the pubic symphysis and the promontory of the sacrum. D

28 **Diagonal conjugate.** Distance between the inferior border of the pubic symphysis and the promontory of the sacrum. D

29 **Straight conjugate.** Distance between the tip of the coccyx and the inferior border of the pubic symphysis. D

30 **Median conjugate.** Distance between the border of the third and fourth sacral vertebrae and the pubic symphysis. D E

31 **External conjugate.** Distance between the last lumbar spinous process and the superior border of the pubic symphysis. It can be measured with a pelvimeter.

32 **Interspinous distance; Interspinous diameter.** Distance between both of the anterior superior iliac spines. C

33 **Intercristal distance; Intercristal diameter.** The greatest distance between the two iliac crests. C

34 **Intertrochanteric distance; Intertrochanteric diameter.** Distance between the greater trochanters of each femur.

35 **Pelvic inclination.** The angle formed by the plane of the pelvic inlet and the horizontal plane (around 65°). F

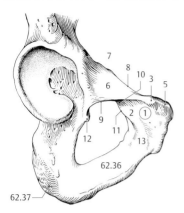

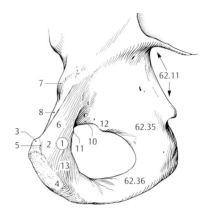

A Lower half of the right hip bone, external surface

B Lower half of the right hip bone, internal surface

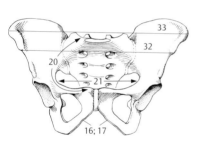

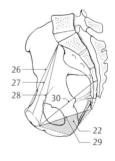

C Female pelvis, anterior view

D Pelvis, medial view

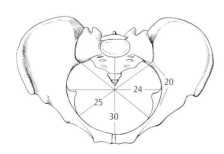

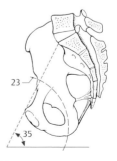

E Pelvis, superior view

F Pelvis, medial view

1 **FREE PART OF LOWER LIMB.**

2 **Femur; Thigh bone.** A B

3 **Head of femur.** A B

4 *Fovea for ligament of head of femur.* Concavity on the head of the femur giving attachment to the ligament of the head of the femur. A B

5 **Neck of femur.** The part of the femur between the head and the greater trochanter. A B

6 **Greater trochanter.** Large prominence on the superolateral aspect of the femur for attachment of the gluteus medius, gluteus minimus, and piriformis muscles. A B

7 *Trochanteric fossa.* Depression medial to the root of the greater trochanter giving attachment to the obturator and gemellus muscles. A B

8 **Lesser trochanter.** Small prominence on the posterior aspect of the femur projecting medially from the junction of the neck and shaft. Attachment site of the iliopsoas muscle. A B

9 [**Third trochanter**]. Projection occasionally found at the base of the greater trochanter at the end of the linea aspera. Attachment site for a portion of the gluteus maximus muscle. B

10 **Intertrochanteric line.** Rough line on the anterior aspect of the femur between the neck and the shaft. It extends from the greater trochanter to the lesser trochanter. A

11 **Intertrochanteric crest.** Bony ridge extending on the posterior aspect of the femur from the greater to the lesser trochanter. B

12 *Quadrate tubercle.* Round eminence on the intertrochanteric crest. B

13 **Shaft of femur; Body of femur.** A B

14 *Linea aspera.* Rough double line on the posterior aspect of the femur. It increases the bending strength of the shaft and gives origin to the vastus medialis and vastus lateralis muscles, the short head of the biceps brachii muscle, as well as attachment to the adductors, gluteus maximus, and pectineus muscles. B

15 *Lateral lip.* Lateral prolongation of the linea aspera. B

16 *Medial lip.* Medial prolongation of the linea aspera. B

17 *Pectineal line, spiral line.* Bony line extending inferiorly from the lesser trochanter, nearly reaching the linea aspera. Attachment site of the pectineus muscle. B

18 *Gluteal tuberosity.* Roughened, elongated area prolonging the lateral lip to superior. It affords insertion to the gluteus maximus muscle. B

19 *Popliteal surface.* Triangular area on the posterior aspect of the femur between the divergent lips of the linea aspera and the intercondylar line. B

20 *Medial supracondylar line.* Continuation of the medial lip of the linea aspera toward the medial condyle. B

21 *Lateral supracondylar line.* Continuation of the lateral lip of the linea aspera toward the lateral condyle. The popliteal surface is situated between the two supracondylar lines. B

22 **Medial condyle.** Rounded projection on the medial aspect of the femur forming part of the knee joint. A B

23 *Medial epicondyle.* Bony prominence on the medial aspect of the medial condyle. A B

24 *Adductor tubercle.* Small protuberance above the medial epicondyle. Attachment site of the adductor magnus muscle. A B

25 **Lateral condyle.** Rounded projection on the lateral aspect of the femur. A B

26 *Lateral epicondyle.* Bony prominence on the lateral aspect of the lateral condyle. A B

27 *Groove for popliteus.* Furrow between the lateral condyle and the lateral epicondyle. B

28 **Patellar surface.** Surface that articulates with the patella. A

29 **Intercondylar fossa.** Notch on the posterior aspect of the femur between the medial and lateral condyles. B

30 **Intercondylar line.** Posterior ridge between the roots of the condyles. B

31 **Tibia.** C D

32 **Superior articular surface.** Articular surfaces of the tibia that form part of the knee joint. C D

33 **Medial condyle.** Medial prominence on the proximal end of the tibia. C D

34 **Lateral condyle.** Lateral prominence on the proximal end of the tibia. C D

35 *Fibular articular facet.* Posterolateral surface articulating with the head of the fibula. C D

36 **Anterior intercondylar area.** Area between the superior articular surfaces of the tibia anterior to the intercondylar eminence. Attachment site of the anterior cruciate ligament. C D

37 **Posterior intercondylar area.** Area between the superior articular surfaces of the tibia posterior to the intercondylar eminence. Attachment site of the posterior cruciate ligament. D

38 **Intercondylar eminence.** Bony prominence between the articular surfaces. Attachment site of the cruciate ligaments and menisci of the knee joint. C D

39 *Medial intercondylar tubercle.* Protuberance from the medial articular surface at the margin facing the intercondylar eminence. D

40 *Lateral intercondylar tubercle.* Protuberance from the lateral articular surface at the margin facing the intercondylar eminence. D

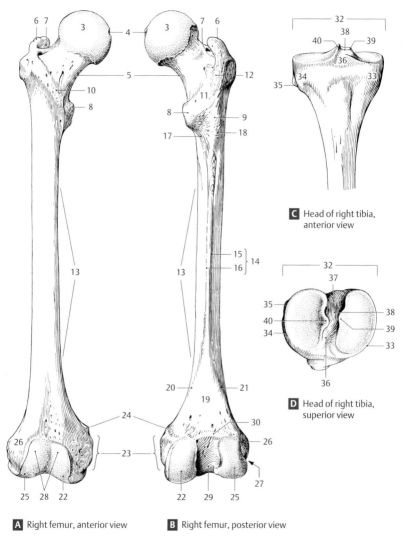

C Head of right tibia, anterior view

D Head of right tibia, superior view

A Right femur, anterior view   **B** Right femur, posterior view

2

1 **Shaft of tibia; Body of tibia.** A B D

2 *Tibial tuberosity.* Roughened area near the upper part of the anterior border of the tibia giving attachment to the patellar ligament. A

3 *Medial surface.* Surface of the tibia facing anteromedially. A D

4 *Posterior surface.* B D

5 *Soleal line.* Bony ridge on the posterior surface of the tibia that extends obliquely from superolateral to inferomedial, giving origin to the soleus muscle. B

6 *Lateral surface.* Surface of the tibia facing anterolaterally. A D

7 *Medial border.* A B D

8 *Anterior border.* A D

9 *Interosseous border.* Border of the tibia that faces the fibula and gives attachment to the interosseous membrane along most of its length. A B D

10 **Medial malleolus.** A B

11 *Malleolar groove.* Small groove on the posterior aspect of the medial malleolus for passage of the tendon of the tibialis posterior muscle. B

12 *Articular facet of medial malleolus.* Lateral cartilage-lined surface of the medial malleolus facing the talus. A B

13 **Fibular notch.** Notch on the lateral aspect of the distal end of the tibia for articulation with the fibula. B

14 **Inferior articular surface.** Inferior joint surface facing the talus. A B

15 **Fibula.** A B D

16 **Head of fibula.** Proximal end of the fibula. A B

17 *Articular facet.* Articular surface on the proximal end of the fibula facing the tibia. A B

18 *Apex of head.* Superiorly directed process on the head of the fibula. A B

19 **Neck of fibula.** A

20 **Shaft of fibula; Body of fibula.** A

21 *Lateral surface.* Surface of the shaft that faces laterally and slightly anteriorly. A D

22 *Medial surface.* Surface of the shaft facing the tibia between the anterior and interosseous borders. A B D

23 *Posterior surface.* Posterior aspect of the shaft between the posterior and interosseous borders. B D

24 *Medial crest.* Bony ridge on the posterior surface of the shaft that forms the boundary between the origins of the tibialis posterior and the flexor hallucis longus muscles. B D

25 *Anterior border.* A D

26 *Interosseous border.* Bony ridge on the shaft between the anterior border and the medial crest. It gives attachment to part of the interosseous membrane. A B D

27 *Posterior border.* Margin facing posterolaterally. B D

28 **Lateral malleolus.** A B

29 *Articular facet of lateral malleolus.* Articular surface facing the talus. A B

30 *Malleolar fossa.* Depression on the posteromedial aspect of the lateral malleolus. Origin of the posterior talofibular ligament. B

31 *Malleolar groove.* Groove lateral to the malleolar fossa for passage of the tendons of the peronei muscles. B

32 **Patella.** The kneecap, which is embedded in the tendon of the quadriceps femoris muscle. C

33 **Base of patella.** Broad, superior border of the patella. C

34 **Apex of patella.** Inferior, pointed border of the patella. C

35 **Articular surface.** Cartilage-covered articular surface facing the femur.

36 **Anterior surface.** Anterior surface of the patella. C

2

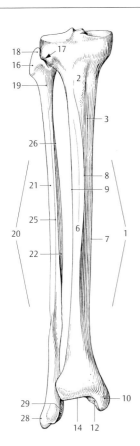

A Right tibia and fibula, anterior view

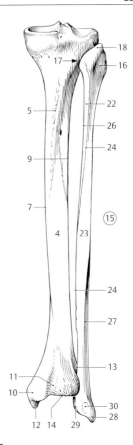

B Right tibia and fibula, posterior view

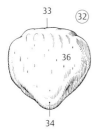

C Patella, anterior view

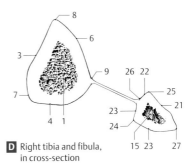

D Right tibia and fibula, in cross-section

2

1 BONES OF FOOT.

2 **Tarsal bones.** The tarsal bones consist of the talus, the calcaneus, the navicular, the cuboid, and the three cuneiform bones. E

3 **Talus.** Bone situated between the tibia, calcaneus, navicular, and fibula. A B E

4 **Head of talus.** The part of the talus that articulates with the navicular. A B

5 *Navicular articular surface.* Anterior surface on the head of the talus for articulation with the navicular. A B

6 *Facet for plantar calcaneonavicular ligament.* Larger articular surface that varies in form located on the medial, anterior, and inferior aspects of the head of the talus. B E

7 *Facet for calcaneonavicular part of bifurcate ligament.* Smaller articular surface that varies in form located on the anterior, inferior, and lateral aspects of the head of the talus. B

8 *Anterior facet for calcaneus.* Anterior articular surface for the calcaneus below the head of the talus. B

9 **Neck of talus.** Tapering part of the talus proximal to its head. A B

10 *Middle facet for calcaneus.* Middle articular surface for the calcaneus. B

11 **Sulcus tali.** Groove between the middle and posterior facets for the calcaneus. B

12 **Body of talus.** B

13 *Trochlea of talus.* Cylindrical projection for articulation with the tibia and fibula. A

14 *Superior facet.* Upper surface of the talus for articulation with the inferior articular surface of the tibia. A

15 *Lateral malleolar facet.* Surface on the lateral aspect of the trochlea of the talus for articulation with the lateral malleolus. A

16 *Lateral process.* Bony projection below the lateral malleolar facet. A

17 *Medial malleolar facet.* Surface that is nearly parallel to the sagittal plane for articulation with the medial malleolus. A

18 *Posterior process.* Broad process below the posterior border of the trochlea of the talus. It bears the medial and lateral tubercles between which passes the groove for the tendon of the flexor hallucis longus. A B

19 *Groove for tendon of flexor hallucis longus.* Groove on the posteromedial aspect of the posterior process for the tendon of the flexor hallucis longus. A B

20 *Medial tubercle.* Bony process medial to the groove for the tendon of the flexor hallucis longus. A B

21 *Lateral tubercle.* Bony process lateral to the groove for the tendon of the flexor hallucis longus. A

22 *Posterior calcaneal articular facet.* Posteroinferior surface that articulates with the calcaneus. B

23 *[Os trigonum].* Accessory lateral tubercle that is occasionally found, arising from a separate ossification center of the posterior process of the body of the talus. E

24 **Calcaneus.** C D E

25 **Calcaneal tuberosity.** Tuberosity on the posterior aspect of the calcaneus. C D

26 *Medial process of calcaneal tuberosity.* Slight projection anterior, inferior, and medial to the calcaneal tuberosity. Origin of the abductor hallucis and the flexor digitorum brevis muscles. D

27 *Lateral process of calcaneal tuberosity.* Slight projection inferolateral to the calcaneus tuberosity. Origin of the adductor digiti minimi muscle. C

28 **Calcaneal tubercle.** Anteriorly projecting eminence on inferior surface of the calcaneus that gives attachment to the plantar calcaneocuboid ligament. C

29 **Sustentaculum tali; Talar shelf.** Shelflike process located inferomedial to the middle talar articular surface. It supports the talus and bears most of its bulk. D E

30 *Groove for tendon of flexor hallucis longus.* Groove on the inferior aspect of the sustentaculum tali for the tendon of the flexor hallucis longus muscle. D

31 **Calcaneal sulcus.** Groove between the middle and posterior talar articular surfaces. C D

32 **Tarsal sinus.** Funnel-shaped prolongation of the calcaneal sulcus and sulcus tali that opens laterally. The subtalar joint is palpable here. B C

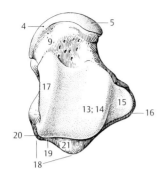

A Right talus, superior view

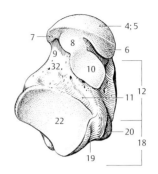

B Right talus, inferior view

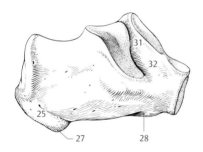

C Right calcaneus, lateral view

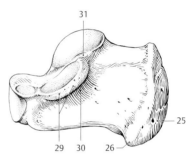

D Right calcaneus, medial view

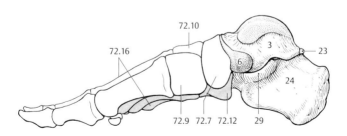

E Right foot, medial view, bones held together

2

1 **Anterior talar articular surface.** Smaller surface on the anterior calcaneus for articulation with the talus. A B

2 **Middle talar articular surface.** Middle surface for articulation with the talus, which is separated from the posterior talar articular surface by the calcaneal sulcus. A B

3 **Posterior talar articular surface.** Largest posterior articular surface for the talus. A B

4 **Groove for tendon of fibularis longus; Groove for tendon of peroneus longus.** Groove on the lateral aspect of the calcaneus below the fibular trochlea. B

5 **Fibular trochlea; Peroneal trochlea; Peroneal tubercle.** Bony projection above the groove for the tendon of the fibularis longus that acts as a pulley for the fibularis longus muscle. Attachment site for part of the peroneal retinaculum. The fibularis brevis muscle passes cranially from the trochlea. B

6 **Articular surface for cuboid.** Surface on the anterior aspect of the calcaneus for articulation with the cuboid. A B

7 **Navicular.** Bone situated medially between the head of the talus and the three cuneiform bones. C D

8 **Tuberosity of navicular bone.** The medial margin of the navicular that gives attachment to the posterior tibialis muscle. It is palpable through the skin. D

9 **Medial cuneiform.** Wedge-shaped bone between the navicular and the first metatarsal. The base of the wedge is directed inferiorly. C D

10 **Intermediate cuneiform; Middle cuneiform.** Cuneiform bone located between the navicular and the second metatarsal. The base of the wedge is directed superiorly. C D

11 **Lateral cuneiform.** Wedge-shaped bone between the navicular and the third metatarsal. Its base is directed superiorly. C D

12 **Cuboid.** Bone located between the calcaneus and the fourth and fifth metatarsals. C D

13 **Groove for tendon of fibularis longus; Groove for tendon of peroneus longus.** Furrow on the inferior and lateral aspect of the cuboid that transmits the tendon of the fibularis longus muscle and is involved in directing the tendon. D

14 **Tuberosity of cuboid.** Bony prominence on the inferior aspect of the cuboid proximal to the groove for the tendon of the fibularis longus. D

15 **Calcaneal process.** Plantar process at the margin of the cuboid that projects proximally and medially. The articular surface on its apex supports the calcaneus. D

16 **Metatarsals (I–V).** The five metatarsal bones. C D

17 **Base of metatarsal.** Thicker, proximal end. D

18 **Shaft of metatarsal; Body of metatarsal.** D

19 **Head of metatarsal.** C D

20 **Tuberosity of first metatarsal bone [1].** Bony protuberance on the inferolateral aspect of the base of the first metatarsal. D

21 **Tuberosity of fifth metatarsal bone [V].** Bony protuberance on the lateral aspect of the base of the fifth metatarsal. Attachment site of the fibularis brevis muscle. C D

22 **Phalanges.** Bones of the toes; digital bones of the foot. C D

23 **Proximal phalanx.** First or proximal phalanx. D

24 **Middle phalanx.** Second phalanx. D

25 **Distal phalanx.** Ungual phalanx of the toe. D

26 *Tuberosity of distal phalanx.* Roughened area on the inferior aspect of the distal phalanx for attachment of the tactile elevation. D

27 **Base of phalanx.** Proximal end of the phalanx with a concave articular surface. D

28 **Shaft of phalanx; Body of phalanx.** D

29 **Head of phalanx.** Distal end of the phalanx with the articular head. D

30 *Trochlea of phalanx.* Trochlea located at the distal end of the proximal phalanx.

31 **Sesamoid bones.** Bones embedded in tendons or ligaments. They are often found below the head of the first metatarsal on either side of the tendon of the flexor hallucis longus muscle. D

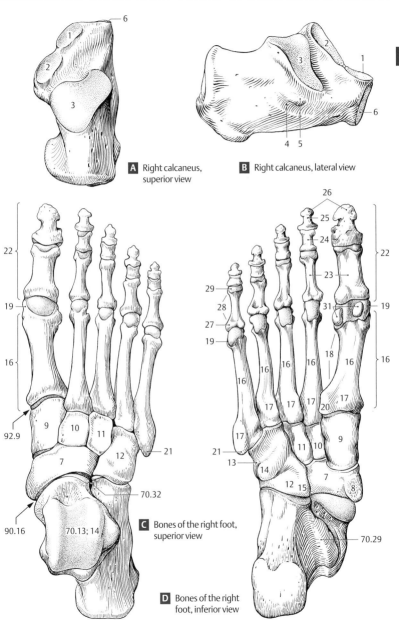

A Right calcaneus, superior view

B Right calcaneus, lateral view

C Bones of the right foot, superior view

D Bones of the right foot, inferior view

1 *JOINTS; ARTICULAR SYSTEM.*

2 *JOINTS OF SKULL.*

3 CRANIAL FIBROUS JOINTS.

4 **Cranial syndesmoses.**

5 **Pterygospinous ligament.** Broad band of fibrous tissue that extends from the superior part of the lateral plate of the pterygoid process to the spine of the sphenoid. p. 77 C

6 **Stylohyoid ligament.** Ligament that extends between the stylohyoid process and the lesser horn of the hyoid bone. Vestige of the second pharyngeal arch. p. 77 C

7 **Cranial sutures.** Articulations in which the cranial bones are joined by connective tissue consisting mainly of collagen fibers.

8 **Coronal suture.** Suture between the frontal bone and the two parietal bones. A C D

9 **Sagittal suture.** Suture that joins the right and left parietal bones in the midline. C

10 **Lambdoid suture.** Suture that unites the occipital bone with the two parietal bones. A D

11 **Occipitomastoid suture.** Continuation of the lambdoid suture to the cranial base. A D

12 **Sphenofrontal suture.** Suture that gradually ascends posteriorly along the lateral aspect of the cranium, joining the greater wing of the sphenoid and the frontal bone. Interior cranium: suture that joins the frontal bone and the lesser wing of the sphenoid. A B D

13 **Spheno-ethmoidal suture.** Short suture in the interior of the cranium in front of the jugum sphenoidale between the body of the sphenoid and the ethmoid. D

14 **Sphenosquamous suture.** Suture between the squamous part of the temporal bone and the greater wing of the sphenoid. A C D

15 **Sphenoparietal suture.** Continuation of the sphenofrontal suture beginning at the coronal suture. A C D

16 **Squamous suture.** Squamous suture between the temporal and parietal bones. A C D

17 **[Frontal suture; Metopic suture].** Frontal suture between the right and left halves of the frontal bone that normally fuses by the second or third year of life. It persists in 7–8% of people of European descent. C

18 **Parietomastoid suture.** Posterior suture that unites the parietal bone and the mastoid process of the temporal bone. A

19 **[Squamomastoid suture].** Suture that fuses early in life, uniting the mastoid process and the squamous part of the temporal bone. A

20 **Frontonasal suture.** Anterior suture that joins the frontal and nasal bones. C

21 **Fronto-ethmoidal suture.** Suture in the interior of the cranium that joins the ethmoidal and frontal bones. B D

22 **Frontomaxillary suture.** Suture located lateral to the nasal bone between the frontal process of the maxilla and the nasal part of the frontal bone. A B C

23 **Frontolacrimal suture.** Suture between the lacrimal and frontal bones. A B C

24 **Frontozygomatic suture.** Suture at the lateral margin of the orbit between the frontal and zygomatic bones. A B C

25 **Zygomaticomaxillary suture.** Suture below the orbit, traversing the floor of the orbit and uniting the maxilla and the zygomatic bone. A B C

26 **Ethmoidomaxillary suture.** Suture in the orbit that unites the orbital plate of the ethmoid with the maxilla. B C

27 **Ethmoidolacrimal suture.** Suture in the orbit that unites the ethmoid and the lacrimal bone. B

28 **Sphenovomerine suture.** Suture in the bony nasal septum that joins the sphenoid and the vomer.

29 **Sphenozygomatic suture.** Suture in the lateral wall of the orbit that joins the greater wing of the sphenoid and the zygomatic bone. B C

30 **Sphenomaxillary suture.** Suture that is occasionally present between the pterygoid process of the sphenoid and the maxilla lateral to the palatine bone. A

31 **Temporozygomatic suture.** Suture on the lateral aspect of the zygomatic arch between the zygomatic bone and the zygomatic process of the temporal bone. A

32 **Internasal suture.** Suture that unites the right and left nasal bones. C

33 **Nasomaxillary suture.** Suture that joins the nasal bone and the frontal process of the maxilla. A C

34 **Lacrimomaxillary suture.** Suture on the anterior aspect of the lacrimal bone, uniting it with the maxilla. A B C

35 **Lacrimoconchal suture.** Suture that is visible from the nasal cavity, joining the lacrimal bone and the inferior nasal concha.

36 **Intermaxillary suture.** Anterior suture that unites the right and left maxillae in the midline. C

37 **Palatomaxillary suture.** Suture in the posterior wall of the orbit and in the lateral wall of the nasal cavity, connecting the palatine bone and the maxilla. B

38 **Palato-ethmoidal suture.** Suture in the posterior wall of the orbit that unites the palatine and ethmoid bones. B

39 **Median palatine suture.** Suture visible from the oral cavity joining the two halves of the palatine bone. E

40 **Transverse palatine suture.** Suture between the palatine process of the maxilla and the palatine bone. E

3

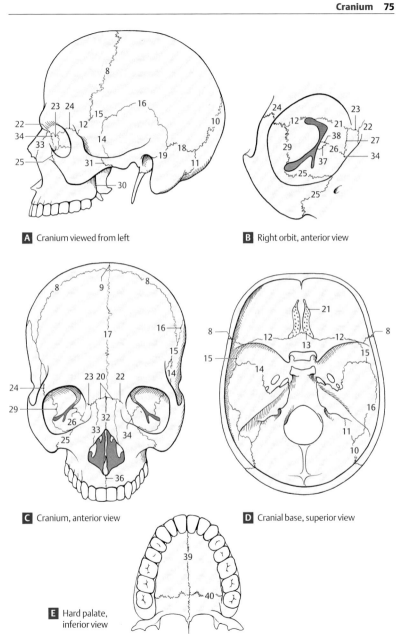

A Cranium viewed from left

B Right orbit, anterior view

C Cranium, anterior view

D Cranial base, superior view

E Hard palate, inferior view

3

1   **Dentoalveolar syndesmosis; Gomphosis.** Joint at the insertion of a tooth in the dental alveoli.

2   CRANIAL CARTILAGINOUS JOINTS.

3   **Cranial synchondroses.** Connections between the cranial bones formed by hyaline cartilage, most of which ossify.

4   **Spheno-occipital synchondrosis.** Cartilaginous union present during development beneath the sella turcica, joining the sphenoid and occipital bones.

5   **Sphenopetrosal synchondrosis.** Cartilaginous union in the lateral continuation of the foramen lacerum, connecting the sphenoid and the petrous part of the temporal bone. Passage of the lesser petrosal nerve. A

6   **Petro-occipital synchondrosis.** Cartilaginous plate that prolongs the jugular foramen to anteromedial. A

7   **[Posterior intra-occipital synchondrosis].** Cartilaginous plate that is present during development between the posterior and the two middle ossification centers of the occipital bone. It usually disappears by the first or second year of life. A

8   **[Anterior intra-occipital synchondrosis].** Cartilaginous plate that is present during development, beginning at the anterior margin of the magnum foramen between the anterior and both middle ossification centers. Disappears by the sixth year of life. A

9   **Spheno-ethmoidal synchondrosis.** Cartilaginous precursor of the sphenoethmoidal suture. p. 74.13

10 CRANIAL SYNOVIAL JOINTS.

11 **Temporomandibular joint.** C E F

12 **Articular disc.** Biconcave disc composed of layers of tough fibrous tissue and fibrocartilage located between the head of the mandible and the mandibular fossa. It is attached around its periphery to the joint capsule, dividing the joint into two cavities, and together they form the disco-capsular system, a single functional unit. E

13 **Lateral ligament.** Inconstant, thick fibers passing from posteroinferior to anterosuperior within or on the lateral surface of the joint capsule. F

14 **Medial ligament.** Thickened portion of the medial wall of the joint capsule that is occasionally present. C

15 **Superior synovial membrane.** Synovial lining of the upper articular cavity. E

16 **Inferior synovial membrane.** Synovial lining of the lower articular cavity. E

17 **Sphenomandibular ligament.** Flat band on the internal aspect of the ramus of the mandible that extends from the spine of the sphenoid to the lingula of the mandibular foramen. It connects with the medial side of the disco-capsular system of the temporomandibular joint. C

18 **Stylomandibular ligament.** Ligament that extends from the anterior surface of the styloid process to the angle of the mandible. C F

19 **Atlanto-occipital joint.** Joint between the atlas and the occipital bone. p. 79 B C

20 **Anterior atlanto-occipital membrane.** Membranous connection between the anterior arch of the atlas and the occipital bone. It is situated in front of the apical ligament of the dens. D

21 **[Anterior atlanto-occipital ligament].** Thickened portion of the anterior atlanto-occipital membrane arising from the anterior tubercle of the atlas.

22 **Posterior atlanto-occipital membrane.** Membrane in the posterior wall of the vertebral canal that extends from the posterior arch of the atlas to the occipital bone. D

23 **Lateral atlanto-occipital ligament.** Band of fibers that extends obliquely from the transverse process of the atlas to the jugular process of the occipital bone.

24 *VERTEBRAL JOINTS.*

25 SYNDESMOSES OF VERTEBRAL COLUMN.

26 **Interspinous ligaments.** Broad ligaments extending between adjacent spinous processes of the vertebrae. D

27 **Ligamenta flava.** Yellow ligaments. A mesh of elastic fibers distorted to form nearly parallel bands running between the vertebral arches. D

28 **Intertransverse ligaments.** Narrow bands extending between the transverse processes of the vertebrae. B

29 **Supraspinous ligament.** Ligaments passing over the spinous processes of the vertebrae from C7 to L4. B

30 **Ligamentum nuchae; Nuchal ligament.** Sagittally widened continuation of the supraspinous ligament that extends from C7 to the external occipital protuberance. In humans it has little elasticity. B

31 **Anterior longitudinal ligament.** Ligament that mainly connects the anterior surfaces of the vertebral bodies. D

32 **Posterior longitudinal ligament.** Ligament that mainly connects the intervertebral discs, traveling along the posterior surfaces of the vertebral bodies within the anterior wall of the vertebral canal. It is continuous with the tectorial membrane from the third cervical vertebra upward. D

33 **Transverse ligaments.** Ligaments passing transversely between the lumbar vertebrae and the sacrum. The last intertransverse ligaments blend with the iliolumbar ligament at the sacrum.

3

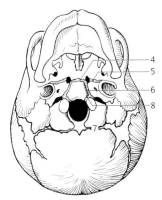

A Cranium of newborn, inferior view

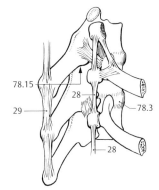

B Ligaments of vertebral column and ribs, lateral view

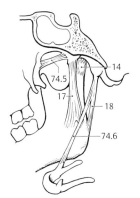

C Temporomandibular joint, medial view

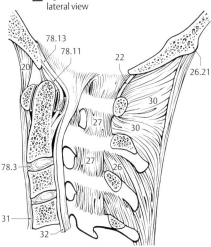

D Ligaments connecting cervical vertebrae, medial view

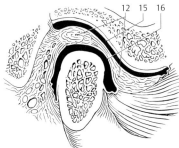

E Temporomandibular joint, longitudinal view

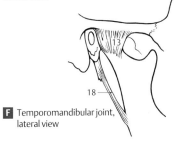

F Temporomandibular joint, lateral view

1 SYNCHONDROSES OF VERTEBRAL COLUMN.

2 **Intervertebral joint.** Fibrocartilaginous connection between the hyaline cartilage of intact epiphysial plates in adjacent vertebral bodies.

3 *Intervertebral disc.* An elastic disc that compresses and rebounds under pressure, consisting of layered rings of fibrous tissue and fibrocartilage around a gelatinous nucleus. It is attached to two adjacent vertebral bodies by their hyaline cartilage plates and by the posterior longitudinal ligament. A

4 *Anulus fibrosus.* Fibrous ring consisting of concentric layers of obliquely oriented fibers running in opposing directions and fibrocartilage. A

5 *Nucleus pulposus.* Semifluid substance at the center of the fibrous anulus. It contains the remains of the notochord. A

6 VERTEBRAL SYNOVIAL JOINTS.

7 **Median atlanto-axial joint.** Joint between the dens of the axis and the atlas. D

8 **Alar ligaments.** Paired ligaments that extend from the dens of the axis to the lateral margin of the foramen magnum. B C

9 *Apical ligament of dens.* Unpaired band extending from the apex of the dens to the anterior margin of the foramen magnum. B D

10 **Cruciate ligament of atlas.** Ligament that comprises the following two ligaments and extends from the dens to the tectorial membrane. C

11 *Longitudinal bands.* Fibrous bands that extend from the body of the axis to the anterior margin of the foramen magnum. They pass posteriorly to the dens and the apical ligament of the dens. C D

12 *Transverse ligament of atlas.* Transverse band that extends from one side of the atlas to the other, passing behind the dens and holding it in position. C D E

13 **Tectorial membrane.** Double-layered continuation of the posterior longitudinal ligament. It extends from the axis to the anterior margin of the foramen magnum where it passes into the periosteal layer of the cranial dura mater. D

14 **Lateral atlanto-axial joint.** Articulation between the inferior articular surface of the atlas and the superior articular facet of the axis. B C

15 **Zygapophysial joints.** Articulations between the articular processes of the vertebrae. Clinically: "small vertebral joints." p. 77 B

16 **Lumbosacral joint.** Articulation between the articular surfaces of the sacrum and L5 (L4). p. 87 A

17 **Iliolumbar ligament.** Strong ligament that chiefly extends from the transverse process of L4 and L5 to the ilium. p. 87 A B

18 **Sacrococcygeal joint.** Articulation between the sacrum and the coccyx. It is often a true joint but can occur as a synchondrosis. F

19 **Superficial posterior sacrococcygeal ligament.** F

20 **Deep posterior sacrococcygeal ligament.** F

21 **Anterior sacrococcygeal ligament.**

22 **Lateral sacrococcygeal ligament.** F

23 *THORACIC JOINTS.*

24 SYNDESMOSES OF THORAX.

25 **External intercostal membrane.** Continuation of the external intercostal muscles at the sternal end of the intercostal space. p. 81 C

26 **Internal intercostal membrane.** Continuation of the internal intercostal muscles near the vertebral end of the intercostal space. p. 81 B

27 SYNCHONDROSES OF THORAX.Thoracic articulations formed by hyaline cartilage.

28 **Costosternal joint.** Cartilaginous joint (usually) between the first, sixth, and seventh ribs and the sternum.

29 **Synchondrosis of first rib.** Cartilaginous connection that is always present at the first rib, directly joining it to the sternum.

30 **Sternal synchondroses.** Remains of hyaline cartilage between developing ossification centers in the sternum that can later ossify.

31 **Xiphisternal joint.** Articulation between the xiphoid process and the sternum. The hyaline cartilage at the ends of each is separated by a plate of fibrocartilage connecting them. p. 53 D

32 *Manubriosternal joint.* Joint between the manubrium and the body of the sternum, which is structured similarly to the xiphisternal joint. p. 53 D

33 *[Manubriosternal synchondrosis].* Connection consisting of merely a plate of hyaline cartilage.

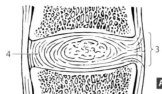

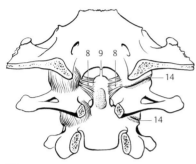

A Intervertebral disc, sagittal section

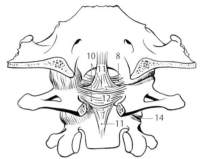

B Dens of axis with ligaments, posterior view

C Atlanto-occipital joint, posterior view

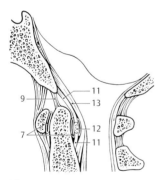

D Ligaments between atlas, axis, and occipital bone

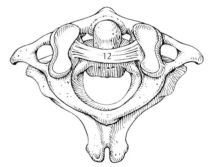

E Atlas and axis, posterosuperior view

F Coccygeal ligaments, posterior view

3

1 SYNOVIAL JOINTS OF THORAX.

2 **Costovertebral joints.** Joints between the ribs and the vertebrae. A

3 **Joint of head of rib.** Articulation between the head of the rib, the vertebral body, and the intervertebral disc. A

4 *Radiate ligament of head of rib.* Ligament that reinforces the anterior surface of the joint capsule. It radiates from the rib in a stellate fashion over the head of the rib to the two adjacent vertebral bodies and the intervertebral disc between them. A B

5 *Intra-articular ligament of head of rib.* Ligament that extends between the crest of the head of the rib and the intervertebral disc, dividing the articular cavity into two chambers. B

6 **Costotransverse joint.** Joint between the articular facet of the tubercle of the rib and the corresponding transverse process of the thoracic vertebra. A

7 *Costotransverse ligament.* Ligament that occupies the space between the body of the transverse process and the neck of the rib. A

8 *Superior costotransverse ligament.* Ligament that connects the neck of the rib to the transverse process of the thoracic vertebra immediately above it. B

9 *Lateral costotransverse ligament.* Ligament that reinforces the joint capsule, extending from the end of the transverse process to the corresponding tubercle of the rib. A

10 *Lumbocostal ligament.* Deep layer of the thoracolumbar fascia. It forms tendinous attachments to the costal processes of the lumbar vertebrae, the twelfth rib, and the border of the pelvis, and serves as the aponeurosis of the transverse abdominal muscle.

11 *Costotransverse foramen.* Opening for the passage of the intercostal nerves between the superior costotransverse ligament and the neck of the rib. B

12 **Sternocostal joints.** Articulations between the costal cartilages and the sternum. C

13 **Intra-articular sternocostal ligament.** Ligament contained in the articular cavity between the costal cartilage and the sternum. It is especially pronounced on the second rib. C

14 **Radiate sternocostal ligaments.** Strengthening ligaments that radiate from the ribs to the joint capsules of the sternocostal joints. C

15 **Sternal membrane.** Membranous covering of the anterior surface of the sternum that is formed by a meshwork of fibers from the radiate sternocostal ligament. C

16 **Costoxiphoid ligaments.** Bands of fibers passing from the seventh costal cartilage downward to the xiphoid process of the sternum.

17 **Costochondral joints.** Articulations between the bony and cartilaginous portions of the ribs without an articular cavity.

18 **Interchondral joints.** Articulations between the costal cartilages, usually of the sixth to the ninth ribs. p. 53 D

19 *JOINTS OF UPPER LIMB.*

20 JOINTS OF PECTORAL GIRDLE.

21 SYNDESMOSES OF PECTORAL GIRDLE; SYNDESMOSES OF SHOULDER GIRDLE.

22 **Coraco-acromial ligament.** Thick band extending from the coracoid process of the scapula to the acromion, forming a roof over the shoulder joint. D

23 **Superior transverse scapular ligament.** Ligament that lies medial to the coracoid process of the scapula and bridges the suprascapular notch. D

24 **[Inferior transverse scapular ligament].** Weak band that extends from the root of the spine of the scapula to the posterior margin of the glenoid cavity. E

25 SYNOVIAL JOINTS OF PECTORAL GIRDLE; SYNOVIAL JOINTS OF SHOULDER GIRDLE.

26 **Acromioclavicular joint.** Joint between the acromion and the clavicle. D

27 **Acromioclavicular ligament.** Ligament that strengthens the superior wall of the joint capsule, holding the acromion and clavicle together. D

28 **(Articular disc).** Fibrocartilage interarticular disc. D

29 **Coracoclavicular ligament.** Ligament that consists of two parts and connects the coracoid process of the scapula and the clavicle. It transmits the weight of the arms to the clavicle. D

30 *Trapezoid ligament.* Portion of the coracoclavicular ligament that extends from the coracoid process of the scapula anterolaterally to the clavicle. It lies between the conoid portion of the coracoclavicular ligament and the coraco-acromial ligament. D

31 *Conoid ligament.* Portion of the coracoclavicular ligament medial to the trapezoid ligament. Triangular band, the base of which is attached to the clavicle and the tip to the coracoid process of the scapula. D

32 **Sternoclavicular joint.** Joint between the sternum and the clavicle which is subdivided into two cavities. C

33 **Articular disc.** Interarticular disc which is attached inferiorly to the first rib and superiorly to the clavicle. C

34 **Anterior sternoclavicular ligament.** Ligament that strengthens the anterior wall of the joint capsule. C

35 **Posterior sternoclavicular ligament.** Ligament that runs posterior to the joint and strengthens the joint capsule.

36 **Costoclavicular ligament.** Ligament that passes laterally to the sternoclavicular joint and connects the first rib to the clavicle. C

37 **Interclavicular ligament.** Ligament that extends across the jugular notch and connects the two clavicles. C

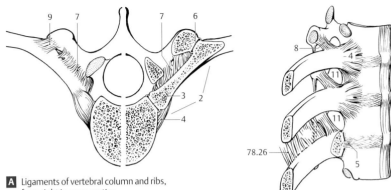

A Ligaments of vertebral column and ribs, from right in cross-section

B Ligaments of vertebral column and ribs

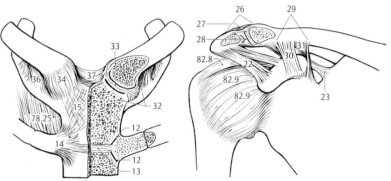

C Sternocostal joints

D Lateral ligaments of shoulder girdle, anterior view

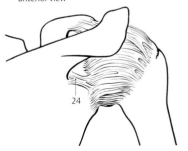

E Shoulder joint, posterior view

3

1 **JOINTS OF FREE UPPER LIMB.**

2 RADIO-ULNAR SYNDESMOSIS. Fibrous joint between the radius and ulna.

3 **Interosseous membrane of forearm.** Membrane that is spread between the interosseous borders of the radius and ulna. A

4 **Oblique cord.** Fibrous ligament that extends from the tuberosity of the ulna obliquely distalward to the radius. It runs opposite to most of the fibers of the interosseous membrane. A

5 SYNOVIAL JOINTS OF FREE UPPER LIMB.

6 **Glenohumeral joint; Shoulder joint.** Ball joint between the scapula and the humerus.

7 **Glenoidal labrum.** Lip of fibrocartilage around the margin of the shoulder joint that augments the bony articular surface. E

8 **Coracohumeral ligament.** Thickened portion of the joint capsule that extends from the root of the coracoid process of the scapula to the superior margins of the lesser and greater tubercles of the humerus. E, p. 81 D

9 **Glenohumeral ligaments.** Three thickened bands (superior, middle, inferior) within the anterior wall of the joint capsule. E, p. 81 D

10 **Transverse humeral ligament.** Transverse band that extends over the intertubercular sulcus, converting it into a canal for the passage of the tendon of the long head of the biceps brachii muscle. p. 56.8

11 **Elbow joint.** Joint formed by the humerus, radius, and ulna.

12 **Humero-ulnar joint.** Joint between the humerus and ulna.

13 **Humeroradial joint.** Joint between the humerus and radius.

14 **Proximal radio-ulnar joint.** Articulation between the articular circumference of the head of the radius and the radial notch of the ulna.

15 **Ulnar collateral ligament.** Triangular plate of fibers, the apex of which is directed superiorly. It is situated on the medial aspect of the arm between the humerus and ulna. A

16 **Radial collateral ligament.** Lateral collateral ligament. Its fibers radiate from the lateral epicondyle of the humerus and blend into the anular ligament of the radius, which continues to the ulna. A

17 **Anular ligament of radius.** Ringlike band that is woven into the joint capsule and encircles a portion of the articular circumference of the head of the radius. It is attached to the anterior and posterior margins of the radial notch of the ulna. A

18 **Quadrate ligament.** Thin band of fibers that extends from the distal margin of the radial notch of the ulna to the neck of the radius.

19 **Sacciform recess.** Thinly walled expansion of the joint capsule deep to the anular ligament encircling the radius. A

20 **Distal radio-ulnar joint.** Inferior part of the elbow joint for articulation between the radius and ulna. B

21 **Articular disc.** Triangular interarticular disc between the ulna and the wrist. It attaches to the radius and the ulnar styloid process, functioning as an interarticular ligament to hold the radius and ulna together. B

22 **Sacciform recess.** Proximal eversion of the loose joint capsule beyond the margin of the articular cartilage. B

23 **Joints of hand.**

24 *Wrist joint.* The proximal wrist joint formed by the proximal row of carpal bones, the radius, and the articular disc. B

25 *Dorsal radiocarpal ligament.* Band on the dorsal surface of the wrist whose fibers mostly extend from the radius to the triquetrum. C

26 *Palmar radiocarpal ligament.* Band on the flexor surface of the radius whose fibers radiate mainly to the lunate and capitate. C

27 *Dorsal ulnocarpal ligament.* Its course corresponds to that of the palmar ulnocarpal ligament.

28 *Palmar ulnocarpal ligament.* Band of fibers that mainly extend from the flexor surface of the head of the ulna to the capitate. It often joins with fibers given off by the palmar radiocarpal ligament. D

29 *Ulnar collateral ligament of wrist joint.* Collateral ligament that extends from the ulnar styloid process to the triquetrum and pisiform. C D

30 *Radial collateral ligament of wrist joint.* Lateral collateral ligament that extends from the radial styloid process to the scaphoid. C D

31 **Carpal joints; Intercarpal joints.** The joints between the carpal bones. B

32 *Midcarpal joint.* The distal wrist joint between the proximal and distal rows of carpal bones. B

33 *Radiate carpal ligament.* Band of fibers that radiate from the capitate to the adjacent bones. D

34 *Dorsal intercarpal ligaments.* Bands on the dorsum of the wrist between the proximal and distal rows of carpal bones. They originate on the triquetrum. C

35 *Palmar intercarpal ligaments.* Group of bands on the palmar aspect of the hand, deep to the radiate carpal ligament, connecting the carpal bones (exception: capitate). D

36 *Interosseous intercarpal ligaments.* Bands that enter the articular cavity between the carpal bones of one row. B

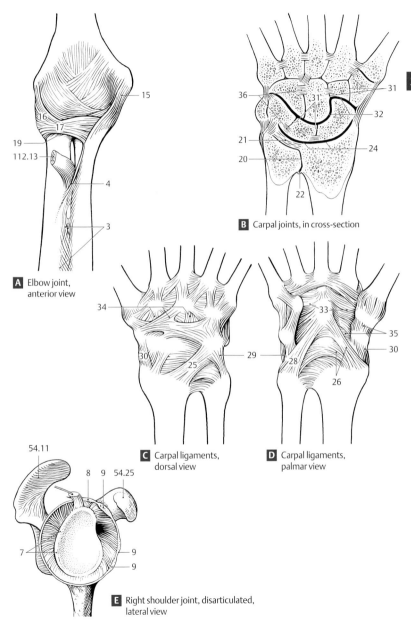

3

A Elbow joint,
anterior view

B Carpal joints, in cross-section

C Carpal ligaments,
dorsal view

D Carpal ligaments,
palmar view

E Right shoulder joint, disarticulated,
lateral view

1 *Pisiform joint.* Joint between the pisiform and triquetrum. A

2 *Pisohamate ligament.* Medial continuation of the tendon of the flexor carpi ulnaris muscle to the hook of hamate. B

3 *Pisometacarpal ligament.* Lateral continuation of the tendon of the flexor carpi ulnaris muscle to the base of the fifth metacarpal. B

4 **Carpal tunnel.** Canal on the palmar aspect between the tubercles of the scaphoid and the trapezium on one side and the pisiform and the hook of hamate on the other. It is bridged by the flexor retinaculum. B

5 **Ulnar canal (Guyon's canal).** Canal between the pisiform and the hook of hamate. Its floor is formed by the pisohamate and pisometacarpal ligaments, along with the flexor retinaculum, and its roof by the palmar ulnocarpal ligament, portions of the forearm fascia, connective-tissue fibers from the flexor carpi ulnaris muscle, and the palmaris brevis muscle. It transmits the ulnar artery and nerve. B

6 **Carpometacarpal joints.** Joints between the distal carpal bones and the metacarpals. Joints II–V are amphiarthroses. A

7 *Dorsal carpometacarpal ligaments.* Tough bands on the dorsum of the hand that connect the distal carpal bones to the metacarpals. C

8 *Palmar carpometacarpal ligaments.* Tough bands on the palmar aspect of the hand that connect the distal carpal bones to the metacarpals. B

9 *Carpometacarpal joint of thumb.* Saddle joint. Independent joint between the first metacarpal and the trapezium. A B

10 **Intermetacarpal joints.** Joints between the bases of the metacarpals. A

11 *Dorsal metacarpal ligaments.* Tough bands between the proximal ends of the metacarpals on the extensor surface of the hand. C

12 *Palmar metacarpal ligaments.* Tough bands on the palmar surface of the hand between the bases of the metacarpals. B

13 *Interosseous metacarpal ligaments.* Short, tough bands on the bases of the metacarpals. They are contained within the joint capsule between the dorsal and palmar metacarpal ligaments. A

14 *Interosseous metacarpal spaces.* Spaces between the metatarsals. A C

15 **Metacarpophalangeal joints.** Basal joints of the fingers located between the heads of the metacarpal bones and the bases of the proximal phalanges. B

16 *Collateral ligaments.* Collateral ligaments of the metacarpophalangeal joints. They become lax when the finger is extended and taut when the fingers form a fist. B

17 *Palmar ligaments.* Fibers in the floor of the tendon sheaths extending from the root of the collateral ligaments to the palmar aspect of the hand. They should not be confused with the anular part of the fibrous sheath. B

18 *Deep transverse metacarpal ligament.* Transverse band on the palmar aspect of the heads of the metatarsals at the height of the articular cavity. It prevents separation of the metatarsals. B

19 **Interphalangeal joints of hand.** Middle and distal joints between the phalanges. B

20 *Collateral ligaments.* Collateral ligaments of the phalangeal joints. B

21 *Palmar ligaments.* Fibers that pass into the floor of the tendon sheaths above the interphalangeal joints of the hand. B

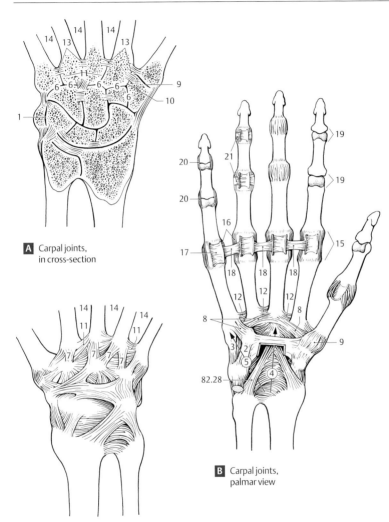

A Carpal joints,
in cross-section

B Carpal joints,
palmar view

C Carpal joints of right hand,
dorsal view

3

1 *JOINTS OF LOWER LIMB.*

2 **JOINTS OF PELVIC GIRDLE.**

3 SYNDESMOSES OF PELVIC GIRDLE.

4 **Obturator membrane.** Membrane that closes the obturator foramen except for a superomedial opening that forms a portion of the obturator canal. Origin of the obturator internus and externus muscles. A B C D

5 **Obturator canal.** Canal formed by the obturator groove of the pubis and the obturator membrane for the passage of the obturator vessels and the obturator nerve. A C D

6 **Pubic symphysis.** Cartilaginous joint between the rami of the pubis. A

7 **Interpubic disc; Interpubic fibrocartilage.** Fibrocartilage plate that in the adult often has a midline cavity. Its lateral surfaces present hyaline cartilage for articulation with the hip bones. A

8 **Superior pubic ligament.** Fibrous band that connects the upper borders of the pubis. A

9 **Inferior pubic ligament.** Ligamentous fibers that line the pubic arch. A

10 **Sacro-iliac joint.** Amphiarthrodial joint between the sacrum and the ilium. It can become synostotic. A

11 **Anterior sacro-iliac ligament.** Ligamentous bands that extend from the anterior aspect of the first and second sacral vertebrae to the ilium. A D

12 **Interosseous sacro-iliac ligament.** Ligamentous bands that pass behind the sacro-iliac joint from the sacral tuberosity to the iliac tuberosity. B

13 **Posterior sacro-iliac ligament.** Group of bands that pass behind the interosseous sacro-iliac ligament connecting the sacrum and ilium. B

14 **Sacrotuberous ligament.** Strong band that extends from the sacrum and the ilium to the ischial tuberosity. B D

15 *Falciform process.* Thin prolongation of the sacrotuberous ligament to the medial aspect of the ischium. B D

16 **Sacrospinous ligament.** Band that extends from the sacrum and the coccyx to the ischial spine, dividing the greater and lesser sciatic foramina. B D

17 **Greater sciatic foramen.** Foramen that is formed by the greater sciatic notch, the sacrospinous ligament, and the sacrotuberous ligament. The piriformis muscle passes from the pelvis through the foramen, producing the following two crevicelike openings. A B D

18 *[[Foramen suprapiriforme]].* Opening giving passage to the superior gluteal artery, vein, and nerve.

19 *[[Foramen infrapiriforme]].* Opening giving passage to the inferior gluteal artery, inferior gluteal nerve, internal pudendal artery and vein, pudendal nerve, sciatic nerve, and posterior femoral cutaneous nerve.

20 **Lesser sciatic foramen.** Foramen that is formed by the lesser sciatic notch, the sacrospinous ligament, and the sacrotuberous ligament. The obturator internus muscle passes from the pelvis through the foramen, which also transmits the internal pudendal artery and vein as well as the pudendal nerve medially to the ischioanal fossa. B D

21 **JOINTS OF FREE LOWER LIMB.**

22 SYNOVIAL JOINTS OF FREE LOWER LIMB.

23 **Hip joint.** Articulation formed by the acetabulum and the head of the femur. A B C

24 **Zona orbicularis.** Ringlike band that encircles the neck of the femur on the inner layer of the joint capsule. It is strengthened by external ligaments and helps secure the head of the femur in the acetabulum. B

25 **Iliofemoral ligament.** Strong anterior band that extends from the anterior inferior iliac spine to the intertrochanteric line. It travels in two main directions. A

26 *Transverse part.* Lateral, transverse portion of the iliofemoral ligament that limits external rotation and abduction. A B

27 *Descending part.* Medial, descending portion of the iliofemoral ligament that limits internal rotation. A

28 **Ischiofemoral ligament.** Ligamentous fibers that spiral from the ischium above the neck of the femur to the trochanteric fossa and also radiate into the zona orbicularis. It limits internal rotation. B

29 **Pubofemoral ligament.** Ligament that extends from the medial surface of the pubis within the joint capsule to the zona orbicularis and to the portion of the femur proximal to the lesser trochanter. It limits abduction. A

30 **Acetabular labrum.** Lip of the acetabulum. Fibrocartilage ring that augments the bony acetabulum. C

31 **Transverse acetabular ligament.** Ligament that spans the acetabular notch and augments the acetabulum. C

32 **Ligament of head of femur.** Intracapsular band that extends from the acetabular notch to the fovea for the ligament of the head of the femur. It transmits vessels and does not directly influence joint mechanics. C

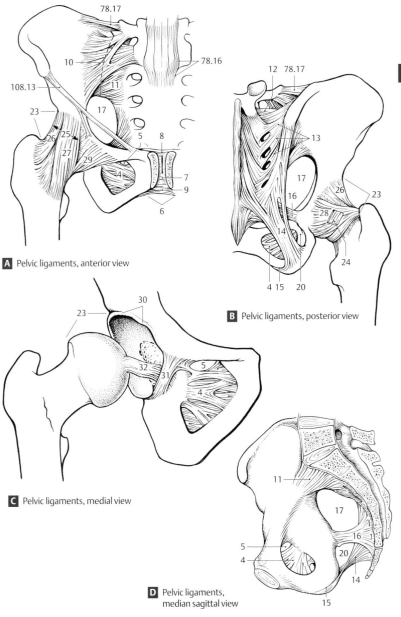

A Pelvic ligaments, anterior view

B Pelvic ligaments, posterior view

C Pelvic ligaments, medial view

D Pelvic ligaments, median sagittal view

3

1   **Knee joint.** A B D C E

2   **Lateral meniscus.** Nearly circular ring below the lateral femoral condyle with close-together attachments. It is not anchored to the fibular collateral ligament and thus is relatively mobile. B D E

3   *Anterior meniscofemoral ligament.* Fibrous band that is occasionally present, extending from the posterior end of the lateral meniscus to the medial condyle of the femur. It lies anterior to the posterior cruciate ligament. D E

4   *Posterior meniscofemoral ligament.* Band that extends posteriorly from the lateral meniscus to the fibular surface of the medial femoral condyle and lies posterior to the posterior cruciate ligament. D E

5   **Medial meniscus.** The crescent-shaped medial meniscus lies beneath the medial femoral condyle and is attached to the tibial collateral ligament. It is highly susceptible to injury. B D E

6   **Transverse ligament of knee.** Transverse band that connects the anterior ends of the two menisci. B D

7   **Anterior cruciate ligament.** Band that extends from the anterior intercondylar area superiorly and posteriorly to the medial aspect of the lateral femoral condyle. B D E

8   **Posterior cruciate ligament.** Band that extends posteriorly from the posterior intercondylar area to anterosuperior to the medial aspect of the medial femoral condyle. B D E

9   **Infrapatellar synovial fold.** Connective tissue fold that often contains adipose tissue extending from the infrapatellar fat pad to the cruciate ligaments. Remnants of an embryonic septum. B

10 *Alar folds.* Pair of pliable projections that are continuous with the infrapatellar fat pad and fill in the spaces in the anterior articular cavity. B

11 **Fibular collateral ligament.** Lateral collateral ligament that extends from the lateral femoral epicondyle to the head of the fibula. It lacks secure attachment to the joint capsule and meniscus. A B C D E

12 **Tibial collateral ligament.** Medial collateral ligament that extends from the medial femoral epicondyle to the tibia. It is attached to the joint capsule and the medial meniscus. A B C D E

13 **Oblique popliteal ligament.** Band of fibers that passes from the insertion of the semimembranosus muscle to superolateral, reinforcing the posterior wall of the joint capsule. C

14 **Arcuate popliteal ligament.** Arched band of fibers that passes from the head of the fibula above the origin of the popliteus muscle to within the posterior wall of the joint capsule which it strengthens. C

15 **Patellar ligament.** Ligamentous continuation of the tendon of the quadriceps femoris muscle that passes from the apex of the patella to the tibial tuberosity. It is 2–3 cm wide and about 0.5 cm thick. A

16 **Medial patellar retinaculum.** Aponeurosis that is derived from a portion of the vastus medialis muscle lying medial to the patella. It inserts medially to the tibial tuberosity, ensures proper patellar tracking by means of muscular contraction, and functions as a back-up extensor mechanism. A

17 **Lateral patellar retinaculum.** Aponeurosis that is derived from portions of the vastus lateralis and rectus femoris muscles as well as fibers from the iliotibial tract. It is situated on the lateral side of the patella and inserts lateral to the tibial tuberosity. See 16 for function. A

18 **Infrapatellar fat pad.** Wedge-shaped mass of adipose tissue that is situated in front of the articular cavity. It includes the alar folds and the infrapatellar synovial fold. A

19 **Tibiofibular joint; Superior tibiofibular joint.** Articulation between the head of the fibula and the lateral condyle of the tibia. E

20 **Anterior ligament of fibular head.** Group of fibers that passes from the head of the fibula to the tibia. It holds the bones together and strengthens the capsule. A

21 **Posterior ligament of fibular head.** Weaker group of fibers passing posteriorly from the head of the fibula to the tibia. See 20 for function. C D E

22 TIBIOFIBULAR SYNDESMOSIS; INFERIOR TIBIOFIBULAR JOINT. Distal articulation between the tibia and fibula.

23 **Interosseous membrane of leg.** Fibrous plate that is attached to the interosseous borders of the fibula and tibia. Origin of the muscles of the tibia and fibula. Stabilizes the mortise formed by the lateral and medial malleoli. A C F G

24 **Anterior tibiofibular ligament.** Ligamentous bands that connect the anterior aspect of the end of the fibula with the lateral malleolus, stabilizing the malleolar mortise. F

25 **Posterior tibiofibular ligament.** Bands that pass on the posterior aspect of the inferior tibiofibular joint, connecting the end of the fibula with the lateral malleolus and stabilizing the malleolar mortise. G

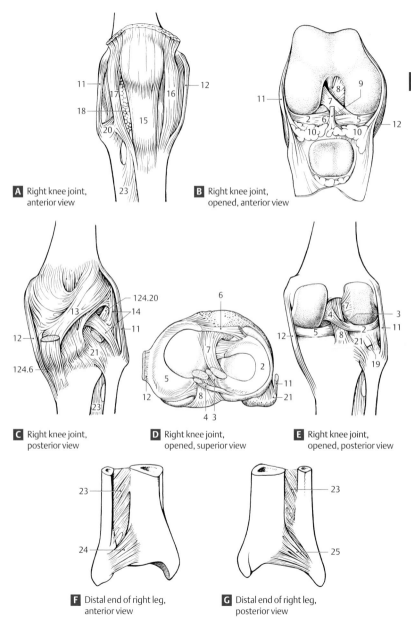

A Right knee joint,
anterior view

B Right knee joint,
opened, anterior view

C Right knee joint,
posterior view

D Right knee joint,
opened, superior view

E Right knee joint,
opened, posterior view

F Distal end of right leg,
anterior view

G Distal end of right leg,
posterior view

1 **Joints of foot.**

2 **Ankle joint.** Talocrural joint formed by the talus, tibia, and fibula. D

3 *Medial ligament*; *Deltoid ligament*. Band on the medial side of the malleolus. It is rather triangular in shape, around 0.5 cm thick, and consists of the following four parts. D

4 *Tibionavicular part.* Group of fibers that pass from the medial malleolus to the dorsal and medial surfaces of the navicular. D

5 *Tibiocalcaneal part.* Fibrous bands that pass from the malleolus to the sustentaculum tali. B D

6 *Anterior tibiotalar part.* Portion of the ligament that extends from the medial malleolus to the medial surface of the neck of the talus. D

7 *Posterior tibiotalar part.* Posterior fibers extending from the medial malleolus and nearly reaching the posterior process of the talus. B D

8 *Lateral ligament.* Band that consists of the following three parts:

9 *Anterior talofibular ligament.* Ligament that passes from the lateral malleolus to the lateral surface of the neck of the talus. A

10 *Posterior talofibular ligament.* Ligament that originates from the malleolar fossa of the lateral malleolus and inserts on the lateral tubercle of the talus. A B

11 *Calcaneofibular ligament.* Ligament that passes from the tip of the lateral malleolus obliquely and posteriorly to the calcaneus. A B

12 **Subtalar joint; Talocalcaneal joint.** Articulation between the talus and calcaneus. Posterior portion of the lower ankle joint with its own joint capsule. A B C D

13 *Lateral talocalcaneal ligament.* Ligament that passes from the trochlea of the talus to the lateral surface of the calcaneus. It is partly covered by the calcaneofibular ligament. A

14 *Medial talocalcaneal ligament.* Ligament on the medial side of the foot that extends from the medial tubercle of the talus to the sustentaculum tali. B D

15 *Posterior talocalcaneal ligament.* Band that passes from the posterior process of the talus to the calcaneus. It spans the groove for the tendon of the flexor hallucis longus.

16 **Transverse tarsal joint.** (Chopart joint). Joint line situated anterior to the talus and calcaneus, but proximal to the cuboid and navicular. It comprises the following two joints. C

17 *Talocalcaneonavicular joint.* Anterior portion of the subtalar joint. It has its own joint capsule in which the talus articulates with the calcaneus and the navicular. A C

18 *Plantar calcaneonavicular ligament*; *Spring ligament.* Ligament that passes from the sustentaculum tali to the plantar and medial surfaces of the navicular, augmenting the articular surface for the head of the talus. p. 92.4

19 *Calcaneocuboid joint.* Joint between the calcaneus and the cuboid which has its own joint capsule. A C

20 **Cuneonavicular joint.** Articulation between the navicular and cuneiform bones. C D

21 **Intercuneiform joint.** Articulations between the cuneiform bones.

22 **Tarsal ligaments.** Bands on the tarsus, most of which strengthen the joint capsules.

23 *Tarsal interosseous ligaments.* Ligaments consisting of the following three bands that pass between the tarsal bones.

24 *Talocalcaneal interosseous ligament.* Strong bands of fibers in the tarsal sinus that divide the upper and lower parts of the ankle joint. A C

25 *Cuneocuboid interosseous ligament.* Tough band that passes from the lateral cuneiform to the cuboid. A C

26 *Intercuneiform interosseous ligaments.* Tough band that connects the three cuneiform bones. C

27 *Dorsal tarsal ligaments.* The following seven dorsal ligaments connecting the tarsal bones.

28 *Talonavicular ligament.* Dorsal band that passes from the head of the talus to the navicular. A D

29 *Dorsal intercuneiform ligament.* Dorsal bands that connect the cuneiform bones. A

30 *Dorsal cuneocuboid ligament.* Dorsal band that extends from the lateral cuneiform to the cuboid. A

31 *Dorsal cuboideonavicular ligament.* Band that connects the cuboid and navicular. A

32 *Bifurcate ligament.* Y-shaped ligament in front of the tarsal sinus on the dorsum of the foot. It passes anteriorly from the calcaneus and consists of the following two parts. A

33 Calcaneonavicular ligament. Medial portion of the bifurcate ligament that passes from the calcaneus to the navicular. A

34 Calcaneocuboid ligament. Portion of the bifurcate ligament that extends from the calcaneus and nearly reaches the middle of the cuboid. A

35 *Dorsal cuneonavicular ligament.* Broad bands on the dorsum of the foot that connect the navicular with the three cuneiform bones. A

36 *Dorsal calcaneocuboid ligament.* Moderately thickened portion of the joint capsule lateral to the bifurcate ligament. A

3

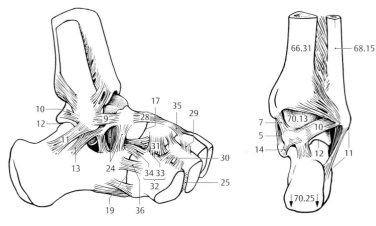

A Ligaments of right tarsus, lateral view

B Ligaments of right ankle joint, posterior view

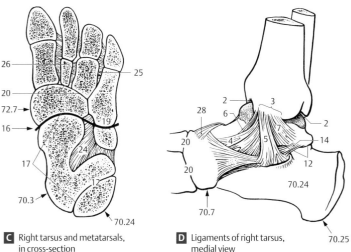

C Right tarsus and metatarsals, in cross-section

D Ligaments of right tarsus, medial view

3

1   *Plantar tarsal ligaments.* Ligaments on the plantar surface of the foot. They are essential to strengthening and supporting the two bony arches of the foot.

2   *Long plantar ligament.* Firm band that passes from the calcaneus just anterior to the calcaneal tuberosity to the cuboid and the bases of metatarsals II–V. It supports the longitudinal arch of the foot.

3   *Plantar calcaneocuboid ligament*; *Short plantar ligament.* Shorter fibers of the long plantar ligament. A

4   *Plantar calcaneonavicular ligament*; *Spring ligament.* A See p. 90.18.

5   *Plantar cuneonavicular ligaments.* Group of ligaments that connect the navicular with the cuneiform bones in front of it. A

6   *Plantar cuboideonavicular ligament.* Band that runs nearly horizontally to the axis of the foot. It connects the plantar surfaces of the cuboid and navicular and supports the transverse arch of the foot. A

7   *Plantar intercuneiform ligaments.* Bands that connect the plantar surfaces of the cuneiform bones and support the transverse arch of the foot. A

8   *Plantar cuneocuboid ligament.* Strengthening ligament that connects the plantar surfaces of the lateral cuneiform and the cuboid. A

9   **Tarsometatarsal joints.** (Lisfranc joint). Articulations between the tarsus and the metatarsals. A B C

10   *Dorsal tarsometatarsal ligaments.* Ligaments on the dorsal side of the foot that connect the tarsus with the metatarsals. B

11   *Plantar tarsometatarsal ligaments.* Ligaments on the plantar side of the foot that connect the tarsus with the metatarsals. A

12   *Cuneometatarsal interosseous ligaments.* Fibrous bands that are located in the articular cavity, connecting the cuneiform bones with the metatarsals. C

13   **Intermetatarsal joints.** Articulations between the bases of the metatarsals. B C

14   *Metatarsal interosseous ligaments.* Fibrous bands that connect the bases of the metatarsals. They form the distal borders of the articular cavities between the metatarsals. C

15   *Dorsal metatarsal ligaments.* Fibrous bands connecting the dorsal surfaces of the bases of the metatarsals. B

16   *Plantar metatarsal ligaments.* Fibrous bands connecting the plantar surfaces of the bases of the metatarsals. A

17   *Intermetatarsal spaces.* Spaces between the shafts of the metatarsals that are occupied by the interossei muscles. A

18   **Metatarsophalangeal joints.** Basal joints of the toes. A

19   *Collateral ligaments.* A

20   *Plantar ligaments.* Fibrous bands that strengthen the joint capsule of the metatarsophalangeal joint. The joint capsule is more firmly attached to the proximal phalanx than to the head of the metatarsal and presents a grooved surface for passage of the flexor tendons. A

21   *Deep transverse metatarsal ligament.* Band that extends horizontally, connecting the heads of the metatarsals. A

22   **Interphalangeal joints of foot.** Proximal and distal articulations between the phalanges of the feet. A

23   *Collateral ligaments.* A

24   *Plantar ligaments.* Fibrous bands that reinforce the plantar side of the interphalangeal joint capsules.

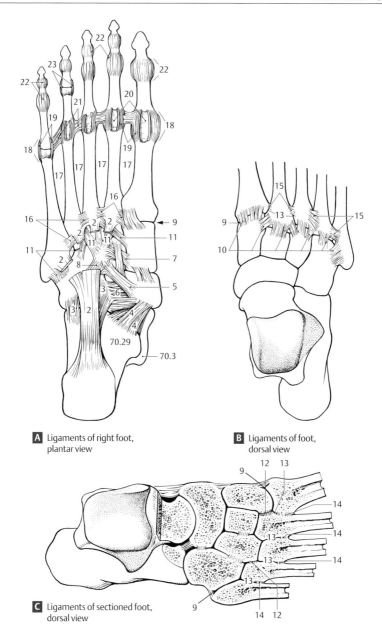

A Ligaments of right foot, plantar view

B Ligaments of foot, dorsal view

C Ligaments of sectioned foot, dorsal view

1 *MUSCLES; MUSCULAR SYSTEM.*

2 *MUSCLES OF HEAD.*

3 **Extra-ocular muscles.** p. 444.9

4 **Muscles of auditory ossicles.** p. 458.1

5 **Muscles of tongue.** p. 140.26

6 **Muscles of soft palate and fauces.** p. 142.16

7 **Facial muscles.**

8 **Epicranius.** Collective term for the muscles inserting into the epicranial aponeurosis. I: Facial nerve. A

9 *Occipitofrontalis.* Muscle that radiates anteriorly and posteriorly into the epicranial aponeurosis. It can move the scalp.

10 *Frontal belly.* Portion of the occipitofrontalis muscle that passes from the eyebrow region and glabella to the epicranial aponeurosis. It elevates the eyebrows and wrinkles the forehead. A

11 *Occipital belly.* Portion of the occipitofrontalis muscle that passes from the highest nuchal line into the epicranial aponeurosis. Antagonist of the frontal belly. A

12 *Temporoparietalis.* Muscle that extends from the auricular cartilage to the epicranial aponeurosis. A

13 *Epicranial aponeurosis.* Hoodlike aponeurosis of both parts of the epicranius that can be moved against the periosteum. Its inferior surface extends from the highest nuchal line to the supraorbital margin and its lateral border nearly reaches the zygomatic arch. A

14 **Procerus.** Muscle that extends from the root of the nose to the skin above the nose. Lowers the skin of the forehead. I: Facial nerve. A

15 **Nasalis.** Collective term for the following two muscles of the nose originating near the canine fossa. I: Facial nerve. B

16 *Transverse part.* Portion of the nasalis muscle that radiates into the aponeurosis on the dorsum of the nose and acts to constrict the nares. B

17 *Alar part.* Portion of the nasalis muscle that extends to the ala of the nose and acts to dilate the nares. B

18 **Depressor septi nasi.** Muscle that passes from the alveolar wall over the medial incisor tooth to the cartilaginous nasal septum and draws the tip of the nose inferiorly. I: Facial nerve.

19 **Orbicularis oculi.** Ringlike sphincter muscle around the eye consisting of various parts. It acts to close the eyelids and support the flow of tears into the lacrimal sac and nose. I: Facial nerve. A

20 *Palpebral part.* Muscle of the eyelid. It arises from the medial palpebral ligament and adjacent bones and comprises the following two parts. A

21 *Ciliary bundle.* Muscle fibers lying on the lid margin that loop around the excretory ducts of the meibomian glands and the eyelash hair follicles.

22 *Deep part.* Bundle of fibers that originate from the posterior lacrimal crest behind the lacrimal sac, encircles the lacrimal canaliculi, and extends to the lacrimal papilla. Its pulling action dilates the lacrimal sac. B

23 *Orbital part.* Portion of the muscle arising from the medial palpebral ligament, the frontal process of the maxilla, and the nasal part of the frontal bone, encircling the eye. A

24 **Corrugator supercilii.** Muscle that passes laterally from the nasal part of the frontal bone into the skin of the eyebrow. It produces vertical wrinkling of the forehead. I: Facial nerve. B, p. 97 A

25 **Depressor supercilii.** Muscle that passes upward from the dorsum of the nose to the skin of the forehead. It produces horizontal folds over the root of the nose. I: Facial nerve. B

26 **Auricularis anterior.** Muscle lying in front of the auricle that passes from the temporal fascia to the spine of the helix. I: Facial nerve. A

27 **Auricularis superior.** Muscle extending from the epicranial aponeurosis to the root of the auricle. I: Facial nerve. A

28 **Auricularis posterior.** Muscle that originates from the mastoid process and attaches to the root of the auricle. I: Facial nerve. A

29 **Orbicularis oris.** Bundles of muscle fibers that surround the oral fissure from both sides. It is the principal muscle of the lips, consisting of two parts. I: Facial nerve.

30 *Marginal part.* Hooklike portion below the vermillion border of the lips. B C

31 *Labial part.* Peripheral main portion of the orbicularis oris muscle. A B C

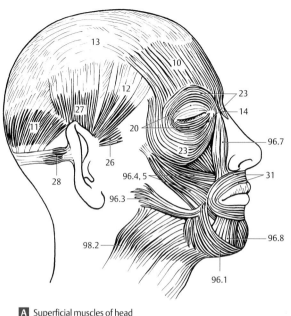

A Superficial muscles of head

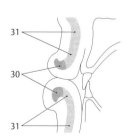

C Sagittal section through the lips

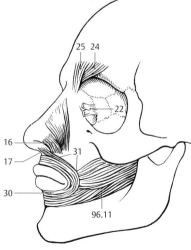

B Deep mimetic muscles

1 **Depressor anguli oris.** Muscle that passes from the anterior and lateral margins of the mandible to the angle of mouth. I: Facial nerve. A, p. 95 A

2 **Transversus menti.** Muscle fibers that cross between the right and left depressor anguli oris below the chin. I: Facial nerve. A

3 **Risorius.** Bundle of muscle fibers that are occasionally present, extending from the parotid fascia and skin of the cheek to the angle of the mouth. I: Facial nerve. A, p. 95 A

4 **Zygomaticus major.** Muscle extending from the zygomatic bone to the angle of the mouth and upper lip. I: Facial nerve. A, p. 95 A

5 **Zygomatic minor.** Muscle passing from the zygomatic bone to the upper lip. I: Facial nerve. A

6 **Levator labii superioris.** Muscle that arises above the infraorbital foramen and whose fibers insert into the orbicularis oris. I: Facial nerve. A

7 **Levator labii superioris alaeque nasi.** Muscle that originates from the frontal process of the maxilla and inserts into the upper lip and ala of the nose. I: Facial nerve. A, p. 95 A

8 **Depressor labii inferioris.** Muscle that lies deep to the depressor anguli oris and passes from the platysma superiorly and medially to the lower lip. I: Facial nerve. A, p. 95 A

9 **Levator anguli oris.** Muscle passing from the canine fossa to the angle of the mouth. I: Facial nerve. A

10 **Modiolus.** Point lateral to the angle of the mouth where adjacent muscles converge and radiate into the orbicularis oris. A

11 **Buccinator.** Muscle arising from the pterygomandibular raphe and adjacent areas of the maxilla and mandible to the height of the first molar teeth, and inserting into the orbicularis oris at the angle of the mouth. It forms the cheek, moves food from the oral vestibule between the dental arcades during mastication, prevents entrapment of the mucous membrane of the mouth, and is active during laughing and crying. I: Facial nerve. A B D, p. 95 B

12 **Mentalis.** Muscle that radiates from the mandible at the height of the roots of the incisor teeth into the skin of the chin (chin cleft). I: Facial nerve. A

13 **Masticatory muscles.**

14 **Masseter.** The most prominent masticatory muscle. It acts to close the mouth and, together with the temporal and medial pterygoid muscles, determines the level of masticatory force. It consists of the following two parts. A F

15 *Superficial part.* o: Anterior two-thirds of the zygomatic arch. i: Angle of mandible; masseteric tuberosity. It passes obliquely from anterosuperior to posteroinferior and draws the mandible slightly forward. A F

16 *Deep part.* Varies in structure. o: Zygomatic arch, disco-capsular system, and sometimes temporal fascia. i: Ramus of mandible. To-

gether with fibers from the temporal muscle coming from anterosuperior, it ensures lateral stabilization of the disco-capsular system during laterotrusion, thus preventing impingement of the disco-capsular system on the balancing side. It can be replaced with parotid or masseteric fascia. F

17 **Temporalis; Temporal muscle.** o: Inferior temporal line, infratemporal crest, temporal fascia [temporal fossa]. i: Its fibers converge at the coronoid process and continue inferiorly to the level of the occlusal plane and near the pterygomandibular raphe. It raises and retracts the mandible, and fixes the pharynx during swallowing. I: Mandibular nerve. B D

18 **Lateral pterygoid.** o: Lateral surface of lateral plate of pterygoid process and inferior surface of greater wing of sphenoid. i: Two-headed (variant: three-headed) at disco-capsular system of temporomandibular joint and pterygoid fovea. I: Mandibular nerve.

19 *Upper head; Superior head.* o: Inferior surface of greater wing of sphenoid. i: Frontal aspect of disco-capsular system or occasionally onto the surface of the bone medial to the pterygoid fovea. Determines repositioning speed of the disco-capsular system. B C

20 *Lower head; Inferior head.* o: Lateral plate of pterygoid process. i: Pterygoid fovea. Variant: Also into the disco-capsular system. Acts in mouth opening. B C

21 **Medial pterygoid.** o: Pterygoid fossa and the maxillary tuberosity. i: Pterygoid tuberosity on inner side of the angle of the mandible, passing obliquely downward and backward. Synergist of the temporal and masseter muscles. I: Mandibular nerve. B

22 **Buccopharyngeal fascia.** Fascia that covers the buccinator muscle and passes over the pterygomandibular raphe to the constrictor muscles of the pharynx as a loose sheath of connective tissue connecting the pharynx with the deep cervical fascia.

23 **Masseteric fascia.** Fascia arising from the zygomatic arch. It invests the masseter muscle and passes over the margin of the mandible, dividing into two portions. One layer passes into the superficial layer of the cervical fascia and the other into the medial pterygoid muscle. E

24 **Parotid fascia.** Sheath of superficial cervical fascia that surrounds the parotid gland. Its deep portion is connected with the masseteric fascia. E

25 **Temporal fascia.** Outer connective-tissue covering of the temporal muscle between the superior temporal line and zygomatic arch. It consists of the following two layers. E

26 *Superficial layer.* Layer of temporal fascia that is attached to the lateral border of the zygomatic arch. E

27 *Deep layer.* Layer of temporal fascia that is attached to the medial border of the zygomatic arch. E

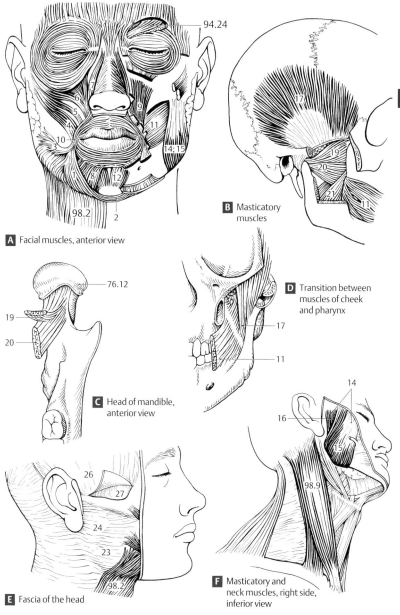

A Facial muscles, anterior view

B Masticatory muscles

C Head of mandible, anterior view

D Transition between muscles of cheek and pharynx

E Fascia of the head

F Masticatory and neck muscles, right side, inferior view

4

1   *MUSCLES OF NECK.*

2   **Platysma.** Cutaneous muscle that extends (with anatomical variations) from above the mandible to the thorax. I: Facial nerve. pp. 95 A; 97 A

3   **Longus colli.** Muscle consisting of three parts that insert into the anterior longitudinal ligament. Superior lateral portion: o: Anterior tubercles of C5–C2. i: Anterior tubercle of atlas, axis. Medial portion: o: Ventral surfaces of vertebral bodies of T3–C5. i: Ventral surface of vertebral bodies of C3–C1. Inferior lateral portion: o: Vertebral bodies of T1–T3. i: Anterior tubercles of C6–C5. Lateral flexion and rotation of the cervical vertebral column as well as anterior flexion of the cervical vertebral column with bilateral action. I: Cervical and brachial plexuses (C2–C8). C

4   **Longus capitis.** o: Anterior tubercles of C3–C6. i: Basilar part of occipital bone. Anterior and lateral flexion of the head and cervical vertebral column. I: Cervical plexus (C1–C3). C

5   **Scalenus anterior; Anterior scalene.** o: Transverse process of C3–C6. i: Scalene tubercle of first rib. Elevation of the first rib, lateral flexion and rotation of the neck; divides anterior and posterior scalene spaces. I: Brachial plexus (C5–C7). C

6   **Scalenus medius; Middle scalene.** o: Transverse processes of C2–C7. i: First rib posterior to the groove for the subclavian artery. Elevation of the first rib and lateral flexion of the neck. I: Cervical plexus and brachial plexus (C4–C8). C

7   **Scalenus posterior; Posterior scalene.** o: Transverse processes of C4–C6. i: Upper margin of second rib. Elevation of the rib. Lateral flexion of the neck. I: Brachial plexus (C7–C8). C

8   **[Scalenus minimus].** Additional muscle that is occasionally present between the anterior and middle scalene muscles. o: Transverse process of C6 or C7. i: First rib and pleural cupula. C

9   **Sternocleidomastoid.** o: Two-headed muscle arising from the sternum and clavicle. i: Mastoid process; superior nuchal line. Rotates the face to the contralateral side and bends the head to the ipsilateral side. Bilateral contraction elevates the face. I: Accessory nerve, cervical plexus (C1–C2). A, p. 97 F.

10 **Suboccipital muscles.** These are the following six muscles. The rectus capitis anterior and lateralis are not autochthonous back muscles.

11 **Rectus capitis anterior.** o: Lateral mass of atlas. i: Basilar part of occipital bone. Forward bending of the head. I: Cervical plexus (C1). C

12 **Rectus capitis lateralis.** o: Transverse process of atlas. i: Jugular process of occipital bone. Lateral bending of the head. I: Anterior ramus of spinal nerve (C1). C

13 **Rectus capitis posterior major.** o: Spinous process of axis. i: Middle of inferior nuchal line. Rotates the face laterally. Posterior flexion. I: Suboccipital nerve. B

14 **Rectus capitis posterior minor.** o: Posterior tubercle of the posterior arch of atlas. i: Medial one-third of inferior nuchal line. Mainly posterior flexion of the head. I: Suboccipital nerve. B

15 **Obliquus capitis superior.** o: Transverse process of atlas. i: Area overlying the insertion of the rectus capitis posterior major. Posterior and lateral bending of the head. I: Suboccipital nerve. B

16 **Obliquus capitis inferior.** o: Spinous process of axis. i: Transverse process of atlas. Lateral rotation of the atlas and face to the ipsilateral side. I: Suboccipital nerve. B

17 **Suprahyoid muscles.** The following muscles situated above the hyoid bone. A

18 **Digastric.** o: Mastoid notch. i: Digastric fossa. It has an intermediate tendon that acts on the lesser horn of the hyoid bone by means of a connective tissue sling. Raises the hyoid bone and opens the mouth. A

19 *Anterior belly.* Portion of the digastric muscle that extends from the mandible to the intermediate tendon. I: Nerve to mylohyoid. A D

20 *Posterior belly.* Portion of the digastric muscle that passes from the mastoid notch to the intermediate tendon. I: Nerve to mylohyoid. A D

21 **Stylohyoid.** o: Styloid process. i: Body of hyoid bone near lesser horn. It accompanies the posterior belly of the digastric muscle and gives it passage through a perforation. It acts to draw the hyoid bone upward and backward during swallowing. I: Facial nerve. A D

22 **Mylohyoid.** o: Mylohyoid line. i: Median fibrous raphe and body of hyoid bone. It forms the muscular floor of the mouth; supports the tongue. Raises the floor of the mouth and the hyoid bone. Draws the mandible inferiorly. I: Nerve to mylohyoid. A E

23 **Geniohyoid.** o: Inferior mental spine. i: Body of hyoid bone. Aids the mylohyoid. I: Anterior rami of spinal nerves (C1–C2). E

24 **Infrahyoid muscles.** Muscles located inferior to the hyoid bone that act to either stabilize it or draw it inferiorly. Accessory muscles of deglutition and respiration. Indirect flexion at head and neck joints. I: Ansa cervicalis (C1–C3). A

25 **Sternohyoid.** o: Posterior surface of manubrium of sternum and sternoclavicular joint. i: Body of hyoid bone. A

26 **Omohyoid.** o: Superior border of scapula. i: Body of hyoid bone. It is divided into two bellies by an intermediate tendon that passes over the jugular vein. Hence it also tenses the pretracheal layer of the cervical fascia. A

27 *Superior belly.* Upper portion of the omohyoid muscle between the hyoid bone and intermediate tendon. A

28 *Inferior belly.* Lower half of the omohyoid muscle that extends from the intermediate tendon to the suprascapular notch. A

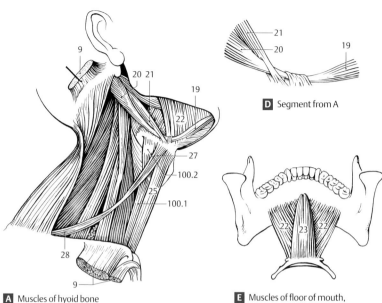

A Muscles of hyoid bone

D Segment from A

E Muscles of floor of mouth, posterosuperior view

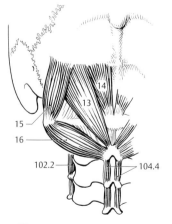

B Short muscles of neck

C Deep neck muscles, anterior view

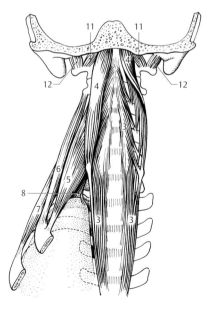

4

1 **Sternothyroid.** o: Posterior surface of manubrium of sternum and first rib. i: Oblique line of thyroid cartilage. p. 99 A

2 **Thyrohyoid.** o: Oblique line of thyroid cartilage. i: Greater horn and lateral one-third of the medial aspect of the hyoid bone. p. 99A

3 **[Levator glandulae thyroideae].** Portion of the thyrohyoid muscle that extends to the thyroid gland.

4 **Cervical fascia.** Collective term for the following three connective tissue layers of the neck.

5 **Investing layer; Superficial layer.** Superficial layer of cervical fascia that surrounds the surface structures of the neck and continues as the nuchal fascia. It ensheathes the sternocleidomastoid and trapezius muscles and is attached to the manubrium of the sternum, the clavicle, hyoid bone, and inferior margin of the mandible. A

6 *Suprasternal space.* Space between the superficial and pretracheal layers of the deep cervical fascia above the sternum.

7 **Pretracheal layer.** Middle layer of cervical fascia that is spread between the two bellies of the omohyoid and encloses the infrahyoid muscles. It is attached to the posterior border of the manubrium of the sternum and to both clavicles, blending laterally into the prevertebral layer of cervical fascia and above the hyoid bone into the superficial layer. It splits to form the outer layer of the fibrous capsule enclosing the thyroid gland. A B

8 *Suspensory ligament of thyroid gland.* Thickened portion of the pretracheal layer of cervical fascia that passes between it and the trachea, thyroid cartilage, cricoid cartilage, and thyroid gland. B

9 **Prevertebral layer.** Deep layer of cervical fascia that extends from the cranial base over the prevertebral and scalene muscles. It encloses the nerve pathways to the arm and passes into the endothoracic fascia. A B

10 **Carotid sheath.** Connective-tissue sheath enclosing a neurovascular bundle (carotid artery, internal jugular vein, vagus nerve). Its fibers blend with the pretracheal layer of cervical fascia. A

11 *MUSCLES OF BACK.* These muscles arise ventrally and cranially and are not innervated by the posterior rami of the spinal nerves.

12 **Trapezius.** Muscle that consists of three parts that act together to position the scapula and clavicle, draw both toward the vertebral column, and brace the shoulder girdle. I: Accessory nerve; brachial plexus C2–C4. D, p. 103 C

13 *Descending part; Superior part.* o: Highest nuchal line, external occipital protuberance, nuchal ligament. i: Usually the lateral one-third of the clavicle. It acts against downward pull and rotates and adducts the scapula. Rotation of the head with fixed scapula. D

14 *Transverse part; Middle part.* o: Spinous processes and supraspinous ligament. C7–T3. i: Acromion including clavicle and spine of scapula. Draws the scapula toward the vertebral column. D

15 *Ascending part; Inferior part.* o: Spinous processes; supraspinous ligament T2–T12. i: Spine of scapula. Rotates and draws the scapula toward the vertebral column. D

16 **[Transversus nuchae].** Muscle occasionally present (25%) between the insertions of the trapezius and sternocleidomastoid muscles. D

17 **Latissimus dorsi.** o: Spinous processes of T7–T12, thoracolumbar fascia, iliac crest, tenth through twelfth ribs. i: Crest of lesser tubercle of humerus. Retraction, medial rotation, adduction of the arm. I: Thoracodorsal nerve. D

18 **Rhomboid major.** o: Spinous processes of T1–T4. i: Medial border of scapula. Draws the scapula medially and cranially and presses it against the ribs. I: Dorsal scapular nerve. D

19 **Rhomboid minor.** Spinous processes of C6–C7. i: Medial border of scapula. See 18 for function and innervation. D

20 **Levator scapulae.** o: Posterior tubercles of cervical vertebrae C1–C4. i: Superior angle of scapula. Raises the scapula; rotates the inferior angle of the scapula medially. I: Dorsal scapular nerve. D, p. 103 C

21 **Serratus posterior inferior.** o: Thoracolumbar fascia at the level of T11–L2. i: Lower four ribs. Draws these ribs inferiorly. I: Intercostal nerves. D

22 **Serratus posterior superior.** o: Spinous processes of C6–T2. i: Second to fifth ribs. Elevates the ribs. I: Intercostal nerves.

23 **Auscultatory triangle; Triangle of auscultation.** Triangular region medial to the scapula between the lateral margin of the trapezius, superior margin of the latissimus dorsi, and medial border of the scapula. The tips of the inferior lobes of the lungs can be auscultated here when the trunk is bent forward with crossed arms. D

24 **Inferior lumbar triangle (Triangle of Petit).** Triangular region bounded by the iliac crest inferiorly and between the borders of the latissimus dorsi and external oblique muscle of the abdomen. Its floor is formed by the internal oblique muscle of the abdomen. D

25 **Superior lumbar triangle.** Inconstant space beneath the latissimus dorsi and external oblique muscle of the abdomen with the thoracolumbar fascia forming its floor. It is limited superiorly by the twelfth rib and posterior inferior serratus, medially by the erector spinae, and laterally by the internal oblique muscle of the abdomen. C

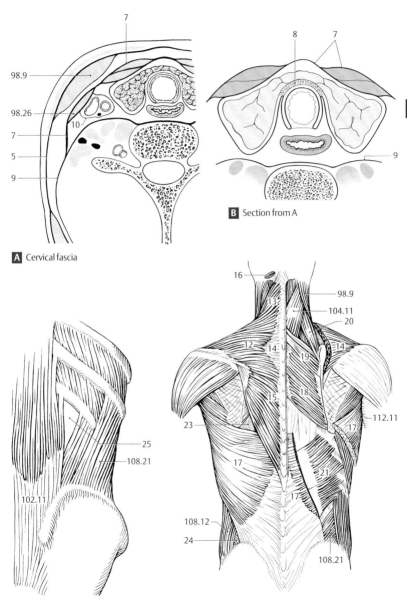

A Cervical fascia

B Section from A

C Superior lumbar triangle

D Superficial muscles of back

1 **Anterior cervical intertransversarii.** Muscles that pass between the anterior tubercles of the cervical vertebrae. I: Anterior rami of spinal nerves.

2 **Lateral posterior cervical intertransversarii.** Muscles that pass between the posterior tubercles of transverse processes of C2–C7. I: Anterior rami of spinal nerves. p. 99 B

3 **Intertransversarii laterales lumborum.** Muscle that consists of two parts and is innervated by the anterior rami of the spinal nerves.

4 *Dorsal parts.* Bands of muscle fibers that pass between the mamillary and accessory processes of the lumbar vertebrae.

5 *Ventral parts.* Bands of muscle fibers extending between the costal processes. p. 105 A

6 **Nuchal fascia.** Continuation of the posterior layer of thoracolumbar fascia to cranial. It ensheathes the splenius and semispinalis capitis muscles. Laterally it blends into the superficial layer of cervical fascia and anteriorly into the prevertebral layer. It is connected medially with the nuchal ligament. C

7 MUSCLES OF BACK PROPER. True (autochthonous) back muscles. They are innervated by the posterior rami of the spinal nerves.

8 **Erector spinae.** Collective term for the iliocostalis, longissimus, and spinalis muscles. A

9 **Erector spinae aponeurosis.** Origin of the erector spinae. Flat sheet of fibers that blends with the thoracolumbar fascia and arises from the spinous processes of the lumbar vertebrae, dorsal surface of the sacrum, and dorsomedial part of the iliac crest. A

10 *Intermuscular septum.* Fibers from the erector spinae aponeurosis that separate muscle parts with various functions.

11 **Iliocostalis.** Muscle composed of the following parts, which are responsible for maintaining erect posture and for lateral bending. I: Posterior rami of spinal nerves of C4–L3. B

12 *Iliocostalis lumborum.* o: Sacrum, iliac crest, erector spinae aponeurosis. i: Angles of all ribs. It can be divided into two parts.

13 *Lumbar part; Lateral division of lumbar erector spinae.* Inferior portion of the muscle that attaches to the six lowest ribs. A B

14 *Thoracic part.* o: Angles of the six lower ribs. i: Angles of the six upper ribs. A B

15 *Iliocostalis cervicis.* o: Angles of sixth to third ribs. i: Posterior tubercles of transverse processes of vertebrae C6–C4. A B

16 **Longissimus.** Muscle that consists of three parts and is responsible for maintaining erect posture. I: Posterior rami of the spinal nerves from C2–L5. B

17 *Longissimus thoracis.* o: Sacrum, spinous processes of lumbar vertebrae, transverse processes of lower thoracic vertebrae. i: Medially on the transverse processes of the lumbar and thoracic vertebrae; laterally on the costal process of the lumbar vertebrae, ribs, and anterior layer of thoracolumbar fascia. A B

18 *Lumbar part; Medial division of lumbar erector spinae.* Inferior portion of the longissimus thoracis muscle. A

19 *Longissimus cervicis.* o: Transverse processes of T6–T1. i: Transverse processes of C7–C2. A B

20 *Longissimus capitis.* o: Transverse processes from T3–T1 and C7–C3. i: Mastoid process. A B

21 **Spinalis.** Group of erector spinae muscles that pass over the spinous processes of the vertebrae. It does not attach to C5 or T9. I: Posterior rami of the spinal nerves of C2–T10. A B

22 *Spinalis thoracis.* o: Spinous processes of L3–T10. i: Spinous processes of T8–T2. B

23 *Spinalis cervicis.* o: Spinous processes of T2–C6. i: Spinous processes of C4–C2. B

24 *Spinalis capitis.* Inconstant muscle with fibers from the cervical and upper thoracic vertebrae. Insertion on the external occipital protuberance.

4

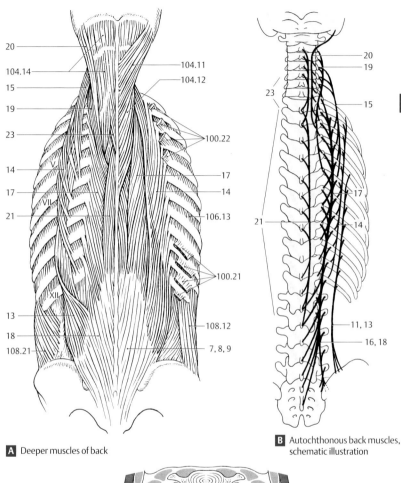

A Deeper muscles of back

B Autochthonous back muscles, schematic illustration

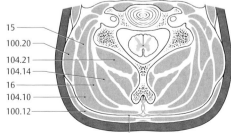

C Cross-section of neck at the level of C5

1 **Interspinales.** Muscles extending between the spinous processes of two adjacent vertebrae. I: Posterior rami of C1–T3 and T11–L5. A

2 **Interspinales lumborum.** Especially strong muscles. A

3 **Interspinales thoracis.** Frequently absent. A

4 **Interspinales cervicis.** Bands of muscle fibers that are attached pairwise to the bifid spinous processes of the vertebrae. A, p. 99 B

5 **Intertransversarii.** Muscles that connect the transverse processes of consecutive vertebrae. I: Posterior rami of spinal nerves of C1–C6; L1–L4.

6 **Medial lumbar intertransversarii.** Muscles that extend between the mamillary and accessory processes of two contiguous vertebrae. A

7 **Thoracic intertransversarii.** Usually absent.

8 **Medial posterior cervical intertransversarii.** Muscles that pass between the posterior tubercles of two contiguous vertebrae. A

9 **Spinotransversales.** Group of oblique bands consisting of only the splenius.

10 **Splenius.** Muscle that covers and fixes the upper portion of the erector spinae. Action on one side produces ipsilateral rotation; bilateral action produces extension. I: Posterior rami of spinal nerves C1–C7. A, p. 103 C

11 *Splenius capitis.* Portion of the splenius extending to the head. o: Spinous processes of T3–C4. i: Lateral part of the superior nuchal line and mastoid process. A, p. 103 A

12 *Splenius cervicis.* Portion of the splenius extending to the neck. o: Spinous processes of T5–T3. i: Posterior tubercles of transverse processes of cervical vertebrae C2–C1. p. 103 A

13 **Transversospinales.** Collective term for the overlapping muscles listed under 18–29, which extend from the transverse process of a vertebra to the spinous process of a higher vertebra, passing over vertebrae in between. Bilateral action produces extension and unilateral action rotation. A B C

14 **Semispinalis.** Superficial layer of the transversospinal muscles. Its fibers span as many as five or more vertebrae. Absent in the lumbar region. A C, p. 103 A

15 *Semispinalis thoracis.* o: Transverse processes of T12–T6. i: Spinous processes of T3–C6. I: Posterior rami of spinal nerves of T4–T6. A B

16 *Semispinalis cervicis.* o: Transverse processes of T6–T2. i: Spinous processes of C6–C2. I: Posterior rami of spinal nerves of C3–C6. A B

17 *Semispinalis capitis.* o: Transverse processes of T6–C3. i: Inferior to the superior nuchal line. I: Posterior rami of spinal nerves of C1–C5. A B

18 **Multifidus.** Muscles passing in transversospinal fashion from the sacrum to the second cervical vertebra. Strong muscle fibers in the lumbar region. I: Posterior rami of spinal nerves of S4–C3. C

19 *Multifidus lumborum.* o: Sacrum, mamillary processes of lumbar vertebrae. i: Spinous processes of L5–L1. A

20 *Multifidus thoracis.* o: Transverse processes of vertebrae. i: Spinous processes of T12–T1. A

21 *Multifidus cervicis.* o: Caudal articular processes. i: Spinous processes of C7–C2. A

22 **Rotatores.** Deepest layer of the transversospinales. It consists of short fibers that pass to the next highest vertebra or second above and thus have stronger rotating action. Usually located in the thoracic region. I: Posterior rami of spinal nerves T11–T1 C, p. 103 C

23 *[Rotatores lumborum].* o: Mammillary processes of lumbar vertebrae. i: Roots of spinous processes of lumbar vertebrae. Short rotatores muscles are absent. A

24 *Rotatores thoracis.* o: Transverse processes of thoracic vertebrae. i: Roots of spinous processes. A B

25 *Rotatores cervicis.* o: Inferior articular processes of cervical vertebrae. i: Vertebral arch or root of the spinous processes. B

26 **Thoracolumbar fascia.** Fascial sheath enclosing the erector spinae. Together with the vertebral column, its spinous processes, and costal surfaces, it forms an osteofascial canal that encases the erector spinae. It consists of three layers that radiate into the following muscles: transverse abdominal, serratus posterior, latissimus dorsi, and sometimes the internal oblique muscle of the abdomen. D

27 **Posterior layer.** Superficial fascial layer that is firmly attached at its sacral end to the erector spinae and blends toward its upper end with the nuchal fascia. D

28 **Middle layer.** Middle fascial layer (previously: deep) that is attached to the tips of the costal processes of the lumbar vertebrae. D

29 **Anterior layer; Quadratus lumborum fascia.** Anterior layer of fascia that encloses the quadratus lumborum. It is attached laterally behind the psoas major to the anterior surface of the costal processes of the lumbar vertebrae. D

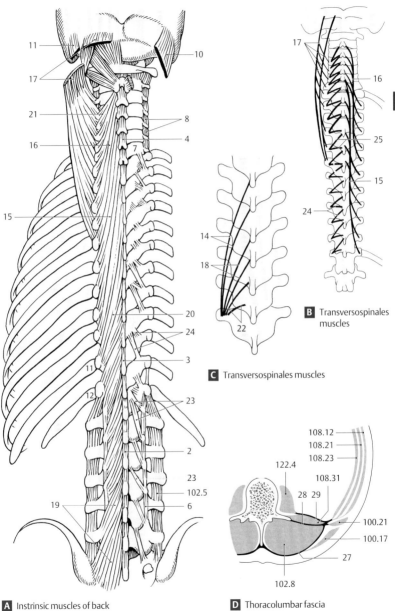

A Instrinsic muscles of back

B Transversospinales muscles

C Transversospinales muscles

D Thoracolumbar fascia

1 *MUSCLES OF THORAX.* Muscles of the chest wall.

2 **[Sternalis].** Anatomical variant present in 4%. It crosses the pectoralis major parallel to the sternum. A

3 **Pectoralis major.** o: Clavicle. Sternum. Second to seventh costal cartilages and rectus sheath. i: Crest of greater tubercle. Adduction and medial rotation of the arm. I: Medial and lateral pectoral nerve. A

4 *Clavicular head.* Portion of the pectoralis major originating from the clavicle. A

5 *Sternocostal head.* Portion originating from the sternum and ribs. A

6 *Abdominal part.* Portion arising from the rectus sheath. A

7 **Pectoralis minor.** Lies deep to the pectoralis major. o: Third to fifth ribs. i: Coracoid process. Rotates the scapula, draws the scapula downward and ribs upward. Accessory respiratory muscle. I: see 3. A

8 **Subclavius.** o: First costal cartilage. i: Inferior surface of clavicle. Stabilizes the sternoclavicular joint against being drawn laterally. I: Subclavian nerve. A

9 **Serratus anterior.** o: First to ninth ribs. i: Inferior surface of medial border of scapula. Fixes, rotates, and lowers the scapula, draws it forward, and assists in raising the arm above the horizontal plane. I: Long thoracic nerve. A

10 **Levatores costarum.** Support rotation of the vertebral column. These muscles are located posteriorly, deep to the long back muscles. o: Transverse processes of thoracic vertebrae. i: Ribs. I: Posterior ramus of spinal nerve. B

11 *Levatores costarum longi.* o: Transverse processes. i: Passes to the second rib beneath its origin. B

12 *Levatores costarum breves.* o: Transverse processes. i: Rib immediately beneath its origin. B

13 **External intercostal muscles.** Muscles that extend obliquely between the ribs from postero-superior to anteroinferior. They are active during inspiration and fix the ribs. I: Intercostal nerves. A E F

14 **External intercostal membrane.** Membrane that replaces the external intercostal muscles between the costal cartilages. A

15 **Internal intercostal muscles.** Muscles that extend between the intercostal spaces from the sternum to the costal angle, passing from anterosuperior to posteroinferior. Expiratory muscles; fixation of the ribs. I: Intercostal nerves. E F

16 **Internal intercostal membrane.** Membrane that replaces the internal intercostal muscles between the costal angle and the vertebrae. E

17 **Innermost intercostal muscles.** Innermost muscle fibers, which are separated from internal intercostal muscles by intercostal vessels. I: Intercostal nerves. F

18 **Subcostales.** Internal intercostal muscles that pass to the second or third rib below. I: Intercostal nerves. E

19 **Transversus thoracis.** o: Medial surface of the body of sternum and xiphoid process. i: Second to sixth costal cartilages. I: Intercostal nerves. C

20 **Pectoral fascia.** Fascial sheet that encloses the pectoralis major, extending to the deltoid muscle and axillary fascia.

21 **Clavipectoral fascia.** Fascial sheet that encloses the pectoralis minor and subclavius muscles and attaches to the axillary fascia. It separates the pectoralis major and minor muscles. A

22 **Thoracic fascia.** Epimysium of the inner thoracic musculature.

23 **Endothoracic fascia; Parietal fascia of thorax.** Sliding layer of loose connective tissue between parietal pleura and chest wall. Continuation of the deep cervical fascia.

24 **Diaphragm.** Dome-shaped musculofibrous septum dividing thoracic and abdominal cavities. I: Phrenic nerve. D

25 **Lumbar part of diaphragm.** Part of the diaphragm that arises from the lumbar vertebrae, intervertebral discs, and tendinous arches. D

26 *Right crus.* Right crus of the lumbar part of the diaphragm. o: L1–3(4). D

27 *Left crus.* Left crus of the lumbar part of the diaphragm. o: L1–2(3). D

28 *Median arcuate ligament.* Tendinous arch over the aortic hiatus. Aortic arcade. D

29 *Medial arcuate ligament.* Psoas arcade. Tendinous arch between the body and transverse process of L1 or L2 that forms a passageway for the psoas muscle. D

30 *Lateral arcuate ligament.* Quadratus arcade. Tendinous arch over the quadratus lumborum between transverse process of L1 or L2 and the twelfth rib. D

31 **Costal part of diaphragm.** Part of diaphragm arising from the costal cartilages of the seventh through the twelfth ribs. C D

32 **Sternal part of diaphragm.** Part of diaphragm that originates from the xiphoid process. C D

33 **Aortic hiatus.** Passageway between the right and left crura of the lumbar part of the diaphragm for the aorta and thoracic duct. D

34 **Esophageal hiatus.** Passageway for the esophageal and vagal nerves. D

35 **Phrenico-esophageal ligament.** Loose connective tissue surrounding the esophagus; it does not fix the esophagus to the diaphragm.

36 **Central tendon.** Convergence of musculature in a central aponeurosis. D

37 **Caval opening.** Opening in the central tendon for passage of the vena cava. D

4

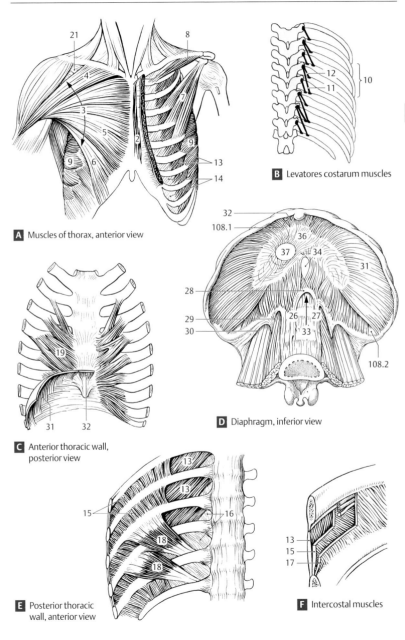

A Muscles of thorax, anterior view

B Levatores costarum muscles

C Anterior thoracic wall, posterior view

D Diaphragm, inferior view

E Posterior thoracic wall, anterior view

F Intercostal muscles

1 **Sternocostal triangle.** Opening between the sternal and costal parts of the diaphragm. p. 107 D

2 **Lumbocostal triangle.** Opening between the lumbar and costal parts of the diaphragm. p. 107 D

3 **Diaphragmatic fascia.** Sheet of fascia covering the ventral side of the diaphragm.

4 *MUSCLES OF ABDOMEN.*

5 **Rectus abdominis.** o: Fifth to seventh costal cartilages, xiphoid process. i: Pubic crest and pubic symphysis. Anterior flexion of the trunk, lowering of the thorax, and elevation of the pelvis. I: Thoracic nerves T7–T12. A D

6 *Tendinous intersections.* Three or four intermediate tendons of the rectus abdominis which are firmly attached to the anterior wall of the rectus sheath. A

7 *Rectus sheath.* Investing layer of the rectus abdominis that is formed by the aponeuroses of the flat abdominal muscles. A

8 *Anterior layer of rectus sheath.* A

9 *Posterior layer of rectus sheath.* A

10 *Arcuate line.* Caudal end of the posterior layer of the rectus sheath. A

11 **Pyramidalis.** Muscle located between two layers in the anterior part of the rectus sheath. o: Pubic crest and pubic symphysis. i: Linea alba. I: Subcostal nerve. A

12 **External oblique.** o: Outer surface of the fifth through twelfth ribs. i: Iliac crest, inguinal ligament, rectus sheath, linea alba. Flexes the trunk, elevates the pelvis, raises intra-abdominal pressure, bends laterally, and rotates the trunk to the contralateral side. I: Intercostal nerves of fifth to twelfth ribs. A C, p. 103 A

13 *Inguinal ligament.* Inferior end of the aponeurosis of the external oblique. It passes from the anterior superior iliac spine to the pubic tubercle. D C

14 *Lacunar ligament.* Arched connective-tissue band that extends inferiorly from the medial attachment of the inguinal ligament to the pubis. C

15 *Pectineal ligament.* Prolongation of the lacunar ligament that extends to the pectineal line of the pubis. C

16 *Reflected ligament.* Expansion of the inguinal ligament that forms the medial part of the floor of the inguinal canal. C

17 **Superficial inguinal ring.** Outer opening of the inguinal canal. C

18 *Medial crus.* Bundle of fibers arising from the aponeurosis of the external oblique medial to the superficial inguinal ring. C

19 *Lateral crus.* Bundle of fibers arising from the aponeurosis of the external oblique lateral to the superficial inguinal ring. C

20 *Intercrural fibers.* Fibers passing in an arch between the medial and lateral crura. C

21 **Internal oblique.** o: Thoracolumbar fascia, iliac crest, anterior superior iliac spine, inguinal ligament. i: Tenth to twelfth ribs and rectus sheath. Flexes the trunk, elevates the pelvis, raises intra-abdominal pressure, bends laterally, and rotates the trunk to the ipsilateral side. I: Intercostal nerves of the eighth through twelfth ribs, iliohypogastric nerve, and ilioinguinal nerve. A, p. 103 A

22 *Cremaster.* Muscle that is usually an expansion of the internal oblique. It encloses the spermatic cord and elevates the testes. A

23 **Transversus abdominis; Transverse abdominal.** Inner surface of the seventh through twelfth costal cartilages, thoracolumbar fascia, iliac crest, anterior superior iliac spine, inguinal ligament. i: Rectus sheath, linea semilunaris. I: Intercostal nerves 7–12, iliohypogastric nerve, ilioinguinal nerve, genitofemoral nerve. A

24 *Inguinal falx; Conjoint tendon.* Tendinous fibers forming an arch that extends from the aponeurosis of the transverse abdominal muscle into the pectineal ligament. A D

25 *Deep inguinal ring.* Inner inguinal ring located at the transition of the transversalis fascia into the internal spermatic fascia. A D

26 **Linea alba.** Strip formed by the fusion of the left and right abdominal aponeuroses between the xiphoid process and pubic symphysis.

27 *Umbilical ring.* Fibrous ring surrounding the umbilical opening in the lineal alba. A

28 *Posterior attachment of linea alba.* Triangular thickening of the linea alba at its attachment to the pubic symphysis. A D

29 **Linea semilunaris.** Arched tendinous border of the transverse abdominal muscle. A

30 **Inguinal canal.** Walls: inguinal ligament, aponeurosis of external oblique, transversalis fascia and its thickened portions, internal oblique, and transverse abdominal muscle. In the male it contains the spermatic cord and in the female the round ligament of the uterus. D

31 **Quadratus lumborum.** o: Iliac crest. i: Twelfth rib, costal processes of lumbar vertebrae L1–L4. Draws ribs inferiorly, lateral flexion. I: Intercostal nerve of twelfth rib, lumbar plexus. B

32 **Abdominal fascia.** Collective term for all abdominal fascia and their respective parts.

33 **Visceral abdominal fascia.** Fascia lying deep to the visceral peritoneum.

34 *Fascia of individual organ.*

35 **Extraperitoneal fascia.** Connective-tissue layer that is not attached to the peritoneum. It can occur as an independent structure or envelop a complex structure.

36 *Extraperitoneal ligament.* Ligament derived from part of the extraperitoneal fascia, e.g., the round ligament of the liver or the median umbilical fold.

4

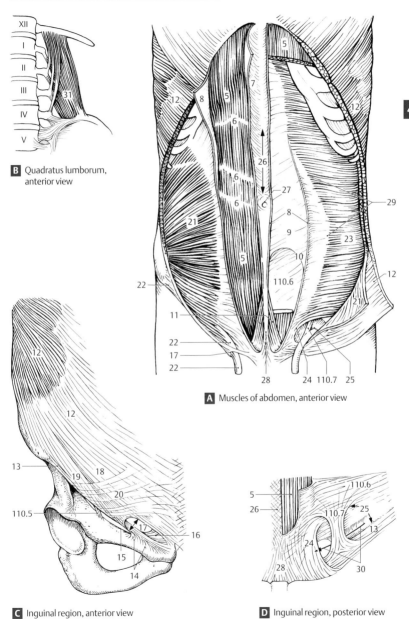

B Quadratus lumborum, anterior view

A Muscles of abdomen, anterior view

C Inguinal region, anterior view

D Inguinal region, posterior view

4

1 **Parietal abdominal fascia; Endo-abdominal fascia.** Term with two uses: fascia of the abdominal wall that lines the entire abdominal cavity; generic term that also includes extraperitoneal and visceral fascia of the abdominal cavity and pelvis.

2 *Fascia of individual organ.*

3 *Iliopsoas fascia*; *Fascia iliaca.* Part of the abdominal wall fascia. Common muscle fascia of the psoas major and iliacus muscles. It becomes thicker as it extends caudally. D

4 **Psoas fascia.** Fascia that surrounds the psoas muscle from the medial arcuate ligament onward. D

5 *Iliac fascia.* Portion extending from the inguinal ligament onward.

6 Iliopectineal arch. Branch of the fascia iliaca that extends from the inguinal ligament to the iliopubic eminence. It divides the vascular space from the muscular space. p. 109 C

7 *Transversalis fascia.* Inner fascial sheath surrounding the flat muscles of the abdomen. D, p. 109 A D

8 *Interfoveolar ligament.* Craniocaudal band of thickened fascia posterior to the inguinal canal. p. 109 A D

9 *Iliopubic tract.* Union of the transversalis fascia and inguinal ligament that forms part of the posterior wall of the inguinal canal.

10 *Umbilical fascia.* Thickening of the transversalis fascia near the umbilical region. D

11 *Investing abdominal fascia.* Collective term for fascial tissue found in the abdominal cavity and lining the abdominal wall.

12 *Deep investing fascia.* Connected fascial coverings of the muscles surrounding the peritoneal cavity. D

13 *Intermediate investing fascia.* Connective-tissue layer that encloses individual abdominal muscles and their aponeuroses. D

14 *Superficial investing fascia.* Outer connective-tissue covering that encloses the abdominal muscles and their aponeuroses. A D

15 Suspensory ligament of clitoris. Fascial and aponeurotic portion of the superficial investing fascia that attaches the body of the clitoris to the pubic symphysis.

16 Suspensory ligament of penis. Fascial and aponeurotic portion of the superficial investing fascia that attaches the body of the penis to the pubic symphysis. A

17 **Loose connective tissue.** It can form subcutaneous tissue devoid of larger quantities of fat; e.g., eyelid, penis, scrotum, labia.

18 **Subcutaneous tissue of abdomen.** Subcutaneous tissue lining the abdominal wall. A

19 *Membranous layer.* Connective-tissue part of subcutaneous abdominal tissue. It becomes denser as it nears the fascia. Caudal to the navel, it is mainly arranged in longitudinal fibers over the rectus abdominis muscle, extending laterally from superolateral to inferomedial (Scarpa's fascia). They pass over the inguinal region and continue as the fascia lata. A

20 *Fundiform ligament of clitoris.* Extension of the membranous layer containing abundant elastic fibers that extends to the clitoris.

21 *Fundiform ligament of penis.* Extension of the membranous layer that forms an elastic band encircling the root of the penis. A

22 *Fatty layer.* Adipose tissue in the subcutaneous tissue of the abdominal wall.

23 *MUSCLES OF UPPER LIMB.*

24 **Compartments.** Muscle compartments, enclosures, and spaces.

25 **Anterior compartment of arm; Flexor compartment of arm.** Boundaries: medial intermuscular septum of arm, humerus, lateral intermuscular septum of arm, brachial fascia. B

26 **Posterior compartment of arm; Extensor compartment of arm.** Boundaries: medial intermuscular septum of arm, humerus, lateral intermuscular septum of arm, brachial fascia. B

27 **Anterior compartment of forearm; Flexor compartment of forearm.** Boundaries: ulna, antebrachial fascia (including fascia investing flexor groups passing to the radius), interosseous membrane. It is divided into two smaller compartments by a connective-tissue septum containing the median nerve. C

28 *Superficial part.* Part of the anterior compartment that contains the superficial flexors originating from the medial epicondyle of the humerus.

29 *Deep part.* Part of the anterior compartment in which the deep flexor muscles originate from the radius, interosseous membrane, and ulna.

30 **Posterior compartment of forearm; Extensor compartment of forearm.** Boundaries: ulna, antebrachial fascia (including fascia investing extensor groups passing to the radius), interosseous membrane. It includes a partially formed lateral compartment. C

31 *Lateral part*; *Radial part.* These muscles originate from above the lateral epicondyle of the humerus, but their attachments are displaced to palmar. They are attached to the radius by fascia investing muscle groups and are covered by the antebrachial fascia. They act to flex the elbow joint. C

4

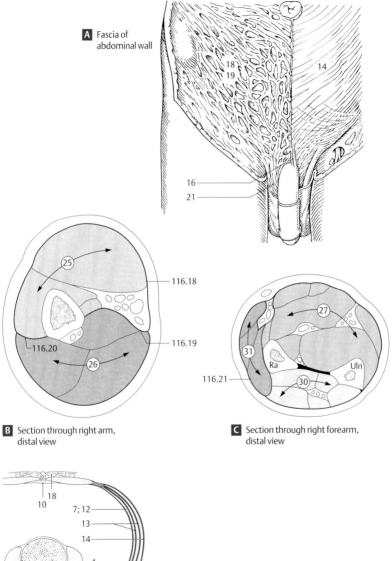

A Fascia of abdominal wall

18
19
14

16
21

B Section through right arm, distal view

25
116.18
116.20
116.19
26

C Section through right forearm, distal view

27
31
Ra
Uln
116.21
30

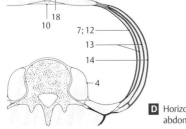

18
10
7; 12
13
14
4

D Horizontal section though abdomen at the level of L2

1 **Muscles.**

2 **Deltoid.** Muscle consisting of three parts, all attaching on the deltoid tuberosity of the humerus and acting together to abduct the arm to about 90°. I: Axillary nerve. A B E F G

3 *Clavicular part.* o: Lateral one-third of clavicle. Adduction, anteversion, medial rotation in various arm positions. A

4 *Acromial part.* o: Acromion. Anteversion, retroversion. A B

5 *Spinal part.* o: Inferior margin of spine of scapula. Adduction, retroversion, lateral rotation in various arm positions. A B

6 **Supraspinatus.** o: Supraspinous fossa, supraspinous fascia. i: Greater tubercle of humerus, capsule of glenohumeral joint. Abduction, tenses the joint capsule, minimal rotational components. I: Suprascapular nerve. A B E F G

7 *Supraspinous fascia.* Fascia enclosing the supraspinatus and giving it origin. A G

8 **Infraspinatus.** o: Infraspinous fossa of scapula, spine of scapula, infraspinous fascia. i: Greater tubercle of humerus. Lateral rotation, strengthens joint capsule. I: Suprascapular nerve. A B F G

9 *Infraspinous fascia.* Fascia enclosing the infraspinatus and giving it origin. A G

10 **Teres minor.** o: Lateral border of scapula. i: Greater tubercle of humerus. Lateral rotation. I: Axillary nerve. A B F G

11 **Teres major.** o: Near the inferior angle of scapula. i: Crest of lesser tubercle of humerus. Retroversion of the arm with adduction and medial rotation. I: Thoracodorsal nerve. A B D E G

12 **Subscapularis.** o: Subscapular fossa. i: Lesser tubercle of humerus. Medial rotation. I: Subscapular nerves. C D E

13 **Biceps brachii.** Two-headed muscle that attaches on the radial tuberosity and extends with the aponeurosis brachii toward the ulna to blend into the antebrachial fascia. It acts in elbow joint flexion and forearm supination. I: Musculocutaneous nerve. D

14 *Long head of biceps brachii.* o: Supraglenoid tubercle. Abduction of shoulder joint. A C D

15 *Short head of biceps brachii.* o: Coracoid process. Adduction of shoulder joint. C D

16 *Bicipital aponeurosis.* Expansion of the tendon of the biceps brachii that blends into the antebrachial fascia near the ulna. Transmits muscle pulling forces to the ulna. D

17 **Coracobrachialis.** o: Coracoid process. i: Anterior surface of the middle of the humerus, provides fixation. It acts to ensure contact at the shoulder joint between the head of the humerus and the glenoid cavity. Anteversion. I: Musculocutaneous nerve. C D E

18 **Brachialis.** o: Anterior surface of the humerus below the deltoid tuberosity. i: Tuberosity of ulna. Flexes the elbow joint. I: Musculocutaneous nerve. A D E F, p. 115 B

19 **Triceps brachii.** Three-headed arm muscle with a common attachment on the olecranon and the posterior wall of the joint capsule. Extends the elbow. I: Radial nerve. G

20 *Long head of triceps brachii.* o: Infraglenoid tubercle. Retroversion and adduction of the shoulder joint. Divides the triangular (medial) and quadrangular (lateral) spaces between the teres major and minor muscles. A B C D G

21 *Lateral head of triceps brachii.* o: Posterior surface of humerus, lateral and proximal to the groove for the radial nerve. A F G

22 *Medial head of triceps brachii; Deep head of triceps brachii.* o: Posterior surface of humerus, medial and distal to the groove for the radial nerve. F G

23 **Anconeus.** o: Posterior surface of epicondyle of lateral humerus. i: Posterior surface of ulna, proximal one-fourth. Extends the elbow joint. I: Radial nerve. G, p. 115 C D F

24 **Articularis cubiti.** Muscle fibers that extend from the triceps brachii and brachialis to the joint capsule. Tenses the joint capsule. I: Radial nerve.

25 **Pronator teres.** Muscle that attaches on the pronator tuberosity of the radius. It flexes the elbow joint, acting as a pronator. I: Median nerve. D, p. 115 A D

26 *Humeral head of pronator teres.* o: Medial epicondyle of humerus, medial intermuscular septum.

27 *Ulnar head of pronator teres.* o: Coronoid process. D E

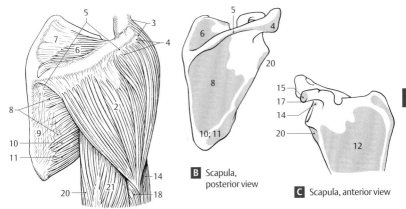

A Muscles of shoulder joint

B Scapula, posterior view

C Scapula, anterior view

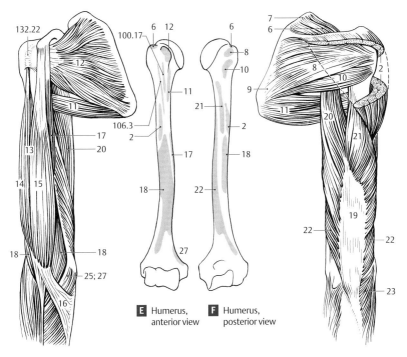

D Arm, anterior view

E Humerus, anterior view

F Humerus, posterior view

G Arm, posterior view

1 **Flexor carpi radialis.** o: Medial epicondyle of humerus, antebrachial fascia. i: Base of second metacarpal. Flexes and pronates elbow joint. Flexion and radial abduction of wrist joint. I: Median nerve. A

2 **Palmaris longus.** o: Medial epicondyle of humerus. i: Palmar aponeurosis. It tenses the aponeurosis and flexes the hand. I: Median nerve. A

3 **Flexor carpi ulnaris.** Muscle that attaches on the pisiform, via the pisohamate ligament on the hamate, via the pisometacarpal ligament on the fifth metacarpal. Flexes and abducts the hand toward the ulna. A

4 *Humeral head of flexor carpi ulnaris.* o: Medial epicondyle of humerus.

5 *Ulnar head of flexor carpi ulnaris.* o: Olecranon, posterior border of ulna. F

6 **Flexor digitorum superficialis.** Muscle that attaches on the middle phalanx of the second through fifth fingers. Flexes the wrist and proximal interphalangeal joints. I: Median nerve. A

7 *Humero-ulnar head of flexor digitorum superficialis.* o: Medial epicondyle of humerus, coronoid process of ulna. A E

8 *Radial head of flexor digitorum superficialis.* o: Anterior surface of radius. A B E

9 **Flexor digitorum profundus.** o: Upper two-thirds of anterior surface of ulna. i: Bases of the distal phalanges of the second through fifth fingers. Flexes wrist and interphalangeal joints. I: Median and ulnar nerves. B E F

10 **Flexor pollicis longus.** o: Anterior surface of the radius, distal to the radial tuberosity. i: Base of distal phalanx of thumb. Flexes hand and phalanges of thumb. Radial abduction. I: Median nerve. B E

11 **Pronator quadratus.** o: Distal one-fourth of the anterior surface of ulna. i: Distal one-fourth of the anterior surface of radius. Forearm pronation. I: Median nerve. A B E

12 **Brachioradialis.** o: Lateral supracondylar ridge of humerus, lateral intermuscular septum. i: Radial styloid process. Flexes the forearm from the intermediate position between pronation and supination. I: Radial nerve. A C E

13 **Extensor carpi radialis longus.** o: Lateral supracondylar ridge of humerus, lateral intermuscular septum. i: Base of second metacarpal. Flexes the elbow joint. Dorsiflexion and radial abduction of the wrist joint. I: Radial nerve. A C

14 **Extensor carpi radialis brevis.** o: Lateral epicondyle of humerus, anular ligament of radius. i: Base of third metacarpal. Dorsiflexion of the hand. C

15 **Extensor digitorum.** o: Lateral epicondyle of humerus, radial collateral ligaments, anular ligament of radius, antebrachial fascia. i: Dorsal aponeuroses of the second through fifth phalanges. Dorsiflexion of the wrist joint, extension of the fingers. I: Radial nerve. C

16 *Intertendinous connections.* Tendinous connections between the extensor tendons of the fingers. C

17 **Extensor digiti minimi.** o: Common origin with extensor digitorum. i: Dorsal aponeurosis of little finger. Extends the little finger. C

18 **Extensor carpi ulnaris.** Attachment on the base of the fifth metacarpal. Abductor. I: Radial nerve. C D F

19 *Humeral head of extensor carpi ulnaris.* o: Lateral epicondyle of humerus, radial collateral ligaments.

20 *Ulnar head of extensor carpi ulnaris.* o: Posterior surface of ulna.

21 **Supinator.** o: Lateral epicondyle of humerus, radial collateral ligaments, anular ligament of radius, and supinator crest of ulna. i: Anterior surface of radius. Supination. I: Radial nerve. B D E F

22 **Abductor pollicis longus.** o: Posterior surface of radius, ulna, and interosseous membrane. i: Base of first metacarpal. Radial abduction and dorsiflexion of the metacarpophalangeal joint of the thumb. I: Radial nerve. C D F

23 **Extensor pollicis brevis.** o: Posterior surface of radius, interosseous membrane. i: Base of metacarpophalangeal joint of thumb. Abduction and extension of the metacarpophalangeal joint of the thumb. I: Radial nerve. C D F

24 **Extensor pollicis longus.** o: Posterior surface of ulna and interosseous membrane. i: Distal phalanx of thumb. Adducts and extends the thumb. I: Radial nerve. C D F

25 **Extensor indicis.** o: Posterior surface of ulna. i: Dorsal aponeurosis of index finger. Extends the index finger, dorsiflexion of the hand. I: Radial nerve. D F

26 **Palmaris brevis.** o: Ulnar side of the palmar aponeurosis. i: Skin of hypothenar eminence. I: Ulnar nerve. A

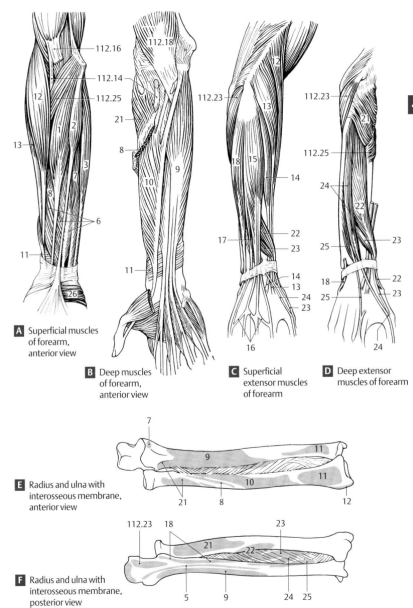

A Superficial muscles of forearm, anterior view

B Deep muscles of forearm, anterior view

C Superficial extensor muscles of forearm

D Deep extensor muscles of forearm

E Radius and ulna with interosseous membrane, anterior view

F Radius and ulna with interosseous membrane, posterior view

4

1 **Abductor pollicis brevis.** o: Scaphoid, flexor retinaculum. i: Thumb, proximal phalanx, radial sesamoid bone, dorsal aponeurosis. Abducts and flexes the thumb. I: Median nerve. B

2 **Flexor pollicis brevis.** Same attachment site as abductor pollicis brevis. Flexion, abduction, adduction, and opposition at the metacarpophalangeal joint of the thumb. B

3 *Superficial head of flexor pollicis brevis.* o: Flexor retinaculum. It lies superficial to the tendon of the flexor pollicis longus. I: Median nerve. B

4 *Deep head of flexor pollicis brevis.* o: Trapezium, trapezoid, capitate. It lies deep to the tendon of the flexor pollicis longus. I: Ulnar nerve. B

5 **Opponens pollicis.** o: Trapezium, flexor retinaculum. i: First metacarpal. Opposition and adduction of the thumb. I: Median nerve. B

6 **Adductor pollicis.** It attaches to the thumb, ulnar sesamoid bone, proximal phalanx, and dorsal aponeurosis. Adduction and opposition. I: Ulnar nerve. B

7 *Oblique head of adductor pollicis.* o: Capitate and second metacarpal. B

8 *Transverse head of adductor pollicis.* o: Third metacarpal. B

9 **Abductor digiti minimi.** o: Pisiform, flexor retinaculum. i: Proximal phalanx of little finger. Abduction. I: Ulnar nerve. B

10 **Flexor digiti minimi brevis.** o: Hook of hamate, flexor retinaculum. i: Palmar surface of the base of the proximal phalanx. Flexion at the metacarpophalangeal joint. I: Ulnar nerve. B

11 **Opponens digiti minimi.** o: Hook of hamate, flexor retinaculum. i: Fifth metacarpal. Opposition of the little finger. I: Ulnar nerve. B

12 **Lumbricals.** o: Tendons of flexor digitorum profundus. i: Doral aponeuroses of second through fifth fingers. Flexion of metacarpophalangeal joint, extension of interphalangeal joints. I: Ulnar nerve. C D E

13 **Dorsal interossei.** o: Two-headed muscle arising from the metacarpal bones. i: Dorsal aponeurosis of proximal phalanges. Flexion of metacarpophalangeal joint, extension of interphalangeal joints. I: Ulnar nerve. C D E

14 **Palmar interossei.** o: Second, fourth, and fifth metacarpals. i: Bases and dorsal aponeuroses of the proximal phalanges of the index, ring, and little fingers. Adduction toward the middle finger. Flexion of metacarpophalangeal joint, extension of interphalangeal joints. I: Ulnar nerve. B D

15 **Axillary fascia.** Connective-tissue sheet with a central perforation covering the fat body of the axilla. It bounds the axilla to lateral and caudal and blends with arm, thoracic, and back fascia. Its deep portion is connected with the clavipectoral fascia. F

16 *Suspensory ligament of axilla.* Connection between the axillary fascia and the clavipectoral fascia below the lateral margin of the pectoralis major. F

17 **Deltoid fascia.** Fascia that encloses the deltoid and forms septa between its fasciculi.

18 **Brachial fascia.** Fascial sheath of the arm that invests extensor and flexor muscles. p. 111 B

19 **Medial intermuscular septum of arm.** Tendinous sheet that attaches the brachial fascia to the medial border of the humerus and gives origin to muscle fibers. p. 111 B

20 **Lateral intermuscular septum of arm.** Tendinous sheet that attaches the brachial fascia to the lateral border of the humerus and gives origin to muscle fibers. p. 111 B

21 **Antebrachial fascia.** Fascial sheath enclosing the forearm muscles. It is firmly attached on its dorsal side to the ulna. A, p. 111 C

22 **Dorsal fascia of hand.** Superficial fascial sheath covering the dorsum of the hand. E

23 **Extensor retinaculum.** Portion of the dorsal fascia that passes over the tendon compartments. E

24 **Superficial transverse metacarpal ligament.** Transverse bands of thickened palmar fascia of the hand at the level of the heads of the metacarpals. A

25 **Palmar aponeurosis.** Aponeurosis between the hypothenar and thenar eminences that is partly formed by the palmaris longus muscle. A

26 **Flexor retinaculum.** Band that passes between the scaphoid and trapezium; triquetrum and hamate. Involved in formation of the carpal tunnel. B

27 **Fibrous sheaths of digits of hand.** Fibrous synovial tunnel for the digital flexor tendons of the fingers. B

28 *Anular part of fibrous sheath.* Very dense circular fibers of the fibrous sheaths between the joints. B

29 *Cruciform part of fibrous sheath.* Fibers crossing over and reinforcing the joints. B

30 **Synovial sheaths of digits of hand.**

31 *Vincula tendinum.* Fibrous bands that convey vessels between the inner and outer layers of the synovial sheath. C

32 *Vinculum longum.* Longer band at the level of the proximal phalanx. C

33 *Vinculum breve.* Shorter band near the tendinous insertions. C

34 **Tendinous chiasm.** Tendinous intersection of the flexor digitorum superficialis and profundus. C

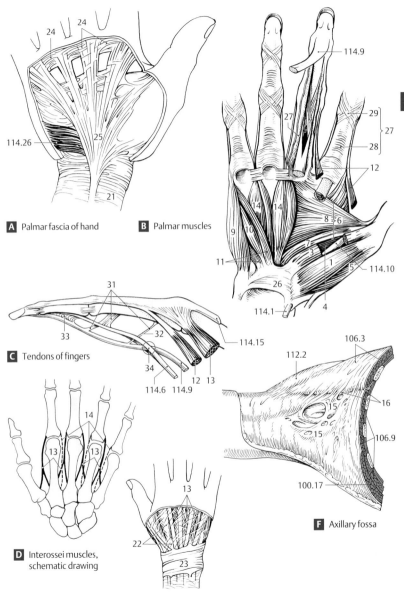

A Palmar fascia of hand

B Palmar muscles

C Tendons of fingers

D Interossei muscles, schematic drawing

E Hand, dorsal view

F Axillary fossa

1 *MUSCLES OF LOWER LIMB.*

2 **Compartments.** Muscle compartments, enclosures, and spaces. A B

3 **Anterior compartment of thigh; Extensor compartment of thigh.** Compartment located anterior and lateral to the femur. It is bounded by the fascia lata, lateral femoral intermuscular septum, femur, and medial femoral intermuscular septum. A

4 **Posterior compartment of thigh; Flexor compartment of thigh.** Compartment located on the posterolateral aspect of the thigh posterior to the lateral femoral intermuscular septum; it is bounded laterally by the fascia lata and posteromedially by the adductor compartment of the thigh. It is connected superiorly with the connective-tissue structures of the lesser pelvis via the greater sciatic foramen and inferiorly with the connective tissue of the popliteal fossa. A

5 **Medial compartment of thigh; Adductor compartment of thigh.** Compartment located on the dorsomedial aspect of the thigh posterior to the medial femoral intermuscular septum. It is bounded laterally by the fascia lata and posterolaterally by the flexor compartment. It is connected to the lesser pelvis via the obturator canal. A

6 **Anterior compartment of leg; Extensor compartment of leg.** It is bounded by the deep fascia of the leg, tibia, interosseous membrane of the leg, fibula, and anterior intermuscular septum of the leg. B

7 **Posterior compartment of leg; Flexor compartment of leg.** It is bounded by the deep fascia of the leg, tibia, interosseous membrane of the leg, fibula, and posterior intermuscular septum of the leg. B

8 *Superficial part.* Part of the posterior compartment containing the superficial flexors, i.e., the gastrocnemius and the soleus muscles.

9 *Deep part.* Part of the posterior compartment containing the deep flexors, which are separated from the superficial flexors by a layer of connective tissue.

10 **Lateral compartment of leg; Fibular compartment of leg; Peroneal compartment of leg.** It is bounded by the deep fascia of the leg, anterior intermuscular septum of the leg, fibula, and posterior intermuscular septum of the leg. B

11 **Fascia lata.** Fascia enclosing the thigh muscles. It is attached anteriorly to the iliac crest and inguinal ligament, splitting into two layers medial to the sartorius muscle and deep to the inguinal ligament. It forms the C-shaped lateral margin of the saphenous opening and covers the femoral vessels with a perforated sievelike sheet. Its deep portion lies posterior to the femoral vessels. Both layers unite with the pectineal fascia. Laterally it thickens to form a tendinous band. It is continuous with the gluteal fascia to posterosuperior and with the deep fascia of the leg to distal. A B C

12 *Iliotibial tract (Maissiat).* Vertically oriented lateral thickening of the fascia lata extending from the anterior part of the iliac crest to the lateral condyle of the tibia. It receives fibers from the tensor muscle of the fascia lata and the gluteus maximus. A C

13 **Lateral femoral intermuscular septum.** Strong layer of connective tissue formed by the fascia lata at the lateral lip of the linea aspera between the biceps femoris and vastus lateralis. A

14 **Medial femoral intermuscular septum.** Strong layer of connective tissue formed by the fascia lata at the medial lip of the linea aspera between the vastus medialis, sartorius, and adductors. A

15 **Saphenous opening.** Large aperture in the fascia lata just below the inguinal ligament for the passage of the great saphenous vein. E

16 *Falciform margin.* Arched margin of the saphenous opening, mainly along its lateral border. E

17 *Superior horn.* Upper arch of the falciform margin. E

18 *Inferior horn.* Lower arch of the falciform margin. E

19 *Cribriform fascia.* Loose, perforated connective-tissue sheet that closes the saphenous opening. E

20 **Femoral triangle (Scarpa's triangle).** Triangular region bounded by the inguinal ligament, sartorius, and adductor longus. D

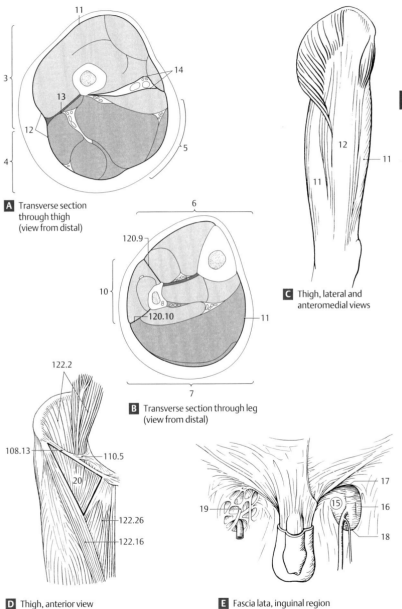

A Transverse section through thigh (view from distal)

B Transverse section through leg (view from distal)

C Thigh, lateral and anteromedial views

D Thigh, anterior view

E Fascia lata, inguinal region

4

1 **Muscular space.** Compartment for the passage of the iliopsoas, femoral nerve, and lateral cutaneous nerve of the thigh between the border of the pelvis, inguinal ligament, and iliopectineal arch. E

2 **Vascular space.** Compartment between the pubis, inguinal ligament, and iliopectineal arch for passage of the femoral vessels, the femoral branch of the genitofemoral nerve, and lymphatic vessels. E F

3 **Femoral ring.** Entrance to the femoral canal, bounded by the femoral vein, inguinal ligament, lacunar ligament, and pectineal ligament. F

4 **Femoral septum.** Connective-tissue covering that closes the femoral ring, consisting of fibers from the transversalis fascia and fascia iliaca. The Rosenmüller's node is situated here. Weak point in the abdominal wall. Hernias can occur in the femoral canal. They appear in the saphenous opening as femoral hernias. E

5 **Adductor canal.** Passageway that is formed by the adductor magnus, vastus medialis, and anteromedial intermuscular septum. It ends at the adductor hiatus. D

6 **Anteromedial intermuscular septum; Subsartorial fascia.** Aponeurotic sheet between the adductor magnus and vastus medialis. D

7 **Adductor hiatus.** Slitlike opening between the insertions of the adductor magnus on the femur. It opens in the popliteal fossa. D, p. 123 B

8 **Deep fascia of leg.** Fascia that is fused with the free margins of the leg bones, and partly giving origin to the muscles of the leg. Thickened, interwoven portions form retinacula, which hold the flexor and extensor tendons in place. A

9 **Anterior intermuscular septum of leg.** Connective-tissue septum between the peroneus and extensor compartments. p. 119 B

10 **Posterior intermuscular septum of leg.** Connective-tissue septum between the peroneus and flexor compartments. p. 119 B

11 **Tendinous arch of soleus.** Tendinous arch extending between the tibia and fibula over the interosseous membrane. Forms part of the origin of the soleus. Passage of the tibial nerve and posterior tibial artery and veins. p. 125 B

12 **Superior extensor retinaculum.** Transverse thickening of the deep fascia of the leg that is about two fingers' width and holds the extensor tendons in place. A B

13 **Flexor retinaculum.** Multilayered band situated over the long flexor tendons passing from the medial malleolus to the calcaneus. Its superficial portion invests the tibial nerve and posterior tibial artery and veins. Its deep portion forms an osteofascial canal with compartments containing the posterior tibial flexor muscles, flexor digitorum longus, and flexor hallucis longus. B

14 **Inferior extensor retinaculum.** Thickened portions of the deep fascia of the leg that extend as cruciate bands from both malleoli to the opposite margins of the foot. A B

15 **Superior fibular retinaculum; Superior peroneal retinaculum.** Upper retinaculum for the peroneus muscles that passes from the lateral malleolus to the calcaneus. A

16 **Inferior fibular retinaculum; Inferior peroneal retinaculum.** Lower retinaculum that holds the peroneus muscles in place. It passes from the extensor retinaculum to the lateral surface of the calcaneus. One band passes to the fibular trochlea, dividing the peroneus brevis and peroneus longus muscles overlying it. It strengthens the dorsal fascia of the foot. A

17 **Dorsal fascia of foot.** Distal expansion of the deep fascia of the leg that extends over the dorsum of the foot and radiates into the dorsal aponeuroses of the toes. A B

18 **Plantar aponeurosis.** Strong, thickened, tendinous fascial sheet on the sole of the foot. It is spread between the calcaneal tuberosity and the plantar ligaments of the metatarsophalangeal joints. It supports the longitudinal arch of the foot. C

19 *Transverse fascicles.* Transverse bundles connecting the distal elongations of the plantar aponeurosis. C

20 **Superficial transverse metatarsal ligament.** Collective term for transverse fibrous bands located peripheral to the transverse fascicles. C

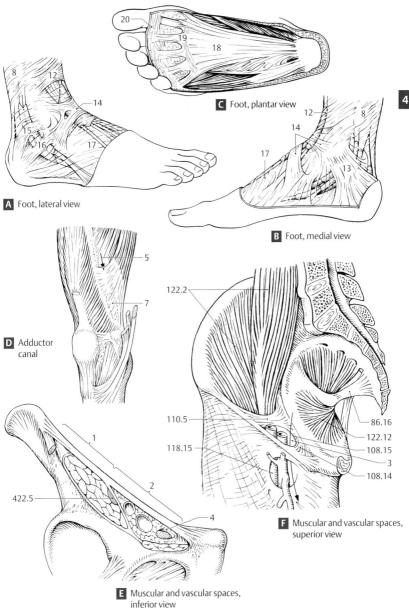

A Foot, lateral view

B Foot, medial view

C Foot, plantar view

D Adductor canal

E Muscular and vascular spaces, inferior view

F Muscular and vascular spaces, superior view

1 **Muscles.**

2 **Iliopsoas.** Muscle comprising the psoas major and iliacus. i: Lesser trochanter. Most important anterior flexor of the leg. Trunk flexion, lateral rotation. B C D

3 *Iliacus.* o: Iliac fossa, hip joint capsule. I: Femoral nerve, lumbar plexus. C

4 *Psoas major.* o: Lateral aspect of vertebral bodies T12 and L1–L4, costal process of L1–L5. I: Lumbar plexus. C

5 **[Psoas minor].** o: Vertebral bodies of T12 and L1. i: Fascia iliaca. I: Lumbar plexus. C

6 **Gluteus maximus.** o: Ilium, behind the posterior gluteal line, sacrum, coccyx, thoracolumbar fascia, sacrotuberous ligament. i: Fascia lata, iliotibial tract, gluteal tuberosity, lateral femoral intermuscular septum, linea aspera. Extension, lateral rotation, abduction, and adduction at the hip joint. I: Inferior gluteal nerve. A D E

7 **Gluteus medius.** o: Lateral surface of ilium. i: Greater trochanter. Abduction, medial and lateral rotation, extension, and flexion at the hip joint. I: Superior gluteal nerve. A D E

8 **Gluteus minimus.** o: Ilium between the anterior and inferior gluteal lines. i: Greater trochanter. Abduction, medial, and lateral rotation, flexion, and extension at the hip joint. I: Superior gluteal nerve. A D E

9 **Gluteal aponeurosis.** Deep, sheetlike tendon of origin of the gluteus maximus lying on the gluteus medius. A

10 **Tensor fasciae latae; Tensor of fascia lata.** o: Near the anterior superior iliac spine. i: Above the iliotibial tract to the lateral tibial condyle. Tenses the fascia lata; flexion, abduction, medial rotation, and extension at the knee joint. I: Superior gluteal nerve. C E

11 **Piriformis.** o: Anterior surface of sacrum. i: Greater trochanter, medial aspect of the apex. Abduction, extension, and lateral rotation at the hip joint. I: Sacral plexus. A D

12 **Obturator internus.** o: Internal surface of obturator membrane and surrounding area. i: Trochanteric fossa of greater trochanter. Lateral rotation, abduction, adduction. I: Sacral plexus. A D

13 **Gemellus superior; Superior gemellus.** o: Ischial spine. i: Tendon of obturator internus muscle and trochanteric fossa. Lateral rotation, adduction, abduction. I: Sacral plexus. A D E

14 **Gemellus inferior; Inferior gemellus.** o: Ischial tuberosity. i: Tendon of obturator internus, trochanteric fossa. Lateral rotation, adduction, abduction. I: Sacral plexus. A D E

15 **Quadratus femoris.** o: Ischial tuberosity. i: Intertrochanteric crest. Lateral rotation and adduction. I: Sacral plexus. A D E

16 **Sartorius.** o: Anterior superior iliac spine. i: Medial to the tibial tuberosity. Flexion, abduction, lateral rotation at the hip joint; flexion and medial rotation at the knee joint. I: Femoral nerve. B C E

17 **Quadriceps femoris.** Muscle group composed of the following four muscles. Its tendon extends to the patella and continues as the patellar ligament to the tibial tuberosity. Extension at the knee joint. I: Femoral nerve.

18 *Rectus femoris.* Two-headed muscle. Also flexes the hip joint. Contributes fibers to the lateral and medial patellar retinacula. B C E

19 *Straight head of rectus femoris.* o: Anterior inferior iliac spine.

20 *Reflected head of rectus femoris.* o: Supra-acetabular groove.

21 *Vastus lateralis.* o: Greater trochanter, lateral lip of linea aspera. A B C D

22 *Vastus intermedius.* o: Anterior surface of femur. B D

23 *Vastus medialis.* o: Medial lip of linea aspera. C D

24 **Articularis genus; Articular muscle of knee.** o: Distal to vastus intermedius. i: Knee joint capsule. Tenses joint capsule. I: Femoral nerve. D

25 **Pectineus.** o: Pectineal line of pubis. i: Pectineal line of femur, linea aspera. Flexion, adduction, and medial rotation at the hip. I: Femoral and obturator nerves. B C D E

26 **Adductor longus.** o: Near the pubic symphysis. i: Medial lip of linea aspera. Adduction, lateral rotation, and flexion at the hip joint. I: Obturator nerve. B C D E

27 **Adductor brevis.** o: Inferior pubic ramus. i: Medial lip of linea aspera. Adduction, flexion, extension, and lateral rotation at the hip. I: Obturator nerve. B D E

28 **Adductor magnus.** o: Inferior pubic ramus, ramus of ischium. i: Medial lip of linea aspera and, via a long tendon, the medial epicondyle. Adduction, lateral rotation, and extension at the hip joint. I: Obturator and tibial nerves. A B C D E

29 **Adductor minimus.** Superior portion of the adductor magnus, taking origin further to anterior from the pelvis. A

30 **Gracilis.** o: Inferior pubic ramus. i: Medial tibial surface. Adduction, flexion, and extension at the hip joint. Flexion and medial rotation at the knee joint. I: Obturator nerve. A B C E

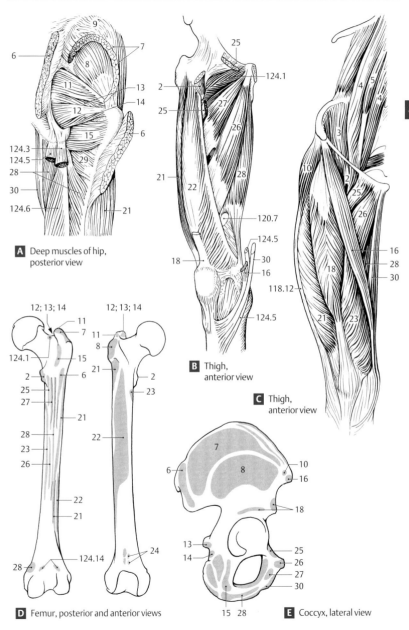

A Deep muscles of hip, posterior view

B Thigh, anterior view

C Thigh, anterior view

D Femur, posterior and anterior views

E Coccyx, lateral view

1 **Obturator externus.** o: External surface of obturator membrane and surrounding area. i: Trochanteric fossa. Lateral rotation and adduction at the hip joint. I: Obturator nerve. A.

2 **Biceps femoris.** Two-headed muscle arising from the pelvis and femur. i: Head of fibula. Flexion at the knee joint, lateral rotation. A B E F

3 *Long head of biceps femoris.* o: Ischial tuberosity. Extension at the hip joint. I: Tibial nerve. A B

4 *Short head of biceps femoris.* o: Lateral lip of linea aspera. I: Common fibular nerve. A B

5 **Semitendinosus.** o: Ischial tuberosity. i: Medial surface of tibia. Extension at the hip joint. Flexion and medial rotation at the knee joint. I: Tibial nerve. A D E

6 **Semimembranosus.** o: Ischial tuberosity. i: Medial condyle of tibia and oblique popliteal ligament. It is partly covered by the semitendinosus muscle. Extension at the hip joint; flexion and medial rotation at the knee joint. Tenses the knee joint capsule. I: Tibial nerve. A B F

7 **Tibialis anterior.** o: Lateral surface of tibia, interosseous membrane, deep fascia of leg. i: Medial aspects of medial cuneiform and first metatarsal. Dorsiflexion and supination of foot. I: Deep fibular nerve. D E

8 **Extensor digitorum longus.** o: Lateral condyle of tibia, interosseous membrane, fibula, deep fascia of leg. i: Dorsal aponeurosis of the second through fifth toes. Dorsiflexion and pronation of foot. Extension of toes. I: Deep fibular nerve. D E

9 **Fibularis tertius; Peroneus tertius.** Part of the extensor digitorum longus muscle with insertion on the base of the fifth metatarsal. Dorsiflexion and pronation. I: Deep fibular nerve. D

10 **Extensor hallucis longus.** o: Interosseous membrane and fibula. i: Distal phalanx of great toe. Dorsiflexion of foot and great toe. I: Deep fibular nerve. D E

11 **Fibularis longus; Peroneus longus.** o: Fibula and deep fascia of leg. i: Passes obliquely under the sole of the foot to insert on the medial cuneiform and first metatarsal. Pronation and plantar flexion. I: Superior fibular nerve. C D E F

12 **Fibularis brevis; Peroneus brevis.** o: Distal two-thirds of fibula. i: Tuberosity of fifth metatarsal bone. Pronation and plantar flexion. I: Superior fibular nerve. C D E F

13 **Triceps surae.** Muscle group consisting of the gastrocnemius and soleus that forms the Achilles tendon. It inserts on the calcaneus tuberosity. I: Tibial nerve.

14 *Gastrocnemius.* Superficial leg muscle composed of the following two heads. Flexion at the knee joint, plantar flexion and supination at the ankle joint. A B C D

15 *Lateral head of gastrocnemius.* o: Proximal to the lateral femoral condyle. i: Achilles tendon. A B C

16 *Medial head of gastrocnemius.* o: Proximal to the medial femoral condyle. i: Achilles tendon. A B C D

17 *Soleus.* o: Head of fibula, upper one-third of the posterior surface of tibia. i: Achilles tendon. Plantar flexion and supination. B F

18 *Calcaneal tendon (Achilles tendon).* Tendon of the triceps surae that attaches on the calcaneal tuberosity. B C

19 **Plantaris.** o: Above the lateral femoral condyle. i: Achilles tendon or calcaneus tuberosity. I: Tibial nerve. B C

20 **Popliteus.** o: Lateral femoral epicondyle. i: Posterior surface of tibia. Medial rotation of the leg with flexed knee joint. I: Tibial nerve. B C F

21 **Tibialis posterior.** o: Tibia, fibula, interosseous membrane. i: Navicular, cuneiform bones I–III, and metatarsals II–IV. Plantar flexion and supination. I: Tibial nerve. C F

22 **Flexor digitorum longus.** o: Tibia. i: Distal phalanges of the second through fifth toes. Plantar flexion, supination, flexion of toes. I: Tibial nerve. C F

23 **Flexor hallucis longus.** o: Fibula. i: Distal phalanx of great toe. Plantar flexion, supination, flexion of great toe. I: Tibial nerve. C F

24 **Extensor hallucis brevis.** o: Dorsal aspect of calcaneus. i: Proximal phalanx of great toe. Extension of great toe. I: Deep fibular nerve. D

25 **Extensor digitorum brevis.** o: Dorsal aspect of calcaneus. i: Dorsal aponeuroses of second through fourth toes. I: Deep fibular nerve. D

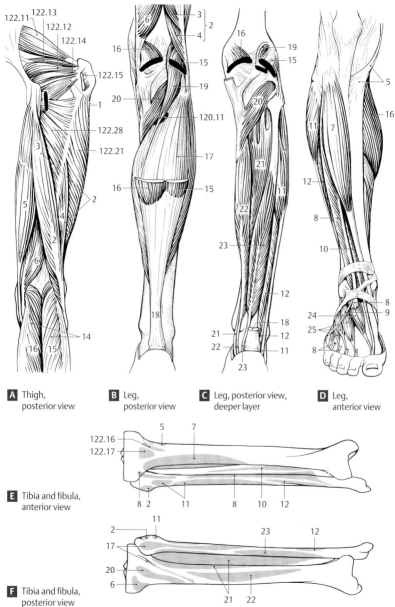

A Thigh,
posterior view

B Leg,
posterior view

C Leg, posterior view,
deeper layer

D Leg,
anterior view

E Tibia and fibula,
anterior view

F Tibia and fibula,
posterior view

1 **Abductor hallucis.** o: Calcaneal tuberosity. i: Medial sesamoid bone and proximal phalanx of great toe. Medial abduction, supports longitudinal arch of foot. I: Medial plantar nerve. A B

2 **Flexor hallucis brevis.** o: Cuneiform (I), long plantar ligament, tendon of tibialis posterior, plantar aponeurosis. Forms the groove for the flexor hallucis longus. Plantar flexion of great toe. I: Medial plantar nerve. A B

3 *Medial head of flexor hallucis brevis.* i: Tendon of abductor hallucis, medial sesamoid bone, proximal phalanx.

4 *Lateral head of flexor hallucis brevis.* i: Tendon of adductor hallucis, lateral sesamoid bone, proximal phalanx.

5 **Adductor hallucis.** Muscle comprised of the following two heads. Supports the arch of the foot. Plantar flexion of proximal phalanx. Adduction of great toe. I: Lateral plantar nerve.

6 *Oblique head of adductor hallucis.* o: Second to fourth metatarsals, lateral cuneiform bone and cuboid. i: Together with the transverse head on the lateral sesamoid bone and proximal phalanx of great toe. B

7 *Transverse head of adductor hallucis.* o: Joint capsules of third to fifth metatarsophalangeal joints. i: Together with the transverse head on the lateral sesamoid bone and proximal phalanx of great toe. Mainly supports transverse arch of foot. A B

8 **Abductor digiti minimi.** o: Calcaneus and plantar aponeurosis. i: Lateral surface of proximal phalanx of fifth toe. Plantar flexion and abduction of fifth toe. Forms the lateral margin of foot. I: Lateral plantar nerve. A B

9 *[Abductor of fifth metatarsal].* Part of abductor digiti minimi that is occasionally present, originating on the tuberosity of the fifth metatarsal.

10 **[Opponens digiti minimi].** Part of the flexor digiti minimi brevis that is occasionally present. o: Distal half of fifth metatarsal.

11 **Flexor digiti minimi brevis.** o: Base of fifth metatarsal and long plantar ligament. i: Proximal phalanx of little toe. Flexion and abduction of little toe. I: Lateral plantar nerve. A B

12 **Flexor digitorum brevis.** o: Calcaneal tuberosity and plantar aponeurosis. i: Its divided tendons insert onto the middle phalanges of the second through fifth toes. Flexion of metatarsophalangeal and middle phalangeal joints, support of longitudinal arch of foot. I: Medial plantar nerve. A B

13 **Quadratus plantae**; **Flexor accessorius.** o: Calcaneus. i: Lateral border of tendon of flexor digitorum longus. Toe flexion and support of longitudinal arch of foot. I: Lateral plantar nerve. B

14 **Lumbricals.** o: Tendons of flexor digitorum longus. i: Bases of proximal phalanges of second through fifth toes. Flexion at metatarsophalangeal joint, movement of toes toward great toe. I: Medial and lateral plantar nerves. A B

15 **Dorsal interossei.** o: Two-headed muscle arising from the metatarsals. i: Proximal phalanges of second through fourth toes, plantar ligament. Abduction and flexion at metatarsophalangeal joint. I: Lateral plantar nerve. C

16 **Plantar interossei.** o: Muscle arising from a single head on third through fifth metatarsals. i: Bases of proximal phalanges. Adduction and flexion at metatarsophalangeal joints. I: Lateral plantar nerve. C

17 *TENDON SHEATHS AND BURSAE.*

18 **Tendinous sheaths of toes.**

19 *Fibrous sheaths of toes.* Rather tough connective-tissue thickening of the tendinous sheaths, mainly on the flexor surface of the toes. D

20 *Anular part of fibrous sheaths.* Ringlike bands of fibrous tissue between the joints. D

21 *Cruciform part of fibrous sheaths.* Bands of fibrous tissue that cross each other over the joints. D

22 *Synovial sheaths of toes.* Synovial part of the tendinous sheaths for the toe flexors. D

23 *Vincula tendinum.* Bands conveying vessels that travel obliquely through the tendinous sheaths. D

5

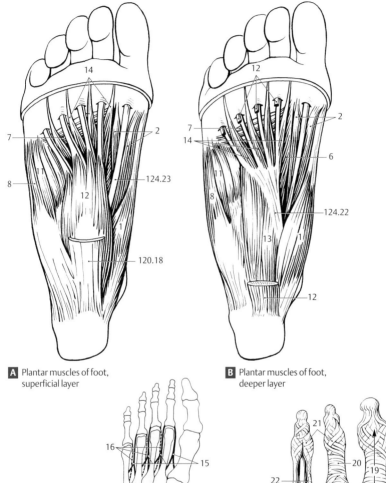

A Plantar muscles of foot,
superficial layer

B Plantar muscles of foot,
deeper layer

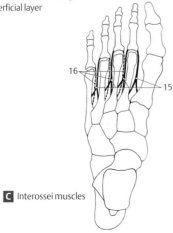

C Interossei muscles

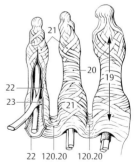

D Toes, plantar view

1 **Bursae of neck.**

2 **Bursa of tensor veli palatini.** Bursa situated between the pterygoid hamulus and the tendon of the tensor veli palatini. p. 143 C

3 **Subcutaneous bursa of laryngeal prominence.** Bursa situated between the skin and the laryngeal prominence of the thyroid cartilage. A

4 **Retrohyoid bursa.** Bursa situated between the body of the hyoid bone and the median thyrohyoid ligament. A

5 **Infrahyoid bursa.** Bursa situated between the superior end of the sternohyoid muscle and the thyrohyoid membrane. A B

6 **Bursae of upper limb.**

7 **Subtendinous bursa of trapezius.** Bursa situated between the trapezius and the spine of the scapula. C

8 **[Subcutaneous acromial bursa].** Bursa situated between the acromion and the skin. D

9 **Subacromial bursa.** Bursa situated between the acromion, coracoacromial ligament, and tendon of the supraspinatus muscle. D E

10 **Subdeltoid bursa.** Bursa situated between the deltoid and the greater tubercle of the humerus. It often communicates with the subacromial bursa. D

11 **[Coracobrachial bursa].** Bursa situated between the tendon of the subscapularis and the coracobrachialis below the apex of the coracoid process. D

12 **Subtendinous bursa of infraspinatus.** Bursa situated between the tendon of insertion of the infraspinatus and the shoulder joint capsule. E

13 **Subtendinous bursa of subscapularis.** Bursa situated between the tendon of insertion of the subscapularis and the shoulder joint capsule that communicates with the articular cavity. D

14 **Subtendinous bursa of teres major.** Bursa situated between the tendon of insertion of the teres major and the humerus. D

15 **Subtendinous bursa of latissimus dorsi.** Bursa situated between the tendons of insertion of the teres major and latissimus dorsi. D

16 **Subcutaneous olecranon bursa.** Bursa situated between the olecranon and the skin. F

17 **[Intratendinous olecranon bursa].** Bursa located within the tendon of the triceps near the olecranon. F

18 **Subtendinous bursa of triceps brachii.** Bursa situated between the tendon of the triceps and the olecranon. F

19 **Bicipitoradial bursa.** Bursa situated between the tendon of insertion of the biceps and the anterior part of the radial tuberosity. F

20 **[Interosseous cubital bursa].** Bursa situated between the tendon of the biceps and the ulna or oblique cord. F

21 **Tendinous sheaths of upper limb.**

22 **Intertubercular tendon sheath.** Expansion of the articular cavity along the tendon of the biceps muscle. D

23 **Carpal tendinous sheaths.**

24 *Dorsal carpal tendinous sheaths.*

25 *Tendinous sheath of abductor longus and extensor pollicis brevis.* Common tendinous sheath for the abductor pollicis longus and extensor pollicis brevis forming the first tendon compartment on the dorsum of the hand. G

26 *Tendinous sheath of extensores carpi radiales.* Common tendinous sheath for the extensor carpi radialis longus and brevis forming the second tendon compartment on the dorsum of the hand. G

27 *Tendinous sheath of extensor pollicis longus.* Tendinous sheath for the extensor pollicis longus forming the third tendon compartment. G

28 *Tendinous sheath of extensor digitorum and extensor indicis.* Tendinous sheath for these muscles forming the fourth tendon compartment on the dorsum of the hand. G

29 *Tendinous sheath of extensor digiti minimi.* Tendinous sheath for the extensor digiti minimi forming the fifth tendon compartment on the dorsum of the hand. G

30 *Tendinous sheath of extensor carpi ulnaris.* Tendinous sheath for the extensor carpi ulnaris forming the sixth tendon compartment on the dorsum of the hand. G

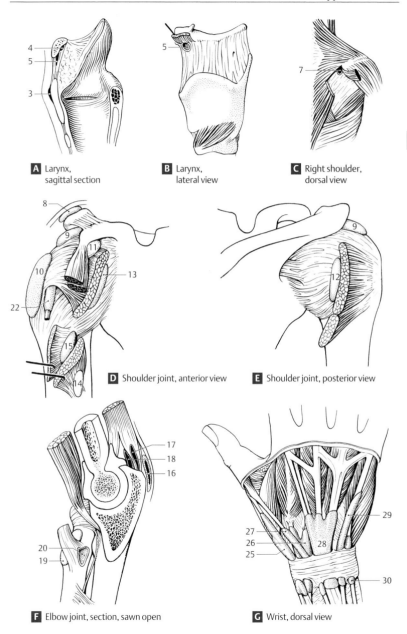

5

A Larynx, sagittal section

B Larynx, lateral view

C Right shoulder, dorsal view

D Shoulder joint, anterior view

E Shoulder joint, posterior view

F Elbow joint, section, sawn open

G Wrist, dorsal view

1 *Palmar carpal tendinous sheaths.* Carpal tendon sheaths for passage of the flexor tendons.

2 *Tendinous sheath of flexor pollicis longus.* Individual tendon sheath for the flexor pollicis longus. A

3 *Tendinous sheath of flexor carpi radialis.* Individual tendon sheath for the flexor carpi radialis at the insertion site of its tendon on the base of the second metacarpal. A

4 *Common flexor sheath.* Common tendon sheath for the two long flexor tendons of the fingers. A

5 *[[Digital synovial tendon sheaths]].* Tendinous sheaths for the flexor tendons along the fingers. A

6 **Bursae of lower limb.**

7 **Subcutaneous trochanteric bursa.** Bursa situated on the tendon of the gluteus maximus between the skin and the greater trochanter. B

8 **Trochanteric bursa of gluteus maximus.** Bursa situated between the tendon of the gluteus maximus and the greater trochanter. B

9 **Trochanteric bursae of gluteus medius.** Term referring to two bursae: the anterior bursa is situated between the tendon of insertion of the gluteus medius and the greater trochanter, and the posterior bursa between the insertion tendon and the piriformis. B C

10 **Trochanteric bursa of gluteus minimus.** Bursa situated between the tendon of insertion of the gluteus minimus and the greater trochanter. B C

11 **Bursa of piriformis.** Bursa situated between the insertion tendon of the piriformis, the bone, and the superior gemellus. B

12 **Sciatic bursa of obturator internus.** Bursa situated between the cartilage-covered surface of the lesser sciatic notch and the tendon of the obturator internus. B

13 **Subtendinous bursa of obturator internus.** Bursa situated beneath the insertion of the obturator internus. B

14 **Intermuscular gluteal bursae.** Two or three bursae situated beneath the insertion of the gluteus maximus on the gluteal tuberosity. B

15 **Sciatic bursa of gluteus maximus.** Bursa situated between the ischial tuberosity and the inferior surface of the gluteus maximus. B

16 **[Iliopectineal bursa].** Bursa situated between the iliopsoas, pelvic bone, and iliofemoral ligament. It overlies the hip joint, with which it often communicates. C

17 **Subtendinous bursa of iliacus.** Bursa situated between the lesser trochanter and the tendon of insertion of the iliopsoas. C

18 **Superior bursa of biceps femoris.** Bursa situated between the origins of the biceps femoris and semimembranosus. B

19 **Subcutaneous prepatellar bursa.** Bursa situated directly between the skin and the fascia anterior to the knee. D

20 **[Subfascial prepatellar bursa].** Bursa situated between the fascia and the tendon fibers of the quadriceps femoris. D

21 **[Subtendinous prepatellar bursa].** Bursa situated directly on the patella, beneath the tendon fibers of the quadriceps femoris. D

22 **Suprapatellar bursa.** Bursa situated between the tendon of the quadriceps and the bone. It nearly always communicates with the articular cavity. D

23 **Subcutaneous infrapatellar bursa.** Bursa situated between the patellar ligament and the skin. D

24 **Deep infrapatellar bursa.** Bursa situated between the patellar ligament and the tibia. D

25 **Subcutaneous bursa of tuberosity of tibia.** Bursa situated between the tibial tuberosity and the skin. Bursa most stressed by kneeling. D

26 **Subtendinous bursa of sartorius.** Bursa situated between the tendon of insertion of the sartorius and the tendons of the gracilis and semitendinosus lying deep to it. E

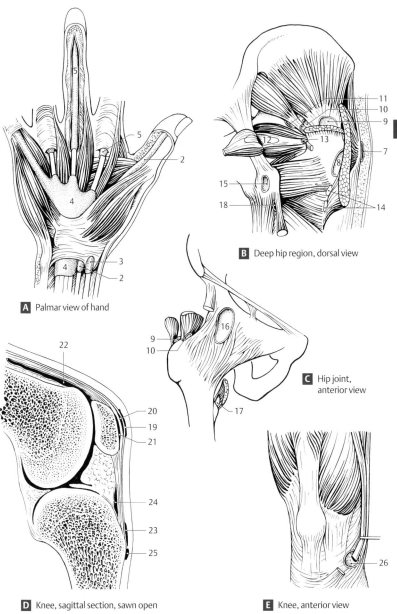

A Palmar view of hand

B Deep hip region, dorsal view

C Hip joint, anterior view

D Knee, sagittal section, sawn open

E Knee, anterior view

5

1 **Anserine bursa.** Bursa located beneath the tendons of the semitendinosus, gracilis, and sartorius on the tibial collateral ligament. It occasionally communicates with the subtendinous bursa of the sartorius. A

2 **Inferior subtendinous bursa of biceps femoris.** Bursa situated beneath the tendon of insertion of the biceps femoris and partly lying on the fibular collateral ligament. B

3 **Subpopliteal recess.** Bursa situated on the lateral femoral condyle beneath the tendon of origin of the popliteus. It always communicates with the articular cavity of the knee and sometimes with the tibiofibular joint. B

4 **Lateral subtendinous bursa of gastrocnemius.** Bursa situated between the lateral femoral condyle and the lateral tendon of origin of the gastrocnemius. B

5 **Medial subtendinous bursa of gastrocnemius.** Bursa situated between the medial femoral condyle and the medial tendon of origin of the gastrocnemius. A B

6 **Semimembranosus bursa.** Bursa situated between the tendon of insertion of the semimembranosus and the superior border of the tibia. A

7 **Subcutaneous bursa of lateral malleolus.** Bursa situated between the skin and the lateral malleolus. C

8 **Subcutaneous bursa of medial malleolus.** Bursa situated between the skin and the medial malleolus. D

9 **Subtendinous bursa of tibialis anterior.** Bursa situated between the tendon and the medial cuneiform. D

10 **Subcutaneous calcaneal bursa.** Bursa situated between the skin and the posterior surface of the calcaneus. D

11 **Bursa of tendo calcaneus; Bursa of calcaneal tendon; Retrocalcaneal bursa. (Achilles bursa).** Bursa between the calcaneus and Achilles tendon. D

12 **Tendinous Sheaths of Lower Limb.**

13 **Anterior tarsal tendinous sheaths.**

14 *Tendinous sheath of tibialis anterior.* Tendon sheath of the tibialis anterior that already begins beneath the extensor retinaculum. D

15 *Tendinous sheath of extensor hallucis longus.* Sheath surrounding the long extensor tendon of the great toe beneath the extensor retinaculum and further to distal. C D

16 *Tendinous sheath of extensor digitorum longus.* Sheath surrounding the long extensor tendons of the toes beneath the extensor retinaculum and further to distal. C

17 **Tibial tarsal tendinous sheaths.**

18 *Tendinous sheath of flexor digitorum longus.* Tendon sheath surrounding the long flexors of the toes, located posterior and inferior to the medial malleolus and covered by the flexor retinaculum. D

19 *Tendinous sheath of tibialis posterior.* Tendon sheath surrounding the tibialis posterior beneath the flexor retinaculum. It begins where it is crossed by the flexor digitorum longus. D

20 *Tendinous sheath of flexor hallucis longus.* Tendon sheath surrounding the long flexor tendon of the great toe, extending to the proximal end of the sole of the foot, where it crosses under the tendon of the flexor digitorum longus. D

21 **Fibular tarsal tendinous sheaths.**

22 *Common tendinous sheath of fibulares; Common tendinous sheath of peronei.* Tendon sheath that extends from beneath the fibular retinacula to the cuboid. C

23 *Plantar tendinous sheath of fibularis longus; Plantar tendinous sheath of peroneus longus.* Tendon sheath on the sole of the foot for passage of the long tendon of the peroneus. D

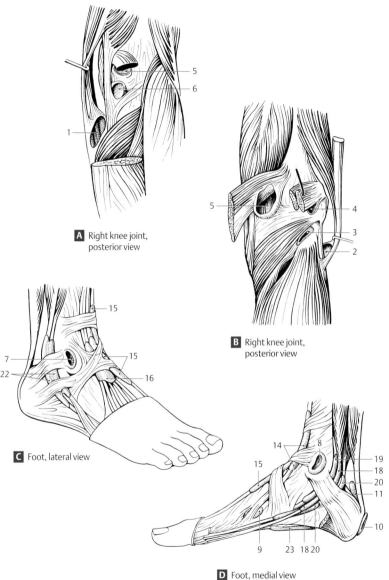

A Right knee joint, posterior view

B Right knee joint, posterior view

C Foot, lateral view

D Foot, medial view

1   *ALIMENTARY SYSTEM.*

2   *Mouth.*

3   **Oral cavity.**

4   **Mucous membrane of mouth.** It is completely covered with nonkeratinized, stratified squamous epithelium and lacks a muscularis mucosae.

5   **Oral vestibule.** Space between the dental arcades and the lips or cheeks. C D

6   **Oral fissure; Oral opening.** A

7   **Lips.**

8   *Upper lip.* A C D

9   *Philtrum.* Groove extending from the nasal septum to the upper lip. A

10 *Tubercle.* Small protuberance on the upper lip at the end of the philtrum. A

11 *Lower lip.* A C D

12 **Frenulum of upper lip.** Midline mucosal fold between the gingiva and upper lip. C

13 **Frenulum of lower lip.** Midline mucosal fold between the gingiva and lower lip. C

14 **Labial commissure.** Junction of the upper and lower lips at the angle of mouth. A C

15 **Angle of mouth.** A

16 **Cheek.** Lateral wall of the oral vestibule. A

17 *Buccal fat pad.* (Bichat's fat pad). Encapsulated fat body situated between the buccinator and masseter. A

18 *Juxta-oral organ.* Presumably a receptor organ in the connective tissue near the buccal fat pad on the buccopharyngeal fascia of the buccinator muscle.

19 **Papilla of parotid duct.** Small mucosal projection at the opening of the parotid duct lateral to the upper second molar tooth. C

20 **Oral cavity proper.** Space bounded anteriorly and laterally by the teeth and extending to the isthmus of fauces. D

21 **Palate.** Partition dividing the oral and nasal cavities.

22 *Hard palate.* Hard, bony part of the palate. D E

23 *Soft palate.* Its posterior border ends with the uvula. D E

24 *Palatine raphe.* Midline mucosal ridge at the union of the right and left bony palatine processes. E

25 *Transverse palatine folds; Palatine rugae.* Transverse mucosal ridges extending across the anterior part of the hard palate. E

26 *Incisive papilla.* Small mucosal eminence located at the anterior end of the palatine raphe above the incisive foramen. E

27 **Gingiva; Gum.** Specific part of the mucous membrane of mouth that surrounds the neck of tooth. It consists of fibrous connective tissue lined with stratified squamous epithelium that is attached to the cement and adjacent alveolar process. B C E

28 *Gingival margin.* Site of the junctional epithelium where the outer and inner parts of the gingiva meet. B C E

29 *Gingival papilla; Interdental papilla.* C E

30 *Gingival sulcus; Gingival groove.* Crevice between the gingival margin and the tooth, which, if widened, can lead to formation of periodontal pockets. B

31 **Sublingual caruncle.** Small mucosal projections, one each on the right and left sides of the frenulum of tongue. The submandibular and major sublingual ducts open here. C

32 **Sublingual fold.** Mucosal prominence overlying the sublingual gland that extends obliquely from the sublingual caruncle to posterolateral. C

33 GLANDS OF MOUTH.

34 **Minor salivary glands.**

35 **Labial glands.** Small salivary glands on the inner side of the lips. C

36 **Buccal glands.** Small salivary glands on the inner side of the cheeks that produce mucous. C

37 **Molar glands.** Buccal glands underneath the mucous membrane of mouth at the level of the molar teeth. C

38 **Palatine glands.** Glands located beneath the mucous membrane. (Two larger masses, one on each side of the midline). C

39 **Lingual glands.** Several mucous, serous, and mixed glands, mainly on the lateral and posterior surfaces of the tongue. C

40 *[Anterior lingual glands (Gland of Nuhn)].* Mixed gland in the tip of tongue with several excretory ducts on the inferior surface of tongue. C

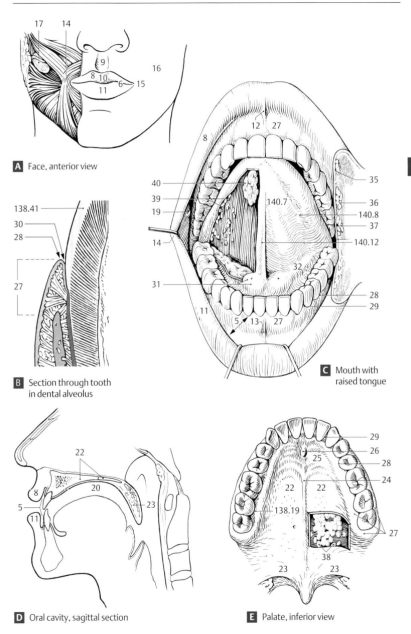

A Face, anterior view

B Section through tooth in dental alveolus

C Mouth with raised tongue

D Oral cavity, sagittal section

E Palate, inferior view

1 **Major salivary glands.**

2 **Sublingual gland.** Predominantly mucous gland contained lying on the floor of the mouth in the mylohyoid muscle with numerous excretory ducts. D

3 *Major sublingual duct.* Main excretory duct of the sublingual gland. It opens next to the submandibular duct at the sublingual caruncle. D

4 *Minor sublingual ducts.* About 40 small ducts that drain the sublingual gland through the sublingual fold and sublingual caruncle. D

5 **Submandibular gland.** Predominantly serous gland that is situated almost entirely beneath the mylohyoid muscle. D G

6 *Submandibular duct.* Excretory duct that drains the submandibular gland. It loops around the posterior border of the mylohyoid, accompanied by glandular tissue and opens at the sublingual caruncle. D

7 **Parotid gland.** It occupies the retromandibular fossa, extending to the temporomandibular joint and the ramus of mandible. G

8 *Superficial part.* Lobe of the parotid gland that lies superficial to the facial nerve branches. G

9 *Deep part.* Lobe of the parotid gland that lies deep to the facial nerve branches. G

10 *Accessory parotid gland.* Accessory lobe situated on the masseter near the parotid duct. G

11 **Parotid duct.** Excretory duct that extends around the anterior border of the masseter, usually over the buccal fat pad, and opens opposite to the upper second molar tooth. G

12 TEETH.

13 **Deciduous teeth.**

14 **Permanent teeth.** Permanent teeth that erupt after loss of deciduous teeth.

15 **Maxillary dental arcade; Upper dental arcade.** Curved dental arcade of the maxilla resembling a parabola of the third degree in shape. p. 135 E

16 **Mandibular dental arcade; Lower dental arcade.** Curved dental arcade of the mandible resembling a parabola of the second degree in shape. p. 139 D

17 **Occlusal curves (Spee curve).** The occlusal surfaces and cusps of teeth in the maxilla form an inferiorly convex curve up to the mesial part of the first molar tooth, which then increases slightly to the third molar tooth. The curvature of the mandible presents the mirror image. H

18 **[Diastema].** Congenital enlargement of the space between the teeth.

19 **Incisor tooth.** Teeth (four) on either side of the midline in the first and second positions in the dental arcade. D H, p. 135 C E

20 **Canine tooth.** Teeth (four) in the third position of the dental arcade. D H, p. 135 C E

21 **Premolar tooth.** Teeth (eight) in the fourth and fifth positions of the dental arcade. D H, p. 135 C E

22 **Molar tooth.** Teeth (twelve) in the sixth, seventh, and eight position of the dental arcade. D H, p. 135 C E

23 *Third molar tooth; Wisdom tooth.* D H, p. 135 C E

24 **Clinical crown.** Part of the tooth protruding from the gum. C

25 **Neck of tooth; Cervix of tooth.** Part of the tooth where the enamel and cement meet. E

26 **Root of tooth.** Part of the tooth covered by cement. E

27 *Root apex.* E

28 **Clinical root.** Part of the tooth situated below the gingival margin. C

29 **Crown of tooth.** Part of the tooth covered by enamel. E

30 *Cusp of tooth; Cuspid of tooth.* Protuberances that divide the occlusal surfaces of the tooth. They are absent on the incisor teeth. E

31 *Apex of cusp.* E

32 *Accessory cusp.* Accessory cusps, especially on the molar teeth.

33 *Transverse ridge.* Inconstant transverse ridge connecting adjacent cusps of teeth. B

34 *Triangular ridge.* Triangular ridge connecting the cusps of molar teeth. B

35 *Oblique ridge.* Inconstant oblique ridge connecting the cusps of the maxillary molar teeth.

36 *Occlusal fissure.* Longitudinal furrow of variable form and with transverse branches on the occlusal surfaces of premolar and molar teeth. B

37 *Occlusal fossa.* Pit in the occlusal surfaces of premolar and molar teeth. E

38 **Mesial fovea.** Pit in the anterior part of the occlusal surface, especially in premolar teeth. F

39 **Distal fovea.** Pit in the posterior part of the occlusal surface, especially in premolar teeth. F

40 **Marginal ridge.** Ridge along the margin of the crown of tooth. A

41 **Cingulum.** Eminence near the neck of tooth that connects the two marginal ridges on the lingual surface of the incisor and canine teeth. A

42 *Tubercle of tooth.* Small protuberance of variable size on the lingual surface of the incisor and canine teeth. A

43 **Incisal margin.** Occlusal margin of the incisor and canine teeth. A

44 **Mammelons.** Small protuberances present at eruption on the incisal margins which are quickly worn down.

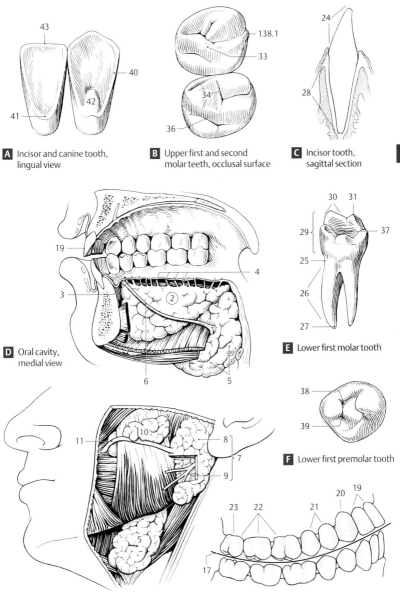

A Incisor and canine tooth, lingual view

B Upper first and second molar teeth, occlusal surface

C Incisor tooth, sagittal section

D Oral cavity, medial view

E Lower first molar tooth

F Lower first premolar tooth

G Salivary glands, lateral view

H Occlusal curves

1 **[Anomalous tubercle].** Protuberance on the palatal surface of the mesial cusp of the upper first molar tooth. p. 137 B

2 **Paramolar cusp; Paramolar tubercle.** Accessory buccal cusp on the second and third molar teeth found in about 1–2 %.

3 **Molar tubercle.** Accessory mesiobuccal cusp predominantly found on the upper first deciduous molar teeth.

4 *Buccal cusp.* Protuberance on the buccal side of premolar teeth. A

5 *Palatal cusp.* Protuberance on the palatal side of maxillary premolar teeth. A

6 *Lingual cusp.* Protuberance on the lingual side of the mandibular premolars.

7 *Mesiobuccal cusp.* Anterior protuberance on the buccal side of the molar tooth. A

8 *Mesiopalatal cusp.* Anterior protuberance on the palatal side of the maxillary molar teeth. A

9 *Mesiolingual cusp.* Anterior protuberance on the lingual side of the mandibular molar teeth. A

10 *Distobuccal cusp.* Posterior protuberance on the buccal side of the molar teeth. A

11 *Distopalatal cusp.* Posterior protuberance on the palatal side of the maxillary molar teeth. A

12 *Distolingual cusp.* Posterior protuberance on the lingual side of the mandibular molar teeth. A

13 *Distal cusp; Hypoconulid.* Posterior protuberance on the lower first molar teeth. A

14 **Occlusal surface.** A

15 **Vestibular surface.** Surface of the crown of the tooth facing the oral vestibule. D

16 *Buccal surface.* Surface of the crown of tooth facing the cheek. D

17 *Labial surface.* Surface of the crown of tooth facing the lip. D

18 **Lingual surface.** Surface of the crown of tooth facing the tongue. D

19 **Palatal surface.** Surface of the crown of tooth facing the palate. p. 135 E

20 **Mesial surface.** Vertical contact area of the teeth facing away from the last molar tooth. D

21 **Distal surface.** Vertical contact area of the teeth facing away from the first incisor tooth. D

22 **Approximal surface; Interproximal surface.** Surface of the crown of tooth facing the adjacent tooth. D

23 **Contact zone.** Area of direct contact between adjacent tooth crowns.

24 **Buccal root.** Root of tooth near the cheek. A

25 **Palatal root.** Root of tooth near the palate. A

26 **Mesial root.** Anterior tooth root.

27 **Distal root.** Posterior tooth root. A

28 **Mesiobuccal root.** Root located anteriorly and near the cheek. A

29 **Mesiolingual root.** Root located anteriorly and near the tongue. A

30 **Accessory root.** Accessory root that is predominantly found in molar teeth.

31 **Canine groove.** Longitudinal groove in the approximal surface of the root of canine tooth. B

32 **Pulp cavity.** Pulp chamber in the dentine that becomes continuous near the root with the root canal. E

33 *Pulp cavity of crown.* Part of the pulp cavity located in the crown of tooth. E

34 *Root canal; Pulp canal.* Part between the pulp cavity and apical foramen. E

35 *Apical foramen.* Opening of the root canal at the apex of the root of tooth. E

36 **Dental pulp.** Contents of the pulp cavity consisting of gelatinous connective tissue, blood vessels, and nerves.

37 *Crown pulp.* Part of the pulp located in the crown of tooth.

38 *Root pulp.* Part of the pulp located in the root of tooth.

39 **Dental papilla.** Term for the mesenchymal component enclosed by the bell-shaped dental organ during tooth development. C

40 **Dentine.** Main component of the tooth consisting of inorganic and organic substance (predominantly collagen fibers). E

41 **Enamel.** Tooth enamel that covers the crown like a mantle. E

42 **Cement.** Substance resembling woven bone that surrounds the tooth from the junction with the enamel to the apex of root. It contains fibers from the desmodontium. E

43 **Periodontium; Periodontal membrane.** Supporting unit for the development of the tooth formed by the alveolar wall, desmodontium, and cement that contains vessels and nerves within loose connective tissue.

44 **Gum; Gingiva.** Part of the gingiva nearest the tooth. Its inner junctional epithelium is partly attached to the enamel thus preserving the continuity of the epithelium of the oral cavity. It closes the roots of teeth off from the oral cavity. Collagen fibers extending from the alveolar process or supra-alveolar root cement into the subepithelial connective tissue, or surrounding the tooth, ensure root enclosure. They stabilize the position of the teeth and align them in an uninterrupted dental arcade. E

45 **Inserting periodontium.** Part of the periodontium in the dental alveolus. E

46 *Desmodontium; Periodontal fiber.* Collection of collagen fibers extending between the cement and alveolar wall of the dental alveolus. E

47 **Dental alveolus.** Tooth socket in the alveolar process. E

6

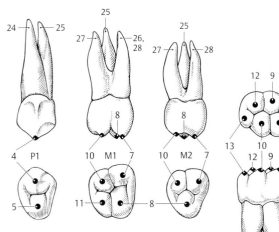

A Buccal and occlusal views of teeth

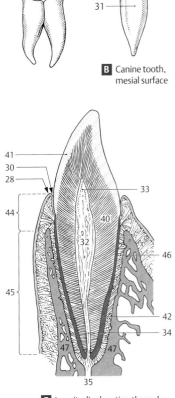

B Canine tooth, mesial surface

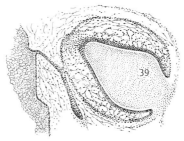

C Tooth development

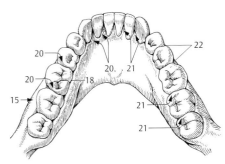

D Mandibular teeth

E Longitudinal section through tooth

1   TONGUE. A B C D E

2   **Body of tongue.** Part of the tongue between the tip and root. E

3   **Root of tongue.** Area of attachment of the tongue to the mandible and hyoid bone. It can also be described as the posterior, vertical portion of the tongue. E

4   **Dorsum of tongue.** E

5   *Anterior part*; *Presulcal part*. Part of the dorsum of tongue anterior to the terminal sulcus. B

6   *Posterior part*; *Postsulcal part*. Vertical part of the dorsum of tongue located between the terminal sulcus and epiglottis. B

7   **Inferior surface of tongue.** p. 135 C

8   *Fimbriated fold.* Fringed fold lateral to the frenulum of tongue. It is a rudiment of a sublingua. C, p. 135 C

9   **Margin of tongue.** Lateral border of the tongue touching the teeth. B

10 **Apex of tongue; Tip of tongue.** B E

11 **Mucous membrane of tongue.** C

12 **Frenulum of tongue.** Mucosal fold extending from the floor of the mouth to the inferior aspect of the tongue. D, p. 135 C

13 **Papillae of tongue; Lingual papillae.** Collective term for the following four different types of mucous membrane formations. A B

14 *Filiform papillae.* Most common form. Epithelial projections, often split at their tips, surrounding a conical connective-tissue core. A

15 *Fungiform papillae.* Scattered, pinhead-sized papillae, occurring in larger numbers on the tip and the margins of tongue. A B

16 *Vallate papillae.* Seven to twelve larger papillae (circular in cross-section) located anterior to the terminal sulcus. The wall of the trench surrounding them contains taste buds. A B

17 *Foliate papillae.* Several parallel mucosal folds containing taste buds on the posterolateral margin of tongue. B D

18 **Midline groove of tongue; Median sulcus of tongue.** Shallow midline longitudinal groove above the lingual septum. B C

19 **Terminal sulcus of tongue.** Bilateral groove that extends obliquely forward from the foramen cecum behind the row of vallate papillae running parallel to it. B

20 **Foramen cecum of tongue.** Groove located at the tip of the terminal sulcus. Remains of the thyroglossal duct present during embryological development. B

21 *[Thyroglossal duct].* Developmental precursor of the thyroid gland that descends as a conical mass of epithelial cells from the base of the tongue at the site of the future foramen cecum.

22 **Lingual tonsil.** Lymphatic tissue aggregations dispersed irregularly along the margin of tongue. B D

23 *Lymphoid nodules.* Nodular mucosal elevations measuring 1–5 mm in diameter that are produced by underlying lymphatic tissue formations. The center of each nodule contains a crypt. A

24 **Lingual septum.** Connective-tissue partition located in the midsagittal plane that partly divides the tongue and gives origin to muscle fibers. C

25 **Lingual aponeurosis.** Tough sheet of connective tissue beneath the dorsal mucous membrane of tongue. Insertion site for muscles of tongue. C

26 **Muscles of tongue.** The following muscles innervated by the hypoglossal nerve (CN XII).

27 **Genioglossus.** o: Mental spine of mandible. i: Fanlike insertion on the lingual aponeurosis from the tip of tongue to the posterior part of tongue. It draws the tongue anteriorly, i.e., toward the chin. I: Hypoglossal nerve. C D

28 **Hyoglossus.** o: Body of hyoid bone and greater horn of hyoid bone. i: It attaches from inferior to the lateral parts of the tongue and extends anteriorly to the lingual aponeurosis. It draws the postsulcal part of tongue posteriorly and inferiorly. I: Hypoglossal nerve. D

29 *Chondroglossus.* Inconstant structure. o: Lesser horn of hyoid bone. i: See hyoglossus. I: Hypoglossal nerve. D

30 *Ceratoglossus.* Inconstant structure. o: Medial aspect of greater horn of hyoid bone. i: See hyoglossus. I: Hypoglossal nerve.

31 *Styloglossus.* o: Styloid process. i: Radiates from posterosuperior into the lateral part of the tongue and merges with the hyoglossus. It draws the tongue backward and upward. I: Hypoglossal nerve. D

32 **Superior longitudinal muscle.** Longitudinal bundle of muscle fibers immediately beneath the mucous membrane. They pass from the tip of tongue to the area near the hyoid bone. o and i: Lingual aponeurosis. I: Hypoglossal nerve. C

33 **Inferior longitudinal muscle.** Longitudinally arranged muscle fibers near the inferior surface of the tongue. They pass from the posterior part of tongue to its tip. I: Hypoglossal nerve. C

34 **Transverse muscle of tongue.** Muscle fibers passing transversely between the longitudinal fibers. They arise from the lingual septum and extend into the mucous membrane of the lateral margins of tongue. Together with the vertical muscle of tongue they act to lengthen the tongue. I: Hypoglossal nerve. C

35 **Vertical muscle of tongue.** Vertically arranged muscle fibers that pass from the dorsum of tongue to its inferior surface. I: Hypoglossal nerve. C

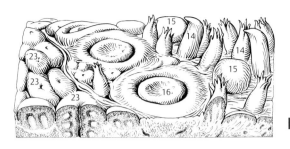

A Surface of the tongue, enlarged image

6

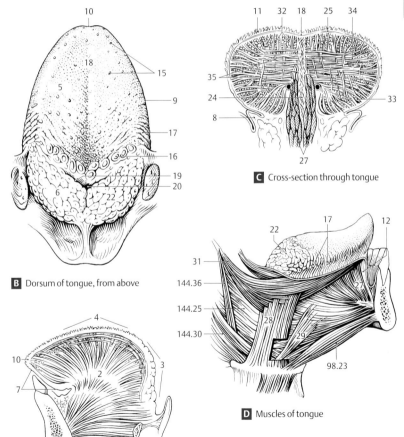

B Dorsum of tongue, from above

C Cross-section through tongue

D Muscles of tongue

E Tongue, sagittal section

1 **FAUCES.** Space between the soft palate, palatoglossal arch, palatopharyngeal arch, and dorsum of tongue. E

2 **Isthmus of fauces; Oropharyngeal isthmus.** Space bounded on the left and right by the palatoglossal and palatopharyngeal arches.

3 **Soft palate.** Its dorsal portion hangs down in front of the posterior wall of the pharynx and assists swallowing by closing off the nasopharynx to the oral cavity like a valve. A D E

4 *Uvula.* Projection that points downward from the posterior border of the soft palate. A D E

5 *Palatoglossal arch*; *Anterior pillar of fauces.* Mucosal fold extending in front of the tonsillar fossa from the palate to the tongue. It overlies the palatoglossus muscle. A

6 *[Triangular fold].* Free posterior margin of the palatoglossal arch that sometimes covers the tonsil. A

7 *Palatopharyngeal arch*; *Posterior pillar of fauces.* Mucosal fold situated behind the tonsillar fossa between the palate and the wall of the pharynx, overlying the palatopharyngeus muscle. A

8 *[Semilunar fold].* Upper border of the tonsillar fossa. Mucosal fold extending between the palatoglossal and palatopharyngeal arches. A

9 **Tonsillar sinus; Tonsillar fossa; Tonsillar bed.** Recess bounded by the palatoglossal and palatopharyngeal arches as well as the triangular and semilunar folds. D

10 *Supratonsillar fossa.* Remnant of the embryonic tonsillar fossa. A

11 **Palatine tonsil.** Tonsil located between the palatoglossal and palatopharyngeal arches. A

12 *Tonsillar capsule.* Fibrous tissue capsule covering the tonsil.

13 *[Tonsillar cleft; Intratonsillar cleft].* Parenchymal depression in the upper part of the tonsil.

14 *Tonsillar pits.* Visible openings to the tonsillar crypts on the surface of the palatine tonsil. B

15 *Tonsillar crypts.* Epithelial recesses that extend from the tonsillar pits to the palatine tonsil. B

16 **Muscles of soft palate and fauces.**

17 **Palatine aponeurosis.** Aponeurosis that is mainly formed by the tendon of the tensor veli palatini and the periosteum of the hard palate. D

18 **Levator veli palatini.** o: Petrous part of temporal bone in front of the inferior opening of the carotid canal. Inferior border of the cartilaginous auditory tube. i: Palatine aponeurosis. It draws the soft palate backward and upward, also moving the dorsomedial cartilaginous part of auditory tube when the pharyngeal opening of auditory tube is opened. I: Vagus nerve. C

19 **Tensor veli palatini.** o: Spine of sphenoid bone, scaphoid fossa, and anterior (lateral) lip of cartilaginous part of auditory tube. i: After changing direction at the pterygoid hamulus, its fibers merge with the palatine aponeurosis, stiffening the anterior (lateral) wall of the membranous lamina of auditory tube and tensing the soft palate. I: Mandibular nerve. C

20 **Musculus uvulae.** o: Palatine aponeurosis. i: Connective tissue of the uvula. I: Vagus nerve. C

21 **Palatoglossus.** o: Palatine aponeurosis. i: Transverse lingual muscle. It elevates the posterior part of tongue and depresses the palate. It forms a ring that constricts around the food bolus to create a suitable size for swallowing. I: Glossopharyngeal nerve. D

22 **Palatopharyngeus.** o: Arises from the palatine aponeurosis in two portions, between which the levator veli palatini inserts, and from the pterygoid hamulus. I: Glossopharyngeal nerve. D

23 *Anterior fascicle.* i: The anterior portion extends predominantly to the posterior border of the thyroid cartilage and underlies the palatopharyngeal arch. C

24 *Posterior fascicle*; *Palatopharyngeal sphincter.* The posterior portion extends circularly to the superior constrictor muscle of pharynx and its oblique fibers pass inferiorly to the posterior wall of the pharynx, joining with fibers from the opposite side. It is involved in formation of [Passavant's ridge]. C

25 **PHARYNX.** Airway and food passageway; 14–16 cm long. It extends from the vault of pharynx to the beginning of the esophagus in front of the sixth cervical vertebra. E

26 CAVITY OF PHARYNX. Space that can be divided into three levels.

27 **Nasopharynx.** Part of the cavity of pharynx behind the choana. E

28 **Vault of pharynx.** Roof of the cavity of pharynx below the sphenoid. E

29 *Pharyngeal hypophysis.* Residual tissue from the adenohypophysis located in the mucous membrane of the vault. It becomes active during middle age with decreased activity of the adenohypophysis.

30 *Pharyngeal tonsil.* Tonsil located in the vault of pharynx. E

31 **Pharyngeal lymphoid nodules.** Lymph nodules near the nasopharynx.

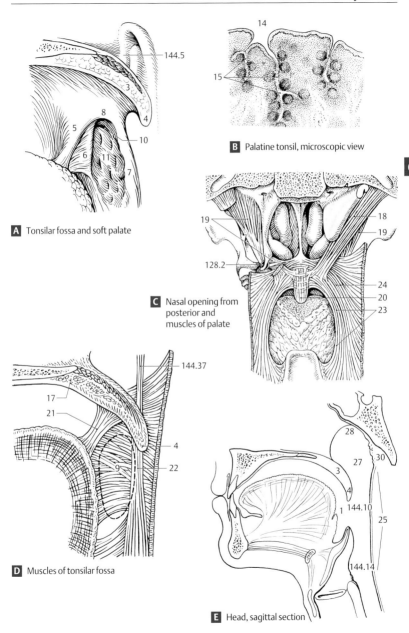

A Tonsilar fossa and soft palate

B Palatine tonsil, microscopic view

C Nasal opening from posterior and muscles of palate

D Muscles of tonsilar fossa

E Head, sagittal section

1   **[Pharyngeal bursa].** Inconstant, deep recess in the pharyngeal tonsil. Anterior end of the notochord during embryonic development.

2   **Pharyngeal opening of auditory tube.** Opening of the auditory tube into the nasopharynx. A

3   **Torus tubarius.** Prominence behind the opening of auditory tube produced by its dorsomedial cartilaginous part. A

4   *Salpingopharyngeal fold.* Fold overlying the salpingopharyngeus muscle that extends obliquely downward from the dorsomedial lip of the cartilaginous part of auditory tube. A

5   *Salpingopalatine fold.* Fold that extends from the anterior lip of the auditory tube in front of the torus tubarius to the soft palate. A

6   **Torus levatorius.** Elevation located below the opening of auditory tube anterior to the dorsomedial lip of its cartilaginous part. It is produced by the levator veli palatini. A

7   **Tubal tonsil.** Submucosal lymphatic tissue near the opening to auditory tube.

8   **Pharyngeal recess.** (Fossa of Rosenmüller). Nasopharyngeal niche situated posterolateral to the auditory tube. A

9   **Palatopharyngeal ridge.** Posterior border of the hard palate.

10 **Oropharynx.** Part of the cavity of the pharynx behind the oral cavity. p. 143 E

11 **Epiglottic vallecula.** Depression between the medial and lateral glosso-epiglottic folds. B

12 **Median glosso-epiglottic fold.** Unpaired mucosal fold situated in the midline between the postsulcal part of tongue and the epiglottis. B

13 **Lateral glosso-epiglottic fold.** Two lateral mucosal folds between the postsulcal part of tongue and the epiglottis. B

14 **Laryngopharynx; Hypopharynx.** Part of the cavity of the pharynx behind the larynx. p. 143 E

15 **Piriform fossa; Piriform recess.** Furrow located between the aryepiglottic fold and the thyrohyoid membrane or thyroid cartilage. B

16 *Fold of superior laryngeal nerve.* Fold in the piriform recess produced by the internal branch of the superior laryngeal nerve and the superior laryngeal artery. B

17 **Pharyngo-esophageal constriction.** Upper narrowing of the esophagus behind the cricoid cartilage.

18 **Pharyngobasilar fascia.** Uppermost, nonmuscular, membranous part of the pharynx. It attaches the wall of the pharynx to the base of the cranium. Corresponds to the submucosa. C D E

19 **Submucosa.** Layer of connective tissue between the mucous membrane and the muscle layer of pharynx. A

20 **Mucosa; Mucous membrane.** Pharyngeal mucous membrane covered with stratified squamous or ciliated (nasopharynx) epithelium.

21 *Pharyngeal glands.* Small subepithelial mixed glands and mucous glands.

22 **Pharyngeal muscles; Muscle layer of pharynx.** Muscular layer of the wall of the pharynx. A

23 **Pharyngeal raphe.** Tendinous seam between the right and left pharyngeal muscles that is located posteriorly in the midline. It extends to the pharyngeal tubercle. C

24 **Pterygomandibular raphe.** Tendinous line between the pterygoid hamulus and the retromolar fossa of the mandible. It divides the buccinator from the constrictor muscles of pharynx. D

25 **Superior constrictor.** Superior constrictor muscle that consists of the following four parts, which insert on the pharyngeal raphe. I: Pharyngeal plexus. C D

26 *Pterygopharyngeal part.* (Passavant's ridge). o: Medial plate of pterygoid process and pterygoid hamulus. D

27 *Buccopharyngeal part.* o: Pterygomandibular raphe. D

28 *Mylopharyngeal part.* o: Posterior end of the mylohyoid line of mandible. D

29 *Glossopharyngeal part.* o: Intrinsic muscles of tongue. D

30 **Middle constrictor.** o: Hyoid bone. i: Pharyngeal raphe. I: Pharyngeal plexus. C

31 *Chondropharyngeal part.* o: Lesser horn of hyoid bone. D

32 *Ceratopharyngeal part.* o: Greater horn of hyoid bone. D

33 **Inferior constrictor.** Lower constrictor muscle arising from the larynx. I: Pharyngeal plexus. C D

34 *Thyropharyngeal part. Thyropharyngeus.* o: Oblique line of thyroid cartilage. D

35 *Cricopharyngeal part; Cricopharyngeus.* o: Cricoid cartilage. D

36 **Stylopharyngeus.** o: Styloid process. i: It extends medially between the superior and middle constrictor muscles and reaches the wall of the pharynx, thyroid cartilage, and epiglottis. I: Glossopharyngeal nerve. C

37 **Salpingopharyngeus.** o: Dorsomedial lip of cartilaginous part of auditory tube, part of the longitudinal muscles of pharynx. i: Lateral wall of pharynx. Prevents the levator veli palatini from sliding posteriorly. I: Pharyngeal plexus. A

38 **Buccopharyngeal fascia.** p. 96.22

39 *Peripharyngeal space.* Connective-tissue space adjoining the pharynx.

40 *Retropharyngeal space.* Connective-tissue space between the pharynx and the prevertebral layer of cervical fascia. A

41 *Parapharyngeal space; Lateral pharyngeal space.* Connective-tissue space lateral to the pharynx.

6

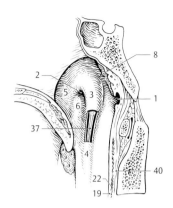

A Pharyngeal opening of auditory tube

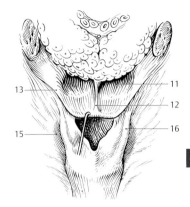

B Posterior part of tongue and opening to larynx

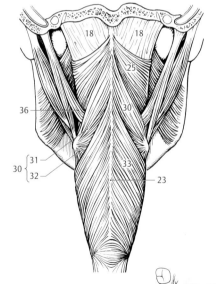

C Pharyngeal muscles, posterior view

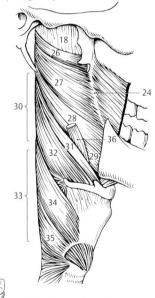

D Pharyngeal muscles, view from right

E Attachment of pharyngobasilar fascia

6

1 **ESOPHAGUS.** Passageway measuring 23–26 cm in length that begins below the cricoid cartilage at the level of the sixth cervical vertebra and ends at the cardia of the stomach. A B

2 **Cervical part of esophagus.** Segment of the esophagus located in front of the cervical vertebral column (C6–T1). A

3 **Thoracic part of esophagus.** Part of the esophagus that extends from the first thoracic vertebra to its passage through the diaphragm (near T11). A

4 *Thoracic constriction*; *Broncho-aortic constriction*. Middle, narrowed part of the esophagus produced by the close proximity of the left main bronchus and aortic arch. A

5 *Diaphragmatic constriction*. Narrowed, inferior part of the esophagus produced by its passage through the diaphragm. A

6 **Abdominal part of esophagus.** Short segment of the esophagus between the diaphragm and stomach. A

7 **Serosa; Serous coat.** Mesothelial lining of the peritoneum enclosing the abdominal part of esophagus.

8 **Subserosa; Subserous layer.** Connective-tissue layer beneath the mesothelium of the peritoneum.

9 **Adventitia.** Loose connective tissue surrounding the esophagus in the mediastinum. It forms a sliding layer that connects it with surrounding structures. C

10 **Muscular layer; Muscular coat.** Double layer of muscle in the wall of the esophagus. In the upper one-third of the esophagus it consists of transverse striated muscle and in the lower one-third of smooth anular (inner) and longitudinal (outer) muscle. C

11 *Crico-esophageal tendon.* Tendinous attachment of the longitudinal muscle fibers of the esophagus to the posterior wall of the cricoid cartilage. B

12 *Broncho-esophageus.* Smooth-muscle fibers that extend from the left main bronchus to the esophagus. B

13 *Pleuro-esophageus.* Smooth-muscle fibers that extend between the esophagus and left mediastinal pleura. B

14 **Submucosa.** Sliding layer between the muscular layer and mucosa consisting mainly of collagenous connective tissue and containing vessels, nerves, and glands. C

15 **Mucosa; Mucous membrane.** It consists of nonkeratinized, stratified squamous epithelium, lamina propria, and muscularis mucosae. C

16 *Muscularis mucosae.* Quite thick layer of smooth muscle situated between the submucosa and lamina propria. C

17 **Esophageal glands.** Individual mucous glands scattered throughout the submucosa. C

18 **STOMACH.** Organ extending from the end of the esophagus to the pylorus. A D

19 **Anterior wall of stomach.** D

20 **Posterior wall of stomach.**

21 **Greater curvature of stomach.** Larger curvature in the contour of the stomach. C

22 **Lesser curvature of stomach.** Smaller curvature in the contour of the stomach. D

23 *Angular incisure.* Notch at the lowermost point of the lesser curvature that is visible on radiographs. D

24 **Cardia; Cardial part of stomach.** Area near the opening of the esophagus. D

25 *Cardial orifice.* Opening of the esophagus into the stomach. D

26 **Fundus of stomach.** Dome-shaped part of the stomach located beneath the diaphragm. D

27 **Fornix of stomach.** Forms the upper border of the fundus of stomach beneath the diaphragm. D

28 *Cardial notch.* Sharp angle formed by the esophagus and the wall of stomach. D

29 **Body of stomach.** Proper body of stomach, bounded superiorly by the cardia and fundus and inferiorly by the pyloric part of stomach. D

30 *Gastric canal.* Passageway in the stomach formed by the longitudinal mucosal folds along the lesser curvature. D

31 **Pyloric part of stomach.** Distal part of the stomach that begins with the angular incisure and extends to and includes the pylorus. D

32 *Pyloric antrum.* Initial segment that begins at the angular incisure, which can be temporarily completely closed off from the rest of the gastric lumen by a peristaltic wave. D

33 *Pyloric canal.* Inferior terminal segment that is around 2–3 cm long. D

34 *Pylorus.* End of the stomach that is reinforced by a ring of muscle. D

35 *Pyloric orifice.* Pyloric lumen connecting the stomach and duodenum. D

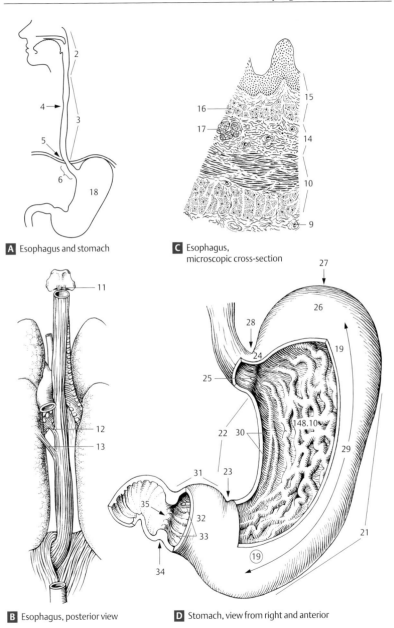

A Esophagus and stomach

C Esophagus, microscopic cross-section

B Esophagus, posterior view

D Stomach, view from right and anterior

1 **Serosa; Serous coat.** Peritoneal covering consisting of simple squamous epithelium. B

2 **Subserosa; Subserous layer.** Connective tissue underlying the serosa. B

3 **Muscular layer; Muscular coat.** Muscular coat of stomach composed of muscle fibers running in three directions. A B

4 *Longitudinal layer.* External layer of longitudinal muscle fibers mainly at the lesser and greater curvatures of stomach. A B

5 *Circular layer.* Middle layer consisting of circular muscle fibers. A B

6 *Pyloric sphincter.* Thickened ring of muscle fibers around the pylorus. A

7 *Oblique fibers.* Innermost layer of the muscular coat with oblique muscle fibers. A B

8 **Submucosa.** Layer between the muscularis mucosae and the muscular coat that consists mainly of collagenous connective tissue and contains vessels and nerves. B

9 **Mucosa; Mucous membrane.** Mucous membrane lining of the stomach that is composed of simple columnar epithelium, connective tissue (lamina propria), and muscularis mucosae. B

10 *Gastric folds*; *Gastric rugae.* Mucosal folds that mainly run longitudinally. p. 147 D

11 *Muscularis mucosae.* Layer of smooth-muscle fibers between the lamina propria and submucosa. Connections to the muscular coat and to the walls of blood vessels. Tightens the mucous membrane of stomach, stiffens the gastric folds, and regulates circulation. B

12 *Gastric areas.* Bumpy areas with a diameter of 1–6 mm bounded by shallow furrows on the mucosal surface. B

13 *Villous folds.* Microscopic folds formed by lamina propria covered with epithelium which contain lymphatic tissue between the gastric pits. B C D

14 *Gastric pits.* Openings of the gastric glands between the villous folds. B C D

15 *Gastric glands.* Tubular glands that are found in the fundus and body of stomach and are composed of four types of cells. B C D

16 *SMALL INTESTINE.* The small intestine consists of the duodenum, jejunum, and ileum.

17 **Serosa: Serous coat.** Peritoneal covering consisting of a single layer of squamous epithelium. F

18 **Subserosa; Subserous layer.** Connective tissue underlying the serous coat. F

19 **Muscular layer; Muscular coat.** It is formed by the two main muscle layers of intestinal wall. F

20 *Longitudinal layer*; *Long pitch helicoidal layer.* Outer layer of longitudinally oriented muscle fibers. Its cells are organized in a helicoidal form in long coils. F

21 *Circular layer*; *Short pitch helicoidal layer.* Inner circular muscle layer. Its cells are coiled tightly in a helicoidal form. F

22 **Circular folds.** (Kerckring's valves). Up to 8 mm high permanent folds containing submucosa that extend transversely to the intestinal axis, encircling around two-thirds of the intestinal lumen. E F

23 **Submucosa.** Sliding layer between the muscularis mucosae and the muscular coat consisting mainly of collagenous connective tissue and containing vessels and nerves. F

24 **Mucosa; Mucous membrane.** It is composed of simple columnar epithelium, connective tissue (lamina propria), and muscularis mucosae.

25 *Muscularis mucosae.* Layer of smooth-muscle cells between the lamina propria and submucosa. It is active in fine adjustments of the mucous membrane for intestinal contents, peristalsis, and villous motility. F

26 *Intestinal villi.* Villi of the small intestine measuring 0.5–1.5 mm in length. F

27 *Intestinal glands.* Cryptlike glands of the small intestine. F

28 *Solitary lymphoid nodules.* Solitary lymphatic follicles in the lamina propria of the stomach and intestinal canals. C D F

29 *Aggregated lymphoid nodules.* (Peyer's patches). Aggregation of lymphatic follicles in the ileum and colon.

6

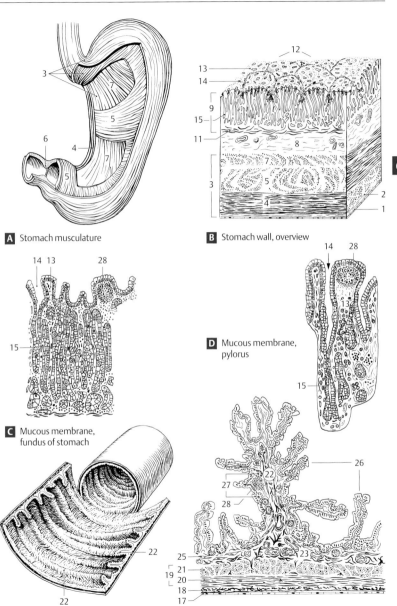

A Stomach musculature

B Stomach wall, overview

C Mucous membrane, fundus of stomach

D Mucous membrane, pylorus

E Intestinal canal

F Intestinal wall, histological section

6

1 **DUODENUM.** The ca. 25–30 cm long segment of the small intestine between the pylorus and duodenojejunal flexure. A

2 **Superior part.** Horizontal initial segment. A

3 *Ampulla; Duodenal cap.* Functional expansion at the beginning of the duodenum; briefly visible on radiographs. A

4 **Superior duodenal flexure.** Flexure between the superior and descending parts of duodenum, medial to the gallbladder. A

5 **Descending part.** Lateral, vertically descending segment. A

6 **Inferior duodenal flexure.** Flexure between the descending and horizontal parts of duodenum. A

7 **Inferior part; Horizontal part; Transverse part.** Horizontal segment below the head of pancreas. A

8 **Ascending part.** Segment to the left of the head of pancreas ascending to the duodenojejunal flexure. A

9 **Duodenojejunal flexure.** Flexure between the duodenum and jejunum. A

10 **Hidden part of duodenum.** Retroperitoneal part of the duodenum.

11 **Suspensory muscle of duodenum; Suspensory ligament of duodenum.** (Ligament of Treitz). Band of muscle and connective tissue fixing the duodenojejunal flexure, ascending, and horizontal parts to the diaphragm and coeliac trunk. It is normally made up of two portions.

12 *Phrenicocoeliac part.* Parts of the diaphragm radiating into the connective tissue around the coeliac trunk. A

13 *Celiacoduodenal part.* Connective tissue fibers with smooth muscle extending from the coeliac trunk to the duodenum and continuing to the duodenojejunal flexure. A

14 **Longitudinal fold of duodenum.** Longitudinal fold caused by the pancreatic duct and bile duct on the left side of the posterior wall of the descending part of duodenum. A

15 **Major duodenal papilla.** Projection at the end of the longitudinal fold with the openings to the bile duct and pancreatic duct. A

16 **Minor duodenal papilla.** Present in most people, the opening of the accessory pancreatic duct above the major duodenal papilla. A

17 **Duodenal glands.** (Brunner's glands). Mucoid glands especially in the duodenal submucosa.

18 **JEJUNUM.** Middle segment of the small intestine, extending about 2.5 m from the duodenojejunal flexure. A, p. 153 A

19 **ILEUM.** Terminal segment of the small intestine, about 3.5 m long. p. 153 A

20 **Terminal ileum.** The terminal ileum is mainly located in the pelvis, ascending into the right iliac fossa where it opens into the medial wall of the large intestine.

21 **[Ileal diverticulum].** (Meckel diverticula). Embryonic vitelline duct, a ca. 5 cm long blind outpouching 0.5–1 m before the ileal papilla.

22 *LARGE INTESTINE.* The large intestine is characterized by tenia, haustra, and omental appendices. It measures 1.5–1.8 m from the cecum to the anus.

23 **Serosa; Serous coat.** Peritoneal covering consisting of a layer of mesothelium. B

24 **Subserosa; Subserous layer.** Connective tissue underlying the serosa. Sometimes contains local deposits of adipose tissue. B

25 **Muscular layer; Muscular coat.** The muscular layer consists of an outer longitudinal and an inner circular muscle layer. The longitudinal muscle layer may be grouped in strands. B

26 **Submucosa.** Its structure is similar to that of the small intestine. B

27 **Mucosa; Mucous membrane.** It is composed of simple columnar epithelium, rich in goblet cells; connective tissue of the lamina propria and the muscularis mucosae. B

28 *Muscularis mucosae.* Comparable to the muscularis mucosae in the small intestine. B

29 *Intestinal glands.* Tubular glands in the colon mucosa. B

30 **CECUM.** Initial segment (ca. 7 cm) of the large intestine below the opening of the ileum. C D

31 **Ileal papilla.** A conical projection, in the living body, around the opening of the ileum into the large intestine which, in the cadaver, becomes a slitlike opening as a result of atonic intestinal musculature. C D

32 **Ileal orifice; Orifice of ileal papilla.** Opening of the ileum into the large intestine. C D

33 *Frenulum of ileal orifice.* Fold formed by the union of the upper and lower borders of the ileal orifice. D

34 *Ileocolic lip; Superior lip.* Upper lip of the margin of the ileal orifice. D

35 *Ileocecal lip; Inferior lip.* Lower lip of the margin of the ileal orifice. D

36 **Appendix; Vermiform appendix.** Cecum appendage that is usually 9 cm long and contains abundant lymphatic tissue. C D

37 *Orifice of vermiform appendix.* Opening of the vermiform appendix into the cecum. D

38 *Aggregated lymphoid nodules.* Lymphatic tissue in the wall of the vermiform appendix.

39 **[Prececocolic fascia].** Inconstant membranous connection between the colon, cecum and anterior, lateral abdominal wall.

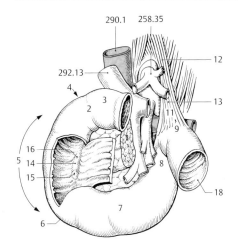

A Hepatic portal vein, inferior vena cava, aorta, and duodenum

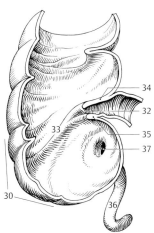

C Cecum in the living body

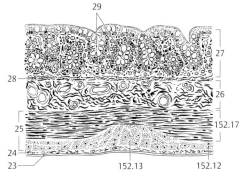

B Colon wall, histological cross-section

D Cecum in the cadaver

6

1 **COLON.** Large intestine segment extending from the ileal orifice to the rectum.

2 **Ascending colon.** Part of the colon that ascends retroperitoneally on the right side of the body. A

3 **Right colic flexure; Hepatic flexure.** Bend in the colon between the ascending and transverse colon. A

4 **Transverse colon.** Intraperitoneal part of the colon between the hepatic and splenic flexures. A

5 **Left colic flexure; Splenic flexure.** Bend in the colon below the left subphrenic space, between the transverse and descending colon. The Cannon–Boehm point is nearby, marking the boundary between the cranial (vagus nerve) and sacral components of the parasympathetic system. A

6 **Descending colon.** Retroperitoneal segment of the colon extending along the left side of the body between the splenic flexure and sigmoid colon. A

7 **Sigmoid colon.** Intraperitoneal segment of the colon between the descending colon and rectum. A

8 **Semilunar folds of colon.** Crescent-shaped folds between two haustra that are composed of all intestinal wall layers and are produced by contractions. A

9 **Haustra of colon.** Sacculation between two semilunar folds. A

10 **Omental appendices; Fatty appendices of colon.** Appendages consisting of adipose tissue in the subserous layer along the free and omental tenia. A

11 **Muscular layer; Muscular coat.** Double-layered muscular wall of the colon. p. 151 B

12 *Longitudinal layer.* Outer layer of varying thickness consisting of longitudinal muscle fibers. p. 151 B

13 *Teniae coli.* Thickened longitudinal muscle bands about 1 cm wide. p. 151 B

14 Mesocolic tenia. Tenia located at the attachment of the mesocolon. It is located in the posteromedial part of the ascending and descending colon. B

15 Omental tenia. Tenia located at the attachment of the transverse colon to the greater omentum. It is located in the posterolateral part of the ascending and descending colon. B

16 Free tenia. Free tenia between the mesocolic and omental teniae. B

17 *Circular layer.* Inner layer of circular muscle fibers of the colon. p. 151 B

18 **RECTUM.** Tenia-free 15 cm long segment extending between the sigmoid colon and anus. C

19 **Sacral flexure.** Anteriorly concave curvature of the rectum that conforms to the sacrum. C

20 **Lateral flexures.** Three lateral flexures formed by the rectum. E

21 *Superodextral lateral flexure; Superior lateral flexure.* Upper flexure with a right-sided convexity. E

22 *Intermediosinistral lateral flexure; Intermediate lateral flexure.* Middle flexure that is convex on the left side. It is the most pronounced of the three. E

23 *Inferodextral lateral flexure; Inferior lateral flexure.* Lower flexure with a right-sided convexity. E

24 **Transverse folds of rectum.** Lateral transverse folds that are usually about 1–2 cm thick consisting of mucosa, submucosa, and the circular layer of the muscular coat. The middle fold (Kohlrausch's fold) is the largest and most constant, palpable on the right side of the rectum 6–8 cm above the anus. A thickened circular layer of muscle forms its base. The other two folds project into the rectum from the left. E C

25 **Rectal ampulla.** Expansion of the rectum below Kohlrausch's fold. E

26 **Muscular layer; Muscular coat.** Muscular wall of the rectum. C

27 *Longitudinal layer.* Layer of longitudinal muscle cells that are evenly distributed over the entire circumference of the rectum. C

28 *Rectococcygeus.* Thin sheet of smooth-muscle cells that passes from the second–third coccygeal vertebrae to the rectum. C D

29 *Anorectoperineal muscles; Recto-urethral muscles.* Bundle of muscle cells arising from the longitudinal muscular layer of rectum and anal canal and passing in males to the male urethra and perineum above the perineal body. D

30 Rectoperinealis; Recto-urethralis superior. Smooth-muscle cells passing from the rectum mainly to the membranous urethra. C D

31 Anoperinealis; Recto-urethralis inferior. Smooth-muscle cells that extend from the anal canal mainly to the perineum. D

32 *Rectovesicalis.* Smooth-muscle cells that extend from the longitudinal layer of rectum in the lateral ligament of bladder to the lateral aspect of the fundus of bladder. D, see p. 188.8

33 *Circular layer.* Inner layer of circular muscle cells which in the rectum do not form semilunar folds. C

34 **Lateral ligament of rectum; Rectal stalk.** Dense connective tissue between the posterolateral pelvic wall and the rectum at the level of S3.

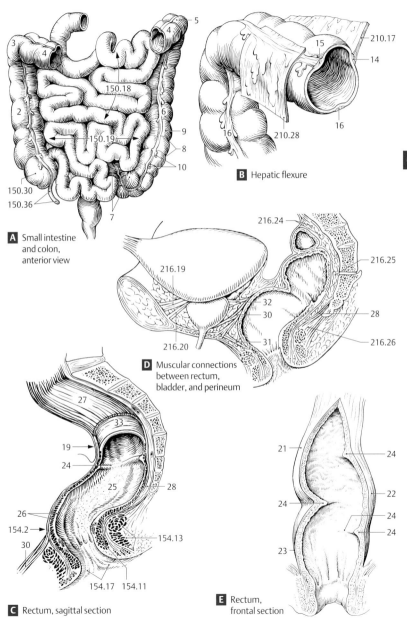

A Small intestine and colon, anterior view

B Hepatic flexure

C Rectum, sagittal section

D Muscular connections between rectum, bladder, and perineum

E Rectum, frontal section

1   **ANAL CANAL.** Terminal segment of the intestinal canal, beginning at the anorectal junction. A

2   **Anorectal flexure; Perineal flexure.** Anteriorly convex bend in the rectum just above the anus. p. 153 C

3   **Anorectal junction.** Beginning of the anorectal flexure, which is situated approximately below the tip of the coccyx and above the anal columns. Site of the levator muscle sling formed by the palpable puborectal muscle. A

4   **Anal columns.** (Columns of Morgagni). Six to ten longitudinal folds containing arteries, venous plexuses, and smooth longitudinal muscle cells. Predominantly columnar epithelium. A

5   **Anal sinuses.** Niches between the anal columns. A

6   **Anal valves.** Small transverse folds that form the inferior boundary of the anal sinuses. A

7   **Anal transition zone.** Histological term that describes transition zone epithelium between the anal columns and anocutaneous line. It is sometimes also used to refer only to the epithelium of the anal pecten. A

8   **Pectinate line.** Inferior line of demarcation of the anal valves. Transition from columnar epithelium to stratified, nonkeratinized squamous epithelium.

9   **Anal pecten.** Lighter stripe between the pectinate line and anocutaneous line where the hairless anal skin is firmly attached to underlying tissues. It is composed of stratified, nonkeratinized squamous epithelium. A

10 **Anocutaneous line.** Lower margin of the internal anal sphincter. Lower border of the anal pecten. Beginning of the external skin, composed of stratified, keratinized squamous epithelium. A

11 **Internal anal sphincter.** Thickened ring of muscle about 1–2 cm high in the circular muscular layer around the anus. A, p. 153 C

12 **Intersphincteric groove.** Palpable groove below the anocutaneous line where connective-tissue fibers from the muscular coat of the rectum end and blend with connective-tissue fibers from the levator ani muscle. A

13 **External anal sphincter.** Muscular ring composed of transversely striated fibers overlying the internal anal sphincter muscle. It comprises the following three parts. I: Pudendal nerve. A, p. 153 C

14 *Deep part of external anal sphincter.* Part of external anal sphincter that is entirely circular in form and measuring 3–4 cm from inferior to superior. A

15 *Superficial part of external anal sphincter.* Muscle fibers extending between the perineal body, anococcygeal ligament, and coccyx. A

16 *Subcutaneous part of external anal sphincter.* Superficial muscle cells that insert on the dermis anteriorly and posteriorly to the anus. It is caudal to the internal anal sphincter muscle and is permeated by connective-tissue fibers from the muscular coat of the rectum and the levator ani muscle. A

17 **Anus.** Inferior opening of the anal canal, encircled by the subcutaneous and superficial parts of external anal sphincter muscle. A, p. 153 C

18 *LIVER.* Organ located in the upper right side of the abdomen in the hypochondrium. Its inferior border runs from the upper left to the lower right through the epigastric region. In healthy subjects its border does not reach below the costal margin. It moves with respiration and is thus palpable. B

19 **Diaphragmatic surface.** Surface of the liver facing the diaphragm. B

20 *Superior part.* Cranially facing part of the diaphragmatic surface. B

21 *Cardiac impression.* Shallow depression below the attachment surface of the pericardium and diaphragm. It extends into the bare area and is bounded by the inferior vena cava. B

22 *Anterior part.* Anteriorly facing part of the diaphragmatic surface. B

23 *Right part.* Right-facing part of the diaphragmatic surface. B

24 *Posterior part.* Posteriorly facing area of the diaphragmatic surface. B

25 *Bare area.* Part of the diaphragmatic surface that lacks a peritoneal covering and presents the attachment surface of the liver and diaphragm. B

26 *Groove for vena cava.* Deep furrow lodging the vena cava. B

27 *Fissure for ligamentum venosum.* Groove that lodges the ligamentum venosum which extends from the porta hepatis to the inferior vena cava between the caudate and left lobes of liver. B

28 *Ligamentum venosum. (Ligament of Arantius).* Connective-tissue vestige of the ductus venosus; embryological anastomosis of the umbilical vein and inferior vena cava.

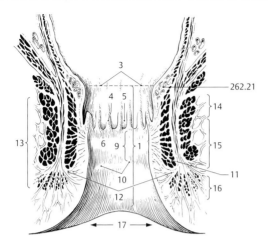

A Anal canal, frontal section

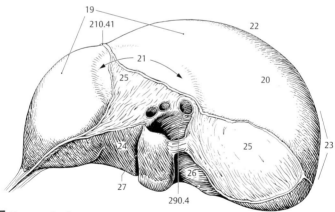

B Liver, superior view

1   **Visceral surface.** Partly concave posteroinferior surface of the liver that faces the viscera. A

2   *Fossa for gallbladder.* Depression on the visceral surface of the liver for the gallbladder. A

3   *Fissure for ligamentum teres; Fissure for round ligament.* Groove on the visceral surface that lodges the round ligament. A

4   *Round ligament of the liver.* Connective tissue remains of the umbilical vein. B

5   *Porta hepatis.* Depression between the caudate and quadrate lobes of liver for the passage of the hepatic artery proper, hepatic portal vein, and hepatic ducts, which unite here to form the common hepatic duct. A B

6   *Omental tuberosity.* Projection on the visceral surface of left lobe of liver to the left of the ligamentum venosum. A B

7   *Esophageal impression.* Groove on left lobe of liver formed by the esophagus. A

8   *Gastric impression.* Impression on the visceral surface of left lobe of liver caused by the stomach. A

9   *Duodenal impression.* Impression on the right lobe of liver to the right of gallbladder produced by the duodenum. A B

10 *Colic impression.* Impression on the right lobe of liver to the right of the fundus of gallbladder produced by the colon. A

11 *Renal impression.* Impression produced by the right kidney on the visceral surface of right lobe of liver. It extends into the bare area. A

12 *Suprarenal impression.* Impression formed by the right suprarenal gland on the bare area of the liver to the right of the inferior vena cava. A

13 **Inferior border.** Border between the diaphragmatic and visceral surfaces of liver. A

14 *Notch for ligamentum teres.* Notch in the inferior border of liver for the passage of the round ligament. A B

15 **Right lobe of liver.** Traditionally the part of the liver to the right of the attachment of the falciform ligament on the diaphragm. A B

16 **Left lobe of liver.** Traditionally the part of the liver to the left of the attachment of the falciform ligament of liver on the diaphragm. A B

17 *Fibrous appendix of liver.* Connective-tissue projection that is occasionally present on the upper end of the left lobe of liver. A

18 **Quadrate lobe.** Lobe of liver situated between the gallbladder, round ligament, and porta hepatis. A B

19 **Caudate lobe.** Lobe of liver situated between the inferior vena cava, porta hepatis, and ligamentum venosum. A B

20 *Papillary process.* Inferiorly directed projection from the caudate lobe. A B

21 *Caudate process.* Parenchymal attachment situated cranial to the porta hepatis between the caudate and right lobes of liver. A B

22 *[[Ligamentum. venae cavae]].* Connective-tissue bridge spanning the inferior vena cava. A B

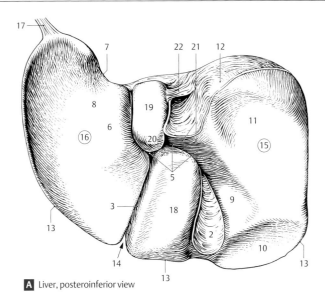

A Liver, posteroinferior view

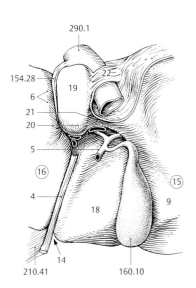

B Porta hepatis

1 **Hepatic segmentation: parts, divisions and segments.** Organization of the internal structures of the liver in parts, divisions, and segments. The term lobe is still used to describe a part. Segmentation is based on the internal distribution of the hepatic portal vein, hepatic arteries, and hepatic ducts. The smallest macroscopically visible units are the portal segments, whose peripheral boundaries are formed by branches of the hepatic veins. Hepatic segmentation is relevant for surgical anatomy.

2 **Umbilical fissure.** Fissure that runs parallel to the falciform ligament along its left side, and follows behind the fissures for the round ligament and ligamentum venosum. Its course corresponds to the projection of the left hepatic vein and its branches to the surface, forming a boundary between hepatic divisions. A B C

3 **Main portal fissure.** Fissure that divides the liver into right and left portions. It corresponds to a plane joining the inferior vena cava and the middle of the fossa for gallbladder and thus the projection of the intermediate hepatic vein to the surface. A B C

4 **Right portal fissure.** Fissure that corresponds to the projection of the right hepatic vein and its branches to the surface. It runs without any surface markings on the visceral side of the liver on the right side of the main portal fissure to the bare area, crossing frontally and coronally to the right, and descending at some distance along the right anterior margin of the liver. It demarcates a boundary between hepatic divisions. A B C

5 **Left liver; Left part of liver.** Part of the liver situated on the left side of the main portal fissure. A

6 *Left lateral division.* Part of the liver that is lateral to the umbilical fissure.

7 *Left posterior lateral segment; Segment II.* A B

8 *Left anterior lateral segment; Segment III.* A B

9 *Left medial division.* Part of the liver between the umbilical fissure and main portal fissure. A

10 *Left medial segment; Segment IV.* A B

11 *Posterior liver; Posterior part of liver; Caudate lobe.* Portion of the liver that is considered an independent part, as it drains directly into the inferior vena cava and receives its blood supply from the left and right hepatic arteries.

12 *Posterior segment; Caudate lobe; Segment I.* Segment that is identical to the posterior part of liver, caudate lobe, or segment I. B

13 **Right liver; Right part of liver.** Part of the liver located on the right side of the main portal fissure. A

14 *Right medial division.* Part of the liver between the main portal fissure and right portal fissure.

15 *Anterior medial segment; Segment V.* A B

16 *Posterior medial segment; Segment VIII.* A

17 *Right lateral division.* Part of the liver situated on the right side of the right portal fissure.

18 *Anterior lateral segment; Segment VI.* A B

19 *Posterior lateral segment; Segment VII.* A B

20 **Serosa; Serous coat.** Peritoneal covering consisting of simple squamous epithelium.

21 **Subserosa; Subserous layer.** Connective-tissue layer underlying the serous coat.

22 **Fibrous capsule.** Immobile connective-tissue capsule containing the liver that is especially thick in the bare area not covered with peritoneum.

23 **Perivascular fibrous capsule.** Connective-tissue sheath that accompanies the hepatic vessels and biliary ducts, extending to their terminal branches. D

24 **Lobules of liver.** Liver lobules measuring 1–2 mm in size.

25 **Interlobular arteries.** Branches of the hepatic artery proper between the lobules of liver. D

26 **Interlobular veins.** Branches of the hepatic portal veins between the liver lobules. D

27 **Central veins.** Veins in the center of the liver lobules for the drainage of blood. D

28 **Interlobular bile ducts.** Biliary ducts located between the lobules of liver. D

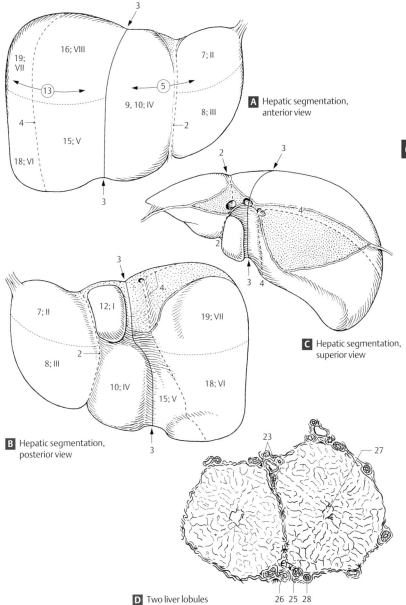

A Hepatic segmentation, anterior view

C Hepatic segmentation, superior view

B Hepatic segmentation, posterior view

D Two liver lobules

1 **Common hepatic duct.** Part of the bile duct between the junction of the right and left hepatic ducts and the cystic duct. A C

2 **Right hepatic duct.** Duct that passes out from the right part of liver. A C

3 *Anterior branch.* Branch from segments V and VI. A

4 *Posterior branch.* Branch from segments VII and VIII. A

5 **Left hepatic duct.** Duct that passes out from the left part of liver. A C

6 *Lateral branch.* Branch emerging from segments II and III. A

7 *Medial branch.* Branch emerging from segment IV. A

8 **Right duct of caudate lobe.** Branch that comes from the right half of the caudate lobe and usually passes to the right hepatic duct. A

9 **Left duct of caudate lobe.** Branch that comes from the left half of the caudate lobe and usually passes to the left hepatic duct. A

10 *GALLBLADDER.* Pear-shaped organ measuring 8-12 cm in length. C

11 **Fundus of gallbladder.** Floor of the gallbladder, which is directed caudally. C

12 **Body of gallbladder.** The body of gallbladder is attached to the liver. C

13 **Infundibulum of gallbladder.** Funnel-shaped part of the body of gallbladder that is not in contact with the liver and which is continuous with the neck of gallbladder. C

14 **Neck of gallbladder.** Part of the gallbladder that is separated from the infundibulum by a bend to the right. C

15 **Serosa; Serous coat.** Peritoneal covering of the gallbladder. D

16 **Subserosa; Subserous layer.** Connective tissue underlying the peritoneal covering. D

17 **Muscular layer; Muscular coat.** Muscular coat in the wall of the gallbladder. D

18 **Mucosa; Mucous membrane.** Mucous membrane of gallbladder composed of simple columnar epithelium. D

19 *Mucosal folds*; *Rugae.* Mucosal folds that project into the lumen, producing a locular relief. C D

20 **Cystic duct.** Duct that drains the gallbladder. It joins the common hepatic duct to form the bile duct. C

21 **Spiral fold.** Spiral-shaped fold in the neck of gallbladder and cystic duct. C

22 **Bile duct.** Duct draining the gallbladder that is formed by the union of the common hepatic and cystic ducts and passes to the major duodenal papilla. C

23 **Sphincter of bile duct.** Autonomous muscle ring that extends to the hepatopancreatic ampulla.

24 *Superior sphincter.* Ring of muscle fibers extending along the bile duct to its junction with the pancreatic duct. Muscular contraction enables filling of the gallbladder. B C

25 *Inferior sphincter.* Ring of muscle fibers above the hepatopancreatic ampulla. Its fibers usually blend with those of the pancreatic duct. B C

26 **Hepatopancreatic ampulla; Biliaropancreatic ampulla.** Expansion located in the wall of the duodenum directly following the opening of the pancreatic duct into the bile duct. B C

27 *Sphincter of ampulla.* (Sphincter of Oddi). Sphincter muscle complex that consists of circular and spiral smooth-muscle cells surrounding the hepatopancreatic ampulla. B

28 **Glands of bile duct.** Mucous glands situated in the bile duct. C

6

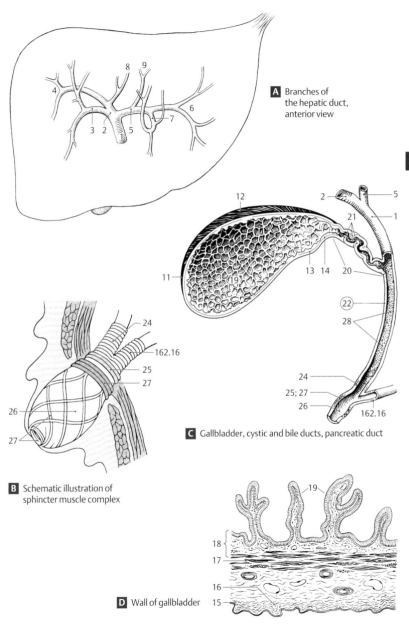

A Branches of the hepatic duct, anterior view

6

C Gallbladder, cystic and bile ducts, pancreatic duct

B Schematic illustration of sphincter muscle complex

D Wall of gallbladder

1 *PANCREAS.* Organ measuring 13–15 cm in length, lying partly in the duodenal loop and partly behind the omental bursa at the level of L1–L2. A B

2 **Head of pancreas.** Part of the pancreas nestled in the duodenal loop. A

3 *Uncinate process.* Hooked process that projects behind the mesenteric vessels. A B

4 *Pancreatic notch.* Groove between the uncinate process and the rest of the pancreas head. A B

5 **Neck of pancreas.** Parenchymal strip anterior to the superior mesenteric veins, which produce a furrow on its posterior aspect. Surgical landmark. A B

6 **Body of pancreas.** Part of the pancreas situated mainly anterior to the vertebral column. It arises from the dorsal pancreatic anlage. A B

7 *Anterosuperior surface.* Surface of the pancreas facing anteriorly and superiorly. A

8 *Posterior surface.* Dorsal surface of the pancreas. B

9 *Antero-inferior surface.* Surface facing anteriorly and inferiorly. Its superior boundary is formed by the root of the transverse mesocolon. A

10 *Superior border.* Upper border between the anterior and posterior surfaces. A B

11 *Anterior border.* Border that corresponds to the line of attachment of the transverse mesocolon and thus the inferior boundary of the omental bursa on the posterior wall of the abdomen. A

12 *Inferior border.* Lower border situated between the anterior and posterior surfaces. A

13 *Omental eminence.* Prominence on the body of pancreas near the head that is produced by the vertebral column and projects into the omental bursa. A B

14 **Tail of pancreas.** Upper left part of the pancreas that is in contact with the spleen. A B

15 **Pancreatic duct.** Main duct draining the pancreas that empties into the major duodenal papilla together with the bile duct. B

16 *Sphincter of pancreatic duct.* Ring of muscle in front of the opening to the pancreatic duct. p. 161 B C

17 **Accessory pancreatic duct.** Additional duct that is usually present and drains into the minor duodenal papilla above the major duodenal papilla. B

18 **[Accessory pancreas].** Diffusely organized pancreatic tissue in the wall of the stomach or small intestine.

19 **Pancreatic islets.** Islets of Langerhans numbering around one million. They produce glucagon and insulin, among other substances.

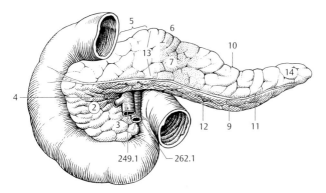

A Duodenum and pancreas,
anterior view,
slightly rotated

6

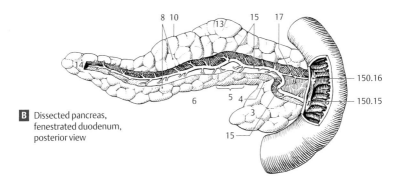

B Dissected pancreas,
fenestrated duodenum,
posterior view

1   *RESPIRATORY SYSTEM.*

2   NOSE.

3   **Root of nose.** Upper part of the nose located between the two orbits. C D

4   **Dorsum of nose.** C

5   **Apex of nose; Tip of nose.** C

6   **Ala of nose.** C

7   **Nasal cartilages.** Cartilaginous parts forming the nonosseous supporting framework of the nose. A B D

8   *Major alar cartilage.* Hook-shaped cartilage surrounding the nasal opening. A

9   *Medial crus.* A B D

10   Mobile part of nasal septum. Mobile anterior and inferior part of the nasal septum. It is composed of skin with a fibrous subcutaneous layer, the membranous part of nasal septum, and the medial crus.

11   *Lateral crus.* Part that curves laterally around the nares. A B

12   *Minor alar cartilages.* Individual smaller cartilage plates that supplement the major alar cartilage. A

13   *Accessory nasal cartilages.* Smaller pieces of cartilage that are occasionally found between the lateral process and the major alar cartilage, supplementing the cartilaginous framework of the nose. A

14   *Septal nasal cartilage.* Larger independent piece of cartilage in the nasal septum between the perpendicular plate of ethmoid and the vomer. A B D

15   *Lateral process.* Cartilaginous part of the septal nasal cartilage that contributes to formation of the lateral wall of the nose. A D

16   *Posterior process; Sphenoid process.* Process of variable length between the vomer and perpendicular plate; it can extend to the sphenoid. D

17   *Vomeronasal cartilage.* Inconstant cartilage plate of variable size lateral to the nasal septum. D

18   Nasal cavity. E

19   **Nares; Nostrils.** Nasal openings that are framed by the ala of nose and the nasal septum. B E

20   **Choanae; Posterior nasal apertures.** Posterior openings of the nasal cavity. D

21   **Nasal septum.** Nasal partition consisting of bony, cartilaginous, and membranous parts. D

22   *Membranous part.* Connective-tissue part of the nasal septum at the tip of nose. D

23   *Cartilaginous part.* Part of the nasal septum between the membranous and bony parts. D

24   *Bony part.* Bony part of nasal septum consisting of the perpendicular plate of ethmoid and the vomer. D

25   *Vomeronasal organ.* (Jacobson's organ). Blind-ending pouch that is occasionally present above the incisive canal, representing an evolutionary vestige of an accessory olfactory organ. D E

26   **Nasal vestibule.** Anterior part of the nasal cavity extending to the limen nasi where its lining of squamous epithelium transitions into ciliated epithelium. E

27   **Limen nasi.** Mucosal ridge at the end of the nasal vestibule produced by the border of the alar cartilage. E

28   **Olfactory groove.** Groove extending from between the root of the middle nasal concha and the dorsum of nose to the olfactory region. E

29   **Highest nasal concha.** Inconstant uppermost nasal concha located at the ethmoid.

30   **Superior nasal concha.** Small upper nasal concha located in front of the sphenoidal sinus. E

31   **Middle nasal concha.** Concha beneath which most of the openings to the paranasal sinuses are located. E

32   **Inferior nasal concha.** Lowest and longest nasal concha. It obscures the opening of nasolacrimal duct. E

33   **Cavernous plexus of conchae.** Venous plexuses near the middle and inferior nasal conchae and the posterior part of the nasal cavity. When full, the mucosa swells by up to 5 mm.

34   **Mucosa; Mucous membrane.** Nasal mucosa of varying structure. Two components are distinguished.

35   **Respiratory region.** Part of the nasal mucosa that is lined with pseudostratified ciliated epithelium. It begins in the nasal vestibule and lines the entire nasal cavity and paranasal sinuses, with the exception of the olfactory region.

36   **Olfactory region.** Olfactory mucosa. Dime-sized region that is lined with olfactory cells located on the upper part of the nasal septum below the cribriform plate and on the lateral wall of the nose. E

37   **Nasal glands.** Mucous and serous glands. Their thin discharge cleanses the olfactory epithelium and is thought to enhance odorants.

38   **Agger nasi.** Prominence directly in front of the middle nasal concha that is a vestige of an accessory nasal concha. E

39   **Spheno-ethmoidal recess.** Niche above the superior nasal concha between the anterior wall of the sphenoidal sinus and the roof of the nasal cavity. E

40   **Superior nasal meatus.** Upper nasal passageway above the middle nasal concha. Opening of the posterior ethmoidal cells. E

41   **Middle nasal meatus.** Middle nasal passageway between the middle and inferior nasal conchae. Opening of the middle ethmoidal cells. E

42   *Atrium of middle meatus.* Area at the beginning of the middle nasal meatus in front of the middle and above the inferior nasal conchae. E

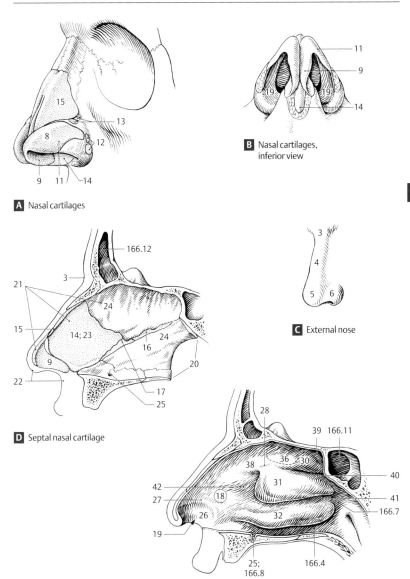

A Nasal cartilages

B Nasal cartilages, inferior view

C External nose

D Septal nasal cartilage

E Lateral nasal wall and sphenoidal sinus

1 *Ethmoidal bulla.* Rudimentary nasal concha below the middle nasal concha that resembles the blisterlike elevation of an ethmoidal cell. C

2 *Ethmoidal infundibulum.* Niche in front of the ethmoidal bulla below the middle nasal concha where the maxillary sinus, frontal sinus, and anterior ethmoidal cells open. C

3 *Semilunar hiatus.* Crescent-shaped crevice between the ethmoidal bulla and the uncinate process. C

4 **Inferior nasal meatus.** Lower nasal passageway between the inferior nasal concha and the floor of the nose. C, p. 165 E

5 *Opening of nasolacrimal duct.* Opening of nasolacrimal canal with a valvelike mucosal fold.

6 **Common nasal meatus.** Space in the nasal cavity between nasal conchae and septum.

7 **Nasopharyngeal meatus.** Junction of the three nasal passageways behind the nasal conchae. C, p. 165 E

8 **[Incisive duct].** Blind pouch that is occasionally present on the floor of the nasal cavity adjacent to the nasal septum and about 2 cm behind the external nasal opening. C, p. 165 E

9 *Paranasal sinuses.*

10 **Maxillary sinus.** Largest of the paranasal sinuses of variable size. It extends in the maxilla to below the orbits and into the maxillary tuberosity. Its deepest point lies above the roots of premolar and first molar teeth. It opens below the middle nasal concha. A

11 **Sphenoidal sinus.** Paired sinus in the body of sphenoid that varies in size. It opens at the spheno-ethmoidal recess. B C, p. 165 E

12 **Frontal sinus.** It can extend beyond the squamous part of frontal bone into the orbital part of frontal bone. It opens below the middle nasal concha above the sphenoidal sinus. A B C, p. 165 D

13 **Ethmoidal cells.** Cavity system of cells of various sizes between the nasal and orbital cavities.

14 *Anterior ethmoidal cells.* Anterior group of ethmoidal cells that open below the middle nasal concha. A B

15 *Middle ethmoidal cells.* Middle group of ethmoidal cells that open below the middle nasal concha. A B

16 *Posterior ethmoidal cells.* Posterior group of ethmoidal cells that open below the superior nasal concha. A B

17 **LARYNX.** The larynx is situated between the pharynx and trachea. D

18 LARYNGEAL CARTILAGES AND JOINTS.

19 **Thyroid cartilage.** Largest laryngeal cartilage partly enclosing the others. D E

20 **Laryngeal prominence.** Prominence in the midline of the neck caused by the thyroid cartilage. It is more pronounced in men (Adam's apple). D E

21 **Right/Left lamina.** Lateral plates of the thyroid cartilage that meet in the midline like the prow of a ship. D E

22 **Superior thyroid notch.** Deep, upper midline notch between the right and left laminae. D E

23 **Inferior thyroid notch.** Shallow, lower midline depression between the right and left laminae. E

24 **Superior thyroid tubercle.** Small lateral protuberance on the outer surface at the superior end of the oblique line. D E

25 **Inferior thyroid tubercle.** Small lateral protuberance on the outer surface at the inferior end of the oblique line. D E

26 **Oblique line.** Oblique ridge on the outer aspect of the thyroid cartilage that gives attachment to the sternothyroid and thyrohyoid muscles and the inferior constrictor muscle of the pharynx. D E

27 **Superior horn.** Upper process projecting from the posterior margin of the thyroid cartilage, giving attachment to the thyrohyoid ligament. D E

28 **Inferior horn.** Lower process projecting from the posterior margin of the thyroid cartilage that articulates with the cricoid cartilage. D E

29 **[Thyroid foramen].** Opening that is occasionally present inferolateral to the superior thyroid tubercle and sometimes gives passage to the superior laryngeal artery and vein. D

30 **Thyrohyoid membrane.** Fibroelastic membrane that extends between the upper medial border of the hyoid bone and the thyroid cartilage. D

31 *Median thyrohyoid ligament.* Medial thickening of the thyrohyoid membrane containing elastic fibers. D

32 *Retrohyoid bursa.* p. 129 A

33 *Infrahyoid bursa.* p. 129 A

34 *Lateral thyrohyoid ligament.* Band that passes from the superior horn to the posterior end of the greater horn of hyoid bone. Lateral thickening of the thyrohyoid membrane. D

35 *Triticeal cartilage.* Elastic cartilage the size of a grain of wheat in the thyrohyoid ligament. D

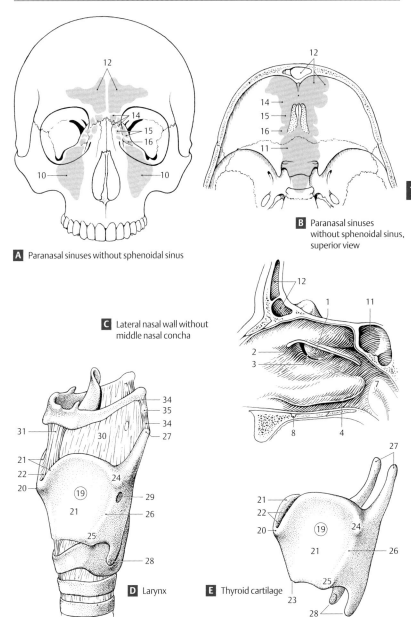

A Paranasal sinuses without sphenoidal sinus

B Paranasal sinuses without sphenoidal sinus, superior view

C Lateral nasal wall without middle nasal concha

D Larynx

E Thyroid cartilage

1 **Cricoid cartilage.** Signet-ring shaped cartilage located at the upper end of the trachea that articulates with the thyroid cartilage. A B D

2 **Arch of cricoid cartilage.** Anterior and lateral part of the cricoid cartilage. A B

3 **Lamina of cricoid cartilage.** Posteriorly directed cricoid cartilage plate. A B

4 *Arytenoid articular surface.* Oblique oval articular facet located laterally on the upper border of the lamina of cricoid cartilage for articulation with the arytenoid cartilage. A

5 *Thyroid articular surface.* Rather prominent articular facet on the lateral aspect of the lamina of cricoid cartilage for articulation with the thyroid cartilage. A

6 **Cricothyroid joint.** Joint formed by the thyroid and cricoid cartilages. It allows tilting movement as well as horizontal and vertical sliding motion of the cricoid cartilage against the thyroid cartilage. B

7 **Capsule of cricothyroid joint.** Thin articular capsule. B

8 **Ceratocricoid ligament.** Thickened portion of the articular capsule that limits translational movement. B D

9 **Median cricothyroid ligament.** Strong vertical band running in the midline between the thyroid and cricoid cartilages. Incision site for cricothyrotomy to establish the airways. B D

10 **Cricotracheal ligament.** Elastic membrane between the cricoid cartilage and first tracheal cartilage. B

11 **Arytenoid cartilage.** Nearly pyramid-shaped cartilage sitting atop the cricoid cartilage. C D

12 **Articular surface.** Cylindrical, concave basal articular surface below the muscular process with which the arytenoid cartilage rides on the cricoid cartilage. C

13 **Base of arytenoid cartilage.** Inferior surface of the arytenoid cartilage. C

14 **Anterolateral surface.** Surface that faces anterolaterally and serves for muscle insertion and origin. C

15 *Vocal process.* Anteriorly projecting process that serves for the attachment of the vocal ligament. C

16 *Arcuate crest.* Ridge of cartilage that begins between the oblong and triangular foveae, curves around the triangular fovea, and ends at the colliculus. C

17 *Colliculus.* Small projection at the end of the arcuate crest. C D

18 *Oblong fovea.* Pit on the anterolateral surface for the attachment of the thyroarytenoid muscle. C

19 *Triangular fovea.* Pit located above the oblong fovea that contains glands. C

20 **Medial surface of arytenoid cartilage.** C

21 **Posterior surface of arytenoid cartilage.** C D

22 **Apex of arytenoid cartilage.** Tip of the arytenoid cartilage that curves posteriorly and bears the corniculate cartilage. C

23 **Muscular process.** Short process on the posterolateral surface for attachment of the posterior and lateral crico-arytenoid muscles. C

24 **Crico-arytenoid joint.** Cylindrical projection for articulation between the arytenoid and cricoid cartilages with a wide capsule and without collateral ligaments. This allows oscillating movement around the oblique axis of the cylinder, gliding movement parallel to the axis, and rotation around the height axis of the arytenoid cartilage. D

25 **Capsule of crico-arytenoid joint.** Thin-walled, lax articular capsule between the arytenoid and cricoid cartilages. It is reinforced, mainly on its medial aspect, by the crico-arytenoid ligament. D

26 **Crico-arytenoid ligament.** Elastic band that is important for closure of the rima glottidis. It passes posteriorly from the lamina of the cricoid cartilage to the medial part of the arytenoid cartilage. D

27 **Cricopharyngeal ligament.** Band that extends from the corniculate cartilage. After attaching to the posterior side of the cricoid cartilage, it passes beneath the pharyngeal mucosa overlying the posterior aspect of the cricoid cartilage. D

28 **[Sesamoid cartilage].** Elastic pieces of cartilage that are occasionally present in the anterior end of the vocal ligaments and near the arytenoid cartilage. D

29 **Corniculate cartilage.** (Santorini's cartilage). Small elastic cartilage on the apex of arytenoid cartilage that produces the corniculate tubercle. C D

30 **Corniculate tubercle.** Mucosa-covered prominence overlying the corniculate cartilage immediately above the apex of the arytenoid cartilage. p. 171B D

7

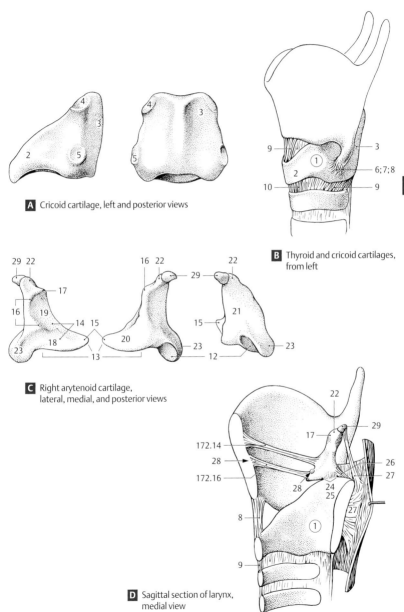

A Cricoid cartilage, left and posterior views

B Thyroid and cricoid cartilages, from left

C Right arytenoid cartilage, lateral, medial, and posterior views

D Sagittal section of larynx, medial view

1 **Cuneiform cartilage.** (Cartilage of Wrisberg). Small cartilage that is occasionally present in the ary-epiglottic fold underneath a fat pad. D

2 **Cuneiform tubercle.** Prominence in the ary-epiglottic fold produced by the cuneiform cartilage or, if the cuneiform cartilage is absent, only by adipose cells. B D

3 **Epiglottis.** Elastic cartilage shaped like a shoe-horn. C

4 **Epiglottic cartilage.** Skeletal framework of the epiglottis composed of elastic cartilage. A C D

5 **Stalk of epiglottis.** Inferiorly directed epiglottis petiolus. It is attached to the prow of the thyroid cartilage by connective tissue. A D

6 **Epiglottic tubercle.** Prominence in the wall of the epiglottis above the stalk. B

7 **Thyro-epiglottic ligament.** Band that attaches the stalk of epiglottis to the posterior surface of the thyroid cartilage. A D

8 **Hyo-epiglottic ligament.** Ligament that extends between the hyoid bone and epiglottis. C

9 **Pre-epiglottic fat body.** Adipose body that fills the space between the epiglottis, thyrohyoid membrane, and hyo-epiglottic ligament. C

10 **Laryngeal muscles.**

11 **Cricothyroid.** o: Anterior and lateral from the cricoid cartilage. i: Inferior margin of the lamina of thyroid cartilage on the inner and outer surface of the inferior horn. If the thyroid cartilage is fixed, it tilts the cricoid cartilage with the arytenoid cartilages posteriorly, thereby tensing the vocal ligaments. I: External branch of superior laryngeal nerve (only one). It is composed in 50% of the following parts. C E

12 *Straight part.* Anterior fibers that run at a rather steep angle. C

13 *Oblique part.* Posterior fibers that run more horizontally. C

14 **Posterior crico-arytenoid.** o: Posterior surface of cricoid cartilage. i: Muscular process of arytenoid cartilage. The only muscle that acts to open the rima glottis, doing so by superolateral rotation of the vocal process. I: Recurrent laryngeal nerve. B D

15 **[Ceratocricoid].** Anatomical variant. o: Inferior horn of thyroid cartilage. i: Inferior margin of cricoid cartilage. I: Recurrent laryngeal nerve. B

16 **Lateral crico-arytenoid.** o: Upper margin and lateral outer surface of cricoid cartilage. i: Lateral margin of muscular process of arytenoid cartilage and adjacent area. Synergist in closing the rima glottidis. I: Recurrent laryngeal nerve. D

17 **Vocalis.** o: Inner surface of thyroid cartilage near the midline. i: Vocal process and oblong fovea of arytenoid cartilage. Its tensing action changes the intrinsic vibration of the vocal ligament. I: Recurrent laryngeal nerve. E

18 **Thyro-arytenoid.** o: Anterior inner surface of thyroid cartilage. i: Anterior lateral surface of arytenoid cartilage. Synergist in closing the rima glottidis. I: Recurrent laryngeal nerve. D E

19 *Thyro-epiglottic part.* o: Anterior inner surface of thyroid cartilage. i: Epiglottis and quadrangular membrane. I: Recurrent laryngeal nerve. D

20 **Oblique arytenoid.** o: Posterior surface of muscular process. i: Apex of the contralateral arytenoid cartilage. Acts to bring the arytenoid cartilages closer together. Synergist in closing the rima glottidis. I: Recurrent laryngeal nerve. B

21 *Ary-epiglottic part.* o: Apex of arytenoid cartilage. i: Epiglottic margin. Forms the ary-epiglottic fold. Draws the epiglottis inferiorly. B

22 **Transverse arytenoid.** Transverse bundle of muscle fibers that connect the lateral margins of the arytenoid cartilages. Acts to bring the arytenoid cartilages closer together. Synergist in closing the rima glottidis. I: Recurrent laryngeal nerve. B

23 **Laryngeal cavity.** Space within the larynx. B E

24 **Laryngeal inlet.** Entrance to the larynx between the epiglottis, ary-epiglottic folds, and interarytenoid notch. E

25 *Ary-epiglottic fold.* Mucosal fold overlying the ary-epiglottic part of oblique arytenoid muscle. It extends from the apex of arytenoid cartilage to the lateral margin of the epiglottis. B D

26 *Interarytenoid notch.* Mucosa-covered notch between the two apexes of arytenoid cartilages. B

27 **Laryngeal vestibule.** It extends from the laryngeal inlet to the vestibular fold. E

28 *Vestibular fold.* Fold produced by the vestibular ligament. It lies between the laryngeal ventricle and the laryngeal vestibule. E

29 *Rima vestibuli.* Space between the two vestibular folds. E

7

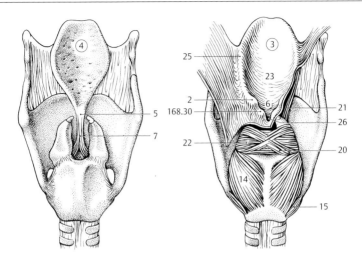

A Laryngeal cartilage, posterior view

B Muscles of larynx, posterior view

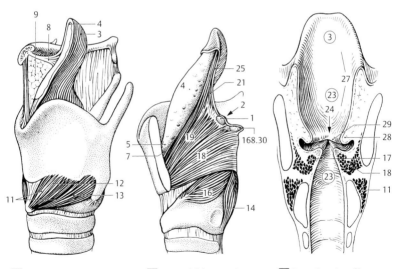

C Larynx, anterolateral view

D Larynx, left lamina of thyroid cartilage removed

E Frontal section of larynx, posterior view

1 **Laryngeal ventricle.** (Ventricle of Morgagni). Lateral outpouching between the vocal folds and vestibular fold. B C D

2 *Laryngeal saccule.* Inconstant, small blind pouch pointing upward from the laryngeal ventricle. B

3 **Glottis.** Part of the larynx composed of the two vocal folds that produce the voice. A

4 *Vocal fold.* The vocal fold overlies the vocal ligament and is supported laterally by the vocalis muscle. A

5 *Rima glottidis.* Fissure between the two arytenoid cartilages and the vocal folds. A

6 **Intermembranous part.** Segment of the rima glottidis that extends from the thyroid cartilage to the tip of the vocal process. A

7 **Intercartilaginous part.** Segment of the rima glottidis between the arytenoid cartilages. A

8 **Interarytenoid fold.** Mucosal fold between the two arytenoid cartilages. A

9 **Infraglottic cavity.** Space enclosed in the conus elasticus between the rima glottidis and the inferior margin of the cricoid cartilage. C

10 **Mucosa; Mucous membrane.** Only on the upper part of the posterior epiglottal surface and the vocal folds is the laryngeal mucosa composed of nonkeratinized, stratified squamous epithelium, while the rest consists of pseudostratified ciliated epithelium. B

11 *Laryngeal glands.* Submucosal mixed glands contained in the laryngeal mucosa. B

12 **Fibro-elastic membrane of larynx.** Submucosal layer of the larynx containing abundant elastic fibers. It begins at the quadrangular membrane and ends at the inferior margin of the conus elasticus. B

13 *Quadrangular membrane.* Membrane extending between the epiglottis, ary-epiglottic fold, and vestibular fold. C D

14 *Vestibular ligament.* Band that reinforces the inferior margin of the quadrangular membrane. C

15 *Conus elasticus; Cricovocal membrane.* Thickened portion of the fibroelastic membrane between the vocal ligament and cricoid cartilage. D

16 *Vocal ligament.* Band extending between the vocal process of arytenoid cartilage and thyroid cartilage. It forms the upper end of the conus elasticus. C

17 **TRACHEA.** Elastic tube between the larynx and bronchi.

18 **Cervical part.** Part of the trachea extending from C6 to C7.

19 **Thoracic part.** Part of the trachea extending from T1 to T4.

20 **Tracheal cartilages.** Horseshoe-shaped cartilages of the trachea that are open posteriorly. E F H

21 **Trachealis.** Smooth-muscle cells that pass between the free ends of the horseshoe-shaped tracheal cartilages in the membranous wall of the trachea. H

22 **Anular ligaments.** Fibrous bridges spanning between and encircling the tracheal cartilages. E F

23 **Membranous wall.** Membranous and muscular posterior wall of the trachea. F

24 **Tracheal bifurcation.** Asymmetrical bifurcation of the trachea at the level of T4. E G

25 **Carina of trachea.** Ridge that protrudes into the tracheal lumen at the tracheal bifurcation and has an aerodynamic effect. G

26 **Mucosa; Mucous membrane.** Mucous membrane lining the trachea composed of pseudostratified ciliated epithelium. H

27 *Tracheal glands.* Mixed glands contained in the submucosa of trachea. H

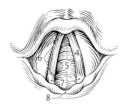

A Laryngeal inlet, superior view

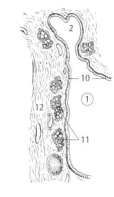

B Laryngeal ventricle

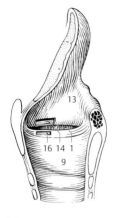

C Larynx, sagittal section

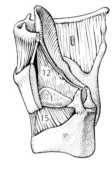

D Larynx, posterolateral view,
left lamina of thyroid cartilage removed

7

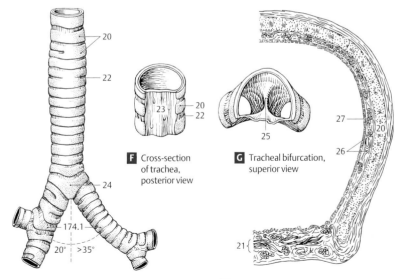

E Trachea and bronchi, anterior view

F Cross-section
of trachea,
posterior view

G Tracheal bifurcation,
superior view

H Cross-section of trachea, histological section

1 **BRONCHI.**

2 **Bronchial tree.** The entire system of bronchial branches.

3 **Right main bronchus.** A

4 **Left main bronchus.** A

5 **Lobar and segmental bronchi.** The bronchi supplying the 5 lobes of lungs and their 20 segments. A B

6 **Right superior lobar bronchus.** Bronchus that branches off shortly after the tracheal bifurcation and supplies the right superior lobe. A B

7 *Apical segmental bronchus (B I).* It supplies the apical segment, extending inferiorly to the third rib. A B

8 *Posterior segmental bronchus (B II).* It supplies the posterior segment, which extends anteriorly to about the midaxillary line. A B

9 *Anterior segmental bronchus (B III).* It supplies the anterior segment, which extends posteriorly to about the midaxillary line. A B

10 **Middle lobar bronchus.** Lobar bronchus supplying the middle lobe of right lung. A

11 *Lateral segmental bronchus (B IV).* It supplies the lateral segment in the dorsal part of the middle lobe. A B

12 *Medial segmental bronchus (B V).* It supplies the anteromedial segment in the middle lobe. A B

13 **Right inferior lobar bronchus.** It supplies the right inferior lobe, which extends posteriorly up to the level of the fourth rib. A B

14 *Superior segmental bronchus (B VI).* Bronchus supplying the apical segment, which borders only on the superior lobe. B

15 *Medial basal segmental bronchus (B VII).* Bronchus supplying the medial segment, which does not reach the outer surface of the inferior lobe. A B

16 *Anterior basal segmental bronchus (B VIII).* Bronchus supplying the wedge-shaped anterior end of the inferior lobe. A B

17 *Lateral basal segmental bronchus (B IX).* Bronchus supplying the small lateral segment located between the anterior and posterior segments. A B

18 *Posterior basal segmental bronchus (B X).* It supplies the segment extending posteriorly to the vertebral column. A B

19 **Left superior lobar bronchus.** Lobar bronchus supplying the superior lobe of left lung. A B

20 *Apicoposterior segmental bronchus (B I + II).* Bronchus supplying the apicoposterior segment of left lung. A B

21 *Anterior segmental bronchus (B III).* It supplies the anterior segment of the superior lobe of left lung, which is anterior to the apical segment. A B

22 *Superior lingular bronchus (B IV).* Bronchus supplying the second lowest segment of the superior lobe of left lung, which extends to the border of the inferior lobe. A B

23 *Inferior lingular bronchus (B V).* Bronchus supplying the lowest segment of the superior lobe, which is mainly situated ventrally. A B

24 **Left inferior lobar bronchus.** Lobar bronchus supplying the inferior lobe of left lung which extends dorsally upward to T4. A B

25 *Superior segmental bronchus (B VI).* Bronchus supplying the apical segment in the posterosuperior part of the inferior lobe. B

26 *Medial basal segmental bronchus (B VII).* It supplies the medial basal segment which does not reach the lateral surface of the lung. A

27 *Anterior basal segmental bronchus (B VIII).* It supplies the anterior basal segment which extends to the anterior boundary of the inferior lobe. A B

28 *Lateral basal segmental bronchus (B IX).* Bronchus supplying the middle basal segment between the anterior and posterior basal segments. A B

29 *Posterior basal segmental bronchus (B X).* Bronchus supplying the posterior basal segment of the inferior lobe located below the apical segment. A B

30 **Intrasegmental bronchi.** Branches of individual segmental bronchi within a segment.

31 **Fibromusculocartilaginous layer.** Outer wall of the intrapulmonary bronchi. It consists of a fibrocartilage covering of connective tissue containing abundant elastic fibers and cartilage embedded within it. Its inner fibrous coat is composed of reticular and circular smooth-muscle cells—expansion of the trachealis muscle—underneath the mucous membrane. C

32 **Submucosa.** Connective-tissue layer beneath the bronchial mucosa. Only in medium-sized and small bronchi is it present beneath the muscular coat. C

33 **Mucosa; Mucous membrane.** Bronchial mucosa composed of columnar ciliated epithelium. C

34 *Bronchial glands.* Mixed glands located underneath the mucosa. C

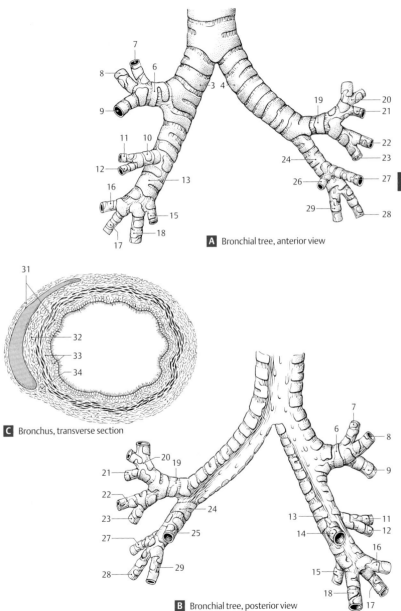

A Bronchial tree, anterior view

C Bronchus, transverse section

B Bronchial tree, posterior view

7

1 **LUNGS.** The lungs occupy the greater part of the thoracic cavity. A B C D

2 **Right lung.** Larger of the two lungs.

3 **Left lung.** The smaller of the two lungs (by 10%).

4 **Base of lung.** Part of the lung facing the diaphragm. A B C D

5 **Apex of lung.** Tip of the lung which extends into the superior thoracic aperture. A B C D

6 **Costal surface.** Surface of the lung adjacent to the ribs. A C

7 *Vertebral part.* Dorsal strip of the costal surface of the lung that is in contact with the vertebral column. B C

8 **Mediastinal surface.** Surface of the lung in contact with the mediastinum, located anterior to the vertebral part of the costal surface. B D

9 *Cardiac impression.* Depression on the medial surface of both lungs produced by the heart. B D

10 **Diaphragmatic surface.** Concave inferior surface of the lung that lies on the diaphragm. A B C D

11 **Interlobar surface.** Surfaces of lung tissue that form the boundary of the lung at the clefts between the lobes.

12 **Anterior border.** Sharp, anterior margin at the junction of the mediastinal and costal surfaces. A B C D

13 *Cardiac notch of left lung.* Notch on the anterior border of the left superior lobe produced by the cardiac impression. C D

14 **Inferior border.** Sharp margin at the junction of the costal and diaphragmatic surfaces. It is less sharp at the transition of the diaphragmatic surface into the mediastinal surface. A B C D

15 **Hilum of lung.** Site of entry and exit of bronchi, vessels, and nerves on the mediastinal surface of the lung. In general, the bronchi are located dorsally, the pulmonary arteries ventral and cranial to the bronchi, and the pulmonary veins ventral and caudal to the bronchi. In the right hilum the superior lobar bronchus is above the pulmonary artery, hence the term "eparterial" bronchus. B D

16 **Root of lung.** It is composed of the main bronchus, blood vessels, lymph vessels and nodes, and autonomic plexuses. B

17 **Superior lobe; Upper lobe.** Superior lobe that extends posteriorly to the fourth rib. In the right lung, its inferior border runs anteriorly at about the level of the fourth rib. In the left, its inferior border extends to the osseocartilaginous border of the sixth rib. A B C D

18 **Lingula of left lung.** Projection between the cardiac notch of the left lung and the inferior border of the left superior lobe. C D

19 **Middle lobe of right lung.** Present only in the right lung. It lies in front of the midaxillary line between the fourth and sixth ribs. A B

20 **Inferior lobe; lower lobe.** It mainly extends dorsally. Its superior border runs obliquely from posterosuperior to anteroinferior. It begins paravertebrally at the fourth rib and ends at the intersection of the midclavicular line and the sixth rib. A B C D

21 **Oblique fissure.** Oblique cleft between the inferior and superior lobes of left lung, and between the lower, middle, and superior lobes of right lung. It runs paravertebrally from the fourth rib to the sixth rib in the midclavicular line. A B C D

22 **Horizontal fissure of right lung.** Cleft that separates the middle and superior lobes. It runs approximately along the level of the fourth rib. A B

23 **Intrapulmonary blood vessels.** Blood vessels within the lung. There are two systems of vascular supply that anastomose in the periphery of the lungs: the vasa publica, i.e., the pulmonary arteries and veins; and the vasa privata, i.e., the bronchial vessels.

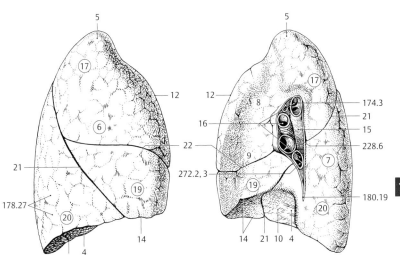

A Right lung, lateral view

B Right lung, medial view

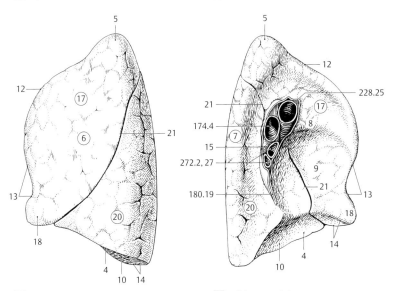

C Left lung, lateral view

D Left lung, medial view

1 **Bronchopulmonary segments.** Lung segments that are bounded from each other peripherally by veins and connective-tissue tracts and that have their own central bronchial and arterial supply. A B

2 **Right lung, superior lobe.** A

3 *Apical segment (S I).* Its inferior part is wedged between the anterior and posterior segments. A

4 *Posterior segment (S II).* Dorsal segment that lies between the apical segment and the inferior lobe of right lung. A

5 *Anterior segment (S III).* Anterior segment located between the apical segment and the middle lobe. A

6 **Right lung, middle lobe.** A

7 *Lateral segment (S IV).* Segment that consists of the dorsal part of the middle lobe and does not reach the hilum. A

8 *Medial segment (S V).* Segment that forms the mediastinal and diaphragmatic surfaces of the middle lobe. A

9 **Right lung, inferior lobe.** A

10 *Superior segment (S VI).* Apical, posterosuperior segment of the inferior lobe. A

11 *Medial basal segment (S VII).* It does not extend to the lateral surface of the lung and is only visible from the medial and inferior surface. A

12 *Anterior basal segment (S VIII).* Segment located between the middle lobe and diaphragm. A

13 *Lateral basal segment (S IX).* Segment located between the posterior and anterior basal segments. A

14 *Posterior basal segment (S X).* Segment located between the vertebral column and lateral basal segment. A

15 **Left lung, superior lobe.** B

16 *Apicoposterior segment (S I + II).* It is composed of two segments that together form a wedge-shaped segment situated between the oblique fissure and anterior segment of the superior lobe. B

17 *Anterior segment (S III).* Anterior segment of the superior lobe that is located between the superior lingular and apicoposterior segments. B

18 *Superior lingular segment (S IV).* It mainly lies on the inferior lingular segment. B

19 *Inferior lingular segment (S V).* It lies between the superior lingular segment and the oblique fissure. B

20 **Left lung, inferior lobe.** B

21 *Superior segment (S VI).* Posterosuperior apical segment of the inferior lobe adjacent to the vertebral column. B

22 *Medial basal segment (S VII).* Often indivisible from the anterior basal segment. B

23 *Anterior basal segment (S VIII).* Segment between the oblique fissure and lateral basal segment. B

24 *Lateral basal segment (S IX).* Segment between the anterior and posterior basal segments. B

25 *Posterior basal segment (S X).* Segment adjacent to the vertebral column below the superior segment of the inferior lobe. B

26 **Bronchioles.** Noncartilaginous segments of the bronchial tree that diverge from the small bronchi and extend to the alveolar ducts. Their lining of simple, ciliated, columnar epithelium transitions into cuboidal epithelium.

27 **Lobule.** Area supplied by a bronchiolus, visible as a polygonal region on the surface of the lung. p. 177 A

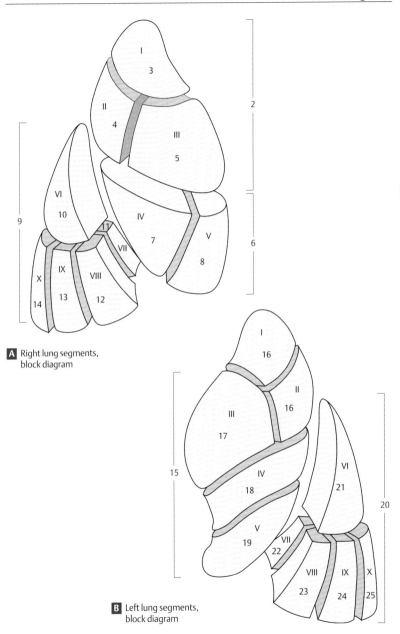

A Right lung segments, block diagram

B Left lung segments, block diagram

7

1   *THORACIC CAVITY; THORAX.* Space inside the thoracic cage enclosed within the ribs and bounded inferiorly by the diaphragm. A B

2   PLEURAL CAVITY. Slitlike space between the parietal and visceral pleura containing a capillary layer and a small amount of serous fluid. A B

3   PLEURA. Serous coat composed of simple serous epithelial cells (mesothelium) and underlying connective tissue. It consists of two sheets that are continuous at the hilum of lung. A

4   **Visceral pleura; Pulmonary pleura.** Part of the pleura that invests the lung and passes into the interlobar spaces. A B

5   *Serosa; Serous coat.* Lining that consists of collagenous fibers and networks of elastic fibers covered with mesothelium.

6   *Subserosa; Subserous layer.* Connective tissue underlying the serous coat containing blood and lymph vessels.

7   **Parietal pleura.** Serous lining of the spaces containing the lungs. A B

8   *Cervical pleura; Dome of pleura; Pleural cupula.* Part of the parietal pleura over the apex of lung at the superior thoracic aperture. A

9   *Costal part.* Part of the parietal pleura that lies on the inner surface of the thoracic wall. A B

10 *Diaphragmatic part.* Part of the parietal pleura that covers the surface of the diaphragm. A

11 *Mediastinal part.* Part of the parietal pleura that lines the mediastinal surfaces of the lung. A B

12 *Serosa; Serous coat.* It is covered with mesothelium. Its connective-tissue layer varies between the costal and diaphragmatic parts, the former having abundant collagenous fibers, and the latter abundant networks of elastic fibers.

13 *Subserosa; Subserous layer.* Connective tissue containing fat as well as blood and lymph vessels.

14 **Pleural recesses.** Cavity-like pockets in the parietal pleura that form additional spaces into which the lungs can expand during inspiration.

15 *Costodiaphragmatic recess.* Pleural recess between the downward-sloping sides of the diaphragm and the lateral wall of the thorax. A

16 *Costomediastinal recess.* Anterior and posterior pleural recess between the costal and mediastinal parts of the pleura. It is larger on the left than on the right. B

17 *Phrenicomediastinal recess.* Dorsal pleural recess between the diaphragm and mediastinum.

18 *Vertebromediastinal recess.* Recess that begins at the costomediastinal recess behind the esophagus. It is also considered a postmortem appearance. B

19 **Pulmonary ligament.** Double fold of pulmonary pleura that passes inferiorly from the right and left sides of the hilum to the mediastinal pleura. Between the two folds, the lung is in contact with the mediastinal connective tissue without a pleural covering. A, p. 177 B D

20 **Endothoracic fascia; Parietal fascia of thorax.** Sliding layer of loose connective tissue between the parietal pleura and the thoracic wall. It represents the continuation of the deep cervical fascia in the thoracic cage. A

21 *Suprapleural membrane.* Thickened portion of the endothoracic fascia at the pleural cupula. A

22 *Phrenicopleural fascia.* Thickened portion of the endothoracic fascia below the diaphragmatic part of parietal pleura. A

23 **Mediastinum.** Part of the thorax between the two pleural sacs. It extends from the anterior surface of the vertebral column to the posterior surface of the sternum and from the superior thoracic aperture to the diaphragm. Its connective tissue is continuous with the cervical connective tissue and it communicates with the abdominal cavity via openings in the diaphragm. A

24 **Superior mediastinum.** Part located above the heart and in the horizontal plane of the sternal angle. It is a structure that gives passage, e.g., to the aortic arch and its branches as well as brachiocephalic veins, superior vena cava, trachea, esophagus, vagus nerves, and thoracic duct. A

25 **Inferior mediastinum.** Collective term for the following three parts.

26 *Anterior mediastinum.* Space between the pericardium and sternum. B

27 *Middle mediastinum.* Space occupied by the heart, pericardium, and phrenic nerves and accompanying vessels. The heart and pericardium displace the lung and pleura asymmetrically to the left. B

28 *Posterior mediastinum.* Space between the pericardium and vertebral column containing the esophagus, vagus nerves, descending aorta, thoracic duct, and azygos and hemiazygos veins. B

29 [[Thymic triangle]]. Pleural boundary between the superior mediastinum and anterior thoracic wall that is shaped like an inverted triangle and contains the thymus. C

30 [[Pericardial triangle]]. Anterior mediastinum posterior to the anterior thoracic wall that is occupied by the heart and pericardium. It does not contain pleura and is shaped like an upright triangle. C

7

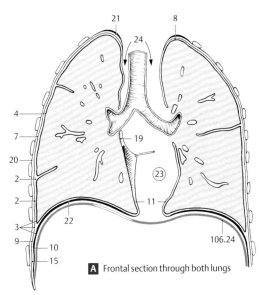

A Frontal section through both lungs

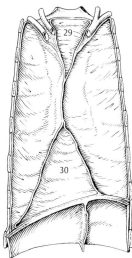

C Anterior thoracic wall,
internal surface

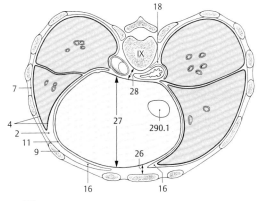

B Horizontal section at the level of T9, inferior view

1   *URINARY SYSTEM.*

2   **KIDNEY.**

3   **Lateral border.** Convex lateral margin of the kidney. A

4   **Medial border.** Medial margin of the kidney with a concave indentation at the hilum. A

5   *Hilum of kidney.* Site of entry and exit of vessels and nerves. The renal pelvis is located here. A

6   *Renal sinus.* Elongated oval indentation in the parenchyma on the medial border of the kidney for the hilum. B D E

7   **Anterior surface.** Highly convex anterior kidney surface. A D

8   **Posterior surface.** Nearly flat posterior kidney surface. B D

9   **Superior pole of kidney; Superior extremity of kidney.** A B

10 **Inferior pole of kidney; Inferior extremity of kidney.** A B

11 **Renal fascia.** Fibrous tissue sheath surrounding the kidney, suprarenal gland, and perirenal fat capsule. It is open medially and inferiorly, allowing access to the hilum of kidney. D

12 *Paranephric fat; Pararenal fat body.* Adipose body between the posterior layer of renal fascia and the transversalis fascia. D

13 **Perinephric fat; Perirenal fat capsule.** Capsule enclosing the kidney and suprarenal gland. Its size depends on nutritional status. D

14 **Fibrous capsule.** Tough fibrous capsule of kidney which is fused with its surface. It can be stripped off. D E

15 **Kidney lobes.** Lobes indicated by furrows in the kidney surface, especially in newborns. Each one is formed by a renal pyramid and its overlying renal cortex.

16 **Renal cortex.** Strip of renal tissue about 6–10 mm wide located beneath the fibrous capsule. It consists of the cortical labyrinth and the medullary rays. C E

17 *Cortical labyrinth.* It mainly consists of renal corpuscles (malpighian corpuscles) and the convoluted renal tubules. E

18 *Cortex corticis.* Part of the labyrinth between the tips of the medullary rays and the capsule. E

19 *Medullary rays.* Medullary components that radiate in bandlike fashion into the renal cortex but do not extend to the capsule. They contain mainly straight parts of the renal tubules and cortical collecting ducts. E

20 **Renal columns.** (Bertin's columns). Part of the labyrinth that encloses the medullary pyramids up to the renal sinus. E

21 **Renal tubule.** Canal system consisting of convoluted and straight segments that belongs to a nephron, the basic unit of the kidney. It begins at the urinary pole and opens via the junctional tubule into a collecting duct.

22 *Proximal convoluted tubule.* Tortuous segment of the proximal tubule. It begins at the urinary pole. C

23 *Proximal straight tubule.* Straight descending limb of the proximal tubule. C

24 *Descending/Ascending thin limb.* Narrow-caliber section between the proximal and distal straight tubule. Narrow part of the loop of Henle. It is supplemented by the straight parts of the proximal and distal tubule. C

25 *Thick ascending limb.* Straight, ascending segment of the distal tubule. C

26 *Distal convoluted tubule.* Tortuous segment of the distal tubule that leads through the junctional tubule into a collecting duct. C

27 **Collecting duct.** Not part of the nephron in terms of embryonic origin. C

28 **Renal medulla.** It contains most of the straight segments of the renal tubules, collecting ducts, and medullary vessels. It can be divided into zones.

29 *Outer zone.* Zone formed by the straight section of the renal tubules and three types of nephrons with variously long loops. It can be divided into two stripes. C

30 *Outer stripe.* Part formed by the straight parts of proximal and distal renal tubules, collecting ducts, and vessel segments. C, p. 185 E

31 *Inner stripe.* Part consisting of thin descending and thick ascending limbs of nephron loops, collecting ducts, and vessel segments. C, p. 185 E

32 Vascular bundles. Bundles of straight arterioles and venules in the renal medulla. p. 185 E

33 Interbundle region. Space in the renal medulla between the fascicles and site of a capillary plexus. It is fed by the descending straight arterioles and gives rise to the ascending straight venules. p. 185 E

34 *Inner zone.* Zone containing thin loops of juxtamedullary renal corpuscles, wide-caliber collecting ducts, and narrow vascular bundles. C, p. 185 E

35 *Renal papilla.* Rounded tip of a renal pyramid projecting into a renal calyx. E

36 *Renal crest.* Adjacent medullary areas fuse during development, forming united papillae that open from a bundle of tips into the calyx. E

37 *Renal pyramids.* Six to twenty renal pyramids separated by the renal columns. They form the medullary substance. E

38 *Cribriform area.* Surface of the renal papillae with sievelike perforations produced by the opening of the uriniferous tubules. E

39 Openings of papillary ducts. Openings of the uriniferous tubules in the cribriform area. C

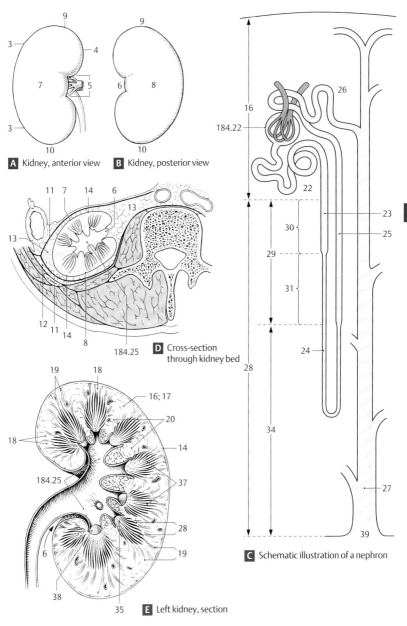

A Kidney, anterior view

B Kidney, posterior view

D Cross-section through kidney bed

C Schematic illustration of a nephron

E Left kidney, section

1 **Renal segments.** Subdivisions of the kidney that correspond to areas supplied by arterial branches.

2 **Superior segment.** Upper segment that extends to the posterior surface of kidney. A B

3 **Anterior superior segment.** A

4 **Anterior inferior segment.** A

5 **Inferior segment.** Lower segment that extends to the anterior and posterior surfaces of kidney. A B

6 **Posterior segment.** B

7 **Intrarenal arteries.**

8 **Interlobar arteries.** Arteries ascending alongside each renal column to the corticomedullary border. E

9 **Arcuate arteries.** Curved arteries arising from the interlobar arteries along the corticomedullary border. E

10 *Cortical radiate arteries; Interlobular arteries.* Branches of the arcuate arteries radiating between medullary rays. E

11 *Afferent glomerular arteriole.* Arteriole originating from an interlobular artery. It passes to the vascular pole of a renal corpuscle where it divides to form a series of capillary loops known as a glomerulus. E

12 *Efferent glomerular arteriole.* Arteriole that leaves the vascular pole of a renal corpuscle. It arises from glomerulus capillaries. E

13 **Perforating radiate arteries.** Branches of the interlobular arteries that lead to the kidney surface. They anastomose with the capsular branches of renal artery. E

14 **Vasa recta; Straight arterioles.** Straight arterioles that extend into the renal medulla from the efferent glomerular arterioles of juxtamedullary renal corpuscle. E

15 **Capsular branches.** Tapering interlobular arteries that, together with branches from the renal artery, form a capillary network in the fibrous capsule. E

16 **Intrarenal veins.**

17 **Interlobar veins.** Veins corresponding to the interlobar arteries. E

18 **Arcuate veins.** Curved veins corresponding to the arcuate arteries that run along the corticomedullary border. E

19 *Cortical radiate veins; Interlobular veins.* Lobular veins corresponding to the interlobular arteries. E

20 **Venulae rectae; Straight venules.** Veins corresponding to the straight arterioles. They drain the capillary plexus of the renal medulla into the interlobular or arcuate veins. E

21 **Stellate veins.** Star-shaped initial segments of the cortical veins beneath the fibrous capsule which drain the superficial renal cortex. E

22 [[**Renal corpuscle**]]. (Malpighian corpuscle). Measuring around 0.25 mm, it is still visible to the naked eye. It consists of two basic structures. p. 183 C

23 *[[Glomerulus]].* Network of anastomosing capillary loops that receive blood via the afferent glomerular arteriole from the urinary pole and convey it via the efferent glomerular arteriole to the vascular pole. E, p. 183 C

24 *[[Glomerular capsule]] [[Bowman capsule]].* Cup-shaped epithelial structure that surrounds the glomerulus up to the vascular pole. It collects ultrafiltrate, which then flows through its floor via the urinary pole to the tubular system. p. 183 C

25 **Renal pelvis.** Funnel-shaped beginning of the urinary excretory duct that is lodged in the renal sinus. It passes into the ureter at the hilum. C D

26 **Branching type.** Tubular renal pelvis into which the three long tubes formed by the major calices open. C

27 *Major calices.* Three large renal calices that are formed by up to 14 minor calices and drain into the respective regions of the kidney.

28 *Superior calyx.* C D

29 *Middle calyx.* C D

30 *Inferior calyx.* C D

31 *Minor calices.* Calices enclosing the tips of the renal papillae. The margin of the calyx is fused with the papillae. The minor calices unite to form the three major calices. C D

32 [**Ampullary type**.] Inconstant form of the renal pelvis. In this type, the minor calices also open into the renal pelvis, forming a large-volume pelvis. D

33 **Adventitia.** Superficial connective tissue that integrates the renal pelvis into the surrounding adipose tissue.

34 **Muscular layer; Muscular coat.** The muscular coat is composed of an inner layer of longitudinal cells and an outer layer of more spirally oriented smooth-muscle cells. They form sphincter-like reinforcements around the margins of the calices and the exit of the ureter.

35 **Mucosa; Mucous membrane.** Mucous membrane of the kidney with transitional epithelium.

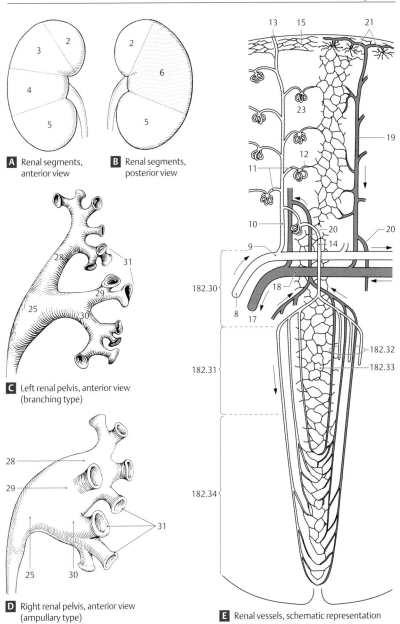

A Renal segments, anterior view

B Renal segments, posterior view

C Left renal pelvis, anterior view (branching type)

D Right renal pelvis, anterior view (ampullary type)

E Renal vessels, schematic representation

8

1 **URETER.** Urinary duct situated in the retroperitoneum. It connects the renal pelvis with the urinary bladder, measures 25–30 cm in length and is about 3 mm thick. A B

2 **Abdominal part.** Part of the ureter located in the abdominal cavity, extending from the renal pelvis to the linea terminalis. During its course it runs on the fascia of the psoas muscle and posterior to the ovarian or testicular vessels. A

3 **Pelvic part.** Part of the ureter located in the pelvis, extending from the linea terminalis to the urinary bladder. At the pelvic inlet it lies in front of the divergence of the common iliac vessels and, in the male lesser pelvis, below the ductus deferens; in the female lesser pelvis below the uterine artery. A

4 **Intramural part.** Part of the ureter located in the wall of the urinary bladder. It is about 2 cm long and runs anteriorly from superolateral to inferomedial. A

5 **Adventitia.** Connective-tissue sheath surrounding the ureter and connecting it to the surrounding structures while allowing for movement. B

6 **Muscular layer; Muscular coat.** Muscular coat in the wall of the ureter. The smooth-muscle cells are arranged in spiral fashion. Due to alternating gradient angles it appears to have two layers (abdomen) or three layers (pelvis). B

7 **Mucosa; Mucous membrane.** The mucous membrane is lined with transitional epithelium. B

8 **URINARY BLADDER.** Organ located beneath the peritoneum in the lesser pelvis posterior to the pubic symphysis. Its size varies depending on fullness, with the urge to evacuate the bladder occurring at about 350 ml. Even at maximum distension it remains below the level of the navel. C D

9 **Apex of bladder.** Tip of the bladder pointing anterosuperiorly and attached to the anterior abdominal wall by the median umbilical ligament. D

10 **Median umbilical ligament.** Remnant of the obliterated allantois in the median umbilical fold. D

11 **Body of bladder.** Part of the bladder between the apex and fundus resting against the peritoneal cavity. D

12 **Fundus of bladder.** Part of the bladder that rests against the pelvic floor and is attached to its subperitoneal connective tissue. It tapers off into the neck of bladder. The ureters open into its posterior wall. D

13 **Neck of bladder.** Part of the bladder from which the urethra emerges. D

14 **Serosa; Serous coat.** Peritoneal covering that mostly surrounds the body of bladder.

15 **Subserosa; Subserous layer.** Layer of connective tissue underlying the peritoneal covering.

16 **Muscular layer; Muscular coat.** The muscular coat of the urinary bladder mainly consists of interwoven bundles of smooth-muscle cells that conform to the degree of its distension. In the trigone region muscle fibers from the urinary bladder overlap with those of the ureter. C D

17 *Trigonal muscles.* Muscles of the trigone of bladder that actively close the opening to the ureter before urination. C D

18 *Superficial trigone.* Continuation of the inner layer of longitudinal muscle of the ureter. Muscle cells from the left and right converge to form a triangular sheet at the trigone of bladder, the apex of which continues into the posterior wall of the urethra, in the male extending to the seminal colliculus. C

19 *Deep trigone.* Continuation of the outer layer of longitudinal muscle of the ureter. It is nearly completely congruent with the overlying superficial trigone. Its apex extends to the opening of the urethra. It also underlies the interureteric crest and is firmly attached to the detrusor. C

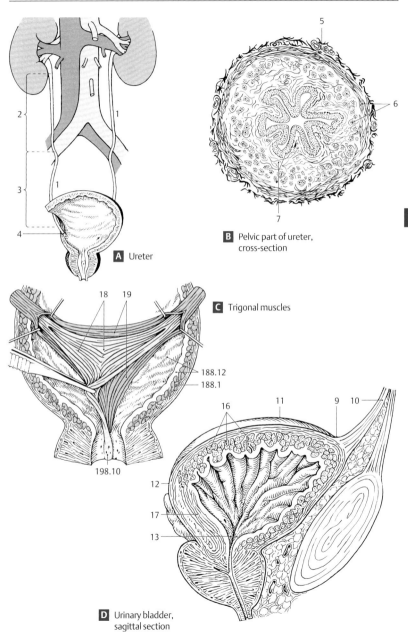

A Ureter

B Pelvic part of ureter, cross-section

C Trigonal muscles

188.12
188.1

198.10

D Urinary bladder, sagittal section

8

1 *Detrusor.* Muscle forming the wall of the urinary bladder excepting the trigone of bladder. It is formed by two differently structured parts that are produced by the spiral arrangement of the cells with alternating gradient angles.

2 *Unstratified part.* Part of the muscle above the neck of bladder. Its muscle cells form a meshwork that is most pronounced at the apex of bladder. B

3 *Bladder neck part.* This part can be divided schematically into three layers:

4 External longitudinal layer. Outer layer of longitudinal muscle cells in the posterior wall of the urinary bladder that loop around the neck of bladder and urethra from anterior. In the male they form a ca. 1 cm wide prepostatic sphincter muscle before continuing to the prostate and its capsule. In the female the muscle cells extend longitudinally and obliquely into the urethra. A

5 Circular layer. Circular muscle layer ending above the neck of bladder. It does not extend to the internal urethral orifice. A

6 Internal longitudinal layer. Inner bundles of longitudinal muscle that run in the ventral part of the neck of bladder. They converge at the internal urethral orifice where they loop around the urethra from behind. A

7 *Pubovesicalis.* Smooth-muscle cells between the posterior wall of the neck of bladder and the pubic symphysis. They can also be viewed as cells given off by the internal longitudinal layer. C

8 *Rectovesicalis.* Smooth-muscle cells extending between the anterior wall of the neck of bladder and the longitudinal layer in the wall of the rectum. They can also be considered fibers given off by the external longitudinal layer. C, p. 153 D

9 *Vesicoprostaticus.* Smooth-muscle cells that pass between the urinary bladder and prostate.

10 *Vesicovaginalis.* Smooth-muscle cells that pass between the urinary bladder and the vagina.

11 **Submucosa.** Easily movable connective-tissue layer underlying the mucosa. It is absent in the trigone of bladder.

12 **Mucosa; Mucous membrane.** The mucous membrane is lined with transitional epithelium.

13 **Trigone of bladder.** Triangular area between the openings of the ureters and the exit site of the urethra, with underlying ureter musculature. It is firmly attached to the mucous membrane and hence does not have any folds. A B

14 *Interureteric crest.* Transverse mucosal fold that forms the posterior boundary of the trigone of bladder. B

15 *[[Fossa retroureterica]].* Transverse depression behind the interureteric crest. It is especially deep in the elderly. Deepest point in the urinary bladder in erect standing posture. Residual urine can accumulate here. B

16 *Ureteric orifice.* Slitlike opening of the ureter. B

17 **Uvula of bladder.** Longitudinally oriented prominence on the tip of the trigone of bladder, produced by a venous plexus beneath the mucous membrane in the posterior wall of the urethral orifice. B

18 *Internal urethral orifice.* Opening to the urethra from the urinary bladder. Due to invagination of the uvula of bladder, its ventral aspect appears convex in cross-section. A

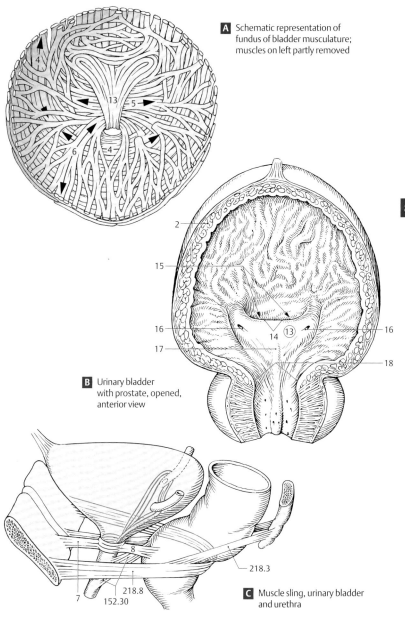

A Schematic representation of fundus of bladder musculature; muscles on left partly removed

B Urinary bladder with prostate, opened, anterior view

C Muscle sling, urinary bladder and urethra

8

1 *GENITAL SYSTEMS.*

2 *MALE GENITAL SYSTEM.*

3 *FEMALE GENITAL SYSTEM.*

4 *MALE INTERNAL GENITALIA.*

5 **TESTIS.** About 5 cm long.

6 **Upper pole of testis; Superior pole of testis.** B

7 **Lower pole of testis; Inferior pole of testis.** B

8 **Lateral surface of testis.** Flattened, lateral-facing surface of the testis. B

9 **Medial surface of testis.** Flattened, medial-facing surface of the testis.

10 **Anterior border.** Free anterior margin of the testis. B

11 **Posterior border.** Posterior margin of the testis, attached to a fold of the serous membrane. B

12 **[[Vaginal process of peritoneum]].** Embryonic peritoneal diverticulum that protrudes through the inguinal canal into the genital torus. The testis descends along its posterior aspect out of the abdominal cavity.

13 **Tunica vaginalis.** Serous covering of the testis. Vestige of the vaginal process of the peritoneum. It consists of the following layers. A

14 *Parietal layer.* Layer that lines the inner surface of the tunica vaginalis and is reflected on the visceral layer at the posterior border of the epididymis and mediastinum of testis. A

15 *Visceral layer.* Layer lying on the tunica albuginea and epididymis. It does not cover the mediastinum of testis. A

16 *Superior ligament of epididymis.* Upper reflection of the tunica vaginalis. A

17 *Inferior ligament of epididymis.* Lower reflection of the tunica vaginalis. A

18 *Sinus of epididymis.* Cleft in the tunica vaginalis between the testis and epididymis that can be accessed from lateral. A

19 *Serosa; Serous coat.* Visceral layer of the tunica vaginalis. It does not have its own subserous layer and cannot be dissected.

20 *Subserosa; subserous layer.* Connective-tissue layer partly consisting of smooth-muscle cells. It underlies the squamous epithelium of the parietal layer and the layer can be dissected.

21 **Tunica albuginea.** Tough connective-tissue capsule surrounding the parenchyma of testis. B

22 **Vascular layer.** Layer surrounding the testis beneath the visceral layer of tunica vaginalis. Blood vessels pass from here through the tunica albuginea into the septa, giving off recurrent vessels to the parenchyma of testis. Veins convey blood from the mediastinum of testis to the pampiniform venous plexus. E

23 **Mediastinum of testis.** Connective tissue protruding from the tunica albuginea into the interior of the testis. B

24 **Septa testis.** Connective tissue partitions between the mediastinum of testis and the tunica albuginea. B C

25 **Lobules of testis.** Lobules that are bounded by the septa testis. B C

26 **Parenchyma of testis.** Specific tissue of the testis comprising the seminiferous tubules. B

27 **Seminiferous tubules; Convoluted seminiferous tubules.** Convoluted seminiferous tubules that form the lobules of testis. C

28 **Straight tubules.** Short transition between the convoluted seminiferous tubules and the rete testis. C

29 **Rete testis.** Network of canals in the mediastinum of testis between the straight tubules and efferent ductules. They are lined with simple cuboidal epithelium. C

30 **Efferent ductules.** Ten to twenty small ducts between the rete testis and the duct of epididymis. B C

31 **EPIDIDYMIS.** Lying on the posteromedial surface of the mediastinum of testis, it serves to store spermatozoa. B D

32 **Head of epididymis.** Part of the epididymis formed by the efferent ductules. D

33 *Lobules of epididymis; Conical lobules of epididymis.* Lobules divided by connective-tissue septa, each of which consists of a coiled, conical efferent ductule of testis. D

34 **Body of epididymis.** Middle part of the epididymis comprising the convolutions of the duct of epididymis. D

35 **Tail of epididymis.** Lower part of the duct of epididymis. D

36 **Duct of epididymis.** Duct that begins at the end of the head of epididymis and passes into the ductus deferens. Uncoiled it measures 5–6 m. D

37 **Aberrant ductules of epididymis.** Vestiges of the caudal mesonephric ducts.

38 *[Superior aberrant ductule].* Upper aberrant ductule at the head of epididymis.

39 *[Inferior aberrant ductule].* Lower aberrant ductule at the tail of epididymis. D

40 *Appendix of testis.* Vesicular appendage of the testis. D

41 *[Appendix of epididymis].* Stalked vesicular appendix at the head of epididymis. D

42 **[PARADIDYMIS].** Remnants of the mesonephric ducts above the head of epididymis in front of the spermatic cord. D

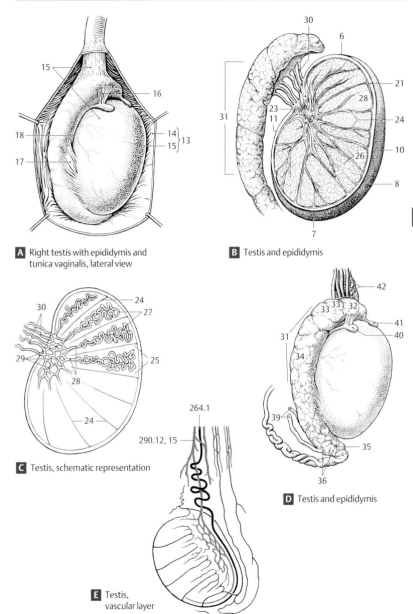

A Right testis with epididymis and tunica vaginalis, lateral view

B Testis and epididymis

C Testis, schematic representation

D Testis and epididymis

E Testis, vascular layer

8

1 **SPERMATIC CORD.** It consists of the ductus deferens, its accompanying vessels, nerves and connective tissues, as well as coverings. A

2 **External spermatic fascia.** Continuation of the superficial fascia of the abdominal wall and the aponeurosis of the external oblique muscle of the abdomen as an outer sheath covering the testes, epididymis, and ductus deferens. A

3 **Cremaster.** Muscle that is mainly derived from the internal oblique abdominal muscle and acts to elevate the testes. A

4 **Cremasteric fascia.** Fascia that surrounds and accompanies the cremaster muscle. It is composed of portions of the fascia of the internal oblique muscle of the abdomen and the transverse abdominal muscle. A

5 **Internal spermatic fascia.** Projection from the transversalis fascia through the inguinal canal that encloses the spermatic cord, epididymis, and testes. A

6 **[Vestige of processus vaginalis].** Partly obliterated remnant of the embryonic vaginal process of the peritoneum. A

7 **DUCTUS DEFERENS; VAS DEFERENS.** The course of the ca. 50 cm long ductus deferens is initially tortuous, then becomes straight. It is a continuation of the duct of epididymis, opening into the urethra. A B C

8 **Scrotal part.** Part of the ductus deferens that passes in the scrotum along the epididymis. A C

9 **Funicular part.** Part of the ductus deferens in the spermatic cord. A C

10 **Inguinal part.** Part of the ductus deferens in the inguinal canal. C

11 **Pelvic part.** Part of the ductus deferens that passes in the lesser pelvis in the retroperitoneum along the lateral wall. C

12 **Ampulla of ductus deferens.** Longitudinal expansion at the fundus of bladder. B C

13 *Diverticula of ampulla.* Lateral outpouchings within the ampulla of ductus deferens. B

14 **Adventitia.** Outer layer of connective tissue surrounding the ductus deferens. E

15 **Muscular layer; Muscular coat.** Muscular coat of the ductus deferens that has three layers in cross-section. The layered appearance is produced by the spiral course of the muscle cell bundles with varying gradient angles. E

16 **Mucosa; Mucous membrane.** The mucous membrane forms longitudinal folds that serve as reservoirs. Its lining contains stereociliated epithelium. E

17 **[[Descent of testis]].** In the final weeks of gestation, the testis normally passes out of the abdominal cavity through the inguinal canal into the scrotum.

18 **[[Gubernaculum testis]].** Connective-tissue band present during fetal development that is derived from the caudal gonadal fold and is involved in testicular descent.

19 **SEMINAL GLAND; SEMINAL VESICLE.** Thin-walled coiled tube about 5 cm in length. B

20 **Adventitia.** Outer layer of connective tissue that fixes the convolutions of the seminal vesicle and attaches it to the fundus of bladder. B

21 **Muscular layer; Muscular coat.** Spirally arranged muscle cell bundles that intersect to form a reticular pattern. D

22 **Mucosa; Mucous membrane.** It is loculated and lined with secretory epithelium. D

23 **Excretory duct.** Duct that opens into the ductus deferens. B

24 **Ejaculatory duct.** Last segment of the ductus deferens, located within the prostate, narrowing similarly to a nozzle. B

8

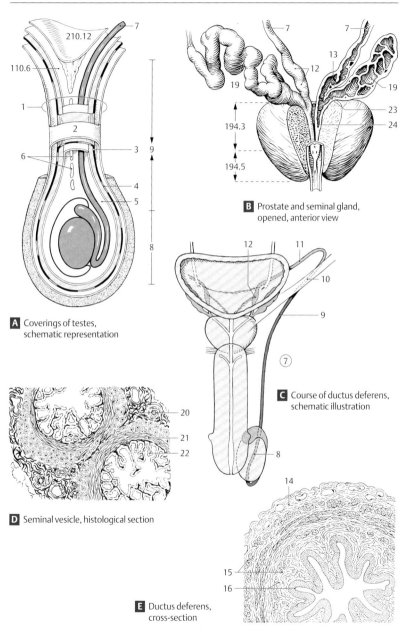

A Coverings of testes, schematic representation

B Prostate and seminal gland, opened, anterior view

C Course of ductus deferens, schematic illustration

D Seminal vesicle, histological section

E Ductus deferens, cross-section

1 **PROSTATE.** Chestnut-sized tubuloalveolar gland below the urinary bladder and having a smooth surface. It surrounds the urethra. A

2 **Base of prostate.** Part of the gland that is fused with the fundus of bladder. A

3 **Proximal part.** Palpable posterosuperior part above the opening to the ejaculatory duct. p. 193 B

4 **Peri-urethral gland zone.** Zone immediately surrounding the urethra in the proximal part of prostate. A

5 **Distal part.** Palpable posteroinferior part of the prostate below the openings of the ejaculatory duct. A, p. 193 B

6 **Apex of prostate.** Anteroinferiorly directed tip of the prostate that surrounds the urethra, close to the superficial transverse perineal muscle. A

7 **Anterior surface.** Surface of the prostate facing the pubic symphysis. A

8 **Posterior surface.** Surface of the prostate facing the rectum. A

9 **Inferolateral surface.** Surface of the prostate facing inferolaterally.

10 **Right and left lobes of prostate.** Separated by a longitudinal furrow, the prostate lobes can be palpated from posteriorly. They can be divided into four lobules each.

11 *Inferoposterior lobule.* Lower posterior lobule. A B

12 *Inferolateral lobule.* Lower lateral lobule. B

13 *Superomedial lobule.* Lobule surrounding the ejaculatory duct. A B

14 *Anteromedial lobule.* Lobule that borders laterally with the proximal urethra. B

15 *[Middle lobe].* Superomedial and anteromedial lobes arise from a middle lobe during development. It tends to undergo hormone-induced hypertrophy in the elderly and can close off the internal urethral orifice like a valve.

16 **Isthmus of prostate; Commissure of prostate.** Anterior connection between the two anteromedial lobules composed of connective tissue and muscle. Glandular elements are seldom present. A B

17 **Capsule of prostate.** Capsule containing smooth-muscle cells surrounding the prostate and firmly attached to it. B

18 **Parenchyma.** Glandular part of the prostate.

19 **Prostatic ducts.** Fifteen to thirty excretory ducts that open into the prostatic urethra. C

20 **Muscular tissue.** Smooth-muscle cells located between the prostatic ducts. C

21 **Trapezoid area.** Area visible on ultrasound between the inferior border of the prostate and the anorectal flexure where the prostate and colon are in contact. p. 217 B

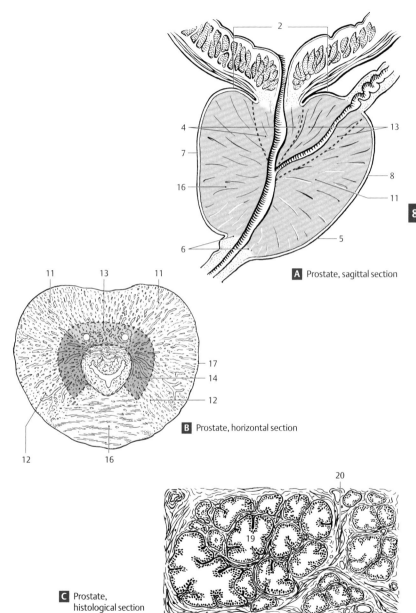

A Prostate, sagittal section

B Prostate, horizontal section

C Prostate,
histological section

8

1 **BULBOURETHRAL GLAND (COWPER'S GLAND).** Pea-sized mucous gland on the posterior end of the bulb of penis at the level of the deep transverse perineal muscle. D

2 **Duct of bulbourethral gland.** The 3–4 cm long excretory duct. D

3 *MALE EXTERNAL GENITALIA.*

4 **PENIS.** Male genital organ consisting of the corpora cavernosa and the male urethra. D

5 **Root of penis.** Part that is attached to the pubis. D

6 **Body of penis.** Shaft situated between the glans and root of penis. D

7 **Crus of penis.** Projection from the corpus cavernosum of penis attached to the inferior pubic ramus. D

8 **Dorsum of penis.** Flattened superior aspect of the penis.

9 **Urethral surface.** Inferior aspect of the penis, along which the male urethra travels through the corpus spongiosum. D

10 **Glans penis.** Enlarged end of the corpus spongiosum of penis. A D

11 *Corona of glans.* Posterior border of the glans penis. A D

12 *Septum of glans.* Partition in the median plane of the glans penis. C

13 *Neck of glans.* Groove behind the corona of glans. A

14 **Prepuce; Foreskin.** Double fold of skin over the glans penis. A

15 *Frenulum of prepuce.* Fold that extends from the foreskin to the inferior aspect of the glans penis. A

16 **Raphe of penis.** Seam on the skin of the inferior surface of the penis that forms during development. B

17 **Corpus cavernosum penis.** Cavernous body that is divided into two halves by the septum penis. A B D

18 **Corpus spongiosum penis.** Cavernous body surrounding the male urethra. A B D

19 *Bulb of penis.* Posterior, thickened end of the corpus spongiosum. D

20 **Tunica albuginea of corpora cavernosa.** Tough connective-tissue sheath consisting of collagen fibers with elastic fiber networks that surrounds the corpus cavernosum. B

21 **Tunica albuginea of corpus spongiosum.** More delicate connective-tissue sheath surrounding the corpus spongiosum. It is mainly composed of an inner circular fiber layer.

22 **Septum penis.** Partition with spaces giving it a pectinate form which divides the right and left corpus cavernosum. It arises from the tunica albuginea. B

23 **Trabeculae of corpora cavernosa.** Connective tissue permeated by smooth-muscle cells in the corpus cavernosum. A B

24 **Trabeculae of corpus spongiosum.** Connective tissue permeated by smooth-muscle cells in the corpus spongiosum. B

25 **Cavernous spaces of corpora cavernosa.** Coarsely meshed, blood-filled, endothelium-lined spaces in the corpus cavernosum. B

26 **Cavernous spaces of corpus spongiosum.** Blood-filled, finely-meshed spongy tissue in the corpus spongiosum. A B

27 **Helicine arteries.** Spiral branches of the deep artery of penis.

28 **Cavernous veins.** Dilated vessels in the cavernous bodies.

29 **Fascia of penis.** Thick fascia that ensheathes the three cavernous bodies and divides the superficial and deep dorsal veins of penis. B

30 **Subcutaneous tissue of penis.** Loose connective tissue containing solitary smooth-muscle cells. It corresponds to the dartos fascia of the scrotum. D

31 **Preputial glands.** Sebaceous glands located mainly on the corona of glans.

8

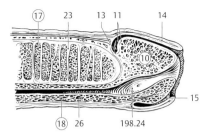

A End of penis, median section

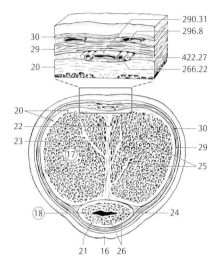

B Penis, cross-section

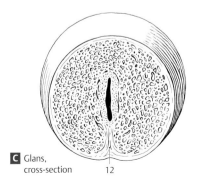

C Glans,
cross-section

D Penis, inferior view

8

1 MALE URETHRA. B

2 **Internal urethral orifice; Internal urinary meatus.** Internal urethral orifice at the anterior tip of the trigone of bladder. The shape of the opening depends on how full the urinary bladder is. A, p. 189 B

3 *Filling internal urethral orifice.* The closed orifice forms a flat sheet together with surrounding structures as the urinary bladder fills. The urethra is long.

4 *Emptying internal urethral orifice.* The urinary bladder descends as the pelvic floor becomes lax. The neck of bladder retracts like a funnel into the male urethra, which appears shortened.

5 **Intramural part; Preprostatic part.** Part of the male urethra located in the muscular wall of the urinary bladder. A B

6 **Prostatic urethra.** Part of the male urethra that passes through the prostate. B

7 *Proximal part.* Part of the male urethra above the seminal colliculus.

8 *Distal part.* Part of the male urethra below the seminal colliculus.

9 *Urethral crest.* Mucosal fold in the posterior wall of the prostatic urethra that is continuous with the uvula of bladder. A

10 *Seminal colliculus.* Elevation on the urethral crest that contains the openings of the ejaculatory ducts. A

11 *Prostatic utricle.* Up to 1 cm long blind-ending sac in the seminal colliculus. It is a vestige of the paramesonephric duct (müllerian duct). A

12 *Prostatic sinus.* Groove on both sides of the seminal colliculus containing the openings of the prostatic ducts. A

13 *Muscular layer; Muscular coat.* Mostly a continuation of the muscular layer in the wall of the urinary bladder, passing over the preprostatic urethra into and onto the proximal part of prostatic urethra.

14 *Circular layer.* Elastic connective tissue interspersed with circular bundles of muscle cells.

15 *Internal urethral sphincter; Supracollicular sphincter; Preprostatic sphincter.* Thickening of the circular layer of the detrusor muscle sling around the preprostatic urethra. Contraction of the muscle prevents retrograde ejaculation into the bladder.

16 *Longitudinal layer.* Longitudinally oriented muscle cell bundles in the male urethra. Parts of the internal longitudinal layer of the urinary bladder. They probably assist in closing the prostatic ducts during urination.

17 *Mucosa; Mucous membrane.* The mucous membrane on up to half of the prostatic urethra is lined with transitional epithelium; later it is lined with pseudostratified columnar epithelium.

18 *External urethral sphincter.* Outer sphincter muscle of the male urethra consisting of transversely striated muscle fibers. Its fibers are derived from the deep transverse perineal muscle and surround most of the distal part of prostatic urethra. It is responsible for voluntary closure of the urethra.

19 **Intermediate part of urethra; Membranous urethra.** Part between the prostatic and spongy urethrae. B

20 *Muscular layer; Muscular coat.* The muscular coat consists of the continuation of bundles of muscle cells from the urinary bladder as well as superficial muscle fiber bundles from the external urethral sphincter.

21 *Longitudinal layer.* Smooth-muscle cells arising from the wall of the urinary bladder.

22 *Mucosa; Mucous membrane.* The mucous membrane is lined with pseudostratified columnar epithelium.

23 **Spongy urethra.** Part of the male urethra surrounded by the corpus spongiosum of penis. B

24 *Navicular fossa.* Elongated expansion of the male urethra before the external urethral orifice. B

25 *[Valve of navicular fossa].* Mucosal fold on the upper wall of the navicular fossa.

26 *Urethral lacunae.* Numerous pits in the mucous membrane of the male urethra that contain the openings of the urethral glands. B

27 *Urethral glands.* Small mucous glands opening into the urethral lacunae.

28 *Para-urethral ducts.* Excretory ducts alongside the urethral glands that open near the external urethral orifice.

29 *Muscular layer; Muscular coat.* Comparable to the muscular layer of the intermediate part of male urethra.

30 *Longitudinal layer.* Comparable to the longitudinal layer in the intermediate part of male urethra.

31 *Mucosa; Mucous membrane.* The mucous membrane contains the veins of the cavernous body. Nonkeratinized stratified epithelium begins at the navicular fossa; keratinized epithelium begins at the external urethral orifice.

32 **External urethral orifice; External urinary meatus.** B

33 **SCROTUM.** Sac containing the two testes and epididymides. C

34 **Raphe of scrotum.** Median line in the skin of the scrotum that forms during development. C

35 **Dartos fascia; Superficial fascia of scrotum.** Dermis of the scrotum that is interspersed with smooth-muscle cells. The dermis and smooth-muscle cells are connected by means of elastic fibers.

36 *Septum of scrotum.* Median connective-tissue septum in the scrotum. C

37 *Dartos muscle.* Smooth muscle of the scrotum. Contraction decreases its surface area, thereby reducing heat loss. C

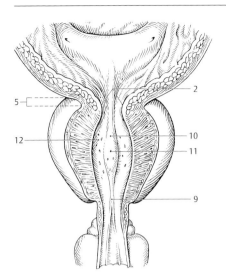

A Male urethra, section

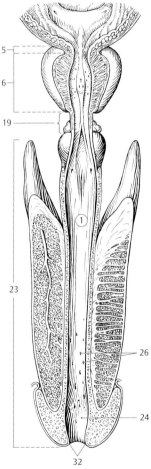

8

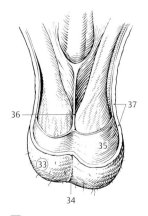

C Scrotum, anterior view

B Penis with prostate and fundus of bladder; dorsal view, opened up to urethra

1 *FEMALE INTERNAL GENITALIA.*

2 **OVARY.** It lies intraperitoneally on the wall of the lesser pelvis in the ovarian fossa. It is 2.5–4.5 cm long and 0.5–1 cm thick. Its long axis is vertical when standing. A

3 **Hilum of ovary.** Site of entry and exit of blood vessels as well as attachment of the mesovarium. B

4 **Medial surface.** Surface of the ovary facing the interior of the pelvis. A

5 **Lateral surface.** Surface of the ovary resting against the wall of the pelvis. A

6 **Free border.** Free border located opposite to the hilum of ovary. A B

7 **Mesovarian border.** Border that gives attachment to the mesovarium, located opposite to the free border of the ovary. A

8 **Tubal extremity.** End of the ovary facing the infundibulum of the uterine tube. A

9 **Uterine extremity.** Pole of the ovary facing the uterus.

10 **Tunica albuginea.** Connective-tissue capsule surrounding the ovary. It is covered with modified peritoneal epithelium ("germinal epithelium"). B

11 **Ovarian stroma.** Structural framework consisting of connective tissue. There are numerous stromal cells in the ovarian cortex. B

12 **Ovarian cortex.** Cortical region containing follicles in various stages of maturity. B

13 **Ovarian medulla.** Region containing nerves as well as blood and lymph vessels. B

14 **Vesicular ovarian follicle (graafian follicle).** Vesicular follicle, tertiary follicle. Mature follicle with fluid-filled space. B

15 **Corpus rubrum.** Remains of the follicle consisting of follicular epithelial cells and theca folliculi with bleeding after ovulation. It develops into the corpus luteum.

16 **[[Theca folliculi]].** Layer of elongated connective-tissue cells around the follicular epithelial cells. B

17 **Corpus luteum.** Gland arising from the corpus rubrum. Fat droplets lend it a yellow appearance. It is an endocrine gland that secretes progesterone and estrogen. B

18 **Corpus albicans.** Remnant of the degenerated corpus luteum. B

19 **Ligament of ovary.** Band that passes between the uterine extremity of the ovary and the uterus, posterior to the tubal angle. It contains smooth-muscle cells and allows for a certain degree of mobility of the ovary, necessary during ovulation. A

20 **Suspensory ligament of ovary; Infundibulopelvic ligament.** Band derived from the superior gonadal fold that passes between the tubal extremity of ovary and the lateral wall of the pelvis. A

21 **UTERINE TUBE.** About 10 cm long tube connecting the region around the ovary with the uterus. A

22 **Abdominal ostium of uterine tube.** Opening of the uterine tube into the peritoneal cavity. A

23 **Infundibulum of uterine tube.** Funnel-shaped beginning of the uterine tube. A

24 **Fimbriae of uterine tube.** Fringelike processes on the infundibulum. A

25 *Ovarian fimbria.* Long fimbria between the infundibulum of uterine tube and ovary. It acts to ensure contact between the end of the tube and the ovary. A

26 **Ampulla of uterine tube.** Lateral enlargement of the uterine tube. Its lumen tapers to form the isthmus of uterine tube. A

27 **Isthmus of uterine tube.** Medial, narrowed one-third of the uterine tube. It adjoins the uterus at the tubal angle. A

28 **Uterine part; Intramural part.** Part of the isthmus situated in the wall of the uterus. A

29 **Uterine ostium of tube.** Opening of the uterine part of the isthmus into the uterine cavity. A

30 **Serosa; Serous coat.** Peritoneal covering of the uterine tube. C

31 **Subserosa; Subserous layer.** Connective-tissue layer underlying the peritoneal covering. C

32 **Muscular layer; Muscular coat.** It is composed of three portions: an internal, longitudinal, and circular layer. It allows peristalsis in the direction of the uterus. Middle transverse bundles of muscle cells. These bundles are connected to vessel walls and compartments in the lumen of the uterine tube. External subperitoneal muscle cells tend to be arranged longitudinally. They act to move the uterine tube and fimbria. C

33 **Mucosa; Mucous membrane.** It contains branching longitudinal folds. It is composed of simple epithelium consisting of ciliated and glandular cells. C

34 *Folds of uterine tube.* Branchlike mucosal folds filling the entire lumen in some sections of the uterine tube. C

35 *[[Primary follicle]].* Each follice of an ovum and a single layer of follicular epithelial cells without a lumen. B

36 *[[Cumulus oophorus]].* Projection consisting of follicular epithelial cells in the fluid-filled space of the follicle. It surrounds the ovum. B

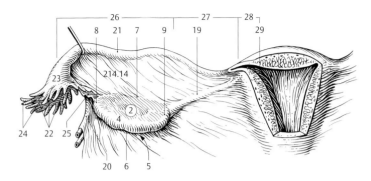

A Uterine tube, ovary, and uterus, posterior view

8

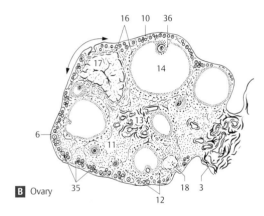

B Ovary

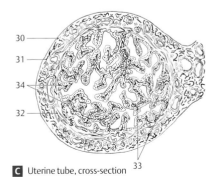

C Uterine tube, cross-section

1 **UTERUS.** Pear-shaped organ measuring about 7.5 cm in length. A B

2 **Fundus of uterus.** Rounded end of the uterus above the openings of the uterine tubes. A B

3 **Body of uterus.** Part of the uterus between the isthmus and fundus. A B

4 **Uterine horn.** Pointed projection from the uterus toward the entrance of the uterine tube. B

5 **Border of uterus.** Blunt lateral borders of the uterus that provide attachment to the broad ligament of the uterus. B C

6 **Intestinal surface; Posterior surface.** Postero-superior surface that is in contact with the intestine. A

7 **Uterine cavity.** Cavity-like space within the uterus that is shaped like an inverted triangle and has a mucosal lining. A

8 **Vesical surface; Anterior surface.** Anteroinferiorly directed surface lying on the urinary bladder. A

9 **Anatomical internal os.** Site of the transition between the flattened lumen of the body of uterus into the round lumen of the cervix of uterus. B

10 **Cervix of uterus.** Rounded inferior one-third of the uterus. A B

11 *Supravaginal part of cervix.* Part of the cervix above the vagina. It is fixed within subperitoneal connective tissues. A

12 *Isthmus of uterus.* Transition between the body of uterus and the cervix of uterus. It widens during pregnancy to form what is referred to in clinical terms as the "lower uterine segment." A B

13 *Histological internal os.* Lower limit of the lumen of the isthmus of uterus. From this point to external, the mucosa no longer undergoes changes during the menstrual cycle. B

14 *Vaginal part of cervix.* Part that projects into the vagina and is lined with vaginal epithelium. Clinical term: "portio." A B

15 **External os of uterus.** Opening of the cervical lumen into the vagina. It has a pitlike shape in nullipara that after childbirth becomes slitlike. A B

16 *Anterior lip.* Anterior border of the external os of uterus. A

17 *Posterior lip.* Posterior border of the external os of uterus. A

18 **Cervical canal.** Tubular lumen of the cervix. A B

19 *Palmate folds.* Mucosal folds that converge in a pattern resembling palm fronds inferiorly in the direction of the lumen. A B

20 *Cervical glands.* Branched tubular glands in the simple epithelium of the mucosa.

21 **Parametrium.** Subperitoneal connective tissue on both sides of the uterus. C

22 *Paracervix.* Subperitoneal connective tissue on both sides of the cervix.

23 **Serosa; Serous coat; Perimetrium.** Peritoneal covering of the uterus. C

24 **Subserosa; Subserous layer.** Connective-tissue layer underlying the peritoneal covering of the uterus. C

25 **Myometrium.** Very thick muscular wall of the uterus composed of three layers. Its middle layer of smooth muscle is arranged as a three-dimensional network in the fundus and body of uterus. The internal and external layers are composed of circular and longitudinal smooth muscle. In the cervix, myometrium cells tend to form circular bands. B C

26 *Recto-uterinus.* Muscle cells in the recto-uterine ligament.

27 **Endometrium.** Mucous membrane lining the uterine cavity. It lies directly on the myometrium. C

28 *Uterine glands.* Branched tubular glands situated in the epithelium of the endometrium. C

29 **Round ligament of uterus.** Ligament derived from the caudal gonadal fold during development. It passes from the tubal angle through the parametrium and inguinal canal into the labia majora. A B

30 **Pubocervical ligament.** Band passing from the posterior aspect of the pubic symphysis to the lateral wall of the neck of bladder and cervix. D

31 **Cardinal ligament; Transverse cervical ligament.** Collection of collagen fibers formed by thickened portions of connective tissue in the paracervix. D

32 **Uterosacral ligament; Recto-uterine ligament.** Bandlike thickening of connective tissue extending between the cervix and rectum. A D

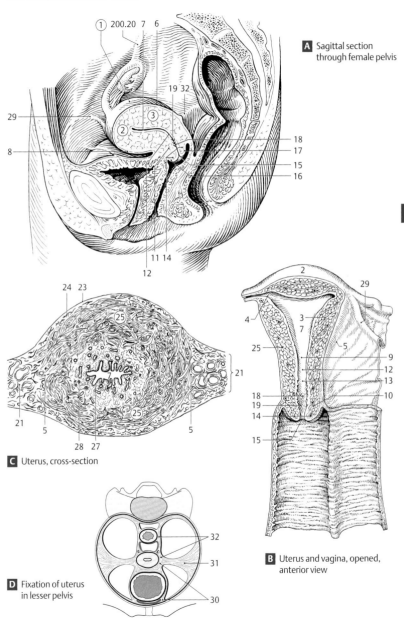

A Sagittal section through female pelvis

8

C Uterus, cross-section

D Fixation of uterus in lesser pelvis

B Uterus and vagina, opened, anterior view

1 **VAGINA.** Fibromuscular canal about 10 cm long that is flattened frontally and appears H-shaped in cross-section. A

2 **Vaginal fornix.** Blind-ending dome surrounding the vaginal part of cervix projecting into the vagina. A

3 *Anterior part.* Flat, anterior part of vaginal fornix. A

4 *Posterior part.* Deeper, posterior part of vaginal fornix. It extends behind the vaginal part of cervix to reach the rectouterine pouch. Clinical puncture site for the peritoneal cavity. A

5 *Lateral part.* Lateral connection between anterior and posterior parts of vaginal fornix.

6 **Anterior wall of vagina.** A

7 **Posterior wall of vagina.** A

8 **Hymen.** Cutaneous fold that usually arises from the posterior wall of the vagina and partially closes the entrance to the vagina as a virginal membrane. C

9 *Carunculae hymenales; Hymenal caruncles.* Remains of the hymen on the wall of the vagina following childbirth. D

10 **Muscular layer; Muscular coat.** Thin muscular coat with smooth-muscle cells that cross each other, forming a network with collagenous and elastic fibers. A

11 **Mucosa; Mucous membrane.** It does not contain any glands and is lined with glycogen-rich nonkeratinized, stratified squamous epithelium. A

12 *Vaginal rugae.* Transverse folds in the vaginal mucosa. A

13 *Vaginal columns.* Two longitudinal ridges in the vaginal wall overlying venous plexuses.

14 Anterior vaginal column. Longitudinal ridge in the anterior vaginal wall. A

15 Posterior vaginal column. Longitudinal ridge in the posterior vaginal wall. A

16 *Urethral carina of vagina.* It is formed by the female urethra in the anterior vaginal wall and represents a prolongation of the vaginal columns to external. A C D

17 **Spongy layer.** Vascular plexuses in the connective tissue outside of the muscular coat. A

18 **Epoophoron.** Vestige of the mesonephros in the mesosalpinx. B

19 **Longitudinal duct.** Remnant of the mesonephric duct in the mesosalpinx. B

20 *Transverse ductules.* Ten to twenty transverse mesonephric ducts that open into the longitudinal duct. B

21 **Vesicular appendices.** Dispersed mesonephric ducts ending in vesicles, usually near the infundibulum of uterine tube. B

22 **Paroophoron.** Tubules arising from the caudal part of the mesonephros between the lowermost branches of the ovarian artery. B

23 **[Vestige of ductus deferens].** Remnant of the wolffian duct.

24 *FEMALE EXTERNAL GENITALIA.*

25 **PUDENDUM; VULVA.** External female genitals.

26 **Mons pubis.** Area of skin overlying a pad of fat and bearing hair in front of and above the pubic symphysis. C

27 **Labium majus.** Longitudinal prominence overlying a pad of fat. It is covered with hair on its external surfaces. It extends from the mons pubis to the perineum and borders with the pudendal cleft. C

28 *Anterior commissure.* Anterior junction of the tissue of the two labia. C

29 *Posterior commissure.* Posterior junction of the tissue of the two labia. C D

30 *Frenulum of labia minora; Fourchette.* Posterior fold with a narrow margin between the labia minora. It can be torn during childbirth. C

31 **Pudendal cleft.** Fissure bounded by the two labia majora. C

32 **Labium minus.** Cutaneous fold that is devoid of fat and hair and contains sebaceous glands. It forms the boundary of the vestibule of vagina. C

33 *Prepuce of clitoris.* Union of the two labia minora above the glans of clitoris. C

34 *Frenulum of clitoris.* Small fold that gives attachment to the two labia minora below the glans of clitoris. D

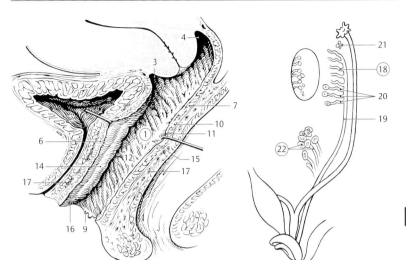

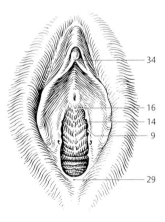

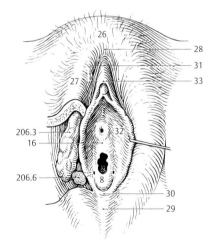

8

A Urinary bladder, urethra, vagina, uterus, and rectum in sagittal section

B Development of female urogenital system

C External virginal genitalia

D Female external genitalia

1 **Vestibule of vagina.** It is enclosed mainly by the labia minora. Site of opening of the female urethra, vagina, and greater and lesser vestibular glands. A

2 *Vestibular fossa.* Small depression between the posterior junction of the labia majora and the frenulum of labia minora. A

3 **Bulb of vestibule.** Erectile tissue corresponding to the corpus spongiosum of penis. It is mainly situated at the roots of the labia majora. p. 205 C

4 *Commissure of bulbs.* Venous bridges passing between the left and right bulbs of the vestibule of vagina in front of the clitoris.

5 **Vaginal orifice.** Opening of the vagina into the vestibule. A

6 **Greater vestibular gland.** Mucous glands on both sides of the posterior end of the bulb of the vestibule. Their long excretory duct opens at the vestibule of vagina between the labia minora and vaginal orifice. A, p. 205 C

7 **Lesser vestibular glands.** Solitary mucous glands near the urethral orifice.

8 **Clitoris.** Erectile part of the vulva on the anterior end of the labia minora. It is composed of the union of two cavernous bodies and is homologous to the corpus cavernosum of penis. A

9 **Crus of clitoris.** Prolongation extending from the clitoris. A

10 **Body of clitoris.** Union of the two crura of clitoris below the pubic symphysis. A

11 *Glans of clitoris.* End of the body of clitoris that can swell. A

12 **Corpus cavernosum of clitoris.** Cavernous body in the body of clitoris. A

13 **Septum of corpora cavernosa.** Incomplete connective-tissue partition between the right and left corpora cavernosa of clitoris.

14 **Fascia of clitoris.** Sheet of connective tissue enclosing the clitoris.

15 **Suspensory ligament of clitoris.** Band that suspends the glans of clitoris from the inferior border of the pubic symphysis. A

16 **Fundiform ligament of clitoris.** Connective-tissue band passing between the clitoris and abdominal fascia.

17 **Female urethra.** It measures 2.5–4 cm in length.

18 **Internal urethral orifice; Internal urinary meatus.** Internal opening of the female urethra at the anterior tip of the trigone of bladder. The shape of the opening depends on how full the urinary bladder is. C

19 *Filling internal urethral orifice.* The closed ostium forms a flat sheet together with surrounding structures as the urinary bladder fills. The urethra appears long.

20 *Voiding internal urethral orifice.* As the pelvic floor becomes lax, the urinary bladder descends. Its neck retracts like a funnel into the urethra, which appears shortened.

21 **Intramural part.** Part of the female urethra situated in the muscular wall of the urinary bladder. C

22 **Urethral crest.** Mucosal fold that forms a prolongation of the uvula of bladder in the posterior wall of the female urethra. B

23 **External urethral orifice.** A C

24 **External urethral sphincter.** It encircles the middle one-third of the female urethra with predominantly circular fibers, consisting of fibers from the deep transverse perineal muscle and cells of the internal urethral sphincter, embedded in connective tissue. Its superior portion blends with the musculature of the urinary bladder and its inferior portion with that of the compressor urethrae. C

25 **Muscular layer; Muscular coat.** Inner muscular coat of the female urethra consisting of smooth-muscle cells. It contains the following two layers.

26 *Circular layer.* Superficial circular muscle cell layers. B

27 *Internal urethral sphincter.* Its muscle cells lie underneath the external urethral sphincter in circular fashion and connect the two sphincter muscles.

28 *Longitudinal layer.* Layer of longitudinal bundles of muscle cells that extends into the subcutaneous adipose tissue around the external urethral orifice. B

29 **Spongy layer.** Submucosal venous plexus. B

30 **Mucosa; Mucous membrane.** It is initially lined with transitional epithelium and pseudostratified columnar epithelium, and later with nonkeratinized, stratified squamous epithelium. B

31 *Urethral glands.* Small mucous glands that open into the female urethra. B

32 *Urethral lacunae.* Mucosal pits containing the openings to the urethral glands. B

33 *[Paraurethral ducts].* (Skene's tubule). Glandular tubes measuring 1–2 cm in length that open next to the urethral orifice. They are homologous to the prostate. B

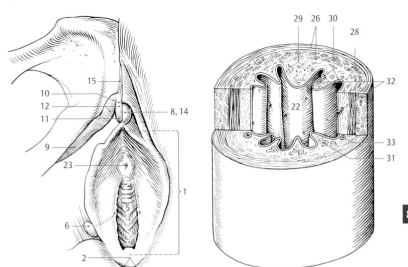

A Female external genitalia and pelvic bones

B Female urethra

8

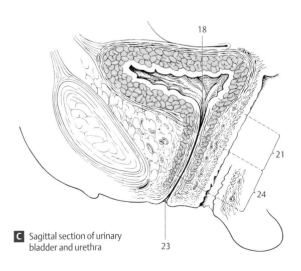

C Sagittal section of urinary
bladder and urethra

1 *PERINEUM.* A term that has different uses: Soft-tissue bridge between the anus and genitalia. In topographic anatomy, a combined region including the urogenital and anal triangles. Space beneath the urogenital and anal triangles between the skin and inferior fascia of pelvic diaphragm.

2 **Perineal raphe.** Continuation of the raphe of scrotum, formed during development.

3 **Perineal muscles.** These can be divided into the following two groups.

4 *Muscle of anal triangle.* The following muscle is the only one found in the anal triangle.

5 *External anal sphincter.* Muscle with transversely striated fibers. A B, p. 218.13

6 *Muscles of urogenital triangle.* These can be divided into muscles of the superficial perineal space and the deep perineal space.

7 **Perineal body.** Elastic sheet of tissue between the rectum and vagina (in the female) or urethra (in the male) composed of fascia and tendons from the levator ani, deep transverse perineal muscle, bulbospongiosus, and external anal sphincter muscle with smooth-muscle cells from the urinary bladder and rectum. It is connected in the male to the prostate capsule and in the female to the vagina. A B

8 **Anococcygeal body; Anococcygeal ligament.** Connective tissue band passing between the anus and coccyx with muscular components. A B, p. 218.17

9 **Subcutaneous tissue of perineum.** Continuation of the subcutaneous tissue of abdomen to the perineum.

10 *Membranous layer.* Continuation of the membranous layer of subcutaneous tissue of abdomen (Scarpa's fascia) into the urogenital triangle. A B C

11 **Subcutaneous perineal pouch.** Potential, closed space in the urogenital triangle between the membranous layer and the perineal fascia. Following injury to the urethra, urine can flow anteriorly from here into the abdominal wall, clitoris, labia, or penis and scrotum. C

12 **Superficial perineal pouch; Superficial perineal compartment; Superficial perineal space.** Closed space between the perineal fascia and the perineal membrane. C

13 **Perineal fascia; Superficial investing fascia of perineum; Deep perineal fascia.** (Colles' fascia). Lower limit of the superficial perineal space. It covers the following three muscles. A B C

14 **Superficial transverse perineal muscle.** Inconstant expansion of the deep transverse perineal muscle that extends from the ischial tuberosity to the perineal body. I: Pudendal nerve. A B

15 **Ischiocavernosus.** Male: Muscle extending from the ramus of ischium over the crus of the penis to the tunica albuginea. Smaller bundles of muscle fibers run over the penis below the pubic symphysis to the contralateral side. A B C
Female: Muscle that originates on the ramus of ischium, attaching to and covering the crus of clitoris. It assists in filling the cavernous bodies with blood. I: Pudendal nerve.

16 **Bulbospongiosus.** Male: Muscle arising from the perineal body and the inferior aspect of the corpus spongiosum of penis, passing to the perineal membrane and dorsum of penis. It is unpaired. It acts to compress the bulb of penis and transport urethral contents further. A B C
Female: Muscle that remains in two parts. The pair of muscles arises from the central tendon of the diaphragm, covering the bulb of vestibule and the greater vestibular gland. It acts to empty the gland and compress the bulb, forcing blood flow anteriorly. I: Pudendal nerve.

17 **Deep perineal pouch; Deep perineal space.** Space above the perineal membrane that is open toward the pelvis due to the oblique upward course of the urethral sphincter muscles. C

18 **Perineal membrane.** Fascia underlying the deep transverse perineal muscle. A B C

19 *Transverse perineal ligament.* Fibrous expansion of the anterior margin of the deep transverse perineal muscle. C D

20 **Deep transverse perineal muscle.** Trapezoidal sheet of muscle spread out in the pubic arch. I: Pudendal nerve. C D E

21 **[[Urogenital diaphragm]].** A term that has been replaced. What was previously conceived of as a unit is now divided into separate terms: perineal membrane, transverse perineal ligament, deep transverse perineal muscle.

22 **External urethral sphincter.** D E, p. 206.24

23 **Compressor urethrae.** Muscle fibers (female) that are continuous with the distal part of the urethral sphincter and pass to the ramus of the ischium. They act to compress the urethra and, due to their course, also elongate it. E

24 **Sphincter urethrovaginalis.** Muscle fibers (female) that are continuous with the distal part of the compressor urethrae and extend to the bulb of vestibule. E

25 **[[Superior fascia of urogenital diaphragm]].** Obsolete term. Current scientific opinion holds that there is no complete boundary to the deep perineal space.

26 **[[Genitofemoral sulcus.]]**. A groove between the thigh and labium majus or scrotum. It is continuous posteriorly with the gluteal fold.

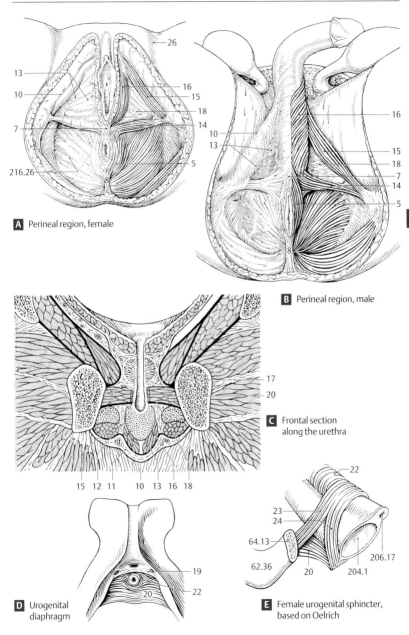

A Perineal region, female

B Perineal region, male

C Frontal section along the urethra

D Urogenital diaphragm

E Female urogenital sphincter, based on Oelrich

8

1   *ABDOMINOPELVIC CAVITY.*

2   **Abdominal cavity.**

3   **Pelvic cavity.**

4   EXTRAPERITONEAL SPACE. Space in the connective tissue with no relation to the peritoneum.

5   **Retroperitoneal space.** Area bounded by connective tissue behind the peritoneal covering.

6   **Retropubic space (Cave of Retzius).** Space behind the pubic symphysis and in front of the urinary bladder. C

7   **Retro-inguinal space.** Space in the connective tissue as the lesser pelvis underneath the peritoneum.

8   PERITONEAL CAVITY. Cavity-like space with a peritoneal lining.

9   PERITONEUM.

10 **Serosa; Serous coat.** It is composed of serous epithelial cells (mesothelium) and their basement membrane.

11 **Subserosa; Subserous layer.** Sliding layer of connective tissue beneath the serous coat that contains vessels.

12 **Parietal peritoneum.** Peritoneum lining the abdominal wall. A

13 **Visceral peritoneum.** Peritoneum covering the abdominal viscera. A

14 **Mesentery.** Dorsal peritoneal fold enclosing vessels and nerves and protecting the supply of the small intestine against vascular torsion. D

15 **Root of mesentery.** Attachment of the mesentery to the posterior wall of the abdominal cavity that extends from the second lumbar vertebra to the right iliac fossa. A

16 **Mesocolon.** Peritoneal fold conveying vessels and nerves that provides attachment and nourishment to the colon.

17 **Transverse mesocolon.** Peritoneal fold attached to the transverse colon. It arises anterior to the head of pancreas and along the inferior border of the body of pancreas. It is fused with the posterior layer of the greater omentum. A B D

18 **[Ascending mesocolon].** Peritoneal fold attached to the ascending colon. It generally fuses with the posterior wall of the abdomen in the fourth month of embryonic development.

19 **[Descending mesocolon].** Peritoneal fold attached to the descending colon. It usually fuses with the posterior wall of the abdomen in the fourth month of embryonic development.

20 **Sigmoid mesocolon.** Peritoneal fold attached to the sigmoid colon. D

21 **Meso-appendix.** Peritoneal fold attached to the vermiform appendix. D

22 **Lesser omentum.** Sheet of peritoneum that is spread mainly between the stomach and liver. It can be subdivided into the following five parts.

23 **Hepatophrenic ligament.** Part of the lesser omentum extending between the right lobe of liver and the diaphragm. A

24 **Hepato-esophageal ligament.** Possible connection between the porta hepatis and the part of the esophagus near the stomach. D

25 **Hepatogastric ligament.** Part of the lesser omentum that passes between the liver and the lesser curvature of stomach. D

26 **Hepatoduodenal ligament.** Part of the lesser omentum passing between the liver and duodenum. It conveys the hepatic artery proper, bile duct, and hepatic portal vein. D

27 **[Hepatocolic ligament].** Occasional continuation of the hepatoduodenal ligament, passing to the right to the hepatic flexure or transverse colon. D

28 **Greater omentum.** It extends from the greater curvature of stomach, draping over the intestinal loops like an apron. It is fused with the transverse colon and mesocolon. D

29 **Gastrophrenic ligament.** Uppermost portion of the gastrosplenic ligament which passes to the diaphragm. A D

30 **Gastrosplenic ligament.** Part of the greater omentum passing from the greater curvature of stomach to the splenic hilum. B D

31 **[Presplenic fold].** Inconstant fanlike fold connecting the gastrosplenic and phrenicocolic ligaments. It can contain branches of the splenic artery or left gastro-omental artery.

32 **[Gastrocolic ligament].** Part of the greater omentum that passes between the greater curvature of stomach and the omental tenia of transverse colon. D

33 **Phrenicosplenic ligament.** Peritoneal fold passing between the diaphragm and spleen. D

34 **Splenorenal ligament; Lienorenal ligament.** Peritoneal fold that passes between the kidney and spleen. It conveys vessels to the splenic hilum. B

35 **Pancreaticosplenic ligament.** Fold of peritoneum passing between the pancreas and spleen. B

36 **Pancreaticocolic ligament.** Peritoneal fold that passes between the pancreas and colon near the splenic flexure of the colon. B

37 **Splenocolic ligament.** Peritoneal fold passing between the spleen and the splenic flexure of the colon. B

38 **Phrenicocolic ligament.** Peritoneal fold passing between the splenic flexure of the colon and diaphragm. Its attachment at the inferior pole of the spleen produces a deep crevice formed by the attachment of the phrenicolic ligament in which the organ rests. B D

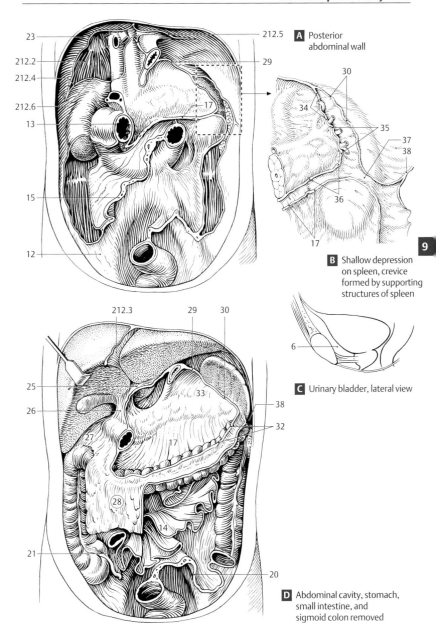

A Posterior abdominal wall

B Shallow depression on spleen, crevice formed by supporting structures of spleen

C Urinary bladder, lateral view

D Abdominal cavity, stomach, small intestine, and sigmoid colon removed

9

1 **Peritoneal attachments of liver.** Ligaments differ from those of the musculoskeletal system.

2 **Coronary ligament.** Parietal peritoneal fold passing from the diaphragm to the visceral peritoneum of the liver at the border of the bare area. p. 211 A

3 *Falciform ligament.* Peritoneal fold passing between the midline of the abdominal wall and the liver. p. 211 D

4 *Right triangular ligament.* Common margin of the hepatophrenic and hepatorenal ligaments. p. 211 A

5 *Left triangular ligament.* Free margin of the left side of the coronary ligament. p. 211 A

6 *Hepatorenal ligament.* Peritoneal fold that passes between the right lobe of liver and the kidney. p. 211 A

7 **Recesses, fossae and folds.**

8 **Omental bursa; Lesser sac.** Largest pocket within the peritoneal cavity, located behind the stomach and lesser omentum. A

9 *Omental foramen; Epiploic foramen.* Entrance to the vestibule of the omental bursa behind the hepatoduodenal ligament. A

10 *Vestibule of omental bursa.* Vestibule situated below the caudate lobe and in front of the inferior vena cava. Its transition into the omental bursa is constricted by the gastropancreatic fold from posterior. A

11 *Superior recess of omental bursa.* Outpouching of the vestibule extending upward between the inferior vena cava and esophagus. A

12 *Inferior recess of omental bursa.* Peritoneal pouch between the stomach and transverse colon. A

13 *Splenic recess of omental bursa.* Left pouch bounded by the gastrosplenic and splenorenal ligaments. A

14 *Gastropancreatic fold.* Fold in the posterior wall of the omental bursa containing the left gastric artery. A

15 *Hepatopancreatic fold.* Fold in the posterior wall of the omental bursa containing the common hepatic artery A

16 **Superior duodenal fold; Duodenojejunal fold.** Peritoneal fold on the left side of the duodenojejunal flexure in front of the superior duodenal fossa. It contains the inferior mesenteric vein. B

17 **Superior duodenal fossa.** Peritoneal recess behind the superior duodenal fold. B

18 **Inferior duodenal fold; Duodenomesocolic fold.** Peritoneal fold below the duodenojejunal flexure. B

19 **Inferior duodenal fossa.** Peritoneal recess behind the inferior duodenal fold. B

20 **[Paraduodenal fold].** Peritoneal fold on the left side of the duodenum. B

21 **[Paraduodenal recess].** Peritoneal recess behind the paraduodenal fold that is open to the right. B

22 **[Retroduodenal recess].** Peritoneal recess between the duodenum and aorta that is open to the left. B

23 **Intersigmoid recess.** Peritoneal recess on the left side of the body in the angle of the root of the sigmoid mesocolon. The ureter can be palpated here. C

24 **Superior ileocecal recess.** Peritoneal recess above the opening of the ileum into the cecum. C

25 **Vascular fold of cecum.** Peritoneal fold in front of the superior ileocecal recess containing a branch of the ileocolic artery. C

26 **Inferior ileocecal recess.** Peritoneal recess below the opening of the ileum into the cecum. C

27 **Ileocecal fold.** Peritoneal fold in front of the inferior ileocecal recess extending downward to the vermiform appendix. C

28 **Retrocecal recess.** Peritoneal recess that is often present on the right side of the body behind the cecum or ascending colon. C

29 **Cecal folds.** Peritoneal folds on the outer surface of the cecum. They are analogous to the semilunar folds of colon. C

30 **Paracolic gutters.** Occasional grooves on the left side of the descending colon. C

31 **Subphrenic space.** Peritoneal pocket between the diaphragm and liver. It is subdivided by the falciform ligament and bounded posterosuperiorly by the coronary ligament. D

32 **Subhepatic space.** Space between the liver and transverse colon; and the stomach and lesser omentum. D

33 *Hepatorenal recess.* Part of the subhepatic space that is bounded by the kidney and suprarenal gland. D

34 **Cystohepatic triangle (Calot's triangle).** Triangular region below the inferior (visceral) border of the liver, bounded by the cystic artery, common hepatic duct, and cystic duct. E

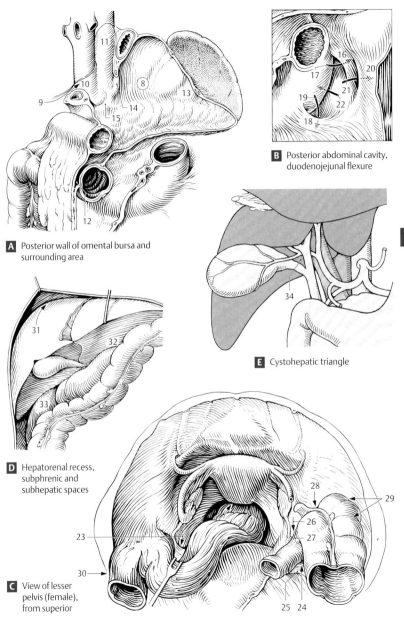

A Posterior wall of omental bursa and surrounding area

B Posterior abdominal cavity, duodenojejunal flexure

D Hepatorenal recess, subphrenic and subhepatic spaces

E Cystohepatic triangle

C View of lesser pelvis (female), from superior

1 **Median umbilical fold.** Fold passing from the apex of bladder to the navel. It contains the remains of the urachus. A B

2 **Supravesical fossa.** Shallow depression in front of the urinary bladder between the median and medial umbilical folds. B

3 **Medial umbilical fold.** Fold corresponding to the obliterated umbilical artery. It is located in the anterior abdominal wall between the median umbilical fold (obliterated urachus) and lateral umbilical fold (inferior epigastric artery). A B

4 **Medial inguinal fossa.** Depression situated opposite to the superficial inguinal ring between the medial and lateral umbilical folds. B

5 **Inguinal triangle.** Triangular region bounded by the lateral border of the rectus abdominis, inguinal ligament, and lateral umbilical fold (inferior epigastric artery). B

6 **Lateral umbilical fold; Epigastric fold.** Fold in the peritoneum produced by the inferior epigastric artery. A B

7 **Lateral inguinal fossa.** Depression lateral to the lateral umbilical fold corresponding to the deep inguinal ring. B

8 **Urogenital peritoneum.** Peritoneum of the urogenital tract.

9 **Paravesical fossa.** Indentation alongside the urinary bladder. It is bounded laterally by the ductus deferens. B

10 **Transverse vesical fold.** Peritoneal fold that passes transversely over the moderately full urinary bladder. It disappears when the urinary bladder is full. B

11 **Vesico-uterine pouch.** Recessed peritoneal pocket between the urinary bladder and uterus. A

12 **Broad ligament of uterus.** Anteriorly situated sheet of connective tissue that is covered with peritoneum and passes between the lateral surface of the uterus and lateral pelvic wall. It divides the female pelvis into two spaces, a vesico-uterine pouch and a rectouterine pouch. A

13 *Mesometrium.* Basal part of the broad ligament of uterus. Its supporting structure is formed by the connective tissue of the parametrium. A

14 *Mesosalpinx.* Superior portion of the broad ligament of uterus containing scant connective tissue; peritoneal fold. A

15 *Mesovarium.* Mesentery of the ovary. Posteriorly directed fold of the broad ligament of uterus. A

16 **Pelvic lateral wall triangle.** Region on the wall of the lesser pelvis between the round ligament of the uterus, external iliac artery, and suspensory ligament of ovary. Access to the extraperitoneal connective-tissue bed of the pelvis. A

17 **Ovarian fossa.** Indentation on the pelvic wall that lodges the ovary, located between the origin of the internal and external iliac arteries.

18 **Recto-uterine fold.** Fold on the right and left sides of the rectouterine pouch. It is composed of connective tissue and smooth-muscle cells connecting the longitudinal layer of muscle of rectum with the uterus. A

19 **Recto-uterine pouch.** Deepest point in the female peritoneal cavity, located between the uterus and rectum. The peritoneal cavity is readily accessible from externally for puncture through the posterior vaginal fornix. A

20 **Recto-vesical pouch.** Deepest point in the male peritoneal cavity, located between the urinary bladder and rectum.

21 **Pararectal fossa.** Shallow indentations alongside the rectum. A

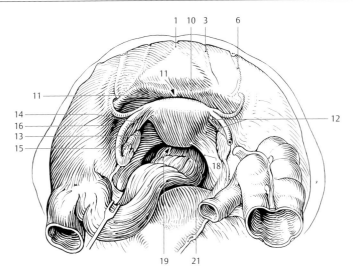

A View of lesser pelvis (female), from superior

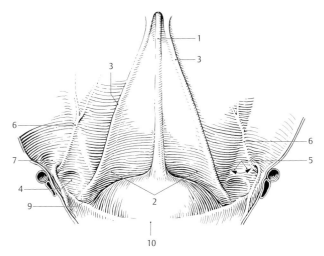

B Anterior abdominal wall, from posterior

1   **Ischio-anal fossa.** Wedged-shaped space that is open posteriorly between the inferior fascia of pelvic diaphragm and the obturator fascia. A

2   **Fat body of ischio-anal fossa.** Fat pad in the ischio-anal fossa. A

3   **Pudendal canal. (Alcock's canal).** Fold of the obturator fascia in the lateral wall of the ischio-anal fossa for the passage of the pudendal vessels and nerves. A

4   **Pelvic fascia.** Continuation of the transversalis fascia into the pelvis. It splits into a visceral layer covering the pelvic viscera and a parietal layer covering the wall of the pelvis.

5   **Visceral pelvic fascia.** Fascial sheath surrounding the pelvic viscera. It is especially thick around the urinary bladder and rectal ampulla. A

6   *Fascia of individual organ.*

7   *Rectoprostatic fascia; Rectovesical septum.* Condensation of visceral fascia in the male that forms a septum between the rectum and prostate or urinary bladder. It contains smooth-muscle cells and extends from the rectovesical pouch to the perineal body. B

8   *Rectovaginal fascia; Rectovaginal septum.* Condensation of visceral fascia in the female that forms a septum between the rectum and vagina. It contains smooth-muscle cells and extends between the rectouterine pouch and perineal body.

9   **Extraperitoneal fascia.** Connective tissue with no relation to the peritoneum. It can form independent structures or invest others. It can also be connected with muscle fibers via the epimysium and can convey vessels and nerves. In the pelvis it is permeated by smooth-muscle cells.

10 *Extraperitoneal ligament.* Bandlike structure formed by extraperitoneal connective tissue, e.g., the round ligament of uterus.

11 **Parietal pelvic fascia; Endopelvic fascia.** Layer of pelvic fascia lining the pelvic wall. It covers the levator ani, coccygeus, piriformis, and, anteriorly, the deep transverse perineal muscle. A

12 *Fascia of individual organ.* Here: Fascia enclosing the pelvic muscles.

13 *Obturator fascia.* Stronger portion of parietal pelvic fascia covering the obturator internus. A C

14 *Tendinous arch of pelvic fascia.* Tendinous thickening of pelvic fascia that passes in an arch from the pubic symphysis to the levator ani and continues posteriorly to the ischial spine. It corresponds to a band giving exit to the visceral vessels and nerves from the lateral pelvic wall and providing an especially firm attachment for the pelvic fascia to the pelvic wall. Formation of the puboprostatic and pubovesical ligaments. C

15 *Piriformis fascia.* Fascia investing the piriformis. It attaches to the sacrum near the anterior sacral foramina and is connected with the nerve sheaths surrounding the sacral nerves. Hence, it represents a prolongation of extraperitoneal connective tissue into the gluteal region. C

16 *Superior fascia of pelvic diaphragm.* Fascial sheath covering the aspect of the levator ani and coccygeus facing the pelvis. A C

17 *Pubovesical ligament; Medial puboprostatic ligament.* Thickening of fascia between the anterior wall of the prostate, urinary bladder, and pubic symphysis. It usually contains smooth-muscle cells (puboprostaticus).

18 *Medial pubovesical ligament.* Fascial thickening in the female passing anteromedially between the urinary bladder and pubic symphysis.

19 *Pubovesicalis.* The pubovesical ligament can be almost entirely composed of smooth-muscle cells. B

20 *Puboprostatic ligament; Lateral puboprostatic ligament.* Fascial thickening lateral to the symphysis between the prostate, urinary bladder, and pelvic wall. Part of the tendinous arch of the pelvic fascia. B

21 *Lateral pubovesical ligament.* Fascial thickening in the female that runs lateral to the pubic symphysis between the urinary bladder and pelvic wall. Part of the tendinous arch of the pelvic fascia.

22 *Lateral ligament of bladder.* Lateral thickening of fascia between the basal part of the bladder and the pelvic wall.

23 *Rectovesicalis.* Smooth-muscle cells arising from the longitudinal muscle layer of rectum and passing to the lateral aspect of the fundus of bladder, usually in the lateral ligament of bladder.

24 *Presacral fascia.* Area of connective tissue in front of the sacrum between the visceral pelvic fascia of the posterior wall of the rectum and the superior fascia of the pelvic diaphragm. It contains the sacral plexus. B

25 *Rectosacral fascia.* Fusion of fascia of the rectal ampulla and sacrum. B

26 *Inferior fascia of pelvic diaphragm.* Caudal fascial sheath covering the levator ani and coccygeus. A

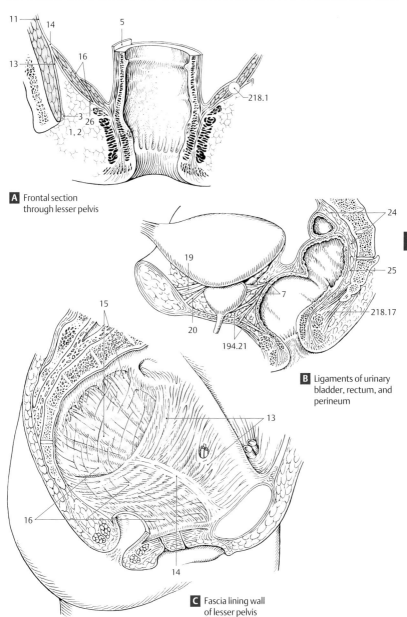

A Frontal section through lesser pelvis

B Ligaments of urinary bladder, rectum, and perineum

C Fascia lining wall of lesser pelvis

1 **Pelvic diaphragm; Pelvic floor.** Funnel-shaped sheet of muscle consisting of the levator ani and coccygeus muscles and covered above and below by fascia, i.e., the superior and inferior fascia of pelvic diaphragm. With the exception of an anterior triangular gap, this sheet of muscle forms the pelvic floor. A B

2 **Levator ani.** Principle muscle of the pelvic diaphragm. It is derived from the abdominal wall musculature and permeated by smooth-muscle cells. I: Sacral plexus, S2–S5. It consists of the following parts. A B

3 *Pubococcygeus.* o: Pubis, near the pubic symphysis, tendinous arch of levator ani. i: Perineal body, anus, anococcygeal ligament, coccyx. A B

4 *Puboperinealis.* Bundle of muscle fibers and cells passing between the pubis and perineal body.

5 *Puboprostaticus; Levator prostatae.* Bundle of muscle fibers and cells passing to the prostate in the pubovesical ligament. A

6 *Pubovaginalis.* Bundle of muscle fibers and cells passing to the wall of the vagina. A

7 *Pubo-analis.* Bundle of muscle fibers and cells passing to the anal sphincter muscle.

8 **Puborectalis.** Bundles of muscle fibers that mostly pass behind the perineal flexure where they blend with fibers from the opposite side. A B

9 *Iliococcygeus.* Bundle of muscle fibers that mostly pass from the tendinous arch of the levator ani to the anococcygeal ligament and lateral wall of the coccyx. A

10 *Tendinous arch of levator ani.* Tendinous arch of variable thickness formed by the obturator fascia at the origin of the levator ani. A B

11 **Urogenital hiatus.** Opening in the pelvic diaphragm for passage of the urethra or urethra and vagina. A

12 **Ischiococcygeus; Coccygeus.** Muscle fibers that fan out from the ischial spine to the lateral surfaces of the sacrum and coccyx. They are joined with the sacrospinal ligament. A

13 **External anal sphincter.** Transversely striated outer sphincter muscle of the anus. It consists of the following three parts. I: Pudendal nerve. B

14 *Subcutaneous part.* Superficial muscle fibers that extend to the dermis in front of and behind the anus. B

15 *Superficial part.* Fibers extending between the perineal body and the anococcygeal ligament. B

16 *Deep part.* Ringlike part of the external anal sphincter extending 3–4 cm along and encircling the anal canal. B

17 **Anococcygeal body; Anococcygeal ligament.** Tough band of connective tissue containing muscle fibers that passes between the anus and coccyx. It is composed of the following parts. A

18 *Pubococcygeal tendon.* Tendinous portion of the pubococcygeus. A

19 *Iliococcygeal raphe.* Line on the lateral side of the muscle where it fuses with the pubococcygeus.

20 *Attachment of superficial external anal sphincter.*

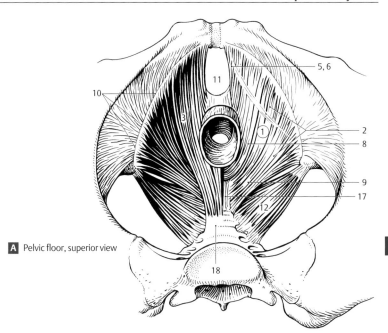

A Pelvic floor, superior view

9

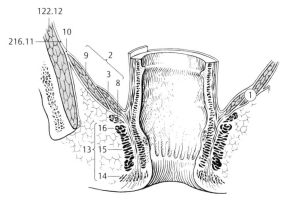

B Frontal section
through lesser pelvis

1 *ENDOCRINE GLANDS.* Ductless glands.

2 PITUITARY GLAND. Gland located in the sella turcica. D

3 **Adenohypophysis; Anterior lobe.** Anterior lobe of the pituitary gland. Embryologically derived from the roof of the pharynx. It is composed of cells with varying functions, mostly regulating other glands. D

4 *Pars tuberalis.* Part of the pituitary gland that covers the infundibulum. D

5 *Pars intermedia.* Intermediate region that borders with the neurohypophysis and contains colloid masses. D

6 *Pars distalis*; *Pars anterior.* Largest, anterior part of the pituitary gland. D

7 **Neurohypophysis; Posterior lobe.** Part derived from the hypothalamus. Serves for storage of hormones. D

8 *Infundibulum.* Funnel-shaped stalk of the pituitary gland. D

9 *Neural lobe*; *Pars nervosa.* True posterior lobe of the pituitary gland. D

10 PINEAL GLAND; PINEAL BODY. It develops from the roof of the diencephalon and overlies the tectal plate. D

11 THYROID GLAND. Produces thyroxine and triiodothyronine, hormones that increase metabolic processes. Pathological enlargement is known as goiter. A B C

12 **Lobe of thyroid gland.** Right and left lobes of the thyroid gland adjacent to the trachea. A

13 **Isthmus of thyroid gland.** Part of the thyroid gland connecting the right and left lobes. A

14 **[Pyramidal lobe].** Remnant forming a medial cord of thyroid tissue. A

15 **Accessory thyroid glands.** Islands of detached thyroid tissue, e.g., in the pharyngeal part of the tongue.

16 **Fibrous capsule.** Double layer of connective tissue forming the capsule around the thyroid gland. The inner layer encloses the organ and the outer layer is composed of the pretracheal layer of cervical fascia.

17 **Stroma.** Connective-tissue framework of the thyroid gland. C

18 **Parenchyma.** Cells specific to the thyroid gland. C

19 **Lobules.** Thyroid gland lobules that are separated by the inner layer of connective tissue from the fibrous capsule. B

20 PARATHYROID GLAND. Small mass of epithelial cells. The parathyroid glands are located posterior to the thyroid gland between the two layers of the fibrous capsule. They secrete parathyroid hormone, which regulates calcium and phosphorus levels by means of osteoclast stimulation.

21 **Superior parathyroid gland.** B

22 **Inferior parathyroid gland.** B

23 **Accessory parathyroid glands.** Number and location vary. They can also lie in the connective tissue above or below the thyroid gland.

24 SUPRARENAL GLAND; ADRENAL GLAND. Gland arising from two components, resting like a cap on the medial part of the superior pole of the kidney. E

25 **Anterior surface of suprarenal gland.** E

26 **Posterior surface of suprarenal gland.**

27 **Renal surface.** Concave, inferolateral surface facing the kidney. E

28 **Superior border.** Upper margin of the suprarenal gland between the anterior and posterior surfaces. E

29 **Medial border.** Medial margin between the anterior and posterior surfaces of the suprarenal gland. E

30 **Hilum.** Exit site of the central vein of the suprarenal gland and lymph vessels. Arteries and nerves enter the gland at various sites.

31 **Central vein.** Main vein of the suprarenal gland that exits at the hilum. E

32 **Cortex.** Cortical region of the suprarenal gland arising from celomic epithelium. It can be divided into three zones. F

33 **Medulla.** Medullary part of the suprarenal gland derived from the neural crest. It is composed of chromaffin cells, sympathetic ganglion cells, and venous sinuses. F

34 **Accessory suprarenal glands.** Masses of detached suprarenal gland tissue.

35 PANCREATIC ISLETS. About one million islets of Langerhans that produce glucagon and insulin.

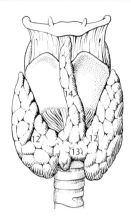

A Thyroid gland, anterior view

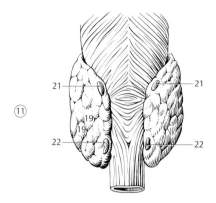

B Thyroid gland, posterior view

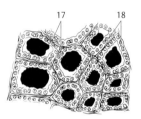

C Thyroid gland, histological section

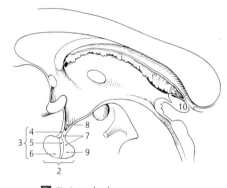

D Pituitary gland

10

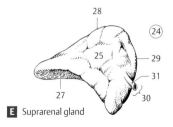

E Suprarenal gland

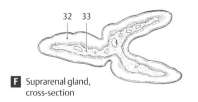

F Suprarenal gland, cross-section

1 *CARDIOVASCULAR SYSTEM.*

2 **Pericardium.** Lubricant-containing sheath enclosing the heart. It consists of a fibrous layer and a double-layered serous coat. A

3 **Fibrous pericardium.** Outer sheath of strong fibrous tissue. Its collagen fibers are arranged in latticelike fashion and it is partly joined with the diaphragm. A

4 *Sternopericardial ligaments.* Bands passing between the pericardium and sternum.

5 **Bronchopericardial membrane.** Frontal layer of connective tissue behind and connected with the pericardium. Crossed by reinforcing collagen fibers, it extends between the tracheal bifurcation, main bronchi, pulmonary ligaments, and diaphragm. It coordinates respiratory movements and posterior tilting of the head. C

6 **Serous pericardium.** Covering consisting of a single layer of cells (mesothelium) lining the inner layer of the pericardium and the surface of the heart.

7 *Parietal layer.* Serous covering of the pericardium. It transitions into the epicardium near the great vessels. A

8 *Visceral layer*; *Epicardium.* Serous covering of the heart. It transitions into the parietal layer near the great vessels. A

9 *Serosa*; *Serous coat.* Single layer of squamous epithelium of mesodermal origin (mesothelium) overlying a delicate layer of connective tissue.

10 *Subserosa*; *Subserous layer.* Sliding layer of well-vascularized connective tissue beneath the serous coat.

11 **Fold of left vena cava.** Pericardial fold in its posterior wall. It is a remnant of the obliterated left superior vena cava, present during embryonic development.

12 **Pericardial cavity.** Space between the layers of the serous pericardium that contains a film of serous fluid.

13 **Transverse pericardial sinus.** Passageway in the pericardial cavity behind the ascending aorta and pulmonary trunk and in front of the veins. A

14 **Oblique pericardial sinus.** Recess in the pericardial cavity between the right pulmonary veins and inferior vena cava on one side and the left pulmonary veins on the other. A

15 *HEART.*

16 **Base of heart.** Broad aspect of the heart facing dorsally and to the right, located opposite to the apex of the nearly conical heart. It is mainly formed by the posterior wall of the left atrium. The pulmonary arteries and vasa privata arise and open here.

17 **Anterior surface; Sternocostal surface.** Anteriorly directed convex surface of the heart. B D

18 **Diaphragmatic surface; Inferior surface.** Inferior, flattened surface of the heart that is in contact with the diaphragm. D

19 **Right/left pulmonary surface.** Surface of the heart beside and touching the lungs. D

20 **Right border.** Right margin that is often sharp in the cadaver. B

21 **Apex of heart.** Part of the heart directed downward and to the left. It is formed by the left ventricle. B

22 *Notch of cardiac apex.* Indentation to the right of the apex where the two interventricular sulci become continuous with each other. B

23 **Anterior interventricular sulcus.** Longitudinal groove on the anterior surface of the heart overlying the interventricular septum. It transmits the anterior branch of the interventricular branch of the left coronary artery. B D

24 **Posterior interventricular sulcus.** Longitudinal groove on the diaphragmatic surface of the heart corresponding to the interventricular septum. It transmits the posterior branch of the interventricular branch of the right coronary artery. D

25 **Coronary sulcus.** Groove that runs around the heart, demarcating the borders between the atria and ventricles. B E

26 **Right/left ventricle.** The wall of the left ventricle is thicker than that of the right ventricle to accommodate functional demands. E

27 **Interventricular septum.** Partition dividing the right and left ventricles of the heart. It can be identified from externally by the anterior and posterior interventricular sulci.

28 *Muscular part.* E

29 *Membranous part.* Short, thin, fibrous portion of the upper part of the interventricular septum near the exit of the aorta. It arises from endocardium. E

30 **Atrioventricular septum.** Portion of the membranous part of interventricular septum between the right atrium and left ventricle above the root of the septal cusp. E

31 **Right/left atrium.** Thin-walled chambers of the heart. E

32 *Auricle.* Outpouching of the atria that resembles a finger of a glove. B E

33 **Interatrial septum.** Partition between the right and left atria of the heart.

34 **Right/left atrioventricular orifice.** Openings between the atria and ventricles. D

35 **Opening of pulmonary trunk.** Opening of the right ventricle to the pulmonary trunk. D

36 **Aortic orifice.** Opening of the left ventricle to the aorta. D

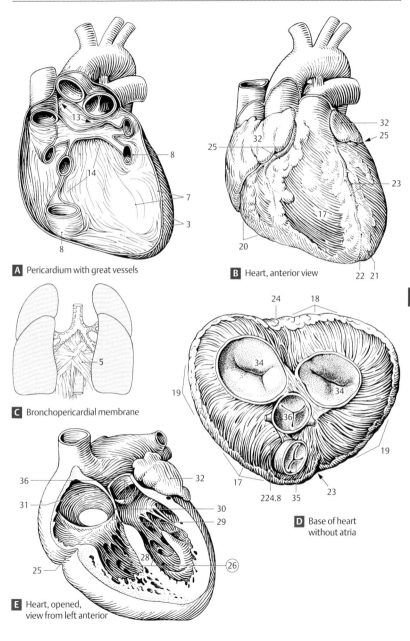

A Pericardium with great vessels

B Heart, anterior view

C Bronchopericardial membrane

D Base of heart without atria

E Heart, opened, view from left anterior

11

1 **Trabeculae carneae.** Muscle columns on the inner surface of the heart that project inward. A

2 **Vortex of heart.** Swirling arrangement of cardiac muscle cells at the apex of the heart. Site of redirection of descending outer longitudinal muscle fibers into ascending inner longitudinal fibers. B

3 **Papillary muscles.** Conical muscles projecting into the heart chambers. They are connected via the chordae tendineae to the atrioventicular valves and prevent eversion of the cusps into the atrium in systole. A D

4 **Chordae tendineae; Tendinous cords.** Tendinous cords passing between the papillary muscles and atrioventicular valves. A D

5 **False chordae tendineae.** Evolutionary vestiges of development of the walls of the heart. Connections vary between the papillary muscles and ventricular wall or parts of the wall. They can be part of the conducting system of heart.

6 **Right/left fibrous trigone.** Connective-tissue gusset located anteriorly and posteriorly between the aorta and atrioventricular orifices. C

7 **Right/left fibrous ring.** Connective-tissue ring between the atria and ventricles from which the atrioventicular valves arise. C

8 **Tendon of infundibulum.** Remnant of the embryonic spiral septum. C, p. 223 D

9 **Tendon of valve of inferior vena cava.** If penetrated, the valve of the inferior vena cava can resemble a free-standing tendon.

10 **Triangle of sinu-atrial node.** Area on the base of the superior vena cava containing the sinu-atrial node. D

11 **Myocardium.** It is composed of transversely striated muscle cells, local collections of smooth-muscle cells, and the conducting system of heart. A D

12 **Conducting system of heart.** It is located in the myocardium beneath the endocardium.

13 *Sinu-atrial node. (Node of Keith–Flack).* Bandlike specialized muscle tissue in front of the entrance of the superior vena cava that functions as the primary center for generating cardiac impulses. D

14 *Atrioventricular node. (Aschoff–Tawara node).* Specialized muscle tissue in the interatrial septum below the fossa ovalis and in front of the opening of coronary sinus. It transmits the myogenically conducted impulse received from the sinu-atrial node after a period of latency to the ventricles via the bundle of His (and right and left bundles of His). If sinu-atrial node function is disrupted, it can act as a secondary center for generation of cardiac impulses. D

15 *Atrioventricular bundle.* Bundle of fibers transmitting cardiac impulses between the atrioventricular node and papillary muscles. D

16 *[Bundle of His].* Initial segment of the atrioventricular bundle extending to the bifurcation at the membranous part of septum where it divides into right and left bundles. D

17 *Right bundle.* Bundle that runs in an arch into the septomarginal trabecula and continues to the anterior papillary muscle. D

18 *Left bundle.* Bundle that expands over the septum and extends to the base of the papillary muscles. D

19 **Subendocardial branches.** (Purkinje fibers). Branches of the conducting system that pass to the myocardium. D

20 **Endocardium.** Serous lining of the heart covered with simple squamous epithelium.

21 RIGHT ATRIUM. A D

22 **Right auricle.** Outpouching of the right atrium. A

23 **Crista terminalis.** Muscular ridge extending from the opening of the superior vena cava anteriorly over the lateral wall of the atrium to the lateral side of the opening of inferior vena cava. Inner border between the atrium and sinus venosus, which is present during embryonic development. A

24 **Openings of smallest cardiac veins.** Openings into the right atrium. A

25 **Fossa ovalis; Oval fossa.** Depression in the interatrial septum, which represents the closed foramen ovale (open during fetal development). A

26 *[Foramen ovale].* Opening in the interatrial septum that is present until birth. Direct flow of blood from the right atrium into the left. A

27 **Limbus fossae ovalis; Border of oval fossa.** Raised border around the fossa ovalis. A

28 **Musculi pectinati; Pectinate muscles.** Muscle columns arising from the crista terminalis in the right atrium. A

29 **Opening of coronary sinus.** A

30 **Opening of inferior vena cava.** A

31 **Opening of superior vena cava.** A

32 **Sinus of venae cavae.** Smooth-walled space bounded by the crista terminalis for the passage of blood from the inferior and superior venae cavae. A

33 **Sulcus terminalis cordis.** Groove visible on the external surface of the right atrium between the embryonic sinus venosus and atrium. It surrounds the region surrounding the openings of the inferior and superior venae cavae. D

34 **Intervenous tubercle.** Prominence on the posterior wall of the right atrium between the openings of inferior and superior venae cavae. A

35 **Valve of inferior vena cava.** (eustachian valve). Semilunar fold in front of the opening of inferior vena cava. During fetal development it directs blood toward the foramen ovale. A

36 **Valve of coronary sinus.** (thebesian valve). Semilunar fold in front of the opening of coronary sinus. A

11

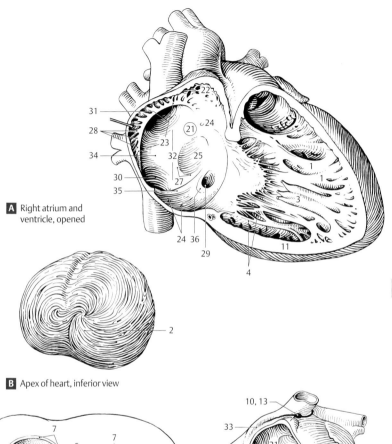

A Right atrium and ventricle, opened

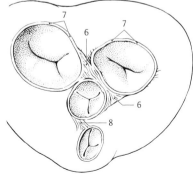

B Apex of heart, inferior view

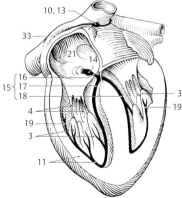

C Heart valves, superior view

D Conducting system of heart

11

1 RIGHT VENTRICLE. C

2 **Tricuspid valve; Right atrioventricular valve.** Valve apparatus between the right atrium and ventricle. It arises from the fibrous ring in three parts which are connected via the chordae tendineae to the papillary muscles. A

3 *Anterior cusp.* Anterior leaflet. A C

4 *Posterior cusp.* Posterior leaflet. A

5 *Septal cusp.* Cusp or leaflet arising from the interventricular septum. A

6 **Supraventricular crest.** Muscular ridge passing obliquely from the interventricular septum to the anterior wall of the ventricle. It separates the outflow tract of the conus arteriosus from the rest of the right ventricle. C

7 **Conus arteriosus; [Infundibulum].** Funnel-shaped smooth-walled outflow tract leading to the pulmonary trunk. A

8 **Pulmonary valve.** Three-part valve apparatus around the opening of pulmonary trunk at the beginning of the pulmonary trunk. A

9 *Anterior semilunar cusp.* A

10 *Right semilunar cusp.* A

11 *Left semilunar cusp.* A

12 *Nodules of semilunar cusps.* Small nodules in the middle of each free margin of the semilunar cusps that seal the wedge-shaped space between the three cusps when closed. C

13 *Lunules of semilunar cusps.* Crescent-shaped areas on both sides of the nodules at the margins of the semilunar cusps. C

14 *Commissures of semilunar cusps.* Ascending projections from adjacent valves that are attached to the pulmonary trunk. C

15 **Anterior papillary muscle.** Largest papillary muscle, located anteriorly and often overlying the septomarginal trabecula. It is connected with the anterior and posterior cusps. C

16 **Posterior papillary muscle.** Muscle connected with the posterior and septal cusps. C

17 **Septal papillary muscle.** Small papillary muscles arising from the interventricular septum. Their chordae tendineae mostly pass to the septal cusp. C

18 **Septomarginal trabecula; Moderator band.** Muscular ridge that extends from the interventricular septum to the root of the anterior papillary muscle. It contains the right bundle of bundle of His. C

19 LEFT ATRIUM. B

20 **Left auricle.** Outpouching of the atrium to the left of the pulmonary trunk. B

21 **Musculi pectinati; pectinate muscles.** Muscular columns in the left atrium that resemble the teeth of a comb.

22 **Valve of foramen ovale.** Floor of the fossa ovalis derived from the septum primum. During fetal development, blood flow forces it into the left atrium. B

23 **Openings of pulmonary veins.** Openings of pulmonary veins into the left atrium. B

24 LEFT VENTRICLE. B

25 **Mitral valve; Left atrioventricular valve.** Valve apparatus between the left atrium and ventricle with two cusps that arise from the fibrous ring and are connected via the chordae tendineae to the papillary muscles of the left ventricle. A

26 *Anterior cusp.* Anterior leaflet situated near the septum. A B D

27 *Posterior cusp.* Posterior leaflet situated near the lateral wall. Its free margin is more deeply grooved than that of the anterior cusp. A B

28 *Commissural cusps.* Two distinct, subdivided lateral margins, one on either side of the middle one-third of the posterior cusp, which is rather smooth and protruding. They can create the appearance of additional cusps.

29 **Anterior papillary muscle.** Larger, anterior papillary muscle arising from the lateral wall of the left ventricle. D

30 **Posterior papillary muscle.** It arises from between the interventricular septum and the lateral wall. D

31 **Aortic vestibule.** Part of the aorta below the aortic valve. In systole it serves as a functional expansion of the left ventricle. D

32 **Aortic valve.** Valve apparatus at the beginning of the aortic outflow tract. D

33 *Right semilunar cusp; Right coronary cusp.* D

34 *Left semilunar cusp; Left coronary cusp.* D

35 *Posterior semilunar cusp; Noncoronary cusp.* D

36 *Nodules of semilunar cusps.* Nodules in the middle of each free margin of a semilunar cusp. They close off the wedge-shaped space between the three cusps on closure. D

37 *Lunules of semilunar cusps.* Crescent-shaped areas on both sides of the nodules of semilunar cusps. D

38 *Commissures of semilunar cusps.* Ascending projections from adjacent valves and their union with the wall of the aorta. D

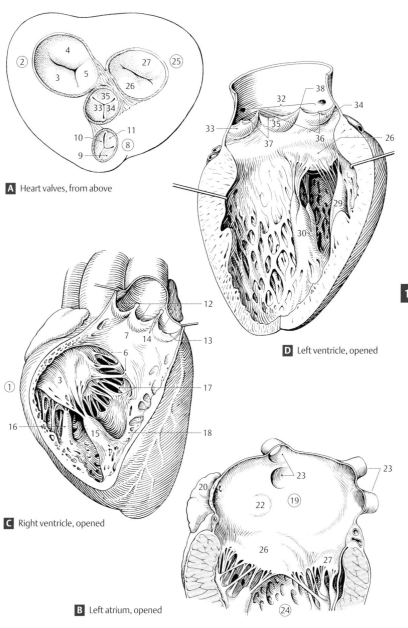

A Heart valves, from above

D Left ventricle, opened

C Right ventricle, opened

B Left atrium, opened

11

1 *ARTERIES.* Blood vessels conveying blood from the heart to the periphery of the body.

2 **PULMONARY TRUNK.** Arterial trunk that ascends in the pericardium. It divides into the right and left pulmonary arteries at the level of the reflection of the serous pericardium. A B

3 **Sinus of pulmonary trunk.** Three dilations in the wall of the pulmonary trunk over the roots of the semilunar cusps. B

4 **Supravalvular ridge.** Ring-shaped prominence in the wall of the pulmonary trunk to which the commissures of the semilunar cusps are attached. p. 231 B

5 **Bifurcation of pulmonary trunk.** Division of the trunk into the two pulmonary arteries. Site of reflection of the serous pericardium. A B

6 RIGHT PULMONARY ARTERY. Artery located behind the ascending aorta. Its ramifications parallel the branches of the bronchial tree. Both form bronchoarterial segments. B

7 **Superior lobar arteries.**

8 *Apical segmental artery.* Artery supplying the apical segment. B

9 *Anterior segmental artery.* Artery supplying the anterior segment.

10 *Ascending branch.* B

11 *Descending branch.* B

12 *Posterior segmental artery.* Artery supplying the posterior segment.

13 *Ascending branch.* B

14 *Descending branch.* B

15 **Middle lobar artery.** B

16 *Medial segmental artery.* Artery supplying the medial segment.

17 *Lateral segmental artery.* Artery supplying the lateral segment. B

18 **Inferior lobar arteries.**

19 *Superior segmental artery.* Artery supplying the superior segment. B

20 *Basal part.* Basal segment of the inferior lobe. B

21 *Anterior basal segmental artery.* Artery supplying the anterior basal segment. B

22 *Lateral basal segmental artery.* Artery supplying the lateral basal segment. B

23 *Medial basal segmental artery.* Artery supplying the medial basal segment. B

24 *Posterior basal segmental artery.* Artery supplying the posterior basal segment. B

25 LEFT PULMONARY ARTERY. Artery lying in front of the descending aorta. On radiographs it appears as a "pulmonary arch" below the "aortic arch." A B

26 **Ligamentum arteriosum [Ductus arteriosus].** (Ligament of Botallo's duct). Connection between the bifurcation of pulmonary trunk and the aortic arch that remains patent until birth. Pulmonary circulation is minimal in the fetus. The ductus arteriosus can remain patent after birth, but is usually replaced by fibrous tissue. A B

27 **Superior lobar arteries.**

28 *Apical segmental artery.* Artery supplying the upper part of the apicoposterior segment. B

29 *Anterior segmental artery.* Artery supplying the anterior segment. B

30 *Ascending branch.* B

31 *Descending branch.* B

32 *Posterior segmental artery.* Artery supplying the lower part of the apicoposterior segment. B

33 *Ascending branch.*

34 *Descending branch.*

35 *Lingular artery.* Branch supplying the lingular segment. B

36 *Inferior lingular artery.* Branch supplying the inferior lingular segment. B

37 *Superior lingular artery.* Branch supplying the superior lingular segment. B

38 **Inferior lobar arteries.**

39 *Superior segmental artery.* Branch supplying the superior segment. B

40 *Basal part.* Basal segment supplying the inferior lobe. B

41 *Anterior basal segmental artery.* Artery supplying the anterior basal segment. B

42 *Lateral basal segmental artery.* Artery supplying the lateral basal segment. B

43 *Medial basal segmental artery.* Artery supplying the medial basal segment. B

44 *Posterior basal segmental artery.* Artery supplying the posterior basal segment. B

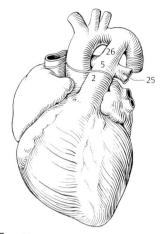

A Fetal heart

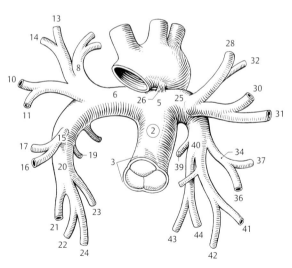

B Pulmonary arteries

12

1   **AORTA.** Main artery supplying the body. A

2   ASCENDING AORTA. Ascending part of the aorta up to its exit from the pericardium. A

3   **Aortic sinus.** Calotte-like dilatations of the aortic lumen at the level of the three aortic valves. B

4   **Supravalvular ridge.** Ring-shaped eminence in the wall to which the commissures of semilunar cusps are attached. B

5   **Aortic bulb.** Onion-shaped dilatation visible on the outer surface of the aorta. It is produced by the aortic sinus. B

6   **Right coronary artery.** It travels in the right coronary sulcus and arises near the right aortic sinus. B C

7   **Atrioventricular branches.** Branches arising in the coronary sulcus and supplying the atrioventricular node. C

8   **Conus branch.** Inferior branch supplying the conus arteriosus. B

9   **Sinu-atrial nodal branch.** Most common branch (55%) passing to a vascular plexus at the entrance of the superior vena cava and via the plexus to the sinu-atrial node. B

10 **Atrial branches.** Branches supplying the right atrium.

11 **Right marginal branch.** Inferior branch on the outer margin of the right ventricle. B C

12 **Intermediate atrial branch.** Superior branch on the posterior side of the right atrium. C

13 **Posterior interventricular branch.** Terminal branch of the right coronary artery lying in the posterior interventricular sulcus. C

14 *Interventricular septal branches.* Branches supplying the interventricular septum. C

15 **Atrioventricular nodal branch.** Branch extending from the beginning of the right posterolateral branch to the atrioventricular node. C

16 **[Right posterolateral branch].** Occasional branch supplying the posterior wall of the left ventricle. C

17 **Left coronary artery.** It arises near the left aortic sinus. B

18 **Anterior interventricular branch.** Branch lying in the anterior interventricular sulcus. B

19 *Conus branch.* Rarely present left branch extending to the conus arteriosus. B

20 *Lateral branch.* Left branch passing to the anterior wall of the left ventricle. B

21 *Interventricular septal branches.* Perforating branches supplying the anterior two-thirds of the interventricular septum. B

22 **Circumflex branch.** Continuation of the left coronary artery that travels in the left coronary sulcus. B C

23 *Atrial anastomotic branch.* Branch of the circumflex branch that supplies the interatrial septum. It anastomoses with branches from the right coronary artery.

24 *Atrioventricular branches.* Distal part of the circumflex branch lying in the coronary sulcus. C

25 *Left marginal artery.* Branch on the outer margin of the left ventricle. B

26 *Intermediate atrial branch.* Branch traveling along the posterior side of the atrium. C

27 *Posterior left ventricular branch.* Occasional branch extending to the posterior side of the left ventricle. C

28 *[Sinu-atrial nodal branch].* Branch most frequently (45%) arising from the beginning of the left coronary artery and passing to the sinu-atrial node. B

29 *[Atrioventricular nodal branch].* Inconstant branch supplying the atrioventricular node.

30 *Atrial branches.* Branches to the left atrium. B

12

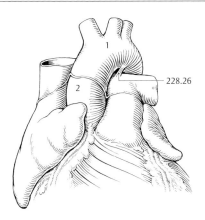

A Aorta and pulmonary trunk, anterior view

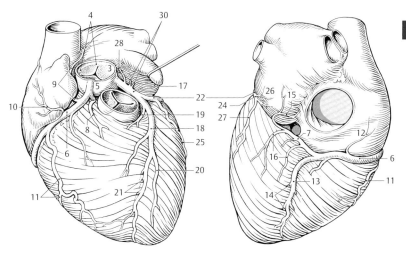

B Coronary arteries, anterior view

C Coronary arteries , posterior view

1 ARCH OF AORTA; AORTIC ARCH. It is located between the ascending and descending aorta. Its roof extends to the first rib at the left border of the sternum. A B

2 **[Aortic isthmus].** Constriction of variable size behind the ligamentum arteriosum. In the fetus it is a narrowed portion of the aortic arch between the exit of the left subclavian artery and the ductus arteriosus. It can remain as an aortic isthmus stenosis. A

3 **Para-aortic bodies; Aortic glomera.** Irregular islands of chromaffin cells lying near the aorta, predominantly on the aortic arch. They are presumably baroreceptors and chemoreceptors.

4 BRACHIOCEPHALIC TRUNK. It arises at the beginning of the aortic arch and divides behind the right sternoclavicular joint into the right subclavian artery and right common carotid artery. A B

5 **[Thyroid ima artery].** Inconstant (10%) unpaired artery supplying the thyroid gland. It usually arises from the brachiocephalic trunk. A

6 COMMON CAROTID ARTERY. Artery of the neck without any branches. It runs on both sides of the trachea and larynx and passes deep to the sternocleidomastoid. It arises on the right from the brachiocephalic trunk and on the left from the aortic arch. A B

7 **Carotid body.** Chromaffin cells in the connective tissue of the carotid bifurcation that presumably form a cluster of chemoreceptors. It is connected via the glossopharyngeal nerve with the circulatory and respiratory center. A

8 **Carotid sinus.** Dilatation of the carotid bifurcation or emerging internal carotid artery. Its walls contain baroreceptors. A

9 **Carotid bifurcation.** Site where the common carotid artery divides in the carotid triangle, usually at the level of the fourth cervical vertebra or laryngeal prominence. A B

10 EXTERNAL CAROTID ARTERY. It extends from the carotid bifurcation to its terminal division into the superficial temporal and maxillary arteries posterior to the neck of mandible. A

11 **Superior thyroid artery.** Usually the first branch of the external carotid artery. It divides into the following seven branches. A D E

12 **Infrahyoid branch.** Branch coursing on the hyoid bone and anastomosing with its counterpart from the opposite side. A

13 **Sternocleidomastoid branch.** Branch supplying the sternocleidomastoid muscle. A

14 **Superior laryngeal artery.** It penetrates the thyrohyoid membrane and lies beneath the mucosa of the piriform recess. It supplies the upper portion of the mucosa and the inner laryngeal muscles. Principle laryngeal artery. It is connected with the inferior laryngeal artery. A C

15 **Cricothyroid branch.** Branch supplying the cricothyroid and the mucosa of the anterior infraglottic cavity. It anastomoses with its counterpart from the opposite side in front of the cricothyroid ligament. A

16 **Anterior glandular branch.** Branch that mainly supplies the anterior portion of the thyroid gland. A

17 **Posterior glandular branch.** Branch that mainly supplies the upper portion, and to a lesser extent, the posterior portion of the thyroid gland. A

18 **Lateral glandular branch.** Branch that mainly supplies the lateral portion of the thyroid gland. A

19 **Ascending pharyngeal artery.** It usually arises from the posterior side of the external carotid artery above the superior thyroid artery. It ascends along the lateral wall of the pharynx, passing medial to the stylohyoid and continuing to the cranial base. A

20 **Posterior meningeal artery.** Artery lying lateral to the internal carotid artery. It usually passes through the jugular foramen to the dura mater and diploe of the posterior cranial fossa. A

21 **Pharyngeal branches.** Branches supplying the wall of the pharynx. They occasionally pass to the auditory tube and palatine tonsil. A

22 **Inferior tympanic artery.** Artery passing via the tympanic canaliculus into the tympanic cavity, reaching the mucosa of the medial wall. It is accompanied by the tympanic nerve. A

23 **[Linguofacial trunk].** Common trunk of the lingual and facial arteries that is occasionally present. E

24 **[[Thyrolingual trunk]].** Common trunk of the lingual and superior thyroid arteries that is occasionally present. D

12

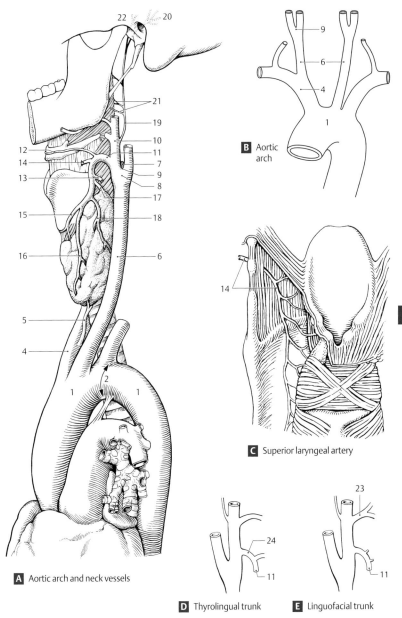

B Aortic arch

C Superior laryngeal artery

A Aortic arch and neck vessels

D Thyrolingual trunk

E Linguofacial trunk

12

1 **Lingual artery.** Second anterior branch of the external carotid artery. It enters the tongue behind the greater horn of hyoid bone, where it is covered by the hyoglossus, and runs near the inferior surface of the tongue to its tip. B C

2 **Suprahyoid branch.** Branch overlying the hyoid bone. It anastomoses with the branch from the opposite side and the infrahyoid branch of the superior thyroid artery. B

3 **Sublingual artery.** Artery arising at the anterior border of the hyoglossus and passing anteriorly between the mylohyoid and sublingual gland. It supplies the gland, muscles, and gingiva. B

4 **Dorsal lingual branches.** Branches supplying the posterior part and dorsum of tongue. B

5 **Deep lingual artery.** Main and terminal branch of the lingual artery. It runs between the genioglossus and inferior longitudinal muscles to the tip of tongue. The arteries on both sides are connected here only by capillaries. B

6 **Facial artery.** Third anterior branch of the external carotid artery. It lies behind the posterior belly of digastric muscle, stylohyoid, and submandibular gland. It crosses the mandible along the anterior border of the masseter and supplies the muscles of facial expression. A B C

7 **Ascending palatine artery.** It ascends on the lateral wall of the pharynx beneath the styloglossus to the palatoglossal and palatopharyngeal arches, soft palate, and palatine tonsil. It can replace or be replaced by the ascending pharyngeal artery. C

8 **Tonsillar branch.** Branch frequently arising from the ascending palatine artery. It penetrates the wall of the pharynx and supplies the palatine tonsil and posterior part of tongue. C

9 **Submental artery.** Lying caudal to the mylohyoid, it supplies the mylohyoid, adjacent muscles, and submandibular gland. It commonly anastomoses with the sublingual artery. C

10 **Glandular branches.** Branches directly supplying the submandibular gland. C

11 **Inferior labial branch.** Branch supplying the lower lip that runs between the orbicularis oris and mucous membrane of mouth. It anastomoses with the artery from the opposite side, the submental artery, and mental branch of inferior alveolar artery. C

12 **Superior labial branch.** Branch supplying the upper lip that runs between the orbicularis oris and mucous membrane of mouth. It anastomoses with the artery from the opposite side, the transverse facial artery, and infraorbital artery. C

13 *Nasal septal branch.* Branch supplying the nasal septum. It is connected with the cavernous body of the septum. C

14 **Lateral nasal branch.** Branch supplying the base of the ala of nose. C

15 **Angular artery.** Terminal branch of the facial artery in the medial angle of eye. It anastomoses with the ophthalmic artery via the dorsal nasal artery. A C

16 **Occipital artery.** Second branch that exits dorsally from the external carotid artery. It runs beneath the posterior belly of digastric muscle, extending medially from the mastoid process to the occiput. It is connected with the superficial temporal artery, vertebral artery, deep cervical artery, and posterior auricular artery. A C D

17 **Mastoid branch.** Branch passing through the mastoid foramen to the diploe and dura mater. It also supplies the mastoid cells. C

18 **Auricular branch.** Branch passing beneath the sternocleidomastoid and running obliquely posterior to the auricle. C

19 **Sternocleidomastoid branches.** Small branches supplying the sternocleidomastoid. C

20 **[Meningeal branch].** Branch that is occasionally present, passing through the parietal foramen to the dura mater. C

21 **Occipital branches.** Usually very tortuous branches that penetrate the trapezius and supply the area of the scalp overlying the occiput. C

22 **Descending branch.** Branch lying beneath the splenius capitis that supplies the neck muscles. C

23 **Posterior auricular artery.** Third branch exiting dorsally from the external carotid artery. It runs beneath the parotid gland and over the stylohyoid posterior to the auricle. It also supplies the muscles attached to the mastoid process and styloid process. C D

24 **Stylomastoid artery.** Thin vessel accompanying the facial artery. It runs with the facial artery from the stylomastoid foramen to the hiatus for greater petrosal nerve, where it supplies the dura mater. Before reaching the hiatus, it distributes branches to the middle and inner ear. D

25 **Posterior tympanic artery.** Artery traveling in the facial canal together with the chorda tympani to the tympanic membrane. D

26 *Mastoid branch.* Branches supplying the mastoid cells. D

27 *[Stapedial branch].* Small branch supplying the stapedius.

28 **Auricular branch.** Branch supplying the posterior side, and with penetrating portions, the anterior side, of the auricle and the small auricular muscles. D

29 **Occipital branch.** Branch that passes over the mastoid process and anastomoses with the occipital artery. D

30 **Parotid branch.** Branch supplying the parotid gland. D

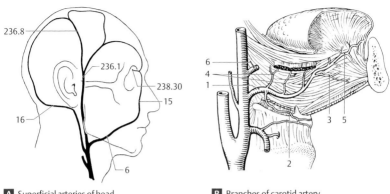

A Superficial arteries of head

B Branches of carotid artery

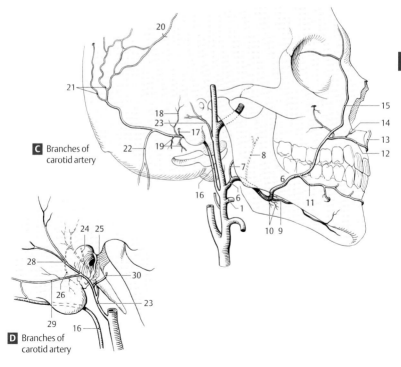

C Branches of carotid artery

D Branches of carotid artery

12

1 **Superficial temporal artery.** Superficial terminal branch of the external carotid artery. It ascends between the external auditory canal and temporomandibular joint, accompanying the auriculotemporal nerve, anterior to the auricle, to the temporal region where it distributes branches. A B, p. 235 A

2 **Parotid branch.** Branch supplying the parotid gland. A

3 **Transverse facial artery.** Covered by the parotid gland, it runs caudally from the zygomatic arch to the cheek. A

4 **Anterior auricular branches.** Smaller branches supplying the auricle and external auditory canal. A

5 **Zygomatico-orbital artery.** It passes superficially above the zygomatic arch to the lateral orbital margin. A

6 **Middle temporal artery.** Artery that enters the temporal muscle through the temporal fascia above the zygomatic arch. A

7 **Frontal branch.** Anterior terminal branch of the superficial temporal artery. It supplies the forehead region of the scalp and anastomoses with its counterpart from the opposite side as well as with the supra-orbital and supratrochlear arteries arising from the internal carotid artery. A

8 **Parietal branch.** Posterior terminal branch of the superficial temporal artery, coursing to the temporal region and supplying the scalp. It anastomoses with its counterpart from the opposite side as well as with the posterior auricular and occipital arteries. A, p. 235 A

9 **Maxillary artery.** Thicker terminal branch of the external carotid artery. It lies beneath the temporomandibular joint and behind the ramus of mandible, running laterally or medially from the lateral pterygoid to the pterygopalatine fossa. A B

10 **Deep auricular artery.** Artery passing backward and upward to the temporomandibular joint, external auditory canal, tympanic membrane, and mucosa of the tympanic cavity. B

11 **Anterior tympanic artery.** Artery accompanying the chorda tympani through the petrotympanic fissure into the tympanic cavity. B

12 **Inferior alveolar artery.** Artery traveling between the ramus of mandible and the medial pterygoid to the mandibular canal where it continues to the mental foramen. B

13 *Dental branches.* Branches supplying the roots of teeth. B

14 *Peridental branches.* Branches supplying the periodontium. B

15 *Mental branch.* Terminal branch of the inferior alveolar artery, supplying the soft tissues around the chin and lower lip. B

16 *Mylohyoid branch.* Branch given off before the artery enters the mandibular canal. It accompanying the mylohyoid nerve in the mylohyoid groove to the mylohyoid muscle. It anastomoses with the submental artery. B

17 **Middle meningeal artery.** Artery passing medial to the lateral pterygoid and through the foramen spinosum into the middle cranial fossa, where it distributes vessels between the dura mater and bone. B C

18 *Accessory branch.* Accessory branch arising from the meningeal or maxillary artery that supplies surrounding muscles and the auditory tube. It sometimes passes through the foramen ovale to the middle cranial fossa, supplying the dura mater up to the trigeminal ganglion. B

19 *Frontal branch.* Thicker anterior, terminal branch of the middle meningeal artery. It supplies the dura mater and bone of the anterior cranial fossa. Its sulcus is sometimes closed to form a canal. C

20 *Orbital branch.* Branch that passes through the superior orbital fissure toward the lacrimal gland. C

21 *Anastomotic branch with lacrimal artery.* Anastomosis of the orbital branch and lacrimal artery. C

22 *Parietal branch.* Branch of the middle meningeal artery supplying the bone and dura mater of the parietal and occipital bones. C

23 *Petrosal branch.* Small branch to the petrous part of temporal bone. It anastomoses with the stylomastoid artery via the hiatus for greater petrosal nerve. C

24 *Superior tympanic artery.* It arises near the petrosal branch and travels with the lesser petrosal nerve to the tympanic cavity. C

25 **Pterygomeningeal artery.** Artery arising from the maxillary or middle meningeal artery. It provides extracranial supply to the pterygoid muscles, tensor veli palatini, and auditory tube. It gives off branches via the foramen ovale to the trigeminal ganglion and dura mater.

26 **Masseteric artery.** Artery passing laterally through the mandibular notch to the masseter muscle. B

27 **Anterior deep temporal artery.** Branch ascending in the temporal fossa to the temporal muscle. B

28 **Posterior deep temporal artery.** Branch ascending in the temporal fossa to the temporal muscle. B

29 *Pterygoid branches.* Branches supplying the pterygoid muscles. B

30 **Buccal artery.** Branch running anteriorly and inferiorly on the buccinator muscle, supplying the buccal mucosa and gingiva. It anastomoses with the facial artery. B

31 **Posterior superior alveolar artery.** Artery that enters the maxilla at the maxillary tuberosity. Site of hemorrhage if the tuberosity is injured during molar extraction. B

32 *Dental branches.* Branches supplying the maxillary molars. B

33 *Peridental branches.* Branches supplying the periodontium and maxillary sinus mucosa. B

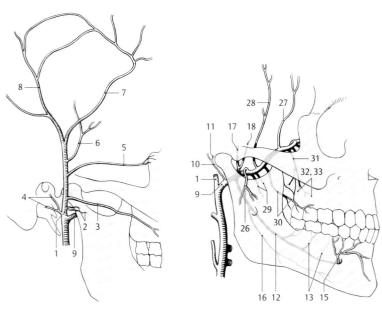

A Superficial temporal artery

B Maxillary artery

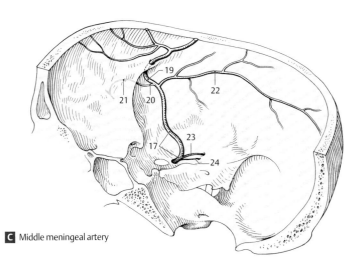

C Middle meningeal artery

1 **Infra-orbital artery.** It enters the orbit through the inferior orbital fissure and travels in the infra-orbital groove and canal to the infra-orbital foramen. A

2 *Anterior superior alveolar arteries.* Arteries that pass from the infra-orbital canal through the maxilla to the incisor teeth. A

3 *Dental branches.* Terminal branches supplying the teeth. A

4 *Peridental branches.* Terminal branches supplying the periodontium. A

5 **Artery of pterygoid canal.** Artery passing through the pterygoid canal to the auditory tube and surrounding area. A B

6 *Pharyngeal branch.* Branch supplying the epipharyngeal mucosa.

7 **Descending palatine artery.** Artery passing near the palate in the greater palatine canal. A B

8 *Greater palatine artery.* Artery emerging from the greater palatine foramen and passing anteriorly to the incisor teeth, supplying the mucous membrane. It lies protected up to the level of the premolar teeth in the palatine grooves. B

9 *Lesser palatine arteries.* Arteries that emerge from the lesser palatine foramina and supply the soft palate. B

10 *Pharyngeal branch.* Branch traveling in the palatovaginal canal that supplies the pharyngeal mucosa up to the level of the tonsil.

11 **Sphenopalatine artery.** Artery emerging from the sphenopalatine foramen into the nasal cavity. B

12 *Posterior lateral nasal arteries.* Arteries supplying the lateral and posterior nasal cavity as well as paranasal sinuses. B

13 *Posterior septal branches.* Branches supplying the inferoposterior nasal septum. B

14 *[[Nasopalatine artery]].* Inferior branch of the posterior septal branches. It travels in the incisive canal and anastomoses with the greater palatine artery.

15 INTERNAL CAROTID ARTERY. It passes from the carotid bifurcation, without any branches, to the cranial base, continuing in the carotid canal to its terminal division into the middle and anterior cerebral arteries. B

16 **Cervical part.** Segment of the artery coursing along the wall of the pharynx to its entrance into the petrous part of temporal bone. B C

17 **Carotid sinus.** Dilation at the beginning of the artery. It commonly involves the carotid bifurcation. Site of baroreceptors. B

18 **Petrous part.** Segment of the artery lying in the carotid canal of the petrous part of temporal bone. C

19 **Caroticotympanic arteries.** Branches to the tympanic cavity. C

20 **Artery of pterygoid canal.** Artery that accompanies the nerve of pterygoid canal along the base of the pterygoid process. C

21 **Cavernous part.** Segment of the artery in the cavernous sinus. Formation of the carotid syphon. C

22 **Tentorial basal branch.** Branch passing over the superior border of petrous part of temporal bone to the tentorium cerebelli. C

23 **Tentorial marginal branch.** Branch passing to the tentorium cerebelli adjacent to the tentorial notch. C

24 **Meningeal branch.** Branch supplying the dura mater of the middle cranial fossa. C

25 **Cavernous branch.** Branch supplying the wall of the cavernous sinus. C

26 **Inferior hypophysial artery.** Branches of the inferior hypophysial artery that form a ring around the neurohypophysis. They anastomose with the superior hypophysial artery. C

27 **Branches to trigeminal ganglion.** C

28 **Branches to nerves.** Branches to the trigeminal and trochlear nerve. C

29 **Cerebral part.** Intradural segment. It extends from the exit of the ophthalmic artery to its division into the anterior and middle cerebral arteries. C

30 **Ophthalmic artery.** Artery arising from the anteriorly convex arch of the internal carotid artery and passing under the optic nerve within the optic canal into the orbit. C

31 **Superior hypophysial artery.** Artery supplying the stalk and infundibulum of pituitary gland, and part of the ventral hypothalamus. C

32 **Posterior communicating artery.** C

33 **Anterior choroidal artery.** p. 242.2

34 **Uncal artery.** Branch supplying the uncus that often arises from the anterior choroidal artery. C

35 **Clivus branches.** Branches supplying the clivus region.

36 **Meningeal branch.** Branch supplying the dura mater of the middle cranial fossa.

37 **Carotid syphon.** Variable convolution in the sagittal plane of the internal carotid artery in the cavernous sinus. It is usually U-shaped or S-shaped with an anteriorly convex curve. Its shape varies with age. C

12

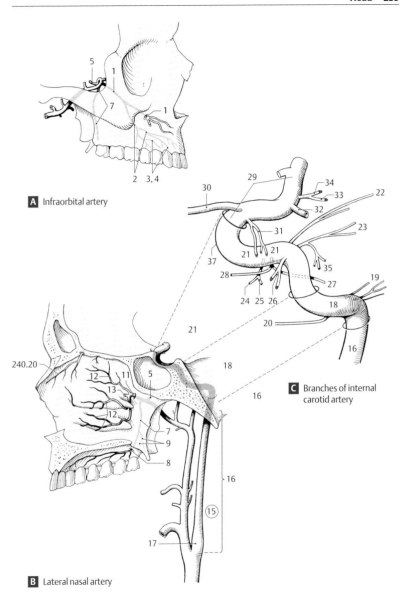

A Infraorbital artery

B Lateral nasal artery

C Branches of internal carotid artery

12

1 **Ophthalmic artery.** Artery arising from the last anterior convexity of the internal carotid artery and traveling beneath the optic nerve within the optic canal to the orbit. A

2 **Central retinal artery.** First branch of the ophthalmic artery. It enters the optic nerve about 1 cm behind the eyeball from inferior and extends with it to the retina. A

3 *Extraocular part.* Segment of the artery in the nerve. C

4 *Intraocular part.* Portion of the artery in the eyeball after it passes through the lamina cribrosa of sclera. C

5 **Lacrimal artery.** Artery branching off the ophthalmic artery laterally and passing with the lacrimal nerve along the upper margin of the lateral rectus muscle to the lacrimal gland. A

6 *Anastomotic branch with middle meningeal artery.* Branch that anastomoses with the orbital branch of middle meningeal artery. It can replace the ophthalmic artery. A

7 *Lateral palpebral arteries.* Terminal branches of the lacrimal artery supplying the lateral parts of the upper and lower lid. A B

8 **Recurrent meningeal branch.** Branch of the lacrimal artery that passes through the superior orbital fissure into the cranial cavity. It anastomoses with the anastomotic branch of middle meningeal artery. A

9 **Short posterior ciliary arteries.** Between 10 and 15 arteries that penetrate the sclera around the optic nerve, supplying the choroid, ciliary body, and passing to the major circulus arteriosus of iris. A C

10 **Long posterior ciliary arteries.** One lateral and one medial artery. They pass from posterior between the sclera and choroid, supply the ciliary body, and terminate at the major circulus arteriosus of iris. A C

11 **Muscular arteries.** Branches supplying the extraocular muscles.

12 *Anterior ciliary arteries.* Arteries arising from the anterior muscular arteries and passing through the sclera to the choroid and ciliary body before opening at the major circulus arteriosus of iris. A C

13 *Anterior conjunctival arteries.* Arteries supplying the conjunctiva of the eyeball. C

14 *Episcleral arteries.* Arteries supplying the superficial sclera. C

15 **Supra-orbital artery.** Artery running beneath the roof of the orbit on the levator palpebrae superioris and through the supra-orbital notch to supply the muscles and skin of the forehead. A B

16 *Diploic branch.* Branch supplying the bone.

17 **Anterior ethmoidal artery.** Together with the anterior ethmoidal nerve it emerges from the anterior ethmoidal foramen, ascends to beneath the dura mater of the anterior cranial fossa, descending through the cribriform plate of the ethmoid into the frontal sinus and nasal cavity as well as anterior and middle ethmoidal cells. A D

18 *Anterior meningeal branch.* Branch supplying the dural portion of the anterior cranial fossa. A D

19 *Anterior septal branches.* Branches supplying to the anterosuperior part of the nasal septum. D

20 *Anterior lateral nasal branches.* Branches supplying the upper part of the lateral wall of the nasal cavity and anterior ethmoidal cells. A

21 **Posterior ethmoidal artery.** Artery coursing together with the posterior ethmoidal nerve beneath the superior oblique muscle through the posterior ethmoidal foramen. It supplies the dura mater overlying the cribriform plate, and passes into the nasal cavity to the mucosa of the posterosuperior part. A

22 **Medial palpebral arteries.** Arteries arising from the ophthalmic artery below the trochlea of the superior oblique and descending behind the lacrimal sac to the upper and lower lid. They form vascular arches with the lateral palpebral arteries of the lacrimal artery. A B

23 *Superior palpebral arch.* Anastomoses between the medial and lateral palpebral arteries on the superior tarsus. B

24 *Inferior palpebral arch.* Anastomoses between the medial and lateral palpebral arteries on the inferior tarsus. B

25 *Posterior conjunctival arteries.* Branches supplying the palpebral conjunctiva. A

26 **Supratrochlear artery.** Ascending terminal branch of the ophthalmic artery traversing the frontal notch to supply the forehead. It anastomoses with the artery from the opposite side, the supra-orbital artery, and superficial temporal artery. A B

27 **Dorsal nasal artery; External nasal artery.** Descending terminal branch of the ophthalmic artery. It exits the orbit between the trochlea of superior oblique and medial palpebral ligament. It gives off a branch to the lacrimal sac, penetrates the nerve of the orbicularis oculi, anastomoses with the angular artery of the facial artery, and proceeds to the dorsum of nose. A B

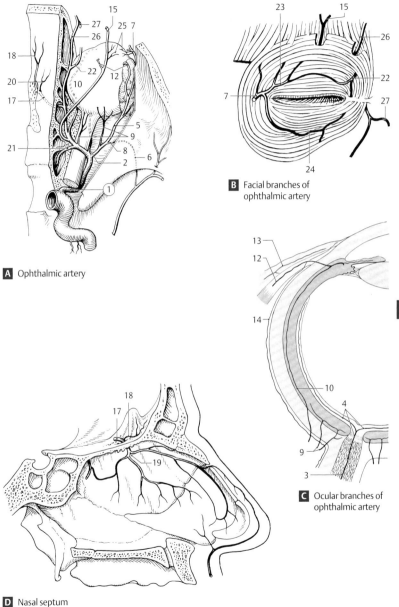

A Ophthalmic artery

B Facial branches of ophthalmic artery

C Ocular branches of ophthalmic artery

D Nasal septum

12

1 ARTERIES OF BRAIN.

2 **Anterior choroidal artery.** Artery usually arising from the internal carotid artery. It follows the optic tract posteriorly, enters the choroid plexus at the inferior horn and passes within it to the interventricular foramen. Its tiny branches are usually not visible on angiography. A B, p. 245 C

3 **Choroidal branches to lateral ventricle.** Branches to the plexus of the lateral ventricle. A B

4 **[Choroidal branches to third ventricle].** Inconstant branches to the plexus of the third ventricle. A

5 **Branches to anterior perforated substance.** Branches that pass through the perforated substance to the internal capsule. B

6 **Branches to optic chiasm; Branches to optic chiasma.** B

7 **Branches to optic tract.** B

8 **Branches to lateral geniculate body.** B

9 **Branches to internal capsule, genu.** B

10 **Branches to internal capsule, posterior limb.**

11 **Branches to internal capsule, retrolentiform limb.** Branches to the terminal portion of the internal capsule.

12 **Branches to globus pallidus.** Branches passing through the anterior perforated substance to the medial part of globus pallidus. B, p. 245 C

13 **Branches to tail of caudate nucleus.** Branches passing from inferior to tail of caudate nucleus.

14 **Branches to hippocampus.**

15 **[Branches to uncus].** Inconstant branches that may also arise directly from the internal carotid artery.

16 **Branches to amygdaloid body.** Branches supplying the medial amygdaloid body. A

17 **[Branches to tuber cinereum].** Inconstant branches supplying the tuber cinereum. B

18 **[Branches to hypothalamic nuclei].** Inconstant branches passing from inferior to the nuclei of the hypothalamus.

19 **Branches to thalamic nuclei.** Branches to the ventrolateral thalamus. p. 245 C

20 **Branches to substantia nigra.** Branches passing through the crus cerebri that supply the substantia nigra. B

21 **Branches to red nucleus.** Branches passing through the crus cerebri that supply the red nucleus. B

22 **Branches to crus cerebri.** Branches passing to the base of the crus cerebri.

23 **Anterior cerebral artery.** Thinner terminal branch of the internal carotid artery. It arises laterally from the division of the internal carotid artery above the anterior clinoid process, passes anteriorly, anastomoses with the artery from the opposite side, and runs between the cerebral hemispheres over the genu of corpus callosum and, on its posterior side, posteriorly toward the splenium. It gives off cortical arteries as well as arteries for subcortical and basal nuclei.

24 **Precommunicating part; A1 segment.** Portion of the artery before the anterior communicating artery. Dysfunction leads chiefly to paralysis of the upper limb. C

25 *Anteromedial central arteries.* The following four groups of vessels that enter the brain.

26 *Proximal medial striate arteries.* Arteries ascending from inferior to supply the brain, parts of the anterior hypothalamus, septum pellucidum, anterior commissure, fornix and striatum. C

27 *[[Artery of Heubner]].* Recurrent artery that runs parallel to the anterior cerebral artery. It is usually considered part of the proximal medial striate arteries. It divides into branches that ascend through the anterior perforated substance to supply parts of the head of caudate nucleus, putamen, and adjacent part of the internal capsule. B C

28 *Supraoptic artery.* Separate branch for the supraoptic nucleus of the hypothalamus.

29 *Anterior perforating arteries.* Arteries passing through the anterior perforated substance and supplying parts of the anterior diencephalon. C

30 *Preoptic arteries.* Separate branches for the preoptic nucleus of the hypothalamus.

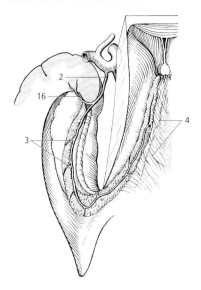

A Anterior choroid artery,
superior view

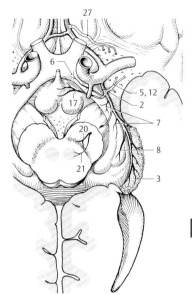

B Anterior choroid artery,
inferior view

12

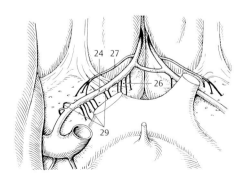

C Branches of anterior cerebral artery

1 **Anterior communicating artery.** Highly variable anterior vessel connecting the two anterior cerebral arteries. Common site of aneurysms. A

2 *Anteromedial central arteries.* The following three groups of vessels that extend from the anterior communicating artery to the brain.

3 *Suprachiasmatic artery.* Separate branch passing to the suprachiasmatic nucleus. A

4 *Median commissural artery.* Usually multiple branches passing to the infundibulum, preoptic region of the hypothalamus, corpus callosum, and anterior commissure. A

5 *Median callosal artery.* Artery that varies in form, extending from the middle of the anterior communicating artery to the rostrum and trunk of corpus callosum. It can assume the role of the pericallosal artery. A

6 **Postcommunicating part; A2 segment.** Segment of the anterior cerebral artery that joins with the anterior communicating artery and passes below the genu of corpus callosum to the vertex of the dorsally convex arch. A B

7 *Distal medial striate artery.* Artery supplying the paraolfactory area and lamina terminalis.

8 *Medial frontobasal artery; Medial orbitofrontal artery.* Branch passing to the inferior surface of the frontal lobe. B

9 *Polar frontal artery.* Branch extending to the anterior pole of the brain.

10 *Callosomarginal artery.* Portion of the artery in the cingulate sulcus that gives off branches to the medial side of the frontal lobe. B

11 *Anteromedial frontal branch.* Branch passing to the inferior half of the medial side of the frontal lobe. B

12 *Intermediomedial frontal branch.* Middle frontal lobe branch. B

13 *Posteromedial frontal branch.* Posterior frontal lobe branch. B

14 *Cingular branch.* Segment that ramifies in the posterior cingulate sulcus. B

15 *Paracentral branches.* Branches supplying the region posterior to the central sulcus. B

16 *Pericallosal artery.* Artery with variable course and ramification. The term is used in various ways. B
Here: Segment of the anterior cerebral artery extending from the exit of the callosomarginal artery along the sulcus of corpus callosum to the splenium.
Angiography: Segment of the anterior cerebral artery extending from the exit of the anterior communicating artery along the segments of the corpus callosum to the splenium.

17 *[Paracentral branches].* Variable branches passing to the paracentral branches of the callosomarginal artery.

18 *Precuneal branches.* Branches passing to the area in front of the cuneus. B

19 *Parieto-occipital branches.* Branches lying in the parieto-occipital sulcus. B

20 **Middle cerebral artery.** Second terminal branch of the internal carotid artery. It passes laterally between the frontal and temporal lobes to the lateral cerebral fossa where it divides. It gives off cortical branches as well as arteries for subcortical and basal nuclear regions. A

21 **Sphenoid part; Horizontal part; M1 segment.** First segment of the artery that travels horizontally and nearly parallel to the lesser wing of the sphenoid. It turns at a right angle at the limen insulae to continue ascending as the insular part. A

22 *Anterolateral central arteries; Lenticulostriate arteries.* Central branches passing to the basal ganglia. They penetrate laterally through the anterior perforated substance, curve upward, and fan out anteroposteriorly within the cerebrum to the internal capsule region. They supply the putamen, globus pallidus, lateral and dorsal parts of the head of caudate nucleus, claustrum, and internal capsule (except for its posterior limb). "Classic" cases of stroke involve these regions, with resulting damage often affecting the entire opposite side of the body. A

23 *Proximal lateral striate branches.* Branches that pass through the lentiform nucleus to the caudate nucleus. C

24 *Distal lateral striate branches.* Branches that pass laterally around the lentiform nucleus to the caudate nucleus. C

25 *[Uncal artery].* Inconstant branch to the uncus.

12

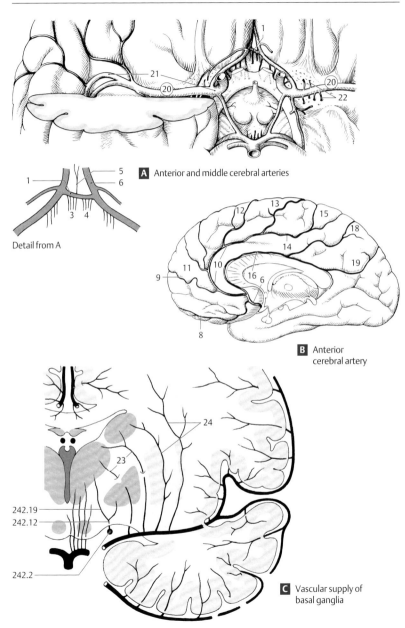

A Anterior and middle cerebral arteries

Detail from A

B Anterior cerebral artery

C Vascular supply of basal ganglia

1 *Polar temporal artery.* Artery to the temporal pole.

2 *Anterior temporal artery.* Additional branch to the temporal pole.

3 **Insular part; M2 segment.** Portion of the vessel on the insula. The middle cerebral artery usually divides into two trunks on the limen insulae that proceed as the terminal branches and supply cortical regions. The convoluted trunks with the initial portions of the terminal branches lie on the insula and are referred to in clinical terminology as the "Sylvian segment". A

4 *Insular arteries.* Arteries arising from the insular part of middle cerebral artery, usually along with initial segments of the terminal branches. They pass to the insular cortex, extreme capsule, claustrum, external capsule, putamen, and the amygdaloid body. A

5 **Inferior terminal branches; Inferior cortical branches; M2 segment.** Branches supplying the cortex of the temporal lobe.

6 *Anterior temporal branch.* Anterior branch supplying the frontal end of the two superior temporal gyri. A B

7 *Middle temporal branch.* A B

8 *Posterior temporal branch.* Branch that usually supplies the inferior temporal lobe and the transverse temporal gyri as well as the sensory region of the brain (Wernicke's area). A B

9 *Temporo-occipital branch.* Longest cortical artery, it supplies the gyri of the occipital lobe. A B

10 *Branch to angular gyrus.* It supplies the angular gyrus and superior occipital gyri. It can also supply the transverse temporal gyri. A B

11 **Superior terminal branches; Superior cortical branches; M2 segment.** Branches supplying the cortex of the frontal and parietal lobes as well as the central region.

12 *Lateral frontobasal artery; Lateral orbitofrontal artery.* Vessel passing anteriorly to the inferior and lateral side of the frontal lobe to the orbital gyri and inferior frontal gyrus. A B

13 *Prefrontal artery.* Artery passing over the insula and ascending along the inferior frontal gyrus, dividing and looping, to the convexity. Its branches supply the head, triangular part of inferior frontal gyrus, and foot of the second and third frontal gyri. On angiography, its branches resemble a candelabra. A B

14 *Artery of precentral sulcus.* Artery exiting the lateral sulcus at the level of the opercular part of inferior frontal gyrus and coursing in the precentral sulcus to the frontal lobe. A B

15 *Artery of central sulcus.* Artery coursing in the central sulcus to the precentral and postcentral gyri. A B

16 *Artery of postcentral sulcus.* Artery coursing in the postcentral sulcus to the parietal lobe. A B

17 *Anterior parietal artery.* Artery supplying the upper half of the posterior gyrus and the anterior parts of the parietal gyri. A B

18 *Posterior parietal artery.* Artery supplying the supramarginal gyrus and the white matter between the temporal horn of lateral ventricle and the insula in which the optic radiation runs. A B

19 **Posterior communicating artery.** Usually bilateral connection between the internal carotid artery or middle cerebral artery and the posterior cerebral artery of the basilar artery. C

20 **Posteromedial central arteries.** Variable branches passing through the posterior perforated substance to the diencephalon. C

21 *Anterior branches.*

22 *Posterior branches.*

23 **Chiasmatic branch.** Branch passing to the optic chiasm. C

24 **Artery of tuber cinereum.** Branches passing to the tuber cinereum. C

25 *Medial branches.*

26 *Lateral branches.*

27 **Thalamotuberal artery; Premammillary artery.** Constant branch passing in front of the mammillary body through the base of the brain mainly to the thalamus. C

28 **Hypothalamic branch.** Branch to the hypothalamus. C

29 **Mammillary arteries.** Branches to the mammillary body. C

30 **Branch to oculomotor nerve.** Branch to the third cranial nerve. C

12

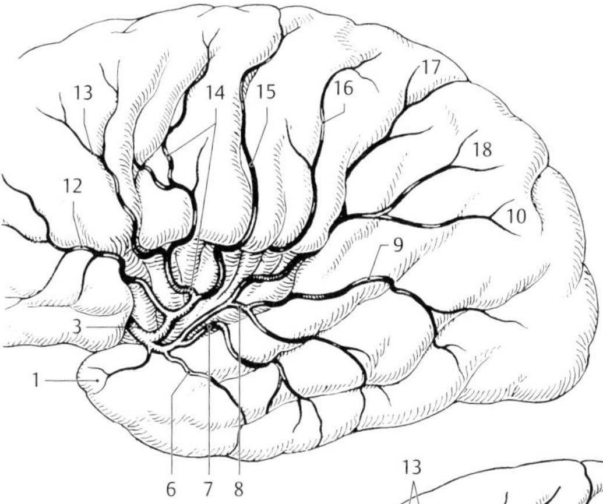

A Insular arteries

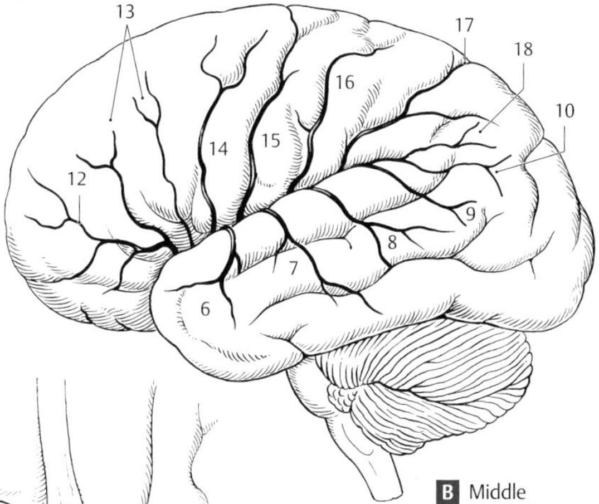

B Middle cerebral artery

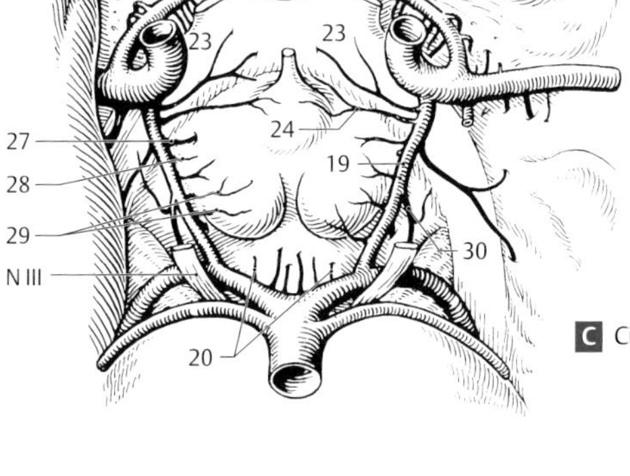

C Circulus arteriosus

1 **Cerebral arterial circle.** (Circle of Willis). Arterial circle on the base of the brain. It connects the carotid and vertebral artery systems and often ensures equilateral blood supply. It mainly supplies the diencephalon via the communicating arteries. B D, p. 247 C

2 **Posterior cerebral artery.** Paired terminal branch of the basilar artery that arises from the union of the right and left vertebral arteries. A B C D, p. 251 C

3 **Precommunicating part; P1 segment.** Portion of the vessel between the bifurcation of the basilar artery and the opening of the posterior communicating artery. It lies in the interpeduncular cistern and crosses over the third cranial nerve. B D

4 *Posteromedial central arteries; Paramedian arteries.* Branches passing through the posterior perforated substance to the mammillary body, thalamus, lateral wall of the third ventricle, and the posterior part of the internal capsule. D

5 *Short circumferential arteries.* Branches ascending along the lateral surface of the mesencephalon. They supply the tegmentum of midbrain and the base of peduncle. D

6 *Thalamoperforating artery.* Branch supplying the medial thalamus nuclei. A

7 *Collicular artery; Quadrigeminal artery.* Vessel distributing branches to the base of peduncle, tegmentum of midbrain, and geniculate bodies. D

8 **Postcommunicating part; P2 segment.** Portion of the vessel between the posterior communicating artery and the origin of the anterior temporal branches. It passes around the midbrain through the ambient cistern and the tentorial notch to the inferior surface of the cerebrum. B

9 *Posterolateral central arteries.* Branches supplying the posterior thalamus, tectal plate, pineal body, and medial geniculate body. C

10 *Thalamogeniculate artery.* Vessel supplying the posterolateral part of the thalamus, posterior portion of the internal capsule, and geniculate bodies. C D

11 *Posterior medial choroidal branches.* Branches passing over the roof of the third ventricle to the choroid plexus. C D, p. 251 C

12 *Posterior lateral choroidal branches.* Branches passing from posterior into the lateral ventricle. C, p. 251 C

13 *Peduncular branches.* Branches supplying the cerebral peduncle, red nucleus, and substantia nigra. p. 251 C

14 **Lateral occipital artery; P3 segment.** Lateral terminal branch of the posterior cerebral artery. It passes to the basilar surface of the posterior lobe and to the posterior temporal lobe. A B

15 *Anterior temporal branches.* Ascending cortical branches that extend to the basilar surface of the temporal lobe. A B

16 *Intermediate temporal branches; Middle temporal branches.* A B

17 *Posterior temporal branches.* A B

18 **Medial occipital artery; P4 segment.** Medial terminal branch of the posterior cerebral artery. It passes to the medial surface of the posterior lobe. A B

19 *Dorsal branch to corpus callosum.* Short branch to the splenium of corpus callosum. It anastomoses on the corpus callosum with the pericallosal artery. A

20 *Parietal branch.* Branch to the superior parietal lobe. A

21 *Parieto-occipital branch.* Branch lying in the parieto-occipital sulcus. It supplies the upper part of the cuneus and a posterior part of the precuneus. A B D

22 *Calcarine branch.* Branch lying in the calcarine sulcus. It supplies the occipital pole and its lateral surface. A B D

23 *Occipitotemporal branch.* Branch that extends as far as the temporal lobe. A B

12

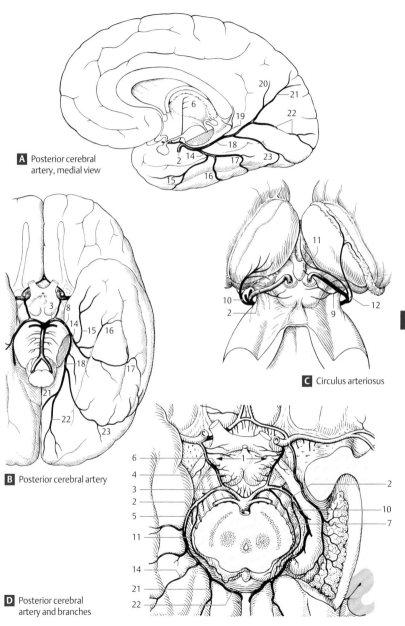

A Posterior cerebral artery, medial view

B Posterior cerebral artery

C Circulus arteriosus

D Posterior cerebral artery and branches

12

1 SUBCLAVIAN ARTERY. Artery that passes with the roots of brachial plexus between the anterior and middle scalene muscles through the scalene space, over the first rib in the groove for the subclavian artery. From the lateral border of the first rib, it continues as the axillary artery. A

2 **Vertebral artery.** Artery arising posterior to the anterior scalene muscle and usually passing from the sixth cervical vertebra through the foramina transversaria, then over the arch of the atlas behind its lateral mass, passing anteriorly through the posterior atlanto-occipital membrane and foramen magnum into the cranial cavity. A

3 **Prevertebral part.** Short portion of the vessel before it enters the foramen transversarium of the sixth cervical vertebra. A

4 **Cervical part.** Portion of the vessel passing through the foramina transversaria of C6–C1. A

5 *Spinal branches.* Transverse segments passing through the intervertebral foramina to the spinal cord, its meninges, and the vertebral bodies. A

6 *Radicular branches.* They extend along the anterior and posterior roots of spinal nerve as far as the spinal cord and provide its main supply. A

7 *Segmental medullary artery.* Artery following the spinal branches, supplying the meninges of the spinal cord and vertebral bodies, and involved in formation of the arterial plexus in the vertebral canal. A

8 *Muscular branches.* Branches to the deep neck muscles. A

9 **Atlantic part.** Tortuous segment of the vessel along the atlas. A

10 **Intracranial part.** Portion of the vessel coursing in the cranium. A

11 *Meningeal branches.* Branches passing along the anterior and posterior rim of the foramen magnum that supply the bone and dura mater of the posterior cranial fossa and falx cerebelli. A

12 *Posterior inferior cerebellar artery.* Artery passing dorsally, around the inferior olive to the inferior surface of the posterior part of the cerebellum. A B C

13 *Posterior spinal artery.* Artery descending in front of and behind the posterior roots of spinal nerve. It anastomoses with the anterior spinal artery. B C

14 *Cerebellar tonsillar branch.* Branch to the cerebellar tonsil.

15 *Choroidal branch to fourth ventricle.* Branch to the choroidal plexus of the fourth ventricle.

16 *Anterior spinal artery.* Right and left arteries join at the inferior border of the inferior olive as an unpaired vessel descending in the anterior median fissure. It anastomoses with the posterior spinal artery and gives off branches to the medulla oblongata, spinal cord, and cauda equina. A B

17 *Medial medullary branches.* Branches to the medulla oblongata.

18 *Lateral medullary branches.* Branches to the inferior cerebellar peduncle.

19 **Basilar artery.** Unpaired vessel that arises from the union of the right and left vertebral arteries and extends in the basilar sulcus of pons to the site where it divides into the posterior cerebral arteries. A B C

20 **Anterior inferior cerebellar artery.** Artery passing to the inferior and lateral surfaces of the cerebellum. B C

21 *Labyrinthine artery.* Artery traveling with the vestibulocochlear nerve to the internal ear. B C

22 **Pontine arteries.** Arteries supplying the pons. B C

23 *Medial branches; Paramedian pontine branches.* Branches arising from the dorsal side of the basilar artery. They penetrate the pons vertically, without reaching the floor of the ventricle.

24 *Lateral branches; Circumferential pontine branches.* Branches arising from the lateral side of the basilar artery and supplying the nuclei of cranial nerves V, VI, VII, and VIII. B C

25 *Mesencephalic arteries.* Branches to the midbrain. B

26 **Superior cerebellar artery.** Artery passing through the ambient cistern and traveling around the midbrain to the cerebellar surface beneath the tentorium cerebelli. B C

27 *Medial branch; Medial superior cerebellar artery.* Branch to the dorsal surface of the cerebellum and branches to the superior cerebellar peduncle.

28 *Superior vermian branch.* Terminal portion of the medial branch. C

29 *Lateral branch; Lateral superior cerebellar artery.* It turns lateralward at the anterior border of the cerebellum and supplies the superolateral portion of the cerebellum.

12

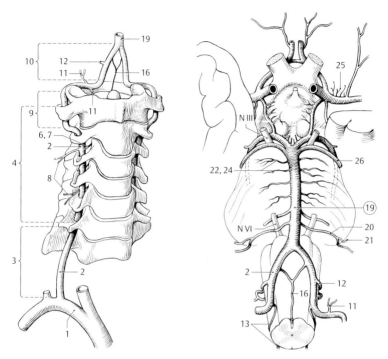

A Vertebral artery

B Arteries of base of brain

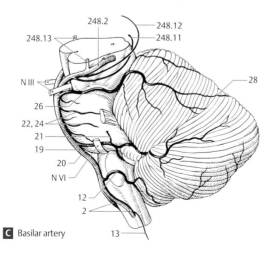

C Basilar artery

1   **Internal thoracic artery.** Artery arising from the subclavian artery and descending along the anterior inner side of the thorax to the diaphragm. A B

2   **Mediastinal branches.** Branches supplying the mediastinum. B

3   **Thymic branches.** Branches supplying the thymus. B

4   **[Bronchial branches].** Branches to the bronchi. B

5   **[Tracheal branches].** Branches to the trachea.

6   **Pericardiacophrenic artery.** It accompanies the phrenic nerve and supplies the pericardium and diaphragm. B

7   **Sternal branches.** Branches to the sternum. B

8   **Perforating branches.** Vessels that penetrate the first through sixth intercostal spaces, passing to the surface of the thorax. B

9   *Medial mammary branches.* Thicker perforating branches passing to the breast. B

10 **[Lateral costal branch].** Anatomical variant arising from the internal thoracic artery and running lateral and parallel to it. B

11 **Anterior intercostal branches.** Anterior tributaries passing into the intercostal spaces. B

12 **Musculophrenic artery.** Artery running posterior to the costal arch and giving off the remaining anterior intercostal branches from the seventh intercostal space onward. B

13 **Superior epigastric artery.** Continuation of the internal thoracic artery after it enters the abdominal cavity between the sternal and costal parts of diaphragm (Larrey's cleft = sternocostal triangle). B

14 **Thyrocervical trunk.** Varying common trunk of the inferior thyroid artery, transverse cervical artery, and suprascapular artery. A B

15 **Inferior thyroid artery.** Artery passing along the anterior border of the anterior scalene muscle to the level of the sixth cervical vertebra and then behind the common carotid artery to the thyroid gland. A B

16 *Inferior laryngeal artery.* Artery ascending behind the trachea, penetrating the inferior constrictor muscle of pharynx, and supplying the inferior part of the larynx. A B

17 *Glandular branches.* Branches supplying the parathyroid gland and the inferior and posterior surfaces of the thyroid gland. A

18 *Pharyngeal branches.* Branches to the wall of the pharynx. A B

19 *Esophageal branches.* Branches supplying the esophagus. A B

20 *Tracheal branches.* Branches supplying the trachea. A B

21 **Ascending cervical artery.** Artery lying medial to the phrenic nerve on the anterior scalene muscle. It can extend as far as the cranial base. A B

22 *Spinal branches.* Branches passing through the intervertebral foramina to the spinal cord. A B

23 **Suprascapular artery.** Artery that usually arises from the thyrocervical trunk, crosses over the anterior scalene muscle, and runs over the superior transverse scapular ligament into the supraspinous and infraspinous fossae. It anastomoses with the circumflex scapular artery. p. 255 A

24 *Acromial branch.* Branch penetrating the insertion of the trapezius and passing to the acromion. p. 255 A

25 **Transverse cervical artery.** Highly variable vessels. The second most common anatomical variant (25%) is presented here. It usually (75%) arises from the subclavian artery, often penetrates the brachial plexus, supplies the superior part of trapezius with its branches, and gives off a branch that accompanies the dorsal scapular nerve. A B

26 *Superficial cervical artery.* Vessel arising either as a superficial branch from the transverse cervical artery or as an autonomous superficial cervical artery from the thyrocervical trunk. It passes alongside the accessory nerve to the superior part of trapezius and the levator scapulae and splenius. A B

27 *Ascending branch.*

28 *Descending branch.*

29 *Deep branch*; *Dorsal scapular artery.* Vessel that arises either as a deep branch of the transverse cervical artery or directly from the subclavian artery (67%) and accompanies the dorsal scapular nerve. It supplies the medial borders of the scapulae and adjacent muscles. A B

30 **[Dorsal scapular artery].** Former term for the deep branch of the transverse cervical artery.

12

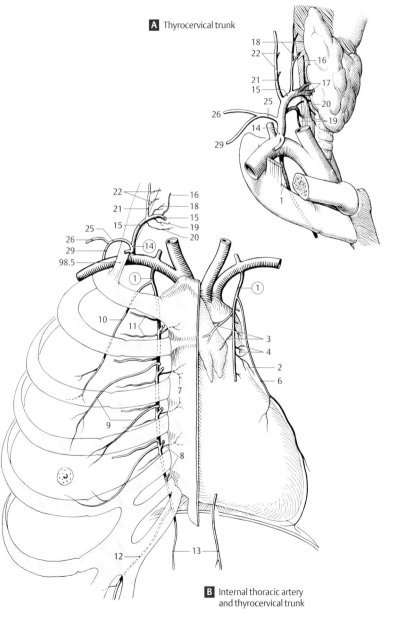

A Thyrocervical trunk

B Internal thoracic artery
and thyrocervical trunk

12

1 **Costocervical trunk.** Origin: posterior wall of subclavian artery, behind the anterior scalene muscle. Trunk of deep cervical artery and supreme intercostal artery. B

2 **Deep cervical artery.** Artery running posteriorly between the transverse processes of C7 and T1, then ascending ventrally on the semispinalis. It supplies the neck muscles. B

3 **Supreme intercostal artery.** Common trunk for the first two intercostal arteries. B

4 *First posterior intercostal artery.* Posterior intercostal artery passing into the first intercostal space. B

5 *Second posterior intercostal artery.* Posterior intercostal artery entering the second intercostal space. B

6 *Dorsal branches.* Branches supplying the muscles and skin of back. B

7 *Spinal branches.* Branches passing through the intervertebral foramen of T1–T2 to the spinal cord. B

8 **ARTERIES OF UPPER LIMB.**

9 **Axillary artery.** Continuation of the subclavian artery that reaches the inferior border of the pectoralis major. A B

10 **Subscapular branches.** Individual branches passing to the subscapularis. A

11 **Superior thoracic artery.** Variable branch passing to the subclavius, first and second intercostal muscles, and serratus anterior. A

12 **Thoraco-acromial artery.** It arises from the superior border of the pectoralis minor and distributes branches in all directions. A

13 *Acromial branch.* Branch that passes superolat. through the deltoid to the acromion. A

14 *Acromial anastomosis.* Arterial rete on the acromion. A

15 *Clavicular branch.* Small branch passing to the clavicle and the subclavius. A

16 *Deltoid branch.* Branch passing posterolat., supplying the deltoid and pectoralis maj. A

17 *Pectoral branches.* Branches passing inferiorly to supply the serratus anterior and pectoralis muscles. A

18 **Lateral thoracic artery.** Vessel descending along the lateral border of the pectoralis minor, supplying the serratus anterior and pectoralis muscles. A

19 *Lateral mammary branches.* Branches passing to the mammary gland. A

20 **Subscapular artery.** Artery originating at the lateral border of the subscapularis that supplies the subscapularis, latissimus dorsi, and teres major. A

21 *Thoracodorsal artery.* Branch to the latissimus dorsi and teres major. A

22 *Circumflex scapular artery.* Artery passing posteriorly through the medial (triangular) space to the infraspinous fossa. It anastomoses with the suprascapular artery. A

23 **Anterior circumflex humeral artery.** Artery that arises beneath the latissimus dorsi, at the same level as or deeper than the posterior circumflex humeral artery. It passes in front of the surgical neck of humerus to the coracobrachialis and biceps brachii and anastomoses with the posterior circumflex humeral art. A

24 **Posterior circumflex humeral artery.** It passes with the axillary nerve through the lateral (quadrangular) space to the shoulder joint and deltoid. It anastomoses with the anterior circumflex humeral artery, suprascapular artery, and thoracoacromial artery. A

25 **Brachial artery.** Continuation of the axillary artery that passes from the inferior border of the pectoralis major in the medial bicipital groove to its division into the radial and ulnar arteries. A

26 **[Superficial brachial artery].** Anatomical variant in which the brachial artery lies on the median nerve rather than beneath it. A

27 **Profunda brachii artery; Deep artery of arm.** Artery accompanying the radial nerve in the groove for radial nerve. A

28 *Humeral nutrient arteries.* Branches supplying the bone marrow of the humerus. A

29 *Deltoid branch.* Branch running superolaterally behind the humerus, passing along its lateral aspect to the deltoid. A

30 *Medial collateral artery.* Vessel passing posteromedially on the arm to the cubital anastomosis. A

31 *Radial collateral artery.* Branch passing with the radial nerve to the cubital anastomosis. An anterior branch continues as the radial recurrent artery. A

32 **Superior ulnar collateral artery.** Artery that often arises near the deep artery of arm. It passes with the ulnar nerve to the cubital anastomosis. A

33 **Inferior ulnar collateral artery.** Artery that often arises above over the medial epicondyle of humerus. It passes on the brachialis through the medial intermuscular septum and to the cubital anastomosis. A

34 **Radial artery.** Continuation of the brachial artery from its bifurcation, or first branch (embryological). It runs on the radial side between the brachioradialis and flexor carpi radialis over the pronator teres to the wrist (pulse palpation site). From there it ascends behind the trapezoid to the lateral aspect of the dorsum of hand where it courses to palmar. It extends between the two heads of the first dorsal interossei to reach to the deep palmar arch. p. 257 B

35 **Radial recurrent artery.** Recurrent artery that extends from the cubital fossa, passing medial to the radial nerve, to the radial collateral artery and cubital anastomosis. p. 257 B

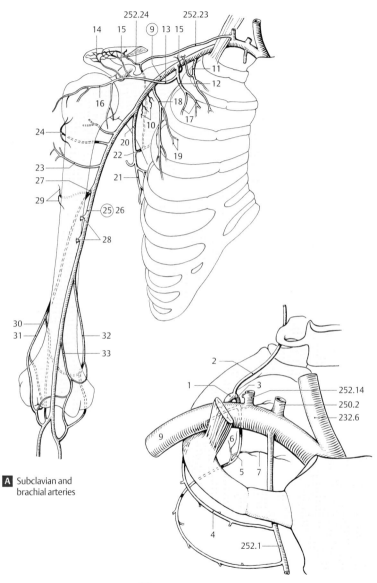

A Subclavian and brachial arteries

B Subclavian artery

1 **Nutrient artery of radius.** It enters the anterior side of the radius between the upper and middle one-third of the bone. B

2 **Palmar carpal branch.** Small branch at the distal border of the pronator quadratus. It contributes to formation of the palmar carpal arch. B

3 **[[Palmar carpal arch]].** Network formed by the palmar carpal branches of radial and ulnar arteries. It mainly supplies the joint capsules of the wrist. B

4 **Superficial palmar branch.** It supplies the muscles of the thenar eminence. It is often connected with the superficial palmar arch. B

5 **Dorsal carpal branch.** It crosses the dorsum of the wrist beneath the long extensor tendons and opening into the dorsal carpal arch. A

6 *Dorsal carpal arch.* Arterial network on the dorsum of the wrist. It receives tributaries from the anterior and posterior interosseous arteries and the dorsal carpal branches of radial and ulnar arteries. A

7 *Dorsal metacarpal arteries.* Vascular branches of the metacarpus, usually arising from the dorsal carpal arch in the interosseous spaces of the metacarpals II–IV. A

8 *Dorsal digital arteries.* Two vessels arising from the bifurcation of the dorsal metacarpal arteries. They supply the adjacent dorsal sides of the fingers. A

9 **Princeps pollicis artery.** Artery lying beneath the oblique head of adductor pollicis that sends two branches to the borders of the thumb. B

10 **Radialis indicis artery.** Variable branch of the princeps pollicis artery, situated radially on the palmar side of the index finger. B

11 **Deep palmar arch.** Continuation of the radial artery beneath the long flexors. It anastomoses with the ulnar artery. B

12 *Palmar metacarpal arteries.* Three or four branches of the deep palmar arch extending to the metacarpus. From there they are connected with the common or proper palmar digital arteries. B

13 *Perforating branches.* Branches that anastomose with the dorsal metacarpal arteries and carpal palmar arch. A B

14 **Ulnar artery.** Branch arising from the bifurcation of the brachial artery. It runs beneath the pronator teres toward the ulna, then accompanies the flexor carpi ulnaris on the flexor digitorum profundus to the wrist; from there it runs radially from the pisiform with the ulnar nerve to the palm, where it forms the superficial palmar arch. B

15 **Ulnar recurrent artery.** Branch of the ulnar artery from the cubital fossa where it supplies the muscle, bone, and joint capsule. B

16 *Anterior branch.* It extends in front of the medial epicondyle to the inferior collateral ulnar artery. B

17 *Posterior branch.* It travels in the groove for the ulnar nerve to the superior ulnar collateral artery and cubital anastomosis. B

18 **Cubital anastomosis.** Arterial plexus encircling the elbow joint. Tributaries from the arteries of the arm: middle and radial collateral arteries, superior and inferior ulnar collateral arteries. Tributaries from the forearm arteries: radial and ulnar recurrent arteries, recurrent interosseous artery. B

19 **Nutrient artery of ulna.** It enters the anterior side of the ulna below the upper one-third of the bone. B

20 **Common interosseous artery.** Trunk formed by the following vessels given off by the ulnar artery or branch arising from the division of the brachial artery (embryological) at the superior border of the pronator teres. B

21 *Anterior interosseous artery.* It runs on the interosseous membrane and beneath the pronator quadratus to the carpal and palmar dorsal arches. It supplies the deep flexors. B

22 *Median artery.* It accompanies the median nerve, which supplies the forearm muscles. B

23 *Posterior interosseous artery.* Artery passing dorsally between the interosseous membrane of forearm and the oblique cord that supplies the extensor muscles of the forearm, extending as far as the carpal dorsal arch. A B

24 *Perforating branch.* Portion of the vessel at its passage through the interosseous membrane of forearm. B

25 *Recurrent interosseous artery.* Recurrent artery passing beneath the anconeus to the cubital anastomosis. B

26 **Dorsal carpal branch.** Branch arising at the level of the pisiform and extending around the wrist to the carpal dorsal arch. A B

27 **Palmar carpal branch.** Branch that arises distal to the pronator quadratus and passes to the palmar carpal arch. B

28 **Deep palmar branch.** Thinner limb of the ulnar artery passing to the deep palmar arch. It leaves the ulnar artery at the level of the pisiform. B

29 **Superficial palmar arch.** It lies on the long flexor tendons. Its main tributary is from the ulnar artery; it anastomoses with the radial artery. B

30 **Common palmar digital arteries.** They pass toward the fingers as three or four arteries from convex palmar arch. B

31 *Proper palmar digital arteries.* Arteries that arise at the level of the bases of proximal phalanges, lie on the lateral flexor sides of the fingers, and branch off dorsally. B

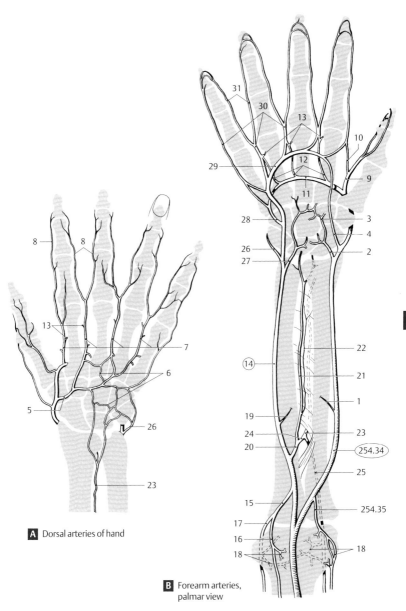

A Dorsal arteries of hand

B Forearm arteries, palmar view

1 DESCENDING AORTA. Portion of the vessel extending from the aortic isthmus at the level of the fourth thoracic vertebra to the aortic bifurcation at the level of the fourth lumbar vertebral body.

2 THORACIC AORTA. Part of the aorta descending to the aortic hiatus of the diaphragm at the level of the twelfth thoracic vertebra. A B

3 **Bronchial branches.** Their origin is highly variable, often at the level of the tracheal bifurcation. They ramify along the bronchi, extend to the bronchioles and supply their walls and the connective-tissue septa of the lungs. They form anastomoses with branches of the pulmonary artery. A

4 **Esophageal branches.** Branches to the wall of the esophagus. A

5 **Pericardial branches.** Small branches passing to the posterior wall of the pericardium. A

6 **Mediastinal branches.** Branches passing to the lymph nodes and connective tissue of the posterior mediastinum. A

7 **Superior phrenic arteries.** Branches passing from the inferior part of the thoracic aorta to the thoracic surfaces of the costal and lumbar parts of diaphragm. A

8 **Posterior intercostal arteries.** Paired tributaries arising from the posterior wall of the aorta, supplying the third through eleventh intercostal spaces. A B

9 *Dorsal branch.* Branch that passes posteriorly between the vertebral bodies and superior costotransverse ligament. It supplies the muscles and skin of back as well as the spinal cord and its meninges. B C

10 *Medial cutaneous branch.* It passes lateral to the spinous process to the skin. B C

11 *Lateral cutaneous branch.* It passes lateral to the transverse process to the skin. B C

12 *Spinal branches.* Branch passing through the intervertebral foramen into the vertebral canal. B C

13 Postcentral branch. Twig lying on the posterior surface of the vertebral body. C

14 Prelaminar branch. Branch lying on the anterior surface of the vertebral arch. C

15 Posterior radicular artery. Branch passing along the posterior root of spinal nerve. C

16 Anterior radicular artery. Branch passing along the anterior root of spinal nerve. C

17 Segmental medullar artery. Anastomosis with the anterior spinal artery. C

18 *Collateral branch.* Parallel branch arising near the angle of rib and passing to the intercostal artery. It travels anteriorly along the superior border of the next lowest rib and anastomoses with the internal thoracic artery. A B

19 *Lateral cutaneous branch.* It ramifies anteriorly and posteriorly, passing into the skin of the breast. B

20 *Lateral mammary branches.* Branches from the lateral cutaneous branches 2–4 that pass to the mammary gland. B

21 **Subcostal artery.** Segmental branch lying below the twelfth rib. It corresponds to an intercostal artery.

22 *Dorsal branch.* Branch supplying the muscles and skin of back. B

23 *Spinal branch.* Branch that passes through the intervertebral foramen, supplying the spinal cord and its meninges. B

24 ABDOMINAL AORTA. Segment of the aorta extending from the aortic hiatus of the diaphragm to its bifurcation at the fourth lumbar vertebral body. A

25 **Inferior phrenic artery.** Paired arteries arising from the anterior surface of the abdominal aorta. They supply the diaphragm from below. A

26 **Superior suprarenal arteries.** Uppermost group of the three suprarenal arteries. A

27 **Lumbar arteries.** Four paired segmental arteries that correspond to the intercostal arteries. A

28 **Dorsal branch.** Branch supplying the muscles and skin of back. A

29 **Spinal branch.** Branch passing through the intervertebral foramen, supplying the spinal cord and its meninges.

30 *Segmental medullary artery.* Anastomosis with the anterior spinal artery.

31 **Median sacral artery.** Median continuation of the aorta over the promontory to the coccygeal body. A

32 **Arteriae lumbales imae.** Paired branches of the median sacral artery. They correspond to a fifth lumbar artery. A

33 **Lateral sacral branches.** Small rectal branches. They anastomose with the lateral sacral branches of the internal iliac artery.

34 **Coccygeal body.** Nodule at the end of the median sacral artery. It lies on the tip of the coccyx and contains arteriovenous anastomoses and epithelioid cells. A

35 **Celiac trunk.** Frequently a common trunk of the left gastric, common hepatic, and splenic arteries at the level of the twelfth thoracic vertebra. The left gastric artery can also branch off of the aorta earlier. A

36 **Left gastric artery.** It ascends in the left gastropancreatic fold to supply the cardia, then passes along the lesser curvature to the pylorus, distributing branches to the anterior and posterior walls of stomach. It anastomoses with the right gastric artery. A

37 *Esophageal branches.* Branches that pass through the esophageal hiatus to the wall of the esophagus above the cardia. A

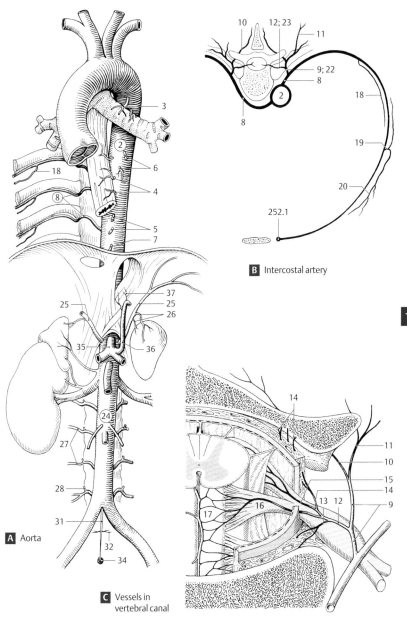

B Intercostal artery

A Aorta

C Vessels in
vertebral canal

12

1 **Common hepatic artery.** Usually a branch from the celiac trunk. It passes in the inferior gastropancreatic fold to the right and divides above the pylorus into the hepatic artery proper and gastroduodenal artery. A C

2 *Hepatic artery proper.* It ascends in the hepatoduodenal ligament and divides at the porta hepatis into two branches. A B C

3 *Right branch.* Right branch of hepatic artery proper supplying the right lobe of liver. It often arises from the superior mesenteric artery. A B

4 Cystic artery. It divides and passes to the anterior and posterior surfaces of the gallbladder. A B

5 Artery of caudate lobe. B

6 Anterior segmental artery. Branch passing to the anterior segment of right lobe. B

7 Posterior segmental artery. Branch passing to the posterior segment of right lobe. B

8 *Left branch.* Left branch of the hepatic artery proper supplying the left lobe of liver. A B

9 Artery of caudate lobe. B

10 Medial segmental artery. Branch passing to the medial liver segment. B

11 Lateral segmental artery. Branch passing to the lateral liver segment. B

12 *Intermediate branch.* Branch passing to the quadrate lobe. B

13 *Gastroduodenal artery.* Branch of the common hepatic artery. It usually lies behind the pylorus and divides at its inferior border. A C

14 *[Supraduodenal artery].* Inconstant first branch. It supplies the anterior two-thirds and posterior one-third of the duodenum.

15 *Posterior superior pancreaticoduodenal artery.* Branch coursing behind the pancreas, approximately following the duodenum. It anastomoses with the inferior pancreaticoduodenal artery. C

16 Pancreatic branches. Branches to the head of pancreas.

17 Duodenal branches. Branches to the duodenum.

18 *Retroduodenal arteries.* Branches of the gastroduodenal artery passing to the posterior surface of the duodenum and head of pancreas. During their course, they cross over the bile duct, distributing a branch to it.

19 *Right gastro-omental artery; Right gastro-epiploic artery.* It arises at the level of the inferior border of the pylorus and passes to the left as the continuation of the gastroduodenal artery in the greater omentum at a variable distance to the greater curvature of stomach. It extends to the left gastro-omental artery, with which it anastomoses. A C

20 Gastric branches. Short branches extending superiorly to the stomach. A

21 Omental branches. Long branches supplying the greater omentum. A

22 *Anterior superior pancreaticoduodenal artery.* Terminal branch descending on the pancreas and anastomosing with an inferior pancreaticoduodenal artery. A C

23 Pancreatic branches. A C

24 Duodenal branches. A C

25 *Right gastric artery.* It passes along the lesser curvature of stomach to the left gastric artery.

26 **Splenic artery.** Third branch of the celiac trunk. It runs along the superior border of the pancreas and then through the splenorenal ligament to the spleen. C

27 *Pancreatic branches.* Numerous smaller and some larger branches passing to the pancreas. A C

28 *Dorsal pancreatic artery.* It arises at the very beginning of the splenic artery and descends behind the neck of pancreas, partly embedded in pancreatic tissue. C

29 *Inferior pancreatic artery.* Branch of the dorsal pancreatic artery. It lies on the left side of the inferoposterior surface of the body of pancreas. C

30 *Prepancreatic artery.* Anastomosis between the main branch of the dorsal pancreatic artery and the anterior superior pancreaticoduodenal artery. C

31 *Greater pancreatic artery.* It passes from about the middle of the splenic artery inferiorly to the posterior surface of the pancreas, dividing and anastomosing with the inferior pancreatic artery. C

32 *Artery to tail of pancreas.* It arises from the distal end of the splenic artery or from one of its terminal branches and anastomoses in the tail of pancreas with the inferior pancreatic artery. C

33 *Left gastro-omental artery; Left gastro-epiploic artery.* It initially lies in the gastrosplenic ligament and then passes in the greater omentum toward the right gastro-omental artery. A C

34 *Gastric branches.* Long branches supplying the stomach.

35 *Omental branches.* Long branches to the greater omentum. A

36 *Short gastric arteries.* Branches of the splenic artery or its branches that mainly pass to the fundus of stomach. A

37 *Splenic branches.* Five or six branches formed by the division of the splenic artery before it enters the spleen. A

38 *Posterior gastric artery.* Branch supplying the posterior wall of stomach. A

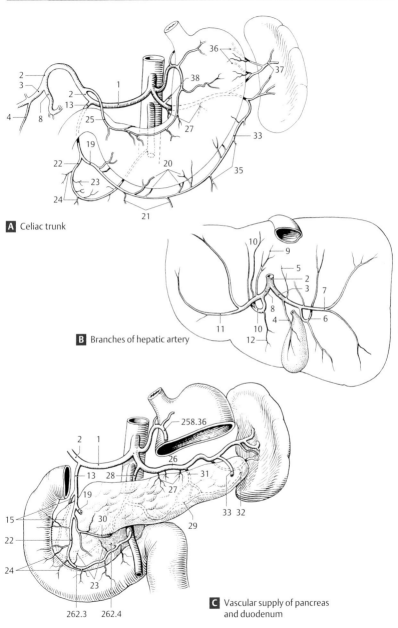

A Celiac trunk

B Branches of hepatic artery

C Vascular supply of pancreas and duodenum

12

1 **Superior mesenteric artery.** Second unpaired aortic branch. It arises about 1 cm below the celiac trunk at the level of the first lumbar vertebra. It initially runs behind the pancreas, then on the uncinate process and gives off branches to the mesentery and mesocolon. It supplies the head of pancreas, the small intestine as far as the superior part of duodenum, and the colon up to the splenic flexure. A B

2 **Inferior pancreaticoduodenal artery.** Artery arising behind the pancreas and running between the duodenum and pancreas to the superior pancreaticoduodenal arteries. It supplies the head of pancreas and duodenum. A

3 *Anterior branch.* It anastomoses with the anterior superior pancreaticoduodenal artery. p. 261 C

4 *Posterior branch.* It anastomoses with the posterior superior pancreaticoduodenal artery. p. 261 C

5 **Jejunal arteries.** Branches running in the mesentery to the jejunum. A

6 **Ileal arteries.** Branches passing in the mesentery to the ileum. A

7 **Ileocolic artery.** Artery coursing near the root of mesentery that passes downward and to the right to the ileocecal junction. A

8 *Colic branch.* Ascending branch to the ascending colon. It anastomoses with the right colic artery. A

9 *Anterior cecal artery.* It runs in the vascular fold of cecum to the anterior surface of the cecum. A

10 *Posterior cecal artery.* It runs behind the opening of the ileum into the cecum to its posterior surface. A

11 *Appendicular artery.* It initially runs behind the ileum, then in the free margin of the meso-appendix. Its exit is highly variable and it sometimes has a dual exit. A

12 *Ileal branch.* Descending branch to the ileum. It anastomoses with the lowermost ileal artery. A

13 **Right colic artery.** Artery passing retroperitoneally to the ascending colon. It anastomoses with the ascending branch of the ileocolic artery and middle colic artery. A

14 **Right flexural artery.** Artery to the right colic flexure. A

15 **Middle colic artery.** Artery passing in the mesocolon to the transverse colon. A

16 **Marginal artery; Juxtacolic artery; Marginal arcade.** Anastomosis between the left colic artery and sigmoid arteries. B

17 **Inferior mesenteric artery.** It arises at the level of the third and fourth lumbar vertebrae and passes leftward to the descending colon, sigmoid colon, and rectum. B

18 **Ascending artery.** Anastomosis between the left colic artery and middle colic artery. A B

19 **Left colic artery.** Artery passing retroperitoneally to the descending colon. B

20 **Sigmoid arteries.** Arteries descending obliquely to the sigmoid colon. B

21 **Superior rectal artery.** Artery passing behind the rectum into the lesser pelvis. It divides into a right and left branch and, after penetrating the muscle, supplies mainly the mucosa up to the anal valves. B

22 **Middle suprarenal artery.** Artery arising directly from the aorta that supplies the suprarenal gland. C

23 **Renal artery.** Artery usually arising in front of the first lumbar vertebra and passing to the kidney after ramifying. C D

24 **Capsular branches.** C

25 **Inferior suprarenal artery.** Branches passing to the suprarenal gland. C

26 **Anterior branch.** Anterior branch for the superior, anterior, and inferior renal segments. C D

27 *Superior segmental artery.* Artery passing to the superior renal segment, extending to the posterior surface of kidney. C

28 *Anterior superior segmental artery.* Artery passing to the anterior, superior renal segment. C

29 *Anterior inferior segmental artery.* Artery passing to the anterior, inferior renal segment. C

30 *Inferior segmental artery.* Artery passing to the inferior renal segment, extending to the posterior surface of kidney. C

31 **Posterior branch.** Posterior branch supplying the larger posterior renal segment. C D

32 *Posterior segmental artery.* Artery passing to the posterior renal segment. D

33 **Ureteric branches.** Small branches supplying the ureter. C

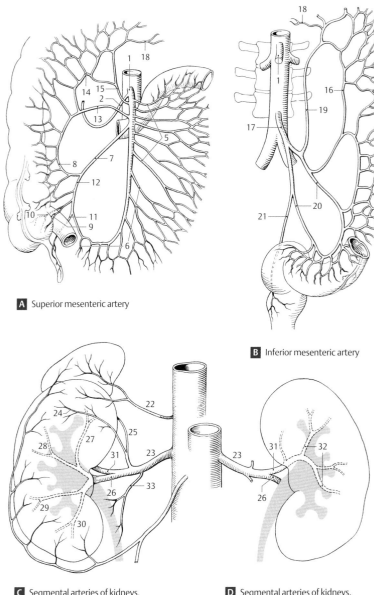

A Superior mesenteric artery

B Inferior mesenteric artery

C Segmental arteries of kidneys, anterior view

D Segmental arteries of kidneys, posterior view

12

1 **Testicular artery.** Artery arising at the level of the second lumbar vertebra. It crosses over the ureter and passes on the ductus deferens through the inguinal canal into the testes. C

2 **Ureteric branches.** Small branches to the ureter. C

3 **Epididymal branches.** Branches to the epididymides.

4 **Ovarian artery.** Artery arising at the level of the second lumbar vertebra. It passes in the suspensory ligament of ovary to the ovary. It anastomoses with the uterine artery. C

5 **Ureteric branches.** Small branches to the ureter. C

6 **Tubal branches.** Branches to the infundibulum of uterine tube. They anastomose with the uterine artery.

7 AORTIC BIFURCATION. Aortic bifurcation in front of the fourth lumbar vertebra, i.e., immediately below the navel. C

8 COMMON ILIAC ARTERY. It extends from the aortic bifurcation at the fourth lumbar vertebra to its division into the internal and external iliac arteries in front of the sacroiliac joint. Its branches are insignificant. C

9 INTERNAL ILIAC ARTERY. Artery beginning at the division of the common iliac artery, passing from here into the lesser pelvis and extending to the upper border of the greater sciatic foramen. Its branches are highly variable. C

10 **Iliolumbar artery.** It passes below the psoas and internal iliac artery into the iliac fossa. C

11 **Lumbar branch.** Branch that passes into the psoas and quadratus lumborum. C

12 **Spinal branch.** Branch that enters the spinal canal between the sacrum and fifth lumbar vertebra. C

13 **Iliacus branch.** Branch to the iliacus that lies parallel to the pelvis and extends to the iliac fossa. It anastomoses with the deep circumflex iliac artery. C

14 **Lateral sacral arteries.** Arteries descending lateral to the median sacral artery. They can also arise from the superior gluteal artery. C

15 **Spinal branches.** Arteries passing through the anterior sacral foramina into the sacral canal. C

16 **Obturator artery.** Artery running in the lateral wall of the pelvis and passing through the obturator foramen to the adductors. B C

17 **Pubic branch.** It anastomoses with the obturator branch of the inferior epigastric artery. C

18 **Acetabular branch.** It passes through the acetabular notch into the ligament of the head of femur. B

19 **Anterior branch.** Anterior branch lying on the adductor brevis. It anastomoses with the medial circumflex femoral artery. B

20 **Posterior branch.** Posterior branch lying beneath the adductor brevis. B

21 **Superior gluteal artery.** Artery passing through the greater sciatic foramen over the piriformis into the gluteal region. A C

22 **Superficial branch.** Branch lying between the gluteus maximus and medius. It anastomoses with the inferior gluteal artery. A

23 **Deep branch.** Branch lying between the gluteus medius and minimus. A

24 *Superior branch.* Branch passing on the upper border of the gluteus minimus to the tensor muscle of fascia lata. A

25 *Inferior branch.* It runs in the gluteus medius as far as the greater trochanter. A

26 **Inferior gluteal artery.** After passing through the greater sciatic foramen, it runs beneath the piriformis, distributing branches beneath the gluteus maximus. It anastomoses with the superior gluteal artery, obturator artery, and circumflex femoral arteries. A C

27 **Artery to sciatic nerve.** Main leg artery from a phylogenetic view. It accompanies and supplies the sciatic nerve. It anastomoses with the medial circumflex femoral artery and perforating branches. A C

28 **Umbilical artery.** First inferior branch arising from the internal iliac artery. It is obliterated postnatally from the exit site of the superior vesical arteries onward. C

29 **Patent part.** Part of the umbilical artery present during fetal development that does not obliterate postnatally. It gives off the following arteries.

30 *Artery to ductus deferens; Artery to vas deferens.* Artery descending in the pelvis to the fundus of bladder and from that point onward accompanying the ductus deferens to the testicular artery. C

31 *Ureteric branches.* Three branches to the ureter. C

32 *Superior vesical arteries.* Branches to the superior and middle segments of the urinary bladder. C

33 **Occluded part.** Part of the fetal umbilical artery that is obliterated postnatally to form the cord of umbilical artery. C

34 **Cord of umbilical artery.** Connective-tissue cord in the medial umbilical fold that is derived from the obliterated umbilical artery. C

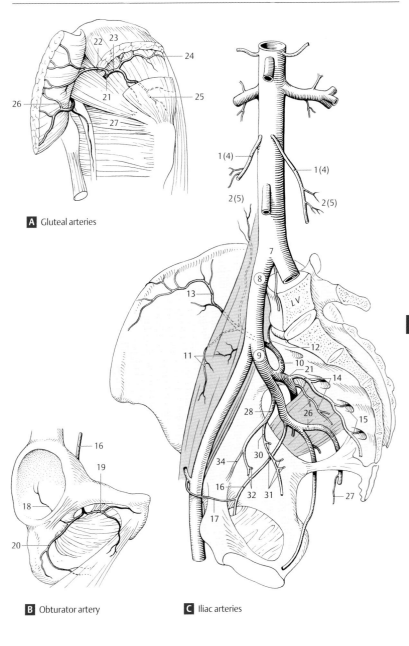

A Gluteal arteries

B Obturator artery

C Iliac arteries

12

1 **Inferior vesical artery.** Artery supplying the inferior portion of the urinary bladder and, in the male, the prostate and seminal vesicle. A

2 **Prostatic branches.** Branches to the prostate and seminal vesicle.

3 **Uterine artery.** Corresponds to the artery of the ductus deferens, passing in the base of the broad ligament of uterus to the cervix of uterus and ascending in a very tortuous course along the side of the uterus. A C

4 **Helicine branches.** Corkscrew-like coiled terminal branches of the uterine artery in the uterine muscles. C

5 **Vaginal branches.** Branches passing to the vagina. They are connected with the vaginal arteries and middle and inferior rectal arteries. A C

6 *[Azygos artery of vagina].* Inconstant unpaired longitudinal anastomoses on the anterior and posterior walls of vagina.

7 **Ovarian branch.** Branch running along the ligament of ovary and through the mesovarium to the ovary. It anastomoses with the ovarian artery and tubal branch. C

8 **Tubal branch.** It passes in the mesosalpinx of the uterine tube to the site of its anastomosis with the ovarian artery. C

9 **Vaginal artery.** Branch supplying the vagina that arises directly from the internal iliac artery. A

10 **Middle rectal artery.** Artery running over the pelvic floor to reach the rectum and supply its musculature. A E

11 **Vaginal branches.** Inferior vaginal branches. A

12 **Prostatic branches.** Branches supplying the prostate.

13 **Internal pudendal artery.** Artery exiting the pelvis through the greater sciatic foramen and passing through the lesser sciatic foramen to the lateral wall of the ischioanal fossa. A D E

14 **Inferior rectal artery.** Artery passing transversely through the ischioanal fossa and supplying both sphincters as well as the skin below the anal valves. D E

15 **Perineal artery.** Artery arising at the posterior margin of the urogenital diaphragm. It supplies the bulbospongiosus and ischiocavernosus. D E

16 **Posterior scrotal branches.** Branches passing to the scrotum. E

17 **Posterior labial branches.** Branches passing to the labia majora. D

18 **Urethral artery.** It enters into the corpus spongiosum at the union of the crura of penis and extends to the glans penis. It anastomoses with the dorsal and deep arteries of penis. E

19 **Artery of bulb of penis.** It supplies the bulb of penis as well as the deep transverse perineal muscle and bulbourethral gland. E

20 **Artery of bulb of vestibule.** D

21 **Deep artery of penis.** Artery passing anteriorly in the corpus cavernosum penis. E

22 **Dorsal artery of penis.** It passes on the dorsum of penis under the fascia to the glans penis. E

23 **Deep artery of clitoris.** Artery to the corpus cavernosum of clitoris. D

24 **Dorsal artery of clitoris.** Its course resembles that of the dorsal artery of penis, supplying the body, glans, and prepuce of clitoris. D

25 **Perforating arteries of penis.** Branches of the dorsal artery that pass through the tunica albuginea to the corpus cavernosum.

26 **ARTERIES OF LOWER LIMB.**

27 EXTERNAL ILIAC ARTERY. Second branch of the common iliac artery, which continues as the femoral artery.

28 **Inferior epigastric artery.** It arises dorsally from the inguinal ligament and ascends to the inner surface of the rectus abdominis, producing the lateral umbilical fold. It anastomoses with the superior epigastric artery. A B

29 *Pubic branch.* Branch extending to the pubis. A

30 *Obturator branch.* Branch anastomosing with the pubic branch of obturator artery. A

31 *[Accessory obturator artery].* Obturator artery arising from the inferior epigastric artery that is seldom present.

32 *Cremasteric artery.* Branch supplying the cremaster and spermatic cord. It corresponds to the artery of round ligament of uterus.

33 *Artery of round ligament of uterus.* Branch supplying the connective tissue and smooth muscles of round ligament of uterus. A C

34 **Deep circumflex iliac artery.** Artery that curves posterolaterally beneath the transversalis fascia along the iliac crest. A

35 *Ascending branch.* Ascending artery that passes between the transverse abdominal and internal oblique muscles of abdomen up to the McBurney's point. It anastomoses with the iliolumbar artery. A

36 **Femoral artery.** Artery extending from the inguinal ligament to the popliteal artery. B

37 **Superficial epigastric artery.** It arises distal to the inguinal ligament and passes on the abdominal muscles toward the navel. B

38 **Superficial circumflex iliac artery.** It runs parallel to the inguinal ligament toward the anterior superior iliac crest. B

39 **Superficial external pudendal artery.** It passes medially through the fascia cribrosa. B

40 **Deep external pudendal artery.** It passes medially along the border of the adductor longus through the fascia lata. B

41 *Anterior scrotal branches.* Branches of the deep external pudendal artery that supply the scrotum. B

42 *Anterior labial branches.* Branches of the deep external pudendal artery that supply the labia. B

43 *Inguinal branches.* Branches in the inguinal region that arise from both external pudendal arteries. B

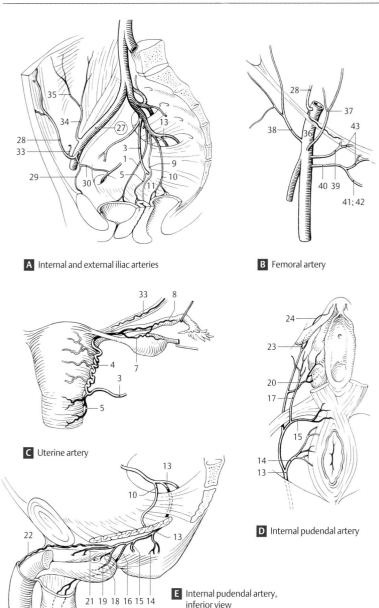

A Internal and external iliac arteries

B Femoral artery

C Uterine artery

D Internal pudendal artery

E Internal pudendal artery, inferior view

1 **Descending genicular artery.** Artery that arises in the adductor canal and passes in the vastus to the genicular anastomosis at the knee joint. A B

2 *Saphenous branch.* Branch accompanying the saphenous nerve and passing to the leg. A B

3 *Articular branches.* Branches traveling through the vastus medialis to the genicular anastomosis. A

4 **Deep artery of thigh.** Thick, deep initially lateral branch of the femoral artery. It crosses under the femoral artery and gives off the following branches.

5 **Medial circumflex femoral artery.** It passes medially and posteriorly between the iliopsoas and pectineus. A

6 *Superficial branch.* Branch running between the pectineus and adductor longus. A

7 *Deep branch.* Branch running below the lesser trochanter to the quadratus femoris, adductor magnus, and hamstrings. It anastomoses with the gluteal arteries. A

8 *Ascending branch.* It passes to the adductor brevis, adductor magnus, and obturator externus. It anastomoses with the obturator artery. A

9 *Descending branch.* It passes between the quadratus femoris and adductor magnus to the hamstrings. A

10 *Acetabular branch.* Branch passing through the acetabular notch into the ligament of the head of femur. It anastomoses with the obturator artery. A

11 **Lateral circumflex femoral artery.** Artery running lateralward beneath the rectus femoris. A

12 *Ascending branch.* Branch ascending beneath the sartorius and rectus femoris and terminating beneath the tensor of fascia lata. It anastomoses with the medial circumflex femoral artery and gluteal arteries. A

13 *Descending branch.* Branch extending beneath the rectus femoris to the knee joint. A

14 *Transverse branch.* Branch that penetrates the vastus lateralis and has numerous anastomoses. A

15 **Perforating arteries.** Terminal branches of the deep artery of thigh that pass through slits in the adductor muscles to run close to the femur posteriorly to the long knee flexors. A

16 *Femoral nutrient arteries.* Arteries arising from the first and third perforating arteries. A

17 **Popliteal artery.** Artery extending from the end of the adductor canal to its division at the inferior border of the popliteus. B

18 **Superior lateral genicular artery.** Artery passing above the lateral femoral condyle and beneath the tendon of the biceps femoris anteriorly to the genicular anastomosis. A B

19 **Superior medial genicular artery.** Artery passing beneath the tendon for the adductor magnus anteriorly to the genicular anastomosis. A B

20 **Middle genicular artery.** It passes inferiorly and posteriorly to the cruciate ligaments and synovial folds. B

21 **Sural arteries.** Branches supplying the calf muscles, and the fascia and skin of the leg. B

22 **Inferior lateral genicular artery.** Artery passing beneath the lateral head of the gastrocnemius and beneath the fibular collateral ligament to the genicular anastomosis. A B

23 **Inferior medial genicular artery.** Artery passing beneath the medial head of the gastrocnemius and tibial collateral ligament to the genicular anastomosis. A B

24 **Genicular anastomosis.** Arterial plexus mainly on the anterior side of the knee joint. A

25 **Patellar anastomosis.** Special arterial plexus situated on the patella. A

26 **Anterior tibial artery.** It extends from its origin at the inferior border of the popliteus to the inferior border of the inferior extensor retinaculum. After penetrating the interosseous membrane, it lies between the tibialis anterior and extensor digitorum longus, then between the tibialis anterior and extensor hallucis longus. A B C

27 **[Posterior tibial recurrent artery].** Inconstant artery that passes beneath the popliteus to the knee joint.

28 **Anterior tibial recurrent artery.** Artery passing through the tibialis anterior to the genicular anastomosis. A B

29 **Anterior lateral malleolar artery.** Artery passing beneath the tendon of the extensor digitorum longus to the lateral malleolar network. C

30 **Anterior medial malleolar artery.** It passes beneath the tendon of the tibialis anterior to the medial malleolar network. C

31 **Lateral malleolar network.** Arterial plexus overlying the lateral malleolus. C

12

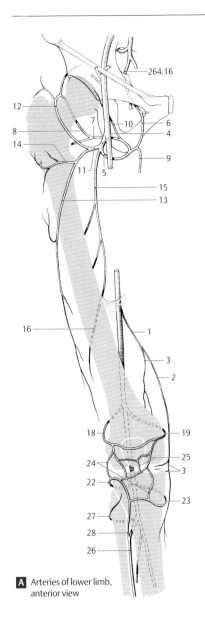

A Arteries of lower limb, anterior view

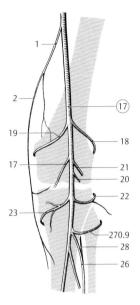

B Popliteal artery

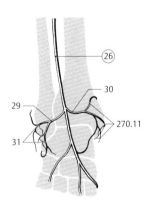

C Ankle joint with arteries, anterior view

12

1 **Dorsalis pedis artery; Dorsal artery of foot.** Continuation of the anterior tibial artery on the dorsum of foot. After crossing under the tendon of the extensor hallucis longus and passage of the extensor retinaculum, it lies lateral to the tendon where it is palpable. B

2 **Lateral tarsal artery.** It arises at the level of the head of talus and passes under the short extensors of the toes toward the cuboid. It anastomoses with the arcuate artery. B

3 **Medial tarsal arteries.** Several free branches passing to the medial border of the foot. B

4 **[Arcuate artery].** It curves laterally over the bases of metatarsals beneath the extensor digitorum brevis. B

5 **Dorsal metatarsal arteries.** Four branches that pass distalward over the intermetatarsal spaces and divide into two dorsal digital arteries each. B

6 **Dorsal digital arteries.** Interdigital arteries that arise from the metatarsal arteries. B

7 **Deep plantar artery.** Especially thick, perforating branch of a dorsal metatarsal artery that anastomoses with the plantar arch. B

8 **Posterior tibial artery.** It passes beneath the tendinous arch of soleus under the superficial flexor group and passes from posterior to the medial malleolus. A C

9 **Circumflex fibular branch; Circumflex peroneal branch.** Branch arising at the very beginning of the posterior tibial artery and traveling anteriorly around the fibula to the genicular anastomosis. A

10 **Medial malleolar branches.** Branches passing behind the medial malleolus to the medial malleolar network. A

11 **Medial malleolar network.** Arterial plexus overlying the medial malleolus. A

12 **Calcaneal branches.** Branches passing to the surface of the calcaneus. A

13 **Tibial nutrient artery.** Artery entering the nutrient foramen below the soleal line. A

14 **Fibular artery; Peroneal artery.** Artery that extends to the calcaneus and is covered for most of its length by the flexor hallucis longus. A

15 **Perforating branch.** It pierces the interosseous membrane immediately above the malleolus and passes to the lateral malleolar network and dorsum of foot. A

16 **Communicating branch.** Transverse branch that anastomoses with the posterior tibial artery. A

17 **Lateral malleolar branch.** Branches that often arise from the communicating branch and pass to the lateral malleolus. A

18 *Calcaneal branches.* Branches that mainly pass to the lateral side of the calcaneus. A

19 **Calcaneal anastomosis.** Arterial network on the posterior calcaneus. A

20 **Fibular nutrient artery.** Branch passing to the fibula. A

21 **Medial plantar artery.** Usually thinner, medial terminal branch of the posterior tibial artery that passes to the abductor hallucis and flexor digitorum brevis. C

22 **Deep branch.** Deep branch that usually anastomoses with the plantar arch. C

23 **Superficial branch.** Branch that courses superficially on the abductor hallucis to the great toe. C

24 **Lateral plantar artery.** Thicker, lateral terminal branch of the posterior tibial artery. It curves anterolaterally from the flexor digitorum brevis to the quadratus plantae. C

25 **Deep plantar arch.** Distal, convex continuation of the lateral plantar artery between the interosseous and oblique head of adductor hallucis. C

26 *Plantar metatarsal arteries.* Four arterial trunks arising from the plantar arch beneath the intermetatarsal spaces. C

27 *Perforating branches.* Usually two vessels each between the metatarsals passing to the dorsum of foot. C

28 *Common plantar digital arteries.* Portion of the distal perforating branch up to its division into the plantar digital arteries proper. C

29 Plantar digital arteries proper. Arteries running along the medial and lateral plantar aspects of the toes. C

30 **[Superficial plantar arch].** Occasional superficial anastomosis between the medial and lateral plantar arteries.

31 **[[Tibiofibular trunk]].** Common trunk formed by the posterior tibial artery and fibular artery, arising after the exit of the anterior tibial artery. Frequent site of occlusion. A

12

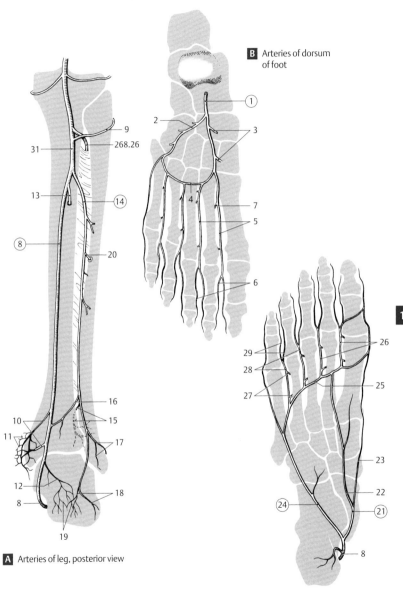

B Arteries of dorsum of foot

1
2
3
4
7
5
6

9
31
268.26
13
14
8
20
16
15
10
11
17
12
8
18
19

A Arteries of leg, posterior view

26
29
28
27
25
23
22
24
21
8

C Arteries of plantar surface of foot

12

1 **VEINS.** Thin-walled blood vessels that return blood to the atrium.

2 PULMONARY VEINS. Blood vessels leading from the lungs to the heart.

3 [[RIGHT PULMONARY VEINS]]. The two right pulmonary veins which occasionally unite to form a single trunk. A B

4 RIGHT SUPERIOR PULMONARY VEIN. Pulmonary vein that drains the superior and middle lobes. A B

5 **Apical vein; Apical branch.** Branch that drains the apical segment. A

6 *Intrasegmental part.* Twig draining the apical segment. A

7 *Intersegmental part.* Twig lying between the apical and posterior segments. A

8 **Anterior vein; Anterior branch.** Anterior branch draining the anterior segment. A

9 *Intrasegmental part.* Twig draining the anterior segment. A

10 *Intersegmental part.* Twig lying between the anterior and lateral segments. A

11 **Posterior vein; Posterior branch.** Branch that drains the posterior segment. A

12 *Infralobar part.* Twig draining the posterior segment. A

13 *Intralobar part.* Twig lying between the posterior segment and the apical segment of the inferior lobe. A

14 **Middle lobe vein; Middle lobe branch.** Branch that drains the middle lobe. A

15 *Lateral part.* Twig that drains the lateral segment of the middle lobe. A

16 *Medial part.* Twig that drains the medial segment of the middle lobe. A

17 RIGHT INFERIOR PULMONARY VEIN. Pulmonary vein that drains the right inferior lobe. A B

18 **Superior vein; Superior branch.** Branch that drains the apical segment of the inferior lobe. A

19 *Intrasegmental part.* Twig draining the apical segment of the inferior lobe. A

20 *Intersegmental part.* Twig lying between the apical segment and posterior basal segment. A

21 **Common basal vein.** Common vein draining the basal segments of the lung. A

22 *Superior basal vein.* Vein that drains blood from the lateral and anterior basal segments. A

23 *Anterior basal vein; Anterior basal branch.* Branch that drains the anterior segment and part of the lateral basal segment. A

24 Intrasegmental part. Twig draining the anterior basal segment. A

25 Intersegmental part. Twig lying between the anterior and lateral basal segments. A

26 *Inferior basal vein.* Vein draining the posterior basal segment. A

27 [[LEFT PULMONARY VEINS]]. The two left pulmonary veins which occasionally unite to form a single trunk. B

28 LEFT SUPERIOR PULMONARY VEIN. Pulmonary vein that drains the left superior lobe. B C

29 **Apicoposterior vein; Apicoposterior branch.** Branch that drains the apicoposterior segment. C

30 *Intrasegmental part.* Twig draining the apicoposterior segment. C

31 *Intersegmental part.* Twig lying between the apicoposterior and anterior segments. C

32 **Anterior vein; Anterior branch.** Branch draining the anterior segment. C

33 *Intrasegmental part.* Twig draining the anterior segment. C

34 *Intersegmental part.* Twig lying between the anterior segment and superior lingular segment. C

13

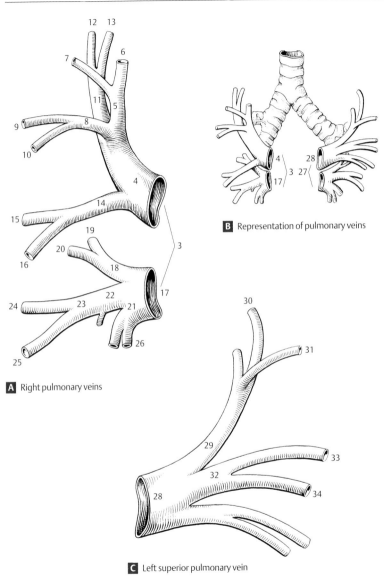

A Right pulmonary veins

B Representation of pulmonary veins

C Left superior pulmonary vein

13

1 **Lingular vein; Lingular branch.** Common branch draining the two lingular segments. A

2 *Superior part.* Twig draining the superior lingular segment. A

3 *Inferior part.* Twig draining the inferior lingular segment. A

4 LEFT INFERIOR PULMONARY VEIN. Pulmonary vein that drains the left inferior lobe. A

5 **Superior vein; Superior branch.** Branch draining the apical segment of the inferior lobe. A

6 *Intrasegmental part.* Twig draining the apical segment of the left inferior lobe. A

7 *Intersegmental part.* Twig lying laterally between the apical segment and anterior basal segment and medially between the apical segment and posterior basal segment. A

8 **Common basal vein.** Common trunk of the inferior and superior basal veins. A

9 **Superior basal vein.** Vein lying between the anterior basal branch and the common basal vein. A

10 *Anterior basal vein; Anterior basal branch.* Branch draining the anterior basal segment. A

11 *Intrasegmental part.* Twig draining the anterior basal segment. A

12 *Intersegmental part.* Twig lying between the medial and lateral segments. A

13 **Inferior basal vein.** Vein draining the posterior basal segment. A

14 VEINS OF HEART. Veins draining the walls of the heart. Their course and size varies. B

15 **Coronary sinus.** Collecting vein situated on the posterior wall of the left atrium that opens into the right atrium. It begins at the opening of the oblique vein of left atrium into the great cardiac vein. B

16 **Great cardiac vein.** Continuation of the anterior interventricular vein to the left coronary sulcus. Main venous outflow tract of the heart. B

17 *Anterior interventricular vein.* It lies in the anterior interventricular sulcus and collects blood from the anterior wall of the two ventricles. B

18 *Left marginal vein.* Vein situated closer to the lateral border of the left ventricle. B

19 **Posterior vein(s) of left ventricle.** It passes beyond the left margin of the heart upward to the great cardiac vein or coronary sinus. Number of vessels varies. B

20 **Oblique vein of left atrium.** Rudimentary vein on the posterior wall of the left atrium. Remnant of the embryonic left [[Duct of Cuvier]]. B

21 *Ligament of left vena cava.* Pericardial fold formed by the connective-tissue cord of the obliterated embryonic left superior vena cava. It lies in front of the left pulmonary vessels, which it can connect with one another. B

22 **Middle cardiac vein; Posterior interventricular vein.** It lies in the posterior interventricular sulcus and opens into the coronary sinus. B

23 **Small cardiac vein.** It lies on the right margin of the heart and in the right coronary sulcus and opens into the coronary sinus. B

24 *Right marginal vein.* It runs on the lateral border of the right ventricle and continues as the small cardiac vein. B

25 *Anterior vein(s) of right ventricle; Anterior cardiac veins.* One to three smaller veins on the right anterior wall. They open either into the small cardiac vein or directly into the right atrium. B

26 **Small cardiac veins [thebesian veins].** Small veins opening directly into the heart chambers, mainly into the right atrium. B

27 *Right atrial veins.* Small branches draining the wall of the right atrium. B

28 *Right ventricular veins.* Small branches draining the wall of the right ventricle. B

29 *[Left atrial veins].* Small branches draining the wall of the left atrium. B

30 *[Left ventricular veins].* Small branches draining the wall of the left ventricle. B

31 **SUPERIOR VENA CAVA.** C

32 RIGHT AND LEFT BRACHIOCEPHALIC VEIN. Right and left branches to the superior vena cava which give off the jugular and subclavian veins. C

33 **Inferior thyroid vein.** Vein passing from the unpaired thyroid plexus beneath the thyroid gland to the left (occasionally also right) brachiocephalic vein. C

34 **Unpaired thyroid plexus.** Venous plexus situated anterior to the trachea and below the caudal border of the thyroid gland. C

35 **Inferior laryngeal vein.** Vein passing from the larynx to the unpaired thyroid plexus. C

13

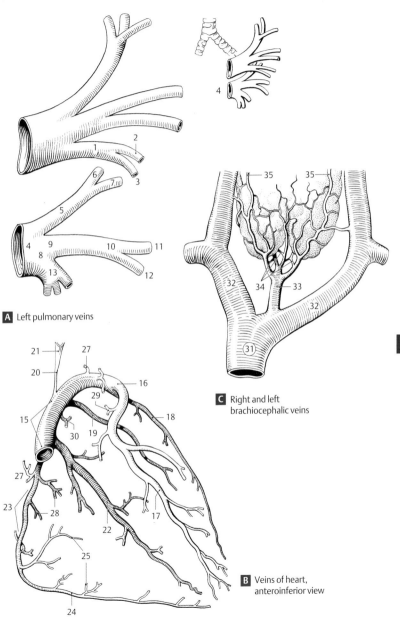

A Left pulmonary veins

C Right and left
brachiocephalic veins

B Veins of heart,
anteroinferior view

13

1 **Thymic veins.** Branches draining the thymus. A

2 **Pericardial veins.** Branches draining the pericardium. A

3 **Pericardiacophrenic veins.** Veins accompanying the pericardiacophrenic artery from the surface of the diaphragm and pericardium. A

4 **Mediastinal veins.** Branches draining the mediastinum. A

5 **Bronchial veins.** Branches draining the bronchi. A

6 **Tracheal veins.** Branches draining the trachea. A

7 **Esophageal veins.** Branches draining the esophagus. A

8 **Vertebral vein.** Vein accompanying the vertebral artery. Usually present as a venous plexus. A

9 *Occipital vein.* Vein beginning in the venous plexus of the scalp. It frequently opens into the vertebral vein or also into the internal or external jugular vein. A

10 *Anterior vertebral vein.* Vein accompanying the ascending cervical artery. It opens inferiorly into the vertebral vein. A

11 *[Accessory vertebral vein].* Continuation of the vertebral venous plexus. It often exits via the foramen transversarium of the seventh cervical vertebra. A

12 **Suboccipital venous plexus.** Venous plexus situated between the occipital bone and atlas. A

13 **Deep cervical vein.** Vein accompanying the deep cervical artery beneath the semispinalis capitis and cervicis. A

14 **Internal thoracic veins.** Veins accompanying the internal thoracic artery. They are often present as two veins as far as the third costal cartilage, after which they pass as a single vein medial to the artery. A

15 *Superior epigastric veins.* Veins accompanying the superior epigastric artery. They pass parasternally behind the costal cartilage to the internal thoracic veins. A

16 *Subcutaneous abdominal veins.* Branches that drain blood from the skin and empty into the superior epigastric veins. A

17 *Musculophrenic veins.* Veins that accompany the musculophrenic artery. A

18 *Anterior intercostal veins.* Branches in the intercostal spaces. A

19 **Supreme intercostal vein.** Conveys blood from the first intercostal space to the brachiocephalic or vertebral vein. A

20 **Left superior intercostal vein.** Vein draining the second to third (fourth) left intercostal spaces. It opens from posterior into the left brachiocephalic vein. A

21 INTERNAL JUGULAR VEIN. Main vein of the neck that extends from the jugular foramen to the venous angle. A

22 **Superior bulb of jugular vein.** Dilatation at the beginning of the vein in the jugular foramen. A

23 *Jugular body; Tympanic body.* Aggregation of cells in the adventitia of the superior bulb of jugular vein that are comparable to the carotid body.

24 **Vein of cochlear aqueduct.** Tiny vein accompanying the perilymphatic duct. A

25 **Inferior bulb of jugular vein.** Dilatation at the end of the internal jugular vein that is closed off cranially by a valve. A

26 **Pharyngeal plexus.** Venous plexus on the pharyngeal muscles. A

27 **Pharyngeal veins.** Veins from the pharyngeal plexus. A

28 **Meningeal veins.** Small branches draining the dura mater.

29 **Lingual vein.** Vein of the tongue that mostly lie near the lingual artery. A

30 *Dorsal lingual veins.* Numerous veins draining the dorsum of tongue. A

31 *Vena comitans of hypoglossal nerve.* Vein accompanying the hypoglossal nerve. A

32 *Sublingual vein.* Larger vein coursing lateral to the hypoglossal nerve. A

33 *Deep lingual vein.* Vein accompanying the deep lingual artery lateral to the genioglossus. A

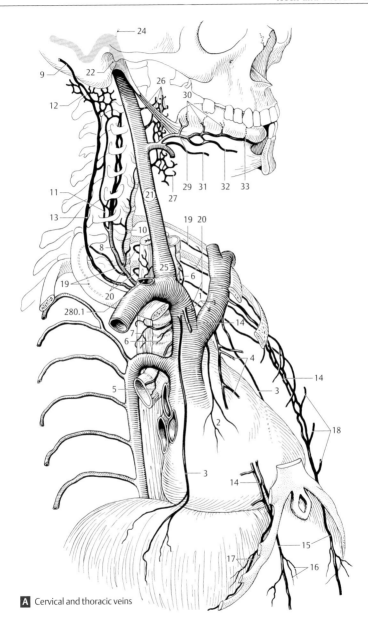

A Cervical and thoracic veins

13

1 **Superior thyroid vein.** Companion vein of the superior thyroid artery. It empties into the facial or internal jugular vein. A B

2 **Middle thyroid veins.** One or more thyroid veins with drainage to the internal jugular vein without corresponding arteries. A

3 **Sternocleidomastoid vein.** Vein from the sternocleidomastoid muscle that empties into the internal jugular vein or superior thyroid vein. A

4 **Superior laryngeal vein.** Companion vein of the superior laryngeal artery that drains into the superior thyroid vein. A

5 **Facial vein.** Vein beginning at the medial angle of eye that lies behind the facial artery and then beneath the submandibular gland. A B

6 **Angular vein.** Beginning of the facial vein at the angle of eye formed by the union of the supratrochlear and supra-orbital veins. It anastomoses with the ophthalmic vein and communicates via the nasofrontal vein with the superior ophthalmic vein. Similar to the latter, it does not have any valves. Potential infection pathway from the face to the orbits and cranial cavity. A B

7 **Supratrochlear veins.** Vein beginning at the coronal suture that drains the medial half of the forehead. It joins the angular vein. A B

8 **Supra-orbital vein.** Vein from the lateral part of the forehead that joins the supratrochlear veins. A

9 **Superior palpebral veins.** Veins draining the upper eyelid. A

10 **External nasal veins.** Veins from the lateral side of the nose. A

11 **Inferior palpebral veins.** Veins draining the lower eyelid. A

12 **Superior labial vein.** Veins draining the upper lip. A

13 **Inferior labial veins.** Usually multiple veins draining the lower lip. A

14 **Deep facial vein.** Vein coming from the pterygoid plexus and passing anteriorly on the maxilla. A B

15 **Parotid veins; Parotid branches.** Branches draining the parotid gland. A

16 **External palatine vein.** Conveys blood from the lateral tonsillar region of the palate and pharyngeal wall to the facial vein. A B

17 **Submental vein.** Companion vein of the submental artery. It anastomoses with the sublingual and anterior jugular veins. A

18 **Retromandibular vein.** It extends from the union of several branches in front of the ear to the facial vein. A B

19 **Superficial temporal veins.** Veins accompanying the superficial temporal artery. A

20 **Middle temporal vein.** Vein from the temporalis that empties into the superficial temporal veins. A

21 **Transverse facial vein.** Vein accompanying the transverse facial artery caudal to the zygomatic arch. A

22 **Maxillary veins.** Veins joining the pterygoid plexus with the beginning of the retromandibular vein. B

23 **Pterygoid plexus.** Venous plexus between the temporalis and medial and lateral pterygoid muscles, mainly around the lateral pterygoid. It has the following tributaries.

24 *Middle meningeal veins.* Veins accompanying the middle meningeal artery. B

25 *Deep temporal veins.* Veins accompanying the deep temporal artery. B

26 *Vein of pterygoid canal.* Vein accompanying the artery of pterygoid canal. B

27 *Anterior auricular veins.* Branches draining the external acoustic meatus and auricle. A B

28 *Parotid veins.* Branches draining the parotid gland. B

29 *Articular veins.* Branches draining the temporomandibular joint. B

30 *Tympanic veins.* Branches draining the tympanic cavity.

31 *Stylomastoid vein.* Vein accompanying the facial nerve from the tympanic cavity. B

13

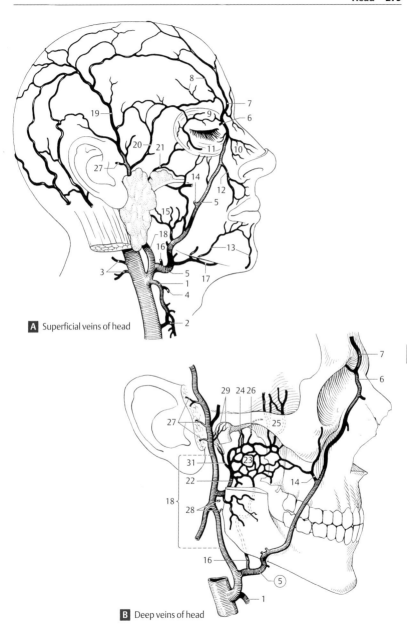

A Superficial veins of head

B Deep veins of head

13

1 **External jugular vein.** Vein lying between the platysma and superficial layer of cervical fascia and usually emptying into the subclavian vein. It is fed by the following veins. A

2 **Posterior auricular vein.** Superficial vein lying behind the ear. A

3 **Anterior jugular vein.** It commences at the level of the hyoid bone and, after crossing under the sternocleidomastoid, often drains into the external jugular vein. A

4 *Jugular venous arch.* Connection between the right and left anterior jugular veins in the suprasternal space. A

5 **Suprascapular vein.** Usually two veins accompanying the suprascapular artery. A

6 **Transverse cervical veins.** Veins accompanying the transverse cervical artery. A

7 **Dural venous sinuses.** Incompressible venous vessels. They lie between the dura mater and cranial periosteum, receive blood from the brain and meninges, and empty into the internal jugular vein. B C

8 **Transverse sinus.** It commences at the confluence of sinuses and passes laterally to the sigmoid sinus. B C

9 **Confluence of sinuses.** Union of the superior sagittal sinus, straight sinus, occipital sinus, and transverse sinus at the internal occipital protuberance. B C

10 **Marginal sinus.** It lies at the entrance to the foramen magnum and connects venous plexuses of the inner cranium with those of the vertebral canal. B

11 **Occipital sinus.** It commences with a venous plexus at the foramen magnum and passes within the root of the falx cerebelli to the confluence of sinuses. B C

12 **Basilar plexus.** Venous plexus on the clivus that is connected with the cavernous and petrosal sinuses, as well as venous plexuses of the vertebral canal. B

13 **Petrosquamous sinus.** Term with two uses. Inconstant sinus.
   1. Sinus lying in the petrosquamous fissure and connecting the transverse sinus and retromandibular vein.
   2. Sinus crossing the floor of the middle cranial fossa between the meningeal veins or sphenoparietal sinus and superior petrosal sinus.

14 **Sigmoid sinus.** It exits the lateral wall of the cranium as a continuation of the transverse sinus and courses in an S-shape to the jugular foramen. B C

15 **Superior sagittal sinus.** It lies within the root of the falx cerebri and extends from the crista galli to the confluence of sinuses. B C

16 *Lateral lacunae.* Small lateral spaces in the superior sagittal sinus. C

17 **Inferior sagittal sinus.** Small sinus at the free margin of the falx cerebri. It terminates in the straight sinus. C

18 **Straight sinus.** It commences at the union of the great cerebral vein and inferior sagittal sinus and runs within the root of the falx cerebri at its junction with the tentorium cerebelli to the confluence of sinuses. C

19 **Inferior petrosal sinus.** It runs from the cavernous sinus along the posterior inferior border of the petrous part of temporal bone to the jugular foramen. B

20 *Labyrinthine veins.* Branches draining the internal acoustic meatus and emptying into the inferior petrosal sinus. C

21 **Superior petrosal sinus.** It passes from the cavernous sinus along the superior border of the petrous part of temporal bone to the sigmoid sinus. B

22 **Cavernous sinus.** Spongy structure of expanded veins on both sides of the sella turcica into which the ophthalmic veins and other veins empty. The carotid artery and abducent nerve lie within it and cranial nerves III, IV, V1, and V2 travel in its lateral side wall. B

23 *Anterior intercavernous sinus.* Connection between the right and left cavernous sinuses anterior to the pituitary gland. C

24 *Posterior intercavernous sinus.* Connection between the right and left cavernous sinuses posterior to the pituitary gland. C

25 **Sphenoparietal sinus.** Sinus that runs beneath the lesser wing of sphenoid to the cavernous sinus. C

26 **Diploic veins.** Veins situated in the diploe of the cranial roof. They receive blood from the dura mater and cranial roof and communicate with both the dural venous sinuses and superficial veins of the head. C

27 **Frontal diploic vein.** Diploic veins running near the midline that empty into the supraorbital vein and superior sagittal sinus. A

28 **Anterior temporal diploic vein.** Anterior diploic vein that empties into the deep temporal vein and sphenoparietal sinus. A

29 **Posterior temporal diploic vein.** Posterior diploic vein that opens into the posterior auricular vein and transverse sinus. A

30 **Occipital diploic vein.** Furthest posterior diploic vein that empties into the occipital vein and transverse sinus. A

31 **[[Occipital vein]].** Vein accompanying the occipital artery. A

13

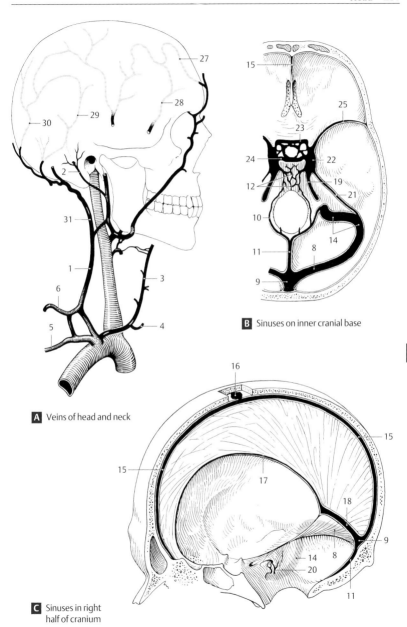

A Veins of head and neck

B Sinuses on inner cranial base

C Sinuses in right half of cranium

13

1 **Emissary veins.** Venous connections between a venous sinus, diploic veins, and superficial cranial veins.

2 **Parietal emissary vein.** Vein connecting the superior sagittal sinus with a superficial temporal vein by way of the parietal foramen. A

3 **Mastoid emissary vein.** Vein connecting the sigmoid sinus with the occipital vein via the mastoid foramen. A

4 **Condylar emissary vein.** Vein connecting the sigmoid sinus with the external vertebral venous plexus through the condylar canal. A

5 **Occipital emissary vein.** Connection between the confluence of sinuses and occipital vein. A

6 **Venous plexus of hypoglossal canal.** Venous plexus in the hypoglossal canal situated between the venous plexus around the foramen magnum and the internal jugular vein. D

7 **Venous plexus of foramen ovale.** Venous plexus in the foramen ovale between the cavernous sinus and pterygoid plexus. D

8 **Internal carotid venous plexus.** Venous plexus in the carotid canal between the cavernous sinus and pterygoid plexus. D

9 **Portal veins of hypophysis.** Veins conveying blood from the arterial capillary networks of the infundibulum and adenohypophysis to the cavernous sinus. E

10 CEREBRAL VEINS. Veins that mostly are located in the subarachnoid space and do not have valves. They mainly empty into the dural venous sinuses.

11 **Superficial cerebral veins.**

12 **Superior cerebral veins.** Superior veins of the cerebral cortex that open into the superior sagittal sinus from the lateral medial, and anterior inferior surface of the cerebrum.

13 *Prefrontal veins.* Veins from the frontal pole and its basal surface. B

14 *Frontal veins.* Veins from the upper one-third of the frontal lobe which extends to the central sulcus. B

15 *Parietal veins.* Sinus vessels from the parietal lobe. B

16 *Temporal veins.* Sinus vessels from the temporal lobe.

17 *Occipital veins.* Sinus vessels from the occipital lobe. B

18 **Superficial middle cerebral vein.** Vein from the inferior two-thirds of the cerebral hemisphere that passes within the lateral cerebral sulcus to the cavernous sinus. B

19 *Inferior anastomotic vein (Trolard's vein).* Inconstant, thicker anastomosis with the superior sagittal sinus. B

20 *Superior anastomotic vein (Vein of Labbé).* Inconstant, thicker anastomosis with the transverse sinus. B

21 **Inferior cerebral veins.** Veins on the cerebral base that open into the cavernous, petrosal, and transverse sinuses. B

22 *Vein of uncus.* Vein from the uncus of the hippocampal gyrus. C

23 *Orbital veins.* Veins from the orbits and surrounding region. D

24 *Temporal veins.* Veins from the temporal lobe. B

25 **Deep cerebral veins.** These are mostly concealed.

26 **Basal vein (Rosenthal's vein).** Vein beginning at the anterior perforated substance, running along the optic tract, and then passing around the brainstem dorsally to the great cerebral vein. C

27 *Anterior cerebral veins.* Veins accompanying the anterior cerebral artery. C

28 *Deep middle cerebral vein.* Vein beginning at the insula and opening into the basal vein. C

29 *Insular veins.* Tributaries to the deep middle cerebral vein.

30 *Inferior thalamostriate veins.* Veins from the caudate and lentiform nuclei as well as thalamus that exit the anterior perforated substance and open into the basal vein or deep middle cerebral vein. C

31 *Vein of olfactory gyrus.* Vein from the olfactory trigone region. C

32 *Inferior ventricular vein.* Vein from the white substance of the temporal lobe that exits at the level of the cerebral crura through the choroidal fissure. C

33 *Inferior choroid vein.* Vein conveying blood from the hippocampus, dentate gyrus, and choroid plexus to the basal vein. C

34 *Peduncular veins.* Veins draining the cerebral peduncle. C

13

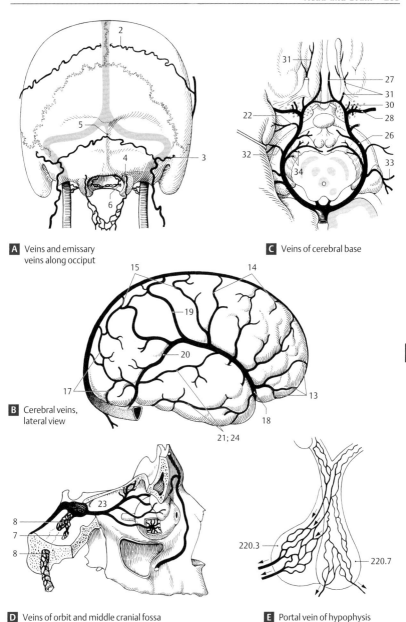

A Veins and emissary veins along occiput

C Veins of cerebral base

B Cerebral veins, lateral view

D Veins of orbit and middle cranial fossa

E Portal vein of hypophysis

1 **Great cerebral vein (Vein of Galen).** Short vein between the union of the two internal cerebral veins and the beginning of the straight sinus. A C

2 *Internal cerebral veins.* Right and left internal cerebral veins. They run in the transverse cerebral fissure, i.e., between the fornix and thalamus or roof of the third ventricle, beginning at the interventricular foramen and ending where they unite from opposite sides to form the great cerebral vein. A C

3 *Superior choroid vein.* It extends the entire length of the choroid plexus to the interventricular foramen and receives branches from the hippocampus, fornix, and corpus callosum. A

4 *Superior thalamostriate vein.* It runs in an angle between the thalamus and caudate nucleus, hence its name. It does not receive any branches from the thalamus, but from the rest of the surrounding region. It ends at its union with superior choroid vein in the interventricular foramen. A

5 *Anterior vein of septum pellucidum.* It passes from its drainage area, the white matter of the frontal lobe and genu of corpus callosum, through the septum pellucidum to the superior thalamostriate vein. A C

6 *Posterior vein of septum pellucidum.* It emerges from the roof of the lateral ventricle and frequently opens into the internal cerebral vein. C

7 *Medial vein of lateral ventricle.* Vein draining the white matter of the parietal and occipital lobes. It courses in the medial wall of the lateral ventricle and opens before the departure of the posterior horn. A

8 *Lateral vein of lateral ventricle.* Vein draining the white matter of the parietal and occipital lobes. It courses in the lateral wall of the lateral ventricle before the departure of the posterior horn. A

9 *Veins of caudate nucleus.* Multiple veins draining the caudate nucleus. A

10 *Lateral direct veins.* Branches from the wall of the lateral ventricle that open directly into the internal cerebral vein. A

11 *Posterior vein of corpus callosum*; *Dorsal vein of corpus callosum.* Branch exiting from inferiorly and from the end of the corpus callosum. A C

12 **Veins of brainstem.**

13 **Pontomesencephalic vein.** Continuation of the veins of medulla oblongata extending into the interpeduncular fossa. It is also an anteromedian anastomosis of both interpeduncular veins, conveying blood from them to the basal or petrosal veins on each side. B C

14 **Interpeduncular veins.** Veins lying in the interpeduncular fossa along the cerebral crura. B

15 **Intercollicular vein.** Vein beneath the median epiphysis between the superior and inferior colliculus. It is involved in formation of the precentral cerebellar vein.

16 **Lateral mesencephalic vein.** In connects the basal vein with the petrosal vein.

17 **Pontine veins.** Veins draining the pons.

18 *Anteromedian pontine vein.* Vein along the basilar sulcus. It anastomoses with the interpeduncular veins. B C

19 *Anterolateral pontine vein.* Vein that varies greatly in form lying lateral to the basilar sulcus. B

20 *Transverse pontine veins.* Veins lying at the level of the origin of the trigeminal nerve and draining the longitudinal network of veins into the petrosal vein. B

21 *Lateral pontine vein.* Continuation of the posteromedian medullary vein that lies on the lateral corner of the pons. B

22 **Veins of medulla oblongata.** Inferior continuation of the pontomesencephalic vein with tributaries from the medulla oblongata. B

23 *Anteromedian medullary vein.* Continuation of the anterior spinal vein that lies in the anterior median fissure. B C

24 *Anterolateral medullary vein.* It runs laterally between the pyramid and inferior olive. B

25 *Transverse medullary veins.* Connections between the two longitudinally coursing medullary veins which runs longitudinally. B

26 *Dorsal medullary veins.* Veins that mainly empty into the fourth ventricle and join in a dorsal vein that runs longitudinally. B

27 *Posteromedian medullary vein.* Continuation of the posterior spinal vein. B

28 **Vein of lateral recess of fourth ventricle.** It exits the lateral recess and opens into the inferior petrosal sinus. C

29 **Vein of cerebellomedullary cistern.** Vein crossing the cistern and draining into the marginal sinus.

30 **Cerebellar veins.**

31 **Superior vein of vermis.** Vein from the superior portion of the vermis of cerebellum that opens into the great or internal cerebral vein. B C

32 **Inferior vein of vermis.** Vein from the inferior half of the vermis that opens into the straight sinus. C

33 **Superior veins of cerebellar hemisphere.** Veins from the lateral hemisphere that usually open into the transverse sinus. A B

34 **Inferior veins of cerebellar hemisphere.** Veins usually from the inferior lateral parts of the hemispheres that open into the adjacent sinuses. C

35 **Precentral cerebellar vein.** Vein beginning between the lingula and central lobule and emptying into the great cerebral vein. C

36 **Petrosal vein.** Vein that is sometimes quite thick, arising near the flocculus and opening into the superior or inferior petrosal sinus. C

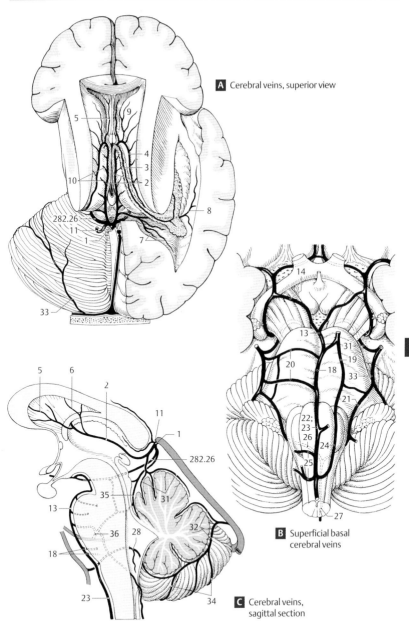

A Cerebral veins, superior view

B Superficial basal cerebral veins

C Cerebral veins, sagittal section

1 ORBITAL VEINS.

2 **Superior ophthalmic vein.** Vein arising medially above the eyeball with the nasofrontal vein and passing through the superior orbital fissure to the cavernous sinus. A

3 **Nasofrontal vein.** Connection between the ophthalmic vein and the union of the supratrochlear vein with the angular vein. A

4 **Ethmoidal veins.** Branches draining the ethmoidal cells. A

5 **Lacrimal vein.** Branch draining the lacrimal gland. A

6 **Vorticose veins.** Four or five branches from the choroid of the eyeball that penetrate the sclera laterally. A

7 **Ciliary veins.** Veins draining the ciliary body that pass either to the veins of the ocular muscles or to choroid veins. B

8 **Anterior ciliary veins.** Veins accompanying the anterior ciliary artery that convey blood from the ciliary body to the veins of the ocular muscles at their beginning. B

9 *Scleral veins.* Thin veins that mainly run in the anterior sclera.

10 **Central retinal vein.** Vein accompanying the central retinal artery. It opens either into the superior ophthalmic vein or directly into the cavernous sinus. B

11 *Extraocular part.* Portion coursing outside of the eyeball. B

12 *Intraocular part.* Portion in the retina. B

13 **Episcleral veins.** Branches lying on the sclera that empty into the superior ophthalmic veins. B

14 *Palpebral veins.* Branches from the upper eyelids. B

15 *Conjunctival veins.* Branches from the conjunctiva. A

16 **Inferior ophthalmic vein.** Vein from the lower eyelid and lacrimal gland that unites with the superior ophthalmic vein or passes directly into the cavernous sinus and pterygoid plexus. B

17 AZYGOS VEIN. Vein lying on the vertebral column that begins at the ascending lumbar vein and opens at the level of the fourth to fifth thoracic vertebrae into the superior vena cava before it enters the pericardium. C

18 **Arch of azygos vein.** Venous arch before the vein opens into the superior vena cava.

19 **Right superior intercostal vein.** Vein arising from the union of the second and third (fourth) right superior intercostal veins and opening into the azygos vein. C

20 **Hemi-azygos vein; Inferior hemi-azygos vein.** Vein that frequently begins at the left ascending lumbar vein, receives the eleventh through ninth intercostal veins, and usually opens at the level of the ninth to tenth thoracic vertebrae into the azygos vein. C

21 **Accessory hemi-azygos vein; Superior hemi-azygos vein.** It receives the fourth through eighth intercostal veins and opens alone or together with the hemi-azygos vein into the azygos vein. It can also receive the first three intercostal veins and, in this case, anastomose with the left brachiocephalic vein. C

22 **Esophageal veins.** Branches from the esophagus that empty into the azygos vein. C

23 **Bronchial veins.** Branches draining the bronchi into the azygos or hemiazygos vein. C

24 **Pericardial veins.** Branches to the azygos vein, superior vena cava, or brachiocephalic vein. C

25 **Mediastinal veins.** Branches from the mediastinum. Some empty into the superior vena cava. C

26 **Superior phrenic veins.** Small branches from the surface of the diaphragm. C

27 **Ascending lumbar vein.** Abdominal portion that becomes the azygos vein on the right side and the hemi-azygos vein on the left. It opens into the inferior vena cava and anastomoses with the common iliac vein. C D

28 *Lumbar veins.* First and second segmental lumbar veins that open into the ascending lumbar vein. C

29 **Subcostal vein.** Segmental vein lying below the twelfth rib. From this tributary onward, the longitudinally running veins it helps form are referred to as the azygos vein on the right side and the hemi-azygos vein on the left. C D

30 **Posterior intercostal veins.** Posterior portion of the fourth to eleventh intercostal veins that open into the azygos or hemi-azygos vein. C

31 *Dorsal vein; Dorsal branch.* Branch from the muscles and skin of back. C D

32 *Intervertebral vein.* Branch emerging from the intervertebral foramen. D

33 *Spinal vein; Spinal branch.* Branch from the spinal cord and its meninges. D

34 **Veins of vertebral column.**

35 **Anterior external vertebral venous plexus.** Venous plexus lying anterior to the vertebral bodies. D

36 **Posterior external vertebral venous plexus.** Venous plexus lying posterior to the vertebral arches. D

37 **Anterior internal vertebral venous plexus.** Venous plexus lying on the anterior wall of the vertebral canal between the dura mater and periosteum. D

38 *Basivertebral veins.* Veins lying in the vertebral bodies that converge posteriorly and open into the anterior internal vertebral venous plexus. D

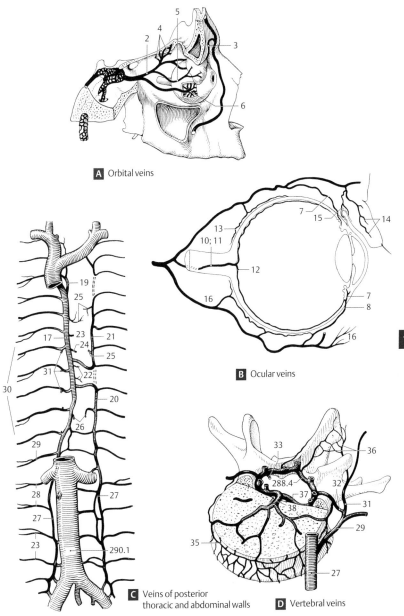

A Orbital veins

B Ocular veins

C Veins of posterior thoracic and abdominal walls

D Vertebral veins

13

1 *Veins of spinal cord.* Venous plexus in the subarachnoid space that drains the spinal cord.

2 *Anterior spinal veins.* Veins that are connected superiorly with the venous network of the pons. They continue inferiorly as the superior thalamostriate vein.

3 *Posterior spinal veins.* Veins terminating superiorly at the rhomboid fossa and inferiorly at the medullary cone.

4 **Posterior internal vertebral venous plexus.** Venous plexus lying on the posterior wall of the vertebral canal between the dura mater and ligaments. p. 286 D

5 **VEINS OF UPPER LIMB.**

6 SUBCLAVIAN VEIN. Vein lying between the anterior scalene muscle and sternocleidomastoid. It extends from the internal jugular vein to the lateral border of the first rib. A

7 **Pectoral veins.** Veins that drain the pectoral muscles and empty into the subclavian vein. A

8 **Dorsal scapular vein.** Companion vein of the dorsal scapular artery that frequently opens into the external jugular vein. A

9 **Axillary vein.** Continuation of the subclavian vein. It extends from the lateral border of the first rib to the inferior border of the tendon of the pectoralis major. A C

10 **Subscapular vein.** Vein accompanying the subscapular artery.

11 **Circumflex scapular vein.** Vein accompanying the circumflex scapular artery.

12 *Thoracodorsal vein.* Vein accompanying the thoracodorsal artery.

13 *Posterior circumflex humeral vein.* Vein accompanying the circumflex humeral artery.

14 *Anterior circumflex humeral vein.* Vein accompanying the anterior circumflex humeral artery.

15 **Lateral thoracic vein.** Vein accompanying the lateral thoracic artery on the serratus anterior. A

16 **Thoraco-epigastric veins.** Subcutaneous veins draining the lateral wall of the trunk. They are collateral veins between the superior and inferior venae cavae. A

17 **Areolar venous plexus.** Venous plexus around the areola. A

18 **Superficial veins of upper limb.**

19 **Cephalic vein.** Epifascial vein arising at the root of the thumb. It courses in the lateral bicipital groove and passes between the deltoid and pectoralis major (deltopectoral triangle; Mohrenheim's fossa) to the axillary vein. B C

20 *Thoraco-acromial vein.* Companion vein of the thoraco-acromial artery that opens into the axillary vein or, occasionally, subclavian vein. A

21 *[Accessory cephalic vein].* It runs from the extensor side of the forearm to the cephalic vein. B C

22 **Basilic vein.** Epifascial vein arising over the distal ulna. It perforates the brachial fascia in the middle of the medial bicipital groove and opens into the brachial vein. A C

23 **Median cubital vein.** Vein running from inferolateral to superomedial, connecting the cephalic and basilic veins. C

24 **Median antebrachial vein; Median vein of forearm.** Epifascial vein occasionally present between the cephalic and basilic veins. C

25 **Cephalic vein of forearm.** Forearm portion of the cephalic vein lying on the flexor aspect of the radius. C

26 **Basilic vein of forearm.** Forearm portion of the basilic vein lying on the flexor aspect of the ulna. C

27 **Dorsal venous network of hand.** Subcutaneous venous plexus on the dorsum of hand. B

28 *Intercapitular veins.* Veins between the heads of metacarpal bones that connect the dorsal and palmar veins of the hand. B C

29 *Dorsal metacarpal veins.* Three of four veins from the ulnar fingers that open into the dorsal venous network of hand. B

30 **Superficial venous palmar arch.** Companion vein of the superficial palmar arch. C

31 *Palmar digital veins.* Veins on the flexor aspect of the fingers. C

32 **Deep veins of upper limb.**

33 **Brachial veins.** Veins accompanying the brachial artery. A

34 **Ulnar veins.** Veins accompanying the ulnar artery. A

35 **Radial veins.** Veins accompanying the radial artery. A

36 **Anterior interosseous veins.** Two companion veins of each anterior interosseous arteries.

37 **Posterior interosseous veins.** Two companion veins of each posterior interosseous arteries.

38 **Deep venous palmar arch.** Vein accompanying the deep palmar arch. A C

39 *Palmar metacarpal veins.* Companion veins of the metacarpal arteries that open into the deep venous palmar arch. A C

13

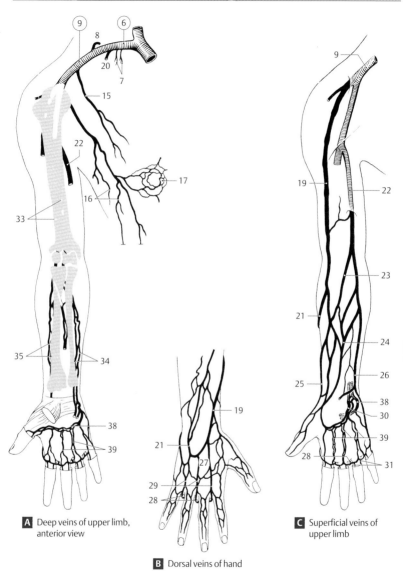

A Deep veins of upper limb, anterior view

B Dorsal veins of hand

C Superficial veins of upper limb

13

1 **INFERIOR VENA CAVA.** It arises at the union of the right and left common iliac veins, lies on the right side of the aorta, and opens into the right atrium of the heart. A

2 **Inferior phrenic veins.** Accompanying veins of the inferior phrenic artery. A

3 **Lumbar veins.** Third and fourth segmental lumbar veins that open directly into the inferior vena cava. A

4 **Hepatic veins.** Short veins of the inner liver.

5 *Right hepatic vein.* Vein from the right lobe of liver. A

6 *Intermediate hepatic vein.* Vein from the caudate lobe. A

7 *Left hepatic vein.* Vein from the left lobe of liver. A

8 **Renal veins.** Right and left veins from the kidney. A

9 *Capsular veins.* Venous network of the perirenal fat capsule. It anastomoses with veins from the surrounding region and the stellate veins of kidney. Collateral circulation. A

10 *Intrarenal veins.* Veins within the kidney.

11 *Left suprarenal vein.* Vein from the left suprarenal gland. A

12 *Left testicular vein.* A

13 *Left ovarian vein.* A

14 **Right suprarenal vein.** Vein from the right suprarenal gland that usually opens directly into the inferior vena cava. A

15 **Right testicular vein.** Right vein from the testis that opens directly into the inferior vena cava. A

16 *Pampiniform plexus.* Venous plexus around the spermatic cord. A

17 **Right ovarian vein.** Vein from the right ovary opening directly into the inferior vena cava. A

18 COMMON ILIAC VEIN. Venous trunk extending from the sacroiliac joint to the fourth lumbar vertebra. It unites with the common iliac vein from the opposite side to form the inferior vena cava. A

19 **Median sacral vein.** Unpaired vein that passes to the common iliac vein. A

20 **Iliolumbar vein.** Companion vein of the iliolumbar artery.

21 INTERNAL ILIAC VEIN. Short venous trunk that receives veins from the pelvic viscera and perineum. B

22 **Superior gluteal veins.** Accompanying veins of the superior gluteal artery that enter the pelvis through the upper part of the greater sciatic foramen. They join to form a trunk which empties into the internal iliac vein. B

23 **Inferior gluteal veins.** Accompanying veins of the inferior gluteal artery that enter the pelvis through the lower part of the greater sciatic foramen. They unite to form a trunk which opens into the internal iliac vein. B C

24 **Obturator veins.** Veins entering the pelvis through the obturator foramen. They usually open into the internal and common iliac veins. B

25 **Lateral sacral veins.** Lateral branches from the sacral venous plexus. B

26 **Sacral venous plexus.** Venous plexus lying in front of the sacrum. B

27 **Rectal venous plexus.** Venous plexus surrounding the rectum. B

28 **Vesical veins.** Veins from the vesical venous plexus. B

29 **Vesical venous plexus.** Venous plexus on the fundus of bladder that is connected with the prostatic or vaginal venous plexus. B C

30 **Prostatic venous plexus.** Venous plexus around the prostate that is connected with the adjacent vesical venous plexus. C

31 **Deep dorsal vein of penis.** Subfascial vein of the dorsum of penis lying below the pubic symphysis between the inferior pubic ligament and transverse perineal ligament that passes to the prostatic venous plexus. It lies between the deep fascia of penis and tunica albuginea and is usually unpaired. C

32 **Deep dorsal vein of clitoris.** Subfascial vein of the corpus of clitoris that passes to the vesical venous plexus. p. 293 B

33 **Uterine veins.** Connecting veins between the uterine venous plexus and internal iliac vein. B

34 **Uterine venous plexus.** Venous plexus mainly at the root of the broad ligament of uterus. It is connected with the vaginal venous plexus. B

35 **Vaginal venous plexus.** Venous plexus around the vagina with numerous connections to the surrounding venous plexuses. B

36 **Middle rectal veins.** Branches of the rectal venous plexus in the lesser pelvis which anastomose with the superior rectal vein and inferior rectal veins. B C

13

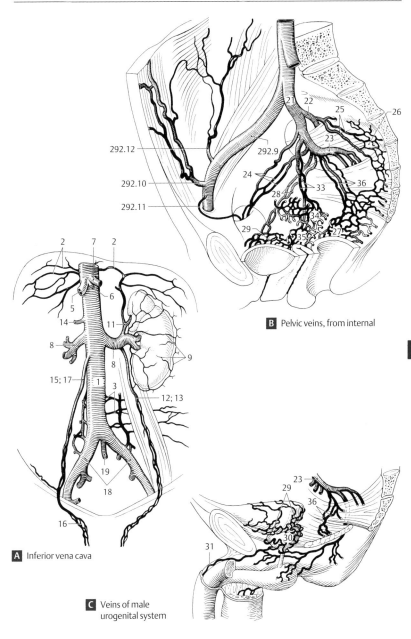

292.12

292.10

292.11

292.9

B Pelvic veins, from internal

A Inferior vena cava

C Veins of male
urogenital system

13

1 **Internal pudendal vein.** Vein running within the lateral wall of the ischiorectal fossa and passing through the lower portion of the greater sciatic foramen into the pelvis. B C

2 *Deep veins of penis.* Veins from the roots of the corpora cavernosa and corpus spongiosum penis. They open via the deep dorsal vein of penis into the prostatic venous plexus. C

3 *Deep veins of clitoris.* Veins emptying the clitoris. They correspond to the deep veins of penis. B

4 *Inferior rectal veins.* Branches from the anal region that pass to the internal pudendal vein. They anastomose with the middle rectal veins and superior rectal vein. B C

5 **Posterior scrotal veins.** Branches passing from the scrotum to the internal pudendal vein. C

6 **Posterior labial veins.** Branches passing from the labia to the internal pudendal vein. B

7 **Vein of bulb of penis.** Vein draining the bulb of penis that conveys blood to the deep dorsal vein of penis or internal pudendal vein. C

8 **Vein of bulb of vestibule.** Vein conveying blood either to the deep dorsal vein of clitoris or internal pudendal vein. B

9 EXTERNAL ILIAC VEIN. It arises at the superior end of the femoral vein below the inguinal ligament and ends where it unites with the internal iliac vein to form the common iliac vein. p. 291 B

10 **Inferior epigastric vein.** Accompanying vein of the inferior epigastric artery from the posterior aspect of the anterior abdominal wall. p. 291 B

11 *Pubic vein*; *Pubic branch [Accessory obturator vein].* Vein that anastomoses on the inner surface of the pubis with the branch of the obturator vein. p. 291 B

12 **Deep circumflex iliac vein.** Accompanying vein of the deep circumflex iliac artery. p. 291 B

13 **Hepatic portal vein.** It conveys blood from the alimentary system to the liver. It forms important anastomoses with the esophageal veins, rectal venous plexus, and superficial veins of the abdominal skin. A

14 **Right branch.** Thick, short right branch. It is divided in the right lobe of liver as far as the interlobular veins. A

15 *Anterior branch.* Branch to the anterior part of the right lobe of liver. A

16 *Posterior branch.* Branch to the posterior part of the right lobe of liver. A

17 **Left branch.** Longer, smaller-caliber branch. It supplies the left lobe of liver as well as the caudate and quadrate lobes. A

18 *Transverse part.* Initial portion of the left branch of portal vein that runs transversely in the porta hepatis. A

19 *Caudate branches.* Twigs to the caudate lobe. A

20 *Umbilical part.* Sagittal continuation of the left branch of portal vein in the left lobe of liver. A

21 *Lateral branches.* Branches to the quadrate lobe and part of caudate lobe.

22 *Umbilical vein.* It conveys blood from the placenta through the umbilical cord to the fetus. After obliteration it forms the round ligament of liver. A

23 *Medial branches.* Branches to the anterior part of the left lobe of liver. A

24 **Cystic vein.** Branch from the gallbladder to the right branch of portal vein. A

25 **Para-umbilical veins.** Small veins in the round ligament of liver that pass to the left branch of portal vein, which anastomoses with subcutaneous abdominal veins. A

26 **Superior posterior pancreaticoduodenal vein.** Vein that empties directly into the portal vein.

27 **Left gastric vein.** Accompanying vein of the left gastric artery. A

28 **Right gastric vein.** Accompanying vein of the right gastric artery. A

29 **Prepyloric vein.** Branch passing in front of the anterior aspect of the pylorus that drains into the right gastric vein or hepatic portal vein. A

13

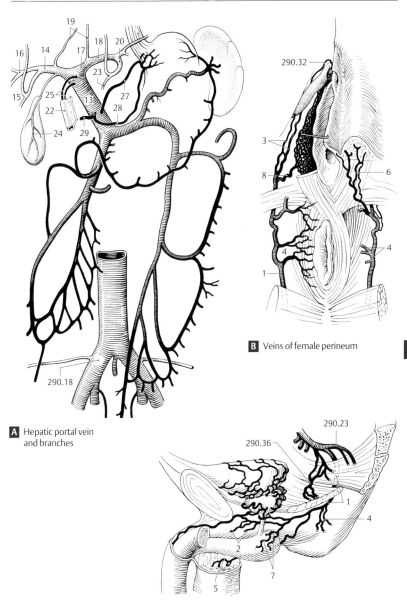

A Hepatic portal vein and branches

B Veins of female perineum

C Veins of male urogenital system

1 **Superior mesenteric vein.** It drains the area from about the inferior half of the duodenum to the splenic flexure. It unites with the splenic vein to form the hepatic portal vein.

2 **Jejunal veins.** Branches from the jejunum and ileum. A

3 **Ileal veins.** Branches from the ileum. A

4 **Right gastro-omental vein; Right gastro-epiploic vein.** Accompanying vein of the right gastro-omental artery. A

5 **Pancreatic veins.** Branches passing directly from the pancreas. A

6 **Pancreaticoduodenal veins.** Accompanying veins of the pancreaticoduodenal arteries. A

7 **Ileocolic vein.** Branch from the ileocecal region. A

8 *Appendicular vein.* Vein from the vermiform appendix. A

9 **Right colic vein.** Vein from the ascending colon. A

10 **Middle colic vein.** Vein draining the transverse colon. It can simultaneously open into the superior and inferior mesenteric veins. A

11 **Splenic vein.** Vein running in the phrenicosplenic ligament and then behind the pancreas. It unites with the superior mesenteric vein to form the hepatic portal vein. A

12 **Pancreatic veins.** Veins emptying directly into the splenic vein. A

13 **Short gastric veins.** Branches running in the gastrosplenic ligament. A

14 **Left gastro-omental vein: Left gastro-epiploic vein.** Accompanying vein of the left gastro-omental artery. A

15 **Inferior mesenteric vein.** Branch extending from the left one-third of the colon to the superior part of the rectum and emptying into the splenic vein. A

16 *Left colic vein.* Vein from the descending colon. A

17 *Sigmoid veins.* Veins from the sigmoid colon. A

18 *Superior rectal vein.* Branch from the superior portion of the rectum. A

13

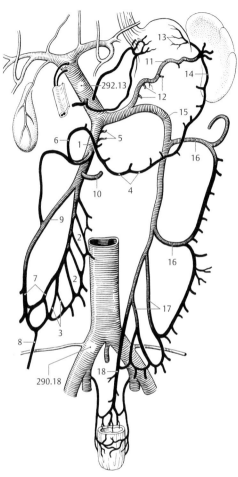

A Hepatic portal vein and branches

1 **VEINS OF LOWER LIMB.**

2 **SUPERFICIAL VEINS OF LOWER LIMB.** Veins that form networks with ventromedial and dorsal longitudinal drainage.

3 **Great saphenous vein; Long saphenous vein.** Vein possessing valves that arises on the medial side of the foot and ascends medially, collecting most of the medial superficial cutaneous veins. It passes through the saphenous opening to empty into the femoral vein. A B C

4 **External pudendal veins.** Individual branches from the external genitalia. A

5 **Superficial circumflex iliac vein.** Subcutaneous companion vein of the superficial circumflex iliac artery. A

6 **Superficial epigastric vein.** Subcutaneous companion vein of the superficial epigastric artery. A

7 **Accessory saphenous vein.** Occasional branch from the small saphenous vein that connects it with the great saphenous vein. Variants collect blood from the thigh, with the exception of the deep and lateral sides. A portion of it runs parallel to the great saphenous vein before joining it. A

8 **Superficial dorsal veins of penis.** Paired epifascial veins that open into the femoral vein or external pudendal veins. A

9 **Superficial dorsal veins of clitoris.** Paired epifascial veins that open into the femoral vein or external pudendal veins.

10 **Anterior scrotal veins.** Veins from the scrotum. See 8 for drainage. A

11 **Anterior labial veins.** Veins from the labia. See 9 for drainage. A

12 **Small saphenous vein; Short saphenous vein.** Vein from the lateral border of the foot that passes over the posterior aspect of the leg to the popliteal vein. A B C D

13 **Dorsal venous network of foot.** Venous plexus on the dorsum of foot that empties into the great and small saphenous veins as well as anterior tibial veins. B

14 **Dorsal venous arch of foot.** Venous arch on the dorsum of foot that receives the dorsal metatarsal veins. It is also the main vein draining the plantar surface of the foot. B C D

15 **Dorsal metatarsal veins.** Veins from the dorsal digital veins of the foot that accompany the dorsal metatarsal artery. B D

16 **Dorsal digital veins.** Veins on the dorsal aspects of the toes. B

17 **Plantar venous network.** Dense, subcutaneous venous plexus on the sole of the foot. C

18 **Plantar venous arch.** Venous arch accompanying the plantar arch. C

19 **Plantar metatarsal veins.** Accompanying veins of the plantar metatarsal arteries. C

20 **Plantar digital veins.** Veins on the flexor aspect of the toes. C

21 **Intercapitular veins.** Connecting veins between the plantar venous arch and dorsal venous arch. D

22 **Lateral marginal vein.** Communicating vein as in 21 that empties into the small saphenous vein. D

23 **Medial marginal vein.** Communicating vein as in 21 that empties into the great saphenous vein. D

24 **DEEP VEINS OF LOWER LIMB.** Usually paired companion veins of the arteries. They have abundant valves and form anastomoses.

25 **Femoral vein.** Accompanying vein of the femoral artery that extends from the adductor hiatus canal to the inguinal ligament. A

26 **Profunda femoris vein; Deep vein of thigh.** Accompanying vein of the deep femoral artery. A

27 **Medial circumflex femoral veins.** Companion veins of the medial circumflex femoral artery. A

28 **Lateral circumflex femoral veins.** Companion veins of the lateral circumflex femoral artery. A

29 **Perforating veins.** Veins from the hamstrings that perforate the adductors and open into the deep femoral vein. A

30 **Popliteal vein.** Vein extending from the union of the anterior and posterior tibial veins to the adductor hiatus. It lies between the popliteal artery and tibial nerve. C

31 **Sural veins.** Accompanying veins of the sural arteries.

32 **Genicular veins.** Usually five veins draining the knee. A

33 **Anterior tibial veins.** Accompanying veins of the anterior tibial artery. A B C

34 **Posterior tibial veins.** Accompanying veins of the posterior tibial artery. C

35 *Fibular veins; Peroneal veins.* Accompanying veins of the fibular artery, lying partly beneath the flexor hallucis longus. C

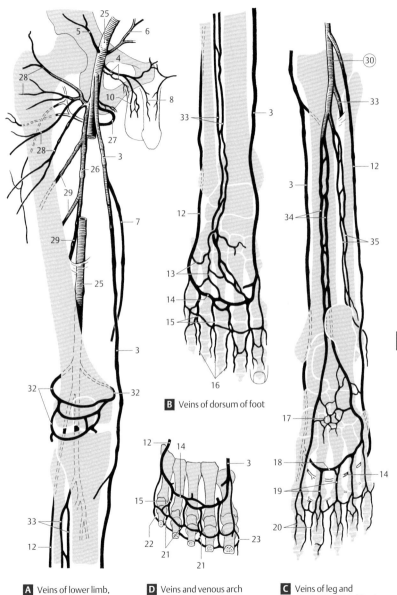

13

A Veins of lower limb, anterior view

B Veins of dorsum of foot

D Veins and venous arch of dorsum of foot

C Veins of leg and plantar surface of foot

1 *LYMPHOID SYSTEM.*

2 **PRIMARY LYMPHOID ORGANS.**

3 **Bone marrow.**

4 **Thymus.** Lymphoid organ situated in the thymic triangle. It regresses during puberty. A

5 **Lobe.** Right and left lobes of thymus. A

6 *Lobules of thymus.* Lobules divided by connective tissue. A

7 *Cortex of thymus.* It contains abundant lymphocytes.

8 *Medulla of thymus.* It has scant lymphocytes and contains the corpuscles of Hassall.

9 **[Accessory thymic lobules].** Scattered islands of thymic tissue.

10 **SECONDARY LYMPHOID ORGANS.**

11 SPLEEN. Lymphoreticular organ assisting the circulatory system. It has mainly filtering and immune functions. B

12 **Fibrous capsule.** C

13 **Splenic trabeculae.** Fibrous tissue trabeculae carrying vessels that extend from the splenic hilum and fibrous capsule into the spleen. B

14 **Splenic pulp.** Parenchyma of the spleen. A fresh cross-section of the spleen reveals the following two components which are visible to the naked eye. C

15 *Red pulp.* Portions of the vessels filled with blood.

16 *White pulp.* Connective-tissue components and lymphocyte aggregations. C

17 **Diaphragmatic surface.** Convex surface facing the diaphragm.

18 **Visceral surface.** Concave surface facing the adjacent viscera. B

19 *Renal impression.* Inferior surface that is in contact with the kidney. B

20 *Gastric impression.* Superior surface that is in contact with the stomach. B

21 *Colic impression.* Surface that is in contact with the colon. B

22 *[Pancreatic impression].* Surface sometimes in contact with the pancreas.

23 **Anterior extremity.** B

24 **Posterior extremity.** B

25 **Inferior border.** Margin between the diaphragmatic surface and renal impression. B

26 **Superior border.** Margin between the gastric impression and diaphragmatic surface. B

27 **Splenic hilum.** Entry and exit site for vessels between the gastric and renal impressions. B

28 **Serosa; Serous coat.** Peritoneal covering. C

29 **Splenic sinus.** Thin-walled blood vessel in the splenic pulp that forms anastomoses. C

30 **Penicilli.** Brushlike branches of the nodular arteries. C

31 **Splenic lymphoid nodules.** Macroscopically visible spheroidal or cylindrical masses of lymphoreticular tissue surrounding an artery. C

32 **[Accessory spleen].** Islands of splenic tissue usually found in the greater omentum or gastrosplenic ligament.

33 PHARYNGEAL LYMPHOID RING. Ring composed of lingual, palatine, pharyngeal, and tubal tonsils. It can also be viewed as an organ, containing tonsillar crypts and pits. D

34 LYMPH NODE. Lymphoreticular filtering organ interposed along the course of lymphoid vessels and measuring 1–25 mm in diameter. Lymph must pass through two lymph nodes before reaching the bloodstream at the venous angle, providing a dual defense against pathogens or tumor cells invading the bloodstream. E

35 **Capsule.** Fibrous tissue capsule. E

36 **Trabeculae.** Fibrous tissue septa. Extensions of the capsule that pass through the lymph node, forming a supporting framework. E

37 **Hilum.** Slightly indented entry site for blood vessels and exit site for blood and lymphatic vessels. E

38 **Cortex.** Densely arranged aggregations of lymphocytes in the lymphoreticular tissue, lying near the capsule. E

39 **Medulla.** Lymphoreticular tissue between the cortex and hilum with low lymphocyte density. E

40 **Solitary lymphoid nodules.** Smallest functional unit of, e.g., a lymph node. E

41 **Aggregated lymphoid nodules.** Group of solitary lymphoid nodules, e.g., in the intestine (Peyer's patches).

42 **Lymph nodules of vermiform appendix.** Aggregation of solitary lymphoid nodules in the vermiform appendix.

14

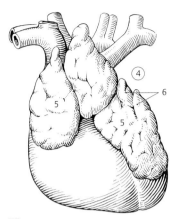

A Thymus

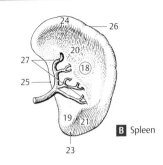

B Spleen

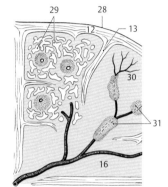

C Spleen, histological representation

14

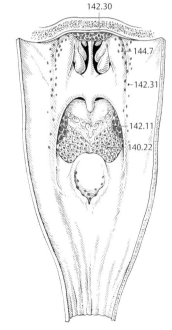

D Pharyngeal lymphoid ring

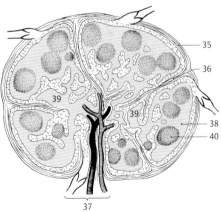

E Lymph node, cross-section

1 *REGIONAL LYMPH NODES.*

2 **Lymph nodes of head and neck.**

3 **Occipital nodes.** Between one and three lymph nodes located near the border of the trapezius. Region drained: scalp, deep muscles of neck. Drain into: deep cervical lymph nodes. A

4 **Mastoid nodes.** Usually two nodes overlying the mastoid process. Region drained: posterior surface of auricle, posterior wall of external acoustic meatus, and corresponding part of scalp. Drain into: deep cervical lymph nodes. A

5 **Superficial parotid nodes.** Lymph nodes located anterior to the tragus, superficial to the parotid fascia. Region drained: adjacent temporal region and anterior surface of the auricle. Drain into: deep cervical lymph nodes. A

6 **Deep parotid nodes.** Group of lymph nodes deep to the parotid fascia. Region drained: tympanic cavity, external acoustic meatus, frontotemporal region, eyelids, root of nose, sometimes also posterior nasal floor and nasopharynx. Drain into: deep cervical lymph nodes. A

7 *Pre-auricular nodes.* Group of lymph nodes situated anterior to the auricle. A

8 *Infra-auricular nodes.* Group of lymph nodes situated below the auricle. A

9 *Intraglandular nodes.* Group of lymph nodes situated within the parotid gland. A

10 **Facial nodes.** Individual nodes are inconstant. Their afferent vessels drain lymph from the eyelids, nose, and rest of the face as well as the buccal mucosa. Drain into: submandibular nodes. Their vessels are located along the course of the facial artery.

11 *Buccinator node.* Deep lymph node situated on the buccinator. A

12 *Nasolabial node.* Lymph node situated deep to the nasolabial fold. A

13 *Malar node.* Superficial lymph node located in the cheek.

14 *Mandibular node.* Lymph node located on the outer surface of the mandible. A

15 **Lingual nodes.** Located on the lateral part of the hyoglossus. Afferent vessels drain the inferior surface of the tongue, its lateral border, and the medial anterior two-thirds of the dorsum of tongue.

16 **Submental nodes.** Nodes located between the anterior bellies of digastric muscles. Region drained: middle part of lower lip, floor of mouth, and tip of tongue. Drain into: deep cervical lymph nodes and submandibular nodes. B

17 **Submandibular nodes.** Lymph nodes located between the mandible and submandibular gland that serve as first and second filtering stations. Directly drain: medial angle of eye, cheek, side of nose, upper lip, lateral part of lower lip, gingiva, and anterior lateral border of the tongue. Indirectly drain: facial and submental nodes. Drain into: deep cervical lymph nodes. B

18 **Anterior cervical nodes.**

19 *Superficial nodes; Anterior jugular nodes.* Lymph nodes located along the anterior jugular vein. Region drained: skin of the anterior side of the neck. Drain into: bilateral deep cervical lymph nodes. A

20 *Deep nodes.* Deep, anterior group of lymph nodes.

21 *Infrahyoid nodes.* Lymph nodes located in the midline below the body of hyoid bone. Afferent vessels drain the laryngeal vestibule, piriform recess, and adjacent hypopharynx. Drain into: deep cervical lymph nodes. B

22 *Prelaryngeal nodes.* Lymph nodes lying on the cricothyroid ligament. Region drained: Inferior half of the larynx. Drain into: deep cervical lymph nodes. B

23 *Thyroid nodes.* Lymph nodes lying on the thyroid gland. Drain into: deep cervical lymph nodes. B

24 *Pretracheal nodes.* Lymph nodes located anterior to the trachea. Region drained: trachea and larynx. Drain into: deep cervical lymph nodes. B

25 *Paratracheal nodes.* Lymph nodes located alongside the trachea. Region drained: trachea and larynx. Drain into: deep cervical lymph nodes. B

26 *Retropharyngeal nodes.* Deep cervical lymph nodes located anterior to the arch of the atlas. p. 302.13

14

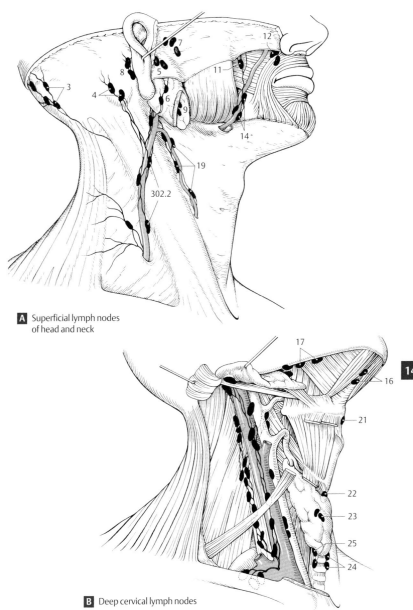

A Superficial lymph nodes
of head and neck

B Deep cervical lymph nodes

14

1 **Lateral cervical nodes.** Group of lymph nodes on the lateral side of the neck that can be grouped as follows:

2 *Superficial nodes.* Lymph nodes located along the external jugular vein. Region drained: inferior auricle and inferior part of parotid gland. Drain into: deep cervical lymph nodes. p. 301 A

3 *Superior deep nodes.* Nodes serving as the second filter station for nearly all lymph nodes of the head. They also receive direct peripheral vessels from the surrounding area. Drain into: jugular trunk. A

4 *Lateral node.* Lymph node located lateral to the internal jugular vein. A

5 *Anterior node.* Lymph node located anterior to the internal jugular vein. A

6 *Jugulodigastric node.* Furthest cranial of the superior deep nodes. It is palpable with inflammation of the tonsils, tongue, or pharynx. A

7 *Inferior deep nodes.* Second filter station for the lymph nodes of the visceral structures of the neck and last filter station for the lymph nodes of the head. They also receive direct tributaries. Drain into: jugular trunk. A

8 *Jugulo-omohyoid node.* Lymph node located between the omohyoid muscle and internal jugular vein. Receives lymph from the tongue. A

9 *Lateral node.* Lymph node located lateral to the internal jugular vein. A

10 *Anterior nodes.* Group of lymph nodes located anterior to the internal jugular vein. A

11 **Supraclavicular nodes.** Group of lymph nodes overlying the clavicle. A

12 **Accessory nodes.** Scattered, accessory lymph nodes.

13 *Retropharyngeal nodes.* Deep cervical lymph nodes located at the level of the lateral mass of atlas and on the lateral border of the longus capitis. A B

14 **Lymph nodes of upper limb.**

15 **Axillary lymph nodes.** Nodes in the region about the axilla. C

16 *Apical nodes.* Lymph nodes extending from the superior border of the pectoralis minor that pass medial to the axillary vein into the apex of the axilla. Afferent vessels from the superior lateral part of the breast and all other axillary lymph nodes. Drain into: on the left side as the subclavian trunk into the thoracic duct or subclavian vein; On the right side directly into the vein or after joining the jugular trunk. C

17 *Humeral nodes; Lateral nodes.* Lymph nodes along the axillary artery draining lymph from the arm. C

18 *Subscapular nodes; Posterior nodes.* Lymph nodes located along the subscapular artery that drain lymph from the posterior part of the thoracic and shoulder regions as well as inferior neck region. C

19 *Pectoral nodes; Anterior nodes.* Lymph nodes located on the lateral border of the pectoralis minor that drain lymph from the anterior and lateral wall of the trunk as far as the navel as well as the central and lateral portions of the breast. C

20 *Central nodes.* Lymph nodes located in the adipose tissue of the axilla. Filter station for lymph from the humeral, subscapular, and pectoral nodes. C

21 **Interpectoral nodes.** Small group of lymph nodes located between the pectoralis major and minor. Region drained: breast. Drain into: apical nodes. C

22 **Deltopectoral nodes; Infraclavicular nodes.** Lymph nodes in the deltopectoral triangle along the cephalic vein that drain lymph from the arm. C

23 **Brachial nodes.** Individual lymph nodes along the brachial vessels.

24 **Cubital nodes.** One or two lymph nodes located along the brachial artery in the cubital fossa. C

25 *Supratrochlear nodes.* One or two lymph nodes located medial to the basilic vein and above the elbow joint. C

26 **Superficial nodes.** Lymph nodes situated along the superficial lymph vessels.

27 **Deep nodes.** Individual lymph nodes that are interposed along the course of the deep lymph vessels.

14

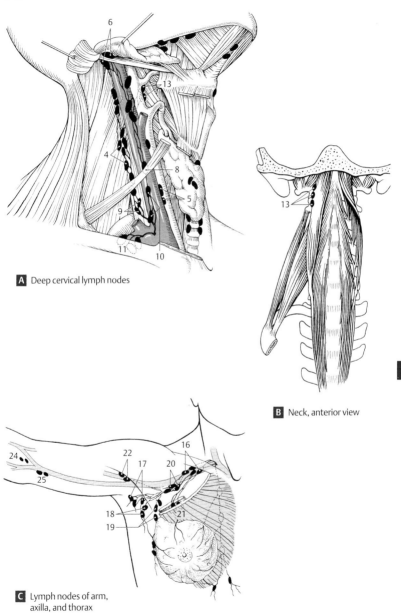

A Deep cervical lymph nodes

B Neck, anterior view

C Lymph nodes of arm, axilla, and thorax

14

1 **Thoracic lymph nodes.**

2 **Paramammary nodes.** Lymph nodes on the lateral border of the mammary gland. A

3 **Parasternal nodes.** Lymph nodes situated in the thorax along the internal thoracic vessels. Region drained: breast, intercostal spaces, parts of liver and diaphragm. Drain into: either directly in the subclavian vein or internal jugular vein or, alternatively, into the thoracic duct or subclavian trunk. A

4 **Intercostal nodes.** Lymph nodes situated in the paravertebral portions of the intercostal spaces. Region drained: pleura and intercostal spaces. D

5 **Superior diaphragmatic nodes.** Lymph nodes located posterior to the osteochondral junction of the seventh rib, at the passage of the aorta through the diaphragm and at the inferior vena cava. Region drained: liver and diaphragm. D

6 **Prepericardial nodes.** Lymph nodes located between the sternum and pericardium. Region drained: sternum and anterior pericardium. Drain into: parasternal nodes. B

7 **Brachiocephalic nodes.** Lymph nodes located anterior to the aortic arch and its branches along the brachiocephalic veins. Drainage area: thymus, thyroid gland, pericardium, and parasternal lymph nodes. Drain into: bronchomediastinal lymphatic trunk. B

8 **[Node of ligamentum arteriosum].** Occasional lymph node along the ligamentum arteriosum. B

9 **[Node of arch of azygos vein].** Occasional lymph node along the arch that the azygos vein forms around the hilum of the right lung before it passes to the superior vena cava. B

10 **Lateral pericardial nodes.** Lymph nodes located between the pericardium and mediastinal pleura. B

11 **Paratracheal nodes.** Lymph nodes located alongside the trachea. C

12 **Tracheobronchial nodes.** Lymph nodes located on the bronchi at their entrance into the lungs. C

13 *Superior tracheobronchial nodes.* Lymph nodes located cranially on the bronchi and trachea. C

14 *Inferior tracheobronchial nodes.* Lymph nodes located caudal to the tracheal bifurcation. C

15 **Bronchopulmonary nodes.** Lymph nodes located at the divisions of the lobar bronchi. C

16 **Intrapulmonary nodes.** Lymph nodes located at the exit sites of the segmental bronchi and in the lung tissue.

17 **Juxta-esophageal nodes.** Lymph nodes located alongside the esophagus, but belonging to the lung. C

18 **Prevertebral nodes.** Lymph nodes located between the esophagus and vertebral column. Region drained: surrounding regions not served by other vessels. C D

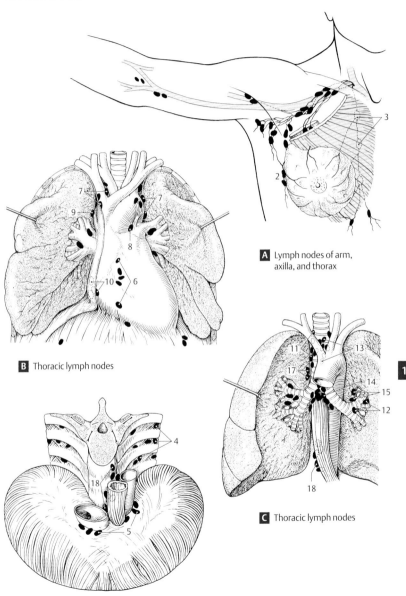

A Lymph nodes of arm, axilla, and thorax

B Thoracic lymph nodes

C Thoracic lymph nodes

D Thoracic lymph nodes

14

1 **Abdominal lymph nodes.**

2 **Parietal lymph nodes.** Lymph nodes in the abdominal wall.

3 *Left lumbar nodes.* Nodes located along the abdominal aorta that, firstly, are secondary filter stations for groups of lymph nodes located further inferiorly and, secondly, also serve as filter stations for the suprarenal glands, kidneys, ureter, testis, ovary, uterine tube, fundus of uterus, and abdominal wall. Drainage: mainly into the lumbar trunk. They can be divided into the following three groups:

4 *Lateral aortic nodes.* Lymph nodes located on the left side of the aorta. A

5 *Pre-aortic nodes.* Lymph nodes located anterior to the aorta. A

6 *Postaortic nodes.* Lymph nodes located between the aorta and vertebral column. A

7 *Intermediate lumbar nodes.* Nodes located between the aorta and inferior vena cava. See 3 for function. A

8 *Right lumbar nodes.* Nodes located around the inferior vena cava. Same function on right side as described in 3. They can be divided into the following groups:

9 *Lateral caval nodes.* Lymph nodes situated on the right side of the inferior vena cava. A

10 *Precaval nodes.* Lymph nodes situated anterior to the vena cava. A

11 *Postcaval nodes.* Lymph nodes situated posterior to the vena cava. A

12 *Inferior diaphragmatic nodes.* Lymph nodes on the inferior surface of the diaphragm near the aortic hiatus. A C

13 *Inferior epigastric nodes.* Three or four lymph nodes along the inferior epigastric artery draining the area it supplies. B

14 **Visceral lymph nodes.** Nodes of the abdominal viscera.

15 *Celiac nodes.* Lymph nodes located around the celiac trunk that form the secondary filter station for the stomach, duodenum, liver, gallbladder, pancreas, and spleen. Their efferent vessels partly form the intestinal trunk and partly pass directly to the chyle cistern. A C

16 *Right/left gastric nodes.* Lymph nodes located at the lesser curvature of the stomach that follow the course of the right and left gastric arteries. Region drained: stomach. Drain into: celiac nodes. C

17 *[Nodes around cardia].* Occasional ring of lymph nodes around the cardia. C

18 *Right/left gastro-omental nodes.* Lymph nodes located along the course of the right and left gastro-omental arteries along the greater curvature of the stomach that drain lymph from the stomach and greater omentum. Drainage is into the hepatic nodes on the right side and splenic and pancreatic nodes on the left side. C

19 *Pyloric nodes.* Lymph nodes situated around the pylorus that drain into the hepatic or celiac nodes.

20 *[Suprapyloric node].* Lymph node situated above the pylorus. C

21 *[Subpyloric nodes].* Group of lymph nodes situated caudal to the pylorus. C

22 *[Retropyloric nodes].* Group of lymph nodes situated dorsal to the pylorus. C

23 *Pancreatic nodes.* Lymph nodes located along the superior and inferior borders of the pancreas that drain lymph from the organ into the splenic nodes, mesenteric nodes, and pancreaticoduodenal nodes.

24 *Superior nodes.* Group of lymph nodes located on the superior border of the pancreas. A C

25 *Inferior nodes.* Group of lymph nodes located on the inferior border of the pancreas. A C

26 *Splenic nodes.* Lymph nodes located at the splenic hilum that drain into the celiac nodes. A C

27 *Pancreaticoduodenal nodes.* Small lymph nodes located between the head of pancreas and duodenum. Drainage area: duodenum and pancreas.

28 *Superior nodes.* Upper group of lymph nodes. Drain into: hepatic nodes. C

29 *Inferior nodes.* Lower group of lymph nodes. Drain into: mesenteric nodes. C

30 *Hepatic nodes.* Lymph nodes located at the porta hepatis and in the hepatoduodenal ligament. They drain the liver and neighboring lymph nodes into the celiac nodes.

31 *Cystic nodes.* Larger lymph nodes located on the neck of gallbladder. C

32 *Node of anterior border of omental foramen.* Large lymph node at the omental foramen. C

14

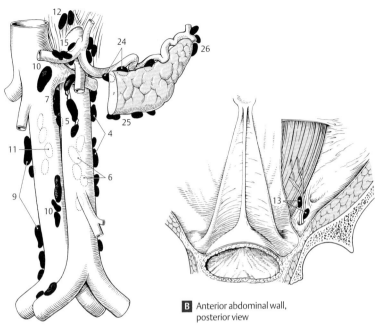

B Anterior abdominal wall, posterior view

A Deep lymph nodes of abdominal cavity

14

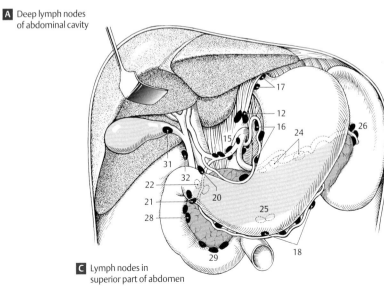

C Lymph nodes in superior part of abdomen

1 *Superior mesenteric nodes.* Numerous (100–150) mesenteric lymph nodes that are important in preventing hyperlipidemia. Drainage via the celiac nodes.

2 *Juxta-intestinal mesenteric nodes.* Subgroup of superior mesenteric nodes located near the small intestine.

3 *Central superior mesenteric nodes.* Part of the group located along the trunk of the mesenteric artery. A

4 *Ileocolic nodes.* Group of lymph nodes located along the ileocolic artery. Drain into: celiac nodes. A

5 *Prececal nodes.* Lymph nodes located along the anterior cecal artery. A

6 *Retrocecal nodes.* Lymph nodes located along the posterior cecal artery. A

7 *Appendicular nodes.* Lymph nodes located along the appendicular artery. They are absent in 33–50%. A

8 *Mesocolic nodes.* Lymph nodes draining the greater portion of the colon. They are mainly located in the mesocolon and drain into the celiac nodes.

9 *Paracolic nodes.* Group of mesocolic nodes located along the colon. A

10 *Right/middle/left colic nodes.* Group of nodes located along the trunks of the left, middle, and right colic arteries. A

11 *Inferior mesenteric nodes.* Lymph nodes located along the inferior mesenteric artery. Drainage area: part of the descending colon, sigmoid colon, and parts of the rectum. Drain into: preaortic nodes at the level of the inferior mesenteric artery. A

12 *Sigmoid nodes.* Lymph nodes located along the sigmoid artery that drain the sigmoid colon and adjoining segment of the colon. A

13 *Superior rectal nodes.* Lymph nodes located along the superior rectal artery that drain the rectum. A

14 **Pelvic lymph nodes.**

15 **Parietal nodes.** Lymph nodes in the wall of the pelvis.

16 *Common iliac nodes.* Group of lymph nodes located along the internal iliac vessels. They serve as a secondary filter station for the lymph nodes of the pelvic organs, genital organs, inner pelvic wall, abdominal wall as far as the navel, and the hip and gluteal muscles. Drain into: lumbar nodes or lumbar trunk. They can be divided into the following groups:

17 *Medial nodes.* Group of lymph nodes located medial to the internal iliac vessels. B

18 *Intermediate nodes.* Lymph nodes located between the medial and lateral group, behind the internal iliac vessels. B

19 *Lateral nodes.* Group located lateral to the internal iliac vessels. B

20 *Subaortic nodes.* Lymph nodes located caudal to the aortic bifurcation, in front of L4. A B

21 *Promontorial nodes.* Group located anterior to the promontory. A B

22 *External iliac nodes.* Lymph nodes located along the external iliac vessels. They are the primary filter station for part of the urinary bladder and vagina and the secondary filter station for the inguinal lymph nodes. Drain into: common iliac nodes. They can be divided into the following groups:

23 *Medial nodes.* Group of nodes located medial to the external iliac vessels. B

24 *Intermediate nodes.* Group of nodes located between the lateral and medial group, posterior to the artery. B

25 *Lateral nodes.* Group located lateral to the external iliac vessels. B

26 *[Medial lacunar node].* Lymph node located medial to the external iliac vessels in the vascular space. B

27 *[Intermediate lacunar node].* Node occasionally present in the middle of the vascular space. B

28 *[Lateral lacunar node].* Node located in the lateral part of the vascular space. B

29 *Interiliac nodes.* Lymph nodes situated at the bifurcation of the internal and external iliac arteries. B

30 *Obturator nodes.* Group located along the obturator artery. B

14

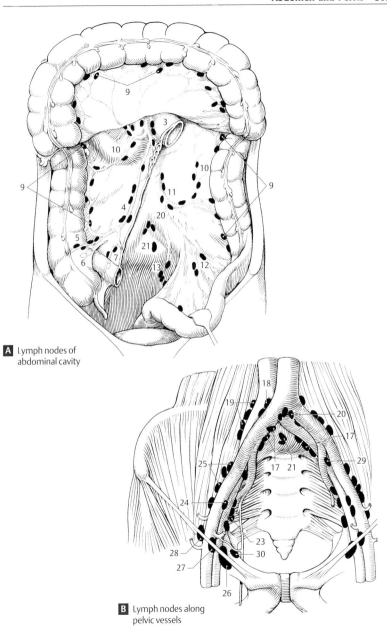

A Lymph nodes of abdominal cavity

B Lymph nodes along pelvic vessels

14

1 *Internal iliac nodes.* Lymph nodes located along the internal iliac artery that drain the pelvic organs, deep perineal region, and outer and inner pelvic wall. Drain into: common iliac nodes.

2 *Gluteal nodes.*

3 Superior nodes. Lymph nodes located along the superior gluteal artery that drain the pelvic wall. A

4 Inferior nodes. Lymph nodes located along the inferior gluteal artery that drain the prostate and proximal part of the urethra. A

5 *Sacral nodes.* Lymph nodes located on the sacrum that drain the prostate or cervix. A

6 **Visceral lymph nodes.**

7 *Paravesical nodes.* Lymph nodes located along the urinary bladder, some of which drain it and some also drain the prostate. A

8 *Prevesical nodes.* Subgroup located between the urinary bladder and pubic symphysis. A

9 Postvesical nodes. Subgroup located posterior to the urinary bladder. A

10 *Lateral vesical nodes.* Lymph nodes located at the inferior end of the median umbilical ligament. A

11 *Para-uterine nodes.* Lymph nodes located alongside the uterus that drain the cervix of uterus. A

12 *Paravaginal nodes.* Lymph nodes located alongside the vagina that drain part of it. A

13 *Pararectal nodes.* Lymph nodes located lateral to the rectum, lying directly on its muscles. They drain it and part of the vagina. A

14 **Lymph nodes of lower limb.**

15 **Inguinal lymph nodes.**

16 *Superficial inguinal nodes.* Group of lymph nodes located in the subcutaneous adipose tissue, i.e., on the fascia lata, that drain the anus, perineum, external genitalia, abdominal wall, and surface of the leg. Drain into: external iliac nodes.

17 *Superomedial nodes.* Medial subgroup of superficial inguinal nodes located along the inguinal ligament. B

18 *Superolateral nodes.* Lateral subgroup of superficial inguinal nodes located below the inguinal ligament. B

19 *Inferior nodes.* Vertical line of nodes at the proximal end of the great saphenous vein that drain the superficial lymphatic vessels of the leg. B

20 *Deep inguinal nodes.* Nodes located deep to the fascia lata at the level of the saphenous opening. The uppermost node is sometimes especially large and located in the femoral canal (Rosenmüller's node). Region drained: deep lymphatic vessels of leg. Drain into: external iliac nodes.

21 *[Proximal node; Rosenmüller's node].* Node usually located in the lateral part of the inguinal ring. It is not always very large. B

22 *[Intermediate node].* Inconstant node located below the inguinal ligament. B

23 *Distal node.* Lymph node located below the junction of the great saphenous vein and femoral vein. B

24 **Popliteal nodes.** Lymph nodes in the popliteal fossa.

25 *Superficial nodes.* Lymph nodes located at the proximal end of the small saphenous vein that drain lymph from the lateral border of foot and calf. Drainage: their afferent vessels pass through the adductor hiatus and run anteriorly to the deep inguinal nodes. C

26 *Deep nodes.* Lymph nodes located between the joint capsule of the knee and popliteal artery. Their afferent vessels drain lymph from the posterior side of the leg, passing anteriorly through the adductor hiatus to the deep inguinal nodes. C

27 **[Anterior tibial node].** Occasional lymph node situated along the anterior tibial artery.

28 **[Posterior tibial node].** Occasional lymph node situated along the posterior tibial artery.

29 **[Fibular node; Peroneal node].** Occasional lymph node situated along the fibular artery.

14

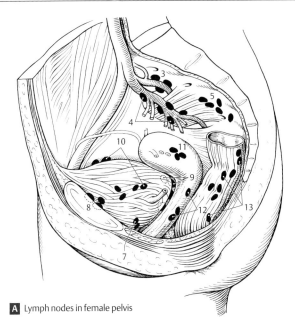

A Lymph nodes in female pelvis

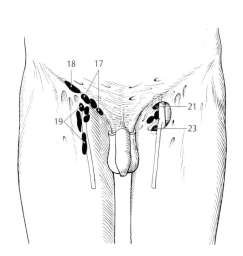

B Lymph nodes in inguinal region

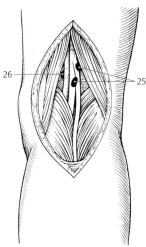

C Lymph nodes in popliteal fossa

1 *LYMPHATIC TRUNKS AND DUCTS.*

2 **Jugular trunk.** Lymphatic trunk accompanying the internal jugular vein to the angle between the internal jugular vein and subclavian vein (venous angle). A

3 **Subclavian trunk.** Lymphatic trunk arising from the arm, accompanying the subclavian vein and often emptying on the right side into the right lymphatic duct and on the left side into the angle between the left subclavian vein and internal jugular vein. A

4 **Axillary lymphatic plexus.** Communicating lymphatic vessels of the 20–30 axillary lymph nodes which may form a network. B

5 **Bronchomediastinal trunk.** Lymphatic trunk that collects lymph from the heart, lung, and mediastinum. It empties on the left side into the thoracic duct and on the right side into the right lymphatic duct, or more commonly, directly into the subclavian vein. A

6 **Right lymphatic duct; Right thoracic duct.** Lymphatic duct formed by the union of the right jugular, subclavian, and bronchomediastinal trunks. It is sometimes absent. A

7 **Thoracic duct.** Duct for breast milk. It arises just below the diaphragm from the chyle cistern, ascends behind the aorta, and empties into the angle between the internal jugular vein and left subclavian vein. A

8 *Arch of thoracic duct.* Arch in front of the opening into the venous angle. A

9 *Cervical part.* Short portion in front of the seventh cervical vertebra. A

10 *Thoracic part.* Part commencing at the aortic hiatus and ending at the superior border of the first thoracic vertebra. A

11 *Abdominal part.* Very short abdominal segment situated in front of the first lumbar vertebra. A

12 **Cisterna chyli; Chyle cistern.** Inconstant dilatation before the beginning of the thoracic duct. It receives the lumbar and intestinal trunks. A

13 **Lumbar trunk.** Main branch that drains lymph from the legs, pelvic viscera, urogenital system, and parts of the abdominal wall as well as abdominal viscera into the chyle cistern. A

14 **Intestinal trunks.** Main branches that drain lymph from the region supplied by the superior and inferior mesenteric arteries into the chyle cistern. A

14

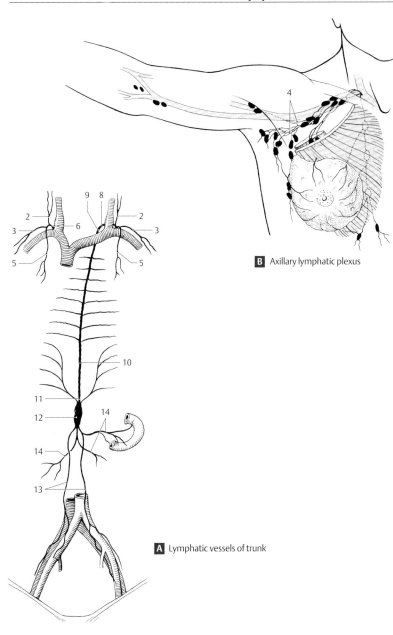

B Axillary lymphatic plexus

A Lymphatic vessels of trunk

1 *NERVOUS SYSTEM.*

2 *CENTRAL NERVOUS SYSTEM.*

3 **MENINGES.** Membranes investing the spinal cord and brain. They consist of the dura mater, arachnoid mater, and pia mater.

4 **Pachymeninx; Dura mater.** Tough, fibrous, hard membrane investing the spinal cord and brain.

5 **Leptomeninx; Arachnoid mater and pia mater.** Soft membrane investing the spinal cord and brain. It consists of two layers: the arachnoid mater and the vascularized pia mater.

6 **Dura mater.** Hard membrane covering the brain and spinal cord.

7 **Cranial dura mater.** Membrane forming a protective capsule around the brain. In the growing body it is firmly attached to the periosteum of the cranial bones. The meningeal and periosteal layers always remain divided at the dural venous sinuses. After growth stops, the periosteal layer separates slightly from the bone, remaining firmly attached at only a few sites, e.g., the crista galli. D

8 *Falx cerebri; Cerebral falx.* Crescent-shaped portion of the dura mater projecting into the longitudinal cerebral fissure. A

9 *Tentorium cerebelli; Cerebellar tentorium.* Dural septum stretched over the cerebellum between the superior border of petrous part of temporal bone and the transverse sinus. It supports the occipital lobe. A

10 *Tentorial notch; Incisura of tentorium.* Opening in the tentorium cerebelli for passage of the brainstem. A

11 *Falx cerebelli; Cerebellar falx.* Small, crescent-shaped dural fold dividing the right and left cerebellar hemispheres. A

12 *Diaphragma sellae; Sellar diaphragm.* Small dural fold stretched horizontally between the clinoid processes over the pituitary gland. A

13 *Trigeminal cave; Trigeminal cavity.* Cavity between the periosteum and dura mater containing the trigeminal ganglion. A

14 *[Subdural space].* Cleft between the dura mater and arachnoid mater containing a capillary layer. It is not considered a naturally-occurring space. D

15 *[Extradural space; Epidural space].* An epidural space is present in the vertebral canal, but not in the cranial cavity.

16 **Spinal dura mater.** Hard membrane forming a protective covering around the spinal cord. It is separated from the wall of the vertebral canal by the epidural space. C

17 *Epidural space.* Space filled with fat and venous plexuses between the spinal dura mater and the wall of the vertebral canal. C

18 **Arachnoid mater.** Transparent fibrocollagenous membrane between the dura mater and pia mater that is covered by epithelioid cells.

19 **Subarachnoid space; Leptomeningeal space.** Space between the arachnoid mater and pia mater that contains arachnoid connective-tissue fibers and cerebrospinal fluid. D

20 *Cerebrospinal fluid.* Fluid containing little protein and consisting of 2–6 cells per mm3. It is secreted mainly by the choroid plexus. C

21 **Cranial arachnoid mater.** Thin, avascular membrane containing connective-tissue fibers that pass to the pia mater. It is attached to the dura mater only by surface adhesion. D

22 *Arachnoid granulations.* Avascular, villus-like protrusions of the arachnoid mater into the sagittal sinus and diploic veins. They become increasingly prominent beginning around age 10 years and are involved in cerebrospinal fluid drainage. D

23 *Arachnoid trabeculae.* Connective-tissue communication between the arachnoid mater and pia mater. D

24 *Subarachnoid cisterns.* Dilatations of the subarachnoid space forming reservoirs for cerebrospinal fluid.

25 *Posterior cerebellomedullary cistern; Cisterna magna.* Dorsal cistern between the cerebellum and medulla oblongata into which the median aperture of the fourth ventricle opens. It can be accessed through the foramen magnum. B

26 *Lateral cerebellomedullary cistern.* Narrow anterolateral portion of the cistern around the medulla oblongata. Its dorsal wall divides it from the posterior cerebellomedullary cistern.

27 *Cistern of lateral cerebral fossa.* Cerebrospinal fluid-filled space that is accessible through the lateral sulcus and is situated between the insula and the temporal, frontal, and parietal lobes. It contains the insular arteries given off by the middle cerebral artery. E

28 *Chiasmatic cistern.* Cerebrospinal fluid-filled space surrounding the optic chiasm. B

29 *Interpeduncular cistern.* Cerebrospinal fluid-filled space behind the chiasmatic cistern and bounded laterally by the temporal lobe and cerebral crura. It contains the oculomotor nerve, bifurcation of the basilar artery, the origin of the superior cerebellar artery, and the posterior cerebral artery. B

30 *Cisterna ambiens; Ambient cistern.* Cistern situated lateral to the cerebral crura. It contains the posterior cerebral artery, superior cerebellar artery, basal vein (Rosenthal's vein), and trochlear nerve. B G

31 *Pericallosal cistern.* Sagittal cistern situated longitudinally along the corpus callosum. G

32 *Pontocerebellar cistern.* Expanded space containing cerebrospinal fluid located in the pontocerebellar angle. Site of the opening of the lateral aperture of the fourth ventricle. F

33 *Cistern of lamina terminalis.* Cisterns along the lamina terminalis. G

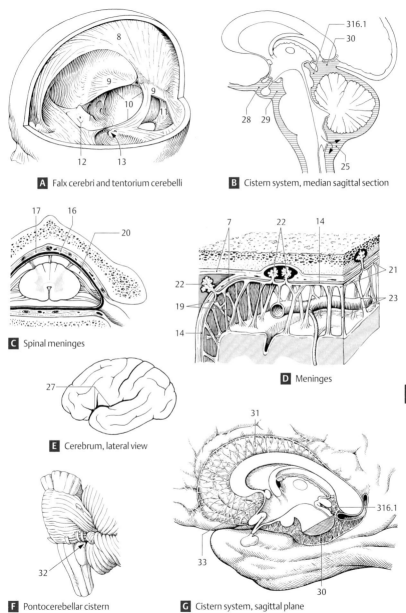

A Falx cerebri and tentorium cerebelli

B Cistern system, median sagittal section

C Spinal meninges

D Meninges

E Cerebrum, lateral view

F Pontocerebellar cistern

G Cistern system, sagittal plane

1 *Quadrigeminal cistern; Cistern of great cerebral vein.* Space spreading out between the splenium of corpus callosum, tectal plate, and superior medullary velum. It contains the great cerebral vein, quadrigeminal arteries, and pineal body. p. 315 B G

2 **Spinal arachnoid mater.** Thin, avascular membrane attached to the spinal dura mater by surface adhesion. Its connective-tissue fibers extend to the pia mater. E

3 *Lumbar cistern.* Dilatation in the lower part of the subarachnoid space containing the terminal filum and cauda equina. E

4 **Pia mater.** Delicate membrane investing the brain and spinal cord.

5 **Cranial pia mater.** Delicate, vascular cranial membrane. It forms a loose connective-tissue sheath lying on the surface of the brain and passing into the sulci, and thus also covering the cranial vessels.

6 *Tela choroidea of fourth ventricle.* Thin layer of pia mater and ependyma forming the inferior part of the ventricle roof. It is attached laterally to the tenia thalami, leaving the lateral and median apertures open. B

7 *Choroid plexus of fourth ventricle.* Paired, garlandlike vascular tuft covered with ependymal cells that projects into the two lateral apertures. B

8 *Tela choroidea of third ventricle.* Thin layer of pia mater covered with ependymal cells extending between the right and left tenia thalami. C

9 *Choroid plexus of third ventricle.* Paired, highly vascularized fringelike projection hanging from the thin roof into the third ventricle. It continues anteriorly through the interventricular foramen as the choroid plexus of the lateral ventricle. C

10 *Choroid plexus of lateral ventricle.* Fringelike, highly vascularized tuft projecting through the choroidal fissure into the lateral ventricle. It extends from the interventricular foramen into the inferior horn. C

11 *Choroidal enlargement.* Thickening of the choroid plexus near the collateral trigone at the root of the posterior horn. C

12 **Spinal pia mater.** Vascularized membrane containing connective-tissue fibers that is firmly attached to the surface of the spinal cord. A

13 *Denticulate ligament.* Sheet of connective tissue running in the frontal plane. It connects the spinal cord with the spinal dura mater and is scalloped at the level of the roots of the spinal nerve. A

14 *Intermediate cervical septum.* Connective-tissue septum located in the cervical spinal cord. It extends from the pia mater into the depths of the posterior funiculus between the gracile and cuneate fasciculi. A F

15 **Filum terminale; Terminal filum.** Tapering, threadlike caudal portion of the spinal cord and its meninges. D E

16 **Dural part; Coccygeal ligament; Filum terminale externum.** Threadlike end of the dura mater that extends from S2 or S3 to the dorsal side of the second coccygeal vertebra. It is attached to the terminal filum. E

17 **Pial part; Pial filament; Filum terminale internum.** Continuation of pia mater within the terminal filum and with intact subarachnoid space, extending to S2. Possible lumbar puncture site. E

18 *SPINAL CORD.* It extends from the end of the medulla oblongata near the exit of the first spinal nerve to the beginning of the terminal filum at L1 or L2. D

19 **EXTERNAL FEATURES.**

20 **Cervical enlargement.** Thickened portion of the spinal cord from C3 to T2 due to greater supply needed for innervation of the upper limb. D

21 **Lumbosacral enlargement.** Thickened portion of the spinal cord from T9 (or T10) to L1 (or L2) due to greater supply needed for innervation of the lower limb. D

22 **Conus medullaris; Medullary cone.** Conical end of the spinal cord that tapers off into the terminal filum at the level of L1 or L2. D

23 **Spinal part of filum terminale.** Part of the terminal filum containing the spinal cord.

24 **Terminal ventricle.** Expansion of the central canal at the end of the medullary cone. D

25 **Anterior median fissure; Ventral median fissure.** Deep, longitudinal, midline fissure on the anterior aspect of the spinal cord. F

26 **Posterior median sulcus; Dorsal median sulcus.** Midline groove between the right and left posterior funiculi. F

27 *Posterior median septum; Dorsal median septum.* Condensation of the subarachnoidal connective tissue as a deeper continuation of the posterior median sulcus. It is less pronounced in the cervical spinal cord and more pronounced in the thoracic region. F

28 **Anterolateral sulcus; Ventrolateral sulcus.** Occasional indistinct groove from which the anterior nerve rootlets emerge. F

29 **Posterolateral sulcus; Dorsolateral sulcus.** Longitudinal groove on the surface of the spinal cord overlying the border between the lateral and posterior funiculi. Entry site of the posterior roots of the spinal nerve. F

30 **Posterior intermediate sulcus; Dorsal intermediate sulcus.** Shallow longitudinal groove on both sides of the posterior median sulcus. It marks the boundary between the gracile and cuneate fasciculi. F

31 **Funiculi of spinal cord.** Three bundles of fiber tracts of the spinal cord, which are divided into groups by the posterior and anterior horns and their root fibers. F

16

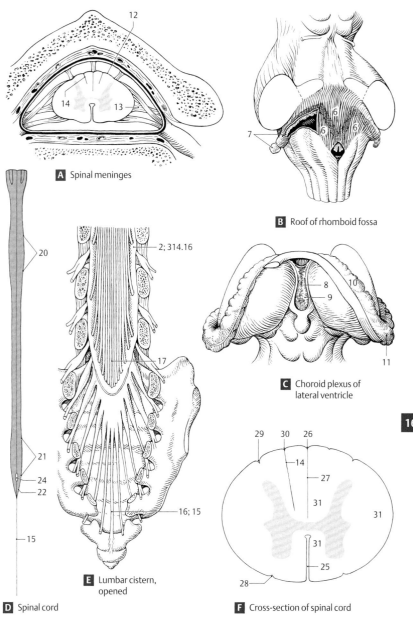

A Spinal meninges

B Roof of rhomboid fossa

C Choroid plexus of lateral ventricle

D Spinal cord

E Lumbar cistern, opened

F Cross-section of spinal cord

16

1 **[[Spinal cord segments]].** "Segment" here refers to a portion of the spinal cord that sends its root fibers through a specific intervertebral foramen. The boundaries cannot be discerned visually.

2 **Cervical Part; Cervical segments [1–8].** There are eight cervical segments for the seven cervical vertebrae. The root fibers of segments 1–7 emerge above the respective vertebrae, while the root fibers of the eighth cervical segment emerge below the seventh cervical vertebra. The cervical part of spinal cord extends from the atlas to the middle of C7. C

3 **Thoracic part; Thoracic segments [1–12].** The twelve thoracic segments of the thoracic part of spinal cord extend from the middle of C7 to the middle of T11. C

4 **Lumbar part; Lumbar segments [1–5].** The five lumbar segments extend from the middle of the body of T11 to the upper border of the body of L1. C

5 **Sacral part; Sacral segments [1–5].** The five sacral segments are located quite far caudally, lying behind the first lumbar vertebral body. C

6 **Coccygeal part; Coccygeal segments [1–3].** The three tiny coccygeal segments. C

7 **INTERNAL FEATURES.**

8 **Central canal.** Remnant of embryonic neural tube lumen. It extends, partially obliterated, from the end of the rhomboid fossa to the terminal filum. A D

9 **Gray substance.** Gray substance of the spinal cord enclosed within the white substance. It mainly consists of a column of multipolar ganglion cells with a channel running down its length (gray columns). Cross-section demonstrates the horns formed by the gray columns. These vary in size in different segments of the spinal cord. A

10 *Anterior horn; Ventral horn.* Anterior column in cross-section. A

11 *Lateral horn.* Lateral projection of gray substance in the thoracic spinal cord, extending from C8 to L2. A

12 *Posterior horn; Dorsal horn.* Posterior column in cross-section. A

13 **White substance.** Portion consisting mainly of myelinated nerve fibers. A

14 **Central gelatinous substance.** Narrow zone of gray substance beneath the ependyma of the central canal. A

15 GRAY COLUMNS. Three-dimensional organization of gray substance into columns. The columns vary in shape and size at different levels of the spinal cord. B

16 **Anterior column; Ventral column.** Its motor neurons are mainly arranged in groups or nuclei. B

17 **Anterior horn; Ventral horn.** Appearance of the anterior column in transverse section. B D

18 **[[Spinal lamina]].** Division of the gray substance of the mammalian spinal cord into ten regions by cytoarchitectural characteristics, which, with the exception of laminae IX and X, form consecutive layers from posterior to anterior. The layers have various configurations along the length of the spinal cord, but are readily distinguishable. This division probably also applies to the human body. p. 321 C

19 *Spinal laminae VII–IX.* Layers of the anterior horn. They are especially thick and varied in shape at the enlargements. They are more simply arranged, for example, in the thoracic spinal cord. The seventh and eighth laminae are presumably zones associated with intrinsic spinal reflexes that are controlled by the mesencephalon or by bulbospinal and propriospinal connections. The seventh lamina is also connected with the cerebellum, which is necessary for regulation of posture and movement. Its cells form an inhibitory center in the enlargements. The ninth lamina is comprised of motor neurons of the spinal cord. p. 321 C

20 *Anterolateral nucleus; Ventrolateral nucleus.* Cell groups with identical function located in the anterolateral part of the anterior horn of segments C4–C8 and L2–S1. They are responsible for innervating muscles of the limbs. D

21 *Anterior nucleus.* Nucleus lying nearly medially that is connected with the anterolateral nucleus of L2–S1. Its function is not well understood.

22 *Anteromedial nucleus; Ventromedial nucleus.* Anteromedial nucleus that extends over the entire length of the spinal cord. It is responsible for innervation of the muscles of the trunk. D

23 *Posterolateral nucleus; Dorsolateral nucleus.* Nucleus located behind the anterolateral nucleus in spinal cord segments C5–T1 and L2–S2. It innervates the muscles of the limbs. D

24 *Retroposterior lateral nucleus; Retrodorsal lateral nucleus.* Nucleus situated behind the posterolateral nucleus in spinal cord segments C8–T1 and S1–S3. It is responsible for innervation of the muscles of the limbs. D

25 *Posteromedial nucleus; Dorsomedial nucleus.* Nucleus situated near the posterior white commissure that extends over spinal cord segments T1–L3. It is responsible for innervation of the muscles of the trunk. D

26 *Central nucleus.* Small group of cells located in a few cervical and lumbar segments. D

27 *Nucleus of accessory nerve.* Nucleus situated in segments C1–C6 near the anterolateral nucleus. It provides the root fibers of the spinal part of the accessory nerve. D

28 *Nucleus of phrenic nerve; Phrenic nucleus.* Nucleus located in the middle of the anterior horn of C4–C7. D

16

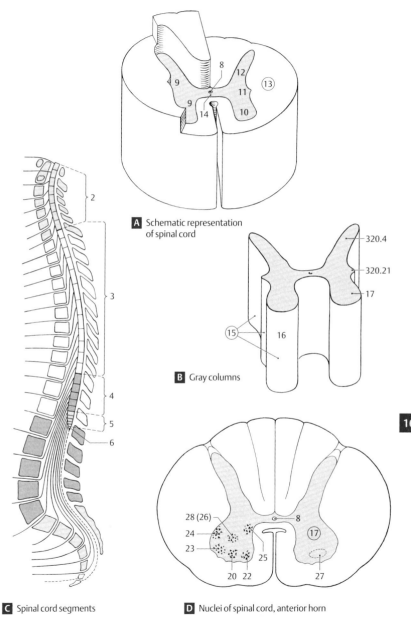

A Schematic representation of spinal cord

B Gray columns

C Spinal cord segments

D Nuclei of spinal cord, anterior horn

16

1   **Posterior column; Dorsal column.**

2   **[[Spinal laminae I–IV]].** Layers serving as the main sites of entry for cutaneous afferents. Their cells also form local closed-loop systems as well as projection neurons of ascending and descending tracts, and are involved in neuropeptidergic systems. C

3   **[[Spinal laminae V–VI]].** Termination site of most proprioceptive afferents. These layers are the target of descending tracts from the motor and sensory cortex as well as subcortical centers and are probably involved in regulation of movement. C

4   **Posterior horn; Dorsal horn.** Appearance of the posterior column in cross-section. Cell morphology varies in different lamina. A, p. 319 B

5   *Apex.* Tip of the posterior horn. It is bounded anteriorly by the Lissauer's tract. A

6   *Marginal nucleus; Spinal lamina I.* Narrow layer of a neural plexus containing various types of neurons along the apex. A

7   *Head.* Part of the posterior horn that is bounded anteriorly by the apex. It is thicker in the cervical and thoracic regions of the spinal cord. A

8   *Gelatinous substance; Spinal lamina II.* Main part of the nerve tissue of the head that has a glassy appearance if unmounted. It contains mainly neurons of various types and unmyelinated nerve fibers. A

9   *Neck.* Narrower part of the posterior horn bounded anteriorly by the head. It contains spinal laminae III–V. A C

10 *Nucleus proprius; Spinal laminae III and IV.* Collection of nerve cells similar to lamina II and mainly containing myelinated fibers. A C

11 *Spinal lamina V.* Layer forming the junction of the neck with the base. Its lateral and medial components are comprised of cells of various morphology. Its lateral portion is not clearly distinct from the reticular formation. C

12 *Base.* Widened base of the posterior horn. A

13 *Spinal lamina VI.* Its structure is similar to that of lamina V, making the two difficult to distinguish. It is only present in upper cervical segments and in segments of the two enlargements. C

14 **Secondary visceral gray substance.** Small region lying anterior to the central intermediate substance that contains ganglion cells of the autonomic nervous system. A

15 **Internal basilar nucleus.** See Note.

16 **Lateral cervical nucleus.** Nucleus that in humans constitutes a rudimentary relay station for impulses from the hair-bearing skin.

17 **Medial cervical nucleus.** Continuation of the [[central cervical nucleus]] into the intermediate Cajal's interstitial nucleus. It is not well-defined in human beings.

18 **Posterior nucleus of lateral funiculus.** See Note.

19 **Intermediate column; Intermediate zone.** Gray substance between the anterior and posterior columns and surrounding the central canal. B

20 **Spinal lamina VII.** Lamina surrounding the greater portion of the intermediate column. C

21 **Lateral horn.** Lateral projection of gray substance. A, p. 319 B

22 *Intermediolateral nucleus.* Group of cells in the lateral horn extending from T1 to L2 that contains sympathetic nerve cells. A

23 **Central intermediate substance.** Gray substance around the central canal.

24 **Posterior thoracic nucleus; Dorsal thoracic nucleus (Stilling–Clarke's column).** Column of nuclei at the base of the posterior horn, generally from C8 to L3. It partly belongs to the posterior spinocerebellar tract. A

25 **Lateral intermediate substance.** Gray substance between the anterior and posterior columns. In the thoracic region of the spinal cord it contains the lateral column. A

26 **Intermediomedial nucleus.** Nucleus lying closer to the central canal that contains sympathetic nerve cells and mainly interneurons from T1 to L2. A

27 **Sacral parasympathetic nuclei.** Parasympathetic nerve cells in sacral segments S2–S4.

28 **Nucleus of pudendal nerve (Onuf's nucleus).** Nucleus of the pudendal nerve located in the anterior horn of S2–S3.

29 **Spinal reticular formation.** Reticulated mixture of gray and white substance. In the thoracic part of the spinal cord it lies between the lateral and posterior horns and in the cervical part of the spinal cord between the posterior and anterior horns. A

30 **Anterior medial nucleus; Ventral medial nucleus.** See Note.

NOTE: Like a number of other terms, internal basilar nucleus (320.15), posterior nucleus of lateral funiculus (320.18), anterior medial nucleus (320.30), and rubronuclear tract (350.14) have been newly added to the existing terminology without accompanying annotation. Our attempts at obtaining information from the commission were unsuccessful.

16

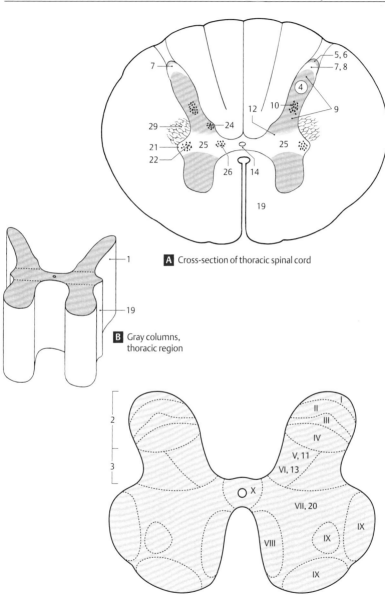

A Cross-section of thoracic spinal cord

B Gray columns, thoracic region

C Spinal laminae, schematic representation

1   WHITE SUBSTANCE. Portion mainly consisting of myelinated nerve fibers.

2   **Anterior funiculus; Ventral funiculus.** White substance between the anterior median fissure and anterior nerve root cells and fibers. A

3   **Anterior fasciculus proprius; Ventral fasciculus proprius.** Ground bundle of the anterior fasciculus. Propriospinal tract. It consists of association fibers and bundled collaterals of projection neurons that lie directly adjacent to the gray substance and allow intersegmental coordination between spinal cord segments. A

4   *Sulcomarginal fasciculus*. Part of the anterior fasciculus proprius lying along the anterior median fissure. A

5   **Anterior corticospinal tract; Ventral corticospinal tract.** Uncrossed part of the pyramidal tract lying lateral to the anterior median fissure. A C

6   **Lateral vestibulospinal tract.** Tract receiving efferent fibers from the Deiters' nucleus which extend to the sacral spinal cord and terminate at the cells of the anterior horn of laminae VII and VIII. Their function in humans has not been clearly shown. B

7   **Medial vestibulospinal tract.** Tract originating in the medial vestibular nucleus, running in the medial longitudinal fasciculus into the middle region of the thoracic spinal cord, and ending mainly in lamina VIII. It influences muscle tone of the neck and upper back. B

8   **Reticulospinal fibers.** Descending fibers from the bulboreticulospinal tract to laminae V–VII. They have not yet been identified in humans

9   **Pontoreticulospinal tract; Medial reticulospinal tract.** Tract originating in the caudal pontine reticular nucleus and caudal part of the oral pontine reticular nucleus and traveling to laminae VII and VIII of the entire spinal cord. It cannot be clearly distinguished in humans. B

10   **Interstitiospinal tract.** Tract running from Cajal's interstitial nucleus in the medial longitudinal fasciculus to laminae VII and VIII of the spinal cord. Its function in humans is not well understood. B

11   **Tectospinal tract.** Efferent fibers arising in the superior colliculi that cross in the posterior tegmental decussation and travel within the longitudinal fasciculus, mostly to the propriospinal system of cervical segments 1–4. They coordinate eye and head movements. A

12   **Anterior raphespinal tract; Ventral raphespinal tract.** Efferent fibers in the medial longitudinal fasciculus that originate in the pallidal and obscurus raphe nuclei and presumably pass to the anterior horns and intermediolateral nucleus. B

13   **Olivospinal fibers.** Not yet identified in humans.

14   **Anterior spinothalamic tract; Ventral spinothalamic tract.** Tract arising from myelinated nerve fibers that cross from the posterior horns via the white commissure to the contralateral anterior funiculus. They transmit perception of crude pressure and tactile sensation. A B

15   **Lateral funiculus.** White substance between the anterior and posterior horn, including their root fibers. A

16   **Lateral fasciculus proprius.** Ground bundle of the lateral funiculus. Its fibers interconnect consecutive segments of the spinal cord. A B

17   **Fastigiospinal tract.** Its existence is not certain in humans.

18   **Interpositospinal tract.** Its existence is not certain in humans.

19   **Lateral corticospinal tract.** Pyramidal tract in the lateral funiculus lying lateral to the posterior horn. Most of its fibers cross below the pyramids of the medulla oblongata to the contralateral side. Its fibers are somatotopically organized. The shortest fibers, which end in the cervical spinal cord, lie medially and the longest, which end in the lower spinal cord, lie furthest lateral. These transmit impulses for voluntary movements and mostly end in laminae VIII–IX, but also in laminae I–VII. A C

20   **Rubrospinal tract (Monakow's tract).** Crossing fibers from the magnocellular part of the red nucleus to the spinal cord. They are poorly developed in humans. A

21   **Bulboreticulospinal tract; Medullary reticulospinal tract; Lateral reticulospinal tract.** Mostly crossed fibers originating in the gigantocellular reticular nucleus and traveling in the lateral funiculus to lamina VII of the spinal cord. It cannot be clearly distinguished in humans. A

22   **Olivospinal fibers.** Not yet identified in humans.

23   **Spinotectal tract.** Ascending fibers of unknown origin. Some travel to the superior colliculus and some to the periaqueductal gray substance and reticular formation of the mesencephalon. It possibly contains pain fibers. B

24   **Lateral spinothalamic tract.** Unmyelinated nerve fibers that arise from the gelatinous substance and cross to the contralateral lateral funiculus via the anterior white commissure. They convey mainly pain and temperature sensations and to a lesser extent exteroceptive and proprioceptive impulses. A

25   **Anterior spinocerebellar tract; Ventral spinocerebellar tract (Gower's tract).** Some of its fibers cross from the posterior horns to the contralateral side, ascend to the superior border of the pons, and bend around to the superior cerebellar peduncle. It transmits information from afferent nerves in the lower half of the body about muscle tone and limb position for coordination of lower limb movement. A B

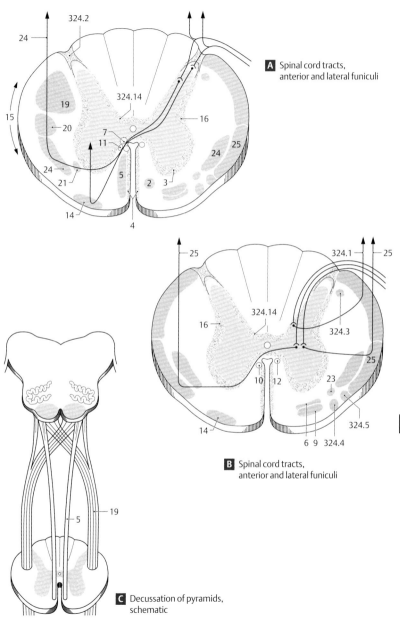

A Spinal cord tracts, anterior and lateral funiculi

B Spinal cord tracts, anterior and lateral funiculi

C Decussation of pyramids, schematic

16

1 **Posterior spinocerebellar tract; Dorsal spinocerebellar tract (Flechsig's tract).** Uncrossed fibers traveling to the inferior cerebellar peduncle. Its function is similar to that of the anterior spinocerebellar tract. A, p. 323 B

2 **Posterolateral tract; Dorsolateral tract (Lissauer's tract).** Tract arising from the short myelinated and unmyelinated fibers between the apex of the posterior horn and the surface. It is part of the lateral fasciculus proprius. A, p. 323 A

3 **Posterior part of lateral funiculus.** Axons originating in lamina IV and traveling to the lateral cervical nucleus. Rudimentary in humans. A, p. 323 B

4 **Spino-olivary tract (Helweg's tract).** Crossed fibers traveling from the posterior horn to the inferior olive that convey cutaneous and proprioceptive impulses. A, p. 323 B

5 **Spinoreticular tract.** Ascending fibers that leave the spinal lemniscus in the medulla oblongata and extend to the reticular formation. A, p. 323 B

6 **Caeruleospinal tract.** Fibers traveling from the caerulean nucleus to the spinal cord. Their existence is not certain in humans.

7 **Hypothalamospinal fibers.** Fibers running between the paraventricular nucleus of the hypothalamus and the intermediolateral nucleus of the spinal cord. They have not yet been identified in humans.

8 **Lateral raphespinal tract.** Fibers traveling from the magnus raphe nucleus to spinal cord laminae I and V. Their existence is not certain in humans.

9 **Solitariospinal tract.** Fibers from the solitary nucleus to the motor neurons of the spinal cord. Their existence is not certain in humans.

10 **Spinocervical tract.** Ascending fibers traveling mainly from lamina IV of the upper cervical spinal cord to the lateral cervical nucleus. Their existence is not certain in humans.

11 **Spinovestibular tract.** Ascending proprioceptive fibers that mostly originate in the caudal portion of the spinal cord and pass to the lateral and medial vestibular nuclei. Their existence is not certain in humans.

12 **Trigeminospinal tract.** Fibers arising from the spinal nucleus of the trigeminal nerve and traveling to the posterior horn of the spinal cord. Their existence is not certain in humans.

13 **Posterior funiculus; Dorsal funiculus.** White substance between the posterior horns including the posterolateral tract (Lissauer's tract). A

14 **Posterior fasciculus proprius; Dorsal fasciculus proprius.** Ground bundle of the posterior funiculus. Tract of varying thickness whose fibers interconnect consecutive spinal segments. A, p. 323 A B

15 **Septomarginal fasciculus (Oval bundle of Flechsig).** Propriospinal fibers that are formed by descending axon collaterals from ascending projection tracts. They lie along the posterior median septum, and in bundles in the lower thoracic spinal cord, lumbar spinal cord (Flechsig's tract), and sacral spinal cord (triangle of Philippe–Gombault). They end in the gray substance of the medullary cone. A

16 **Interfascicular fasciculus (Schultze's comma tract).** Fibers of the propriospinal system that consist of descending axon collaterals of ascending projection tracts. They are grouped in bundles in the cervical and upper thoracic spinal cord between the gracile and cuneate fasciculi. A B

17 **Gracile fasciculus (Goll's tract).** Medial portion of the posterior funiculus. It lies medial to the posterior intermediate sulcus and contains fibers of tactile sensation and deep sensibility from the lower half of the body (coccygeal vertebrae to T5). A, p. 333 A

18 **Cuneate fasciculus (Burdach's tract).** Lateral portion of the posterior funiculus. It lies lateral to the posterior intermediate sulcus and contains fibers of tactile sensation and deep sensibility. It begins at the upper half of the body (T4–C1). A B, p. 333 A

19 **Cuneospinal fibers.** Scattered fibers of the propriospinal system along the cuneate fasciculus. p. 333.A

20 **Gracilespinal fibers.** Scattered fibers of the propriospinal system along the gracile fasciculus.

21 **Spinocuneate fibers.** Ascending fibers that pass from nerve cells in the posterior root of the spinal cord within the cuneate fasciculus to the cuneate nucleus. Together with the spinogracile fibers they are collectively referred to as postsynaptic posterior horn fibers.

22 **Spinogracile fibers.** Ascending fibers from nerve cells in the posterior root of the spinal cord that travel in the gracile fasciculus to the gracile nucleus. See 17.

23 CENTRAL CORD STRUCTURES.

24 **Spinal area X; Spinal lamina X.** Region around the central canal. A

25 **Anterior gray commissure; Ventral gray commissure.** Narrow strip of gray substance anterior to the central canal. A

26 **Posterior gray commissure; Dorsal gray commissure.** Narrow strip of gray substance posterior to the central canal. A

27 **Anterior white commissure; Ventral white commissure.** Part of the fasciculi proprii, it contains crossing fibers of commissural cells that connect opposite sides of the spinal cord. A

28 **Posterior white commissure; Dorsal white commissure.** Part of the fasciculi proprii. A

29 **Central canal.** Remnant of the embryonic neural tube lumen. It sometimes obliterates. A

A Cross-section of spinal cord

B Fasciculus formation

1   *BRAIN.*

2   **Rhombencephalon; Hindbrain.** Genetic, structural, and functional unit. Systematically, it comprises the medulla oblongata, pons, and cerebellum. It surrounds the fourth ventricle. A

3   *Myelencephalon; Medulla oblongata; Bulb.* Rostral continuation of the spinal cord that ends cranially at medullopontine sulcus at the posterior border of the pons. Its agreed-upon caudal border lies along a plane above the root fibers of the first cervical segment. A

4   *Metencephalon; Pons and cerebellum.* Part of the rhombencephalon consisting of the pons and cerebellum. A

5   **Mesencephalon; Midbrain.** Part of the brain that does not form a genetic unit, but rather developed in the region between the rhombencephalon and prosencephalon. This topographical term also includes the tegmentum, red nucleus, tectal plate, cerebral crura, and substantia nigra. A

6   **Prosencephalon; Forebrain.** Origin of the diencephalon and telencephalon, neither of which contain cranial nerve nuclei. A

7   *Diencephalon.* Part of the forebrain comprising the thalamus, epithalamus and pineal body, hypothalamus, and globus pallidus. It encloses the third ventricle and extends from the anterior border of the superior colliculus as far as the interventricular foramen. A

8   *Telencephalon.* Part consisting of two hemispheres that each surround a lateral ventricle and are connected with each other.

9   **Brainstem.** Collective anatomical term for the rhombencephalon and mesencephalon. The clinical definition includes the basal ganglia, diencephalon, and portions of the [[rhinencephalon]].

10 **MEYELENCEPHALON; MEDULLA OLBONGATA; BULB.** Continuation of the spinal cord. See 3.

11 **EXTERNAL FEATURES.**

12 **Anterior median fissure; Ventral median fissure.** Continuation of the anterior median fissure of the spinal cord that is covered by the decussation of pyramids. C

13 **Foramen cecum of medulla oblongata.** Depression on the posterior border of the pons that forms the end of the anterior median fissure. C

14 **Pyramid.** Longitudinal prominence consisting of fibers from the pyramidal tract on both sides of the anterior median fissure. It ends at the decussation of pyramids. C

15 **Decussation of pyramids; Motor decussation.** Between three and five bundles of crossing fibers of the lateral corticospinal tract at the end of the medulla oblongata. C D, p. 331 B

16 **Anterolateral sulcus; Ventrolateral sulcus.** Groove lying lateral to the pyramid that contains the inferior olive. The roots of C1 lie directly below, at the level of the decussation of pyramids. C

17 **Pre-olivary groove.** Indentation between the pyramid and inferior olive. Site of emergence of the root fibers of the hypoglossal nerve. C

18 **Lateral funiculus.** Continuation of the lateral funiculus of the spinal cord to the inferior olive. C

19 **Inferior olive.** Bean-shaped prominence measuring about 1.5 cm in length that is produced by an underlying nucleus. C, p. 329 A B

20 **Anterior external arcuate fibers; Ventral external arcuate fibers.** Fibers from the arcuate nucleus that travel via the caudal end of the inferior olive to the inferior cerebellar peduncle. Scattered fibers of the pontocerebellar tract. C

21 **Retro-olivary groove.** Furrow located posterior to the inferior olive where cranial nerves IX and X emerge. The roots of the accessory nerve arise in its prolongation to the cervical spinal cord. C

22 **Retro-olivary area.** Region posterior to the retro-olivary groove. C

23 **Posterolateral sulcus; Dorsolateral sulcus.** Groove extending anterior to the cuneate fasciculus and ending anterior to the trigeminal tubercle. B

24 **Inferior cerebellar peduncle.** It extends with fibers from the posterior spinocerebellar tract and inferior olive to the cerebellum. There is no clear boundary between it and the middle cerebellar peduncle. B

25 *Restiform body.* It is considered not identical to, but rather a part of, the inferior cerebellar peduncle. B

26 **Trigeminal tubercle.** Elevation produced by the spinal nucleus of trigeminal nerve in the continuation of the spinal cord. D

27 **Cuneate fasciculus.** Lateral part of the posterior funiculus with fibers from the upper half of the body. B

28 **Cuneate tubercle.** Enlargement at the end of the cuneate fasciculus produced by the cuneate nucleus. B D

29 **Gracile fasciculus.** Medial part of the posterior funiculus with fibers from the lower half of the body. B

30 **Gracile tubercle.** Enlargement at the end of the gracile fasciculus that is produced by the gracile nucleus. B D

31 **Posterior median sulcus; Dorsal median sulcus.** Continuation of the posterior median sulcus of the spinal cord. B

32 **Obex.** Transverse medullary layer where the posterior median sulcus terminates and the central canal opens into the fourth ventricle. B

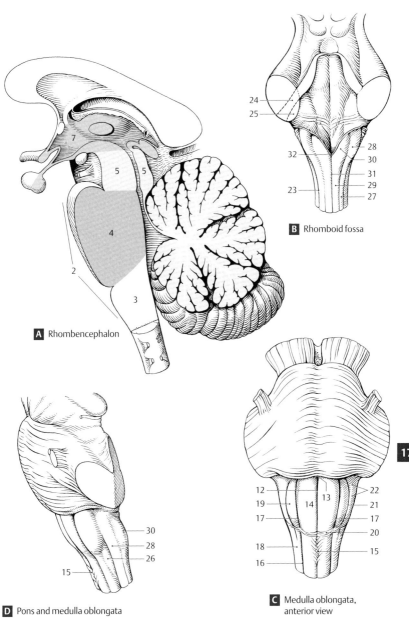

A Rhombencephalon

B Rhomboid fossa

C Medulla oblongata, anterior view

D Pons and medulla oblongata

1 **INTERNAL FEATURES.**

2 **WHITE SUBSTANCE.**

3 **Pyramidal tract.** Tract arising from the cerebral cortex, especially from regions in the frontal and parietal lobes. It transmits activating and inhibiting impulses for voluntary motor function. A B C, p. 333 A

4 *Corticospinal fibers.* Fibers forming the pyramids of medulla oblongata. About 80% cross to the opposite side at the decussation of pyramids where they form the lateral corticospinal tract. The remainder are uncrossed and form the anterior corticospinal tract. A B C

5 *Bulbar corticonuclear fibers.* Fibers ending at the motor nuclei of cranial nerves, the spinal nucleus of accessory nerve, the nucleus of hypoglossal nerve, and the nucleus ambiguus. They leave the pyramidal tract at the level of the respective nuclei.

6 *Corticoreticular fibers.* Fibers extending to the nuclei of the reticular formation. Here: bilaterally to the gigantocellular reticular nucleus.

7 **Decussation of pyramids; Motor decussation.** Crossing of the pyramids. p. 327 C D

8 **Gracile fasciculus.** Medial part of the posterior funiculus with fibers from the lower half of the body. C, p. 325 A 17

9 **Cuneate fasciculus.** Lateral part of the posterior funiculus with fibers from the upper half of the body. C, p. 325 A 18

10 **Internal arcuate fibers.** Portion of fibers from the nuclei of the posterior funiculus that form the medial lemniscus. They consist of axons of second-order neurons from the posterior fasciculus. B C, p. 333 A

11 **Decussation of medial lemniscus; Sensory decussation.** Midline crossing of the majority of internal arcuate fibers at the level of the inferior olive. B C

12 **Medial lemniscus.** Ascending fibers passing from the decussation of medial lemniscus through the brainstem to the thalamus. They convey impulses of general cutaneous sensation. A B C, p. 333 A

13 **Tectospinal tract.** Portion of the tract between the superior colliculus and propriospinal system of the spinal cord. C

14 **Medial longitudinal fasciculus.** Bundle of various fiber systems that enter and leave at different levels. Its fibers interconnect the motor nuclei of cranial nerves and also connect the vestibular apparatus with ocular muscles, neck muscles, and the extrapyramidal system. This serves to coordinate muscle groups, e.g., masticatory, tongue, and pharyngeal muscles when swallowing or speaking; or ocular muscles for movements of the globe. B, p. 333 A

15 **Posterior longitudinal fasciculus; Dorsal longitudinal fasciculus (Fasciculus of Schütz; Bundle of Schütz).** Important tract of efferent fibers from the hypothalamus to secretory and motor nuclei in the floor of rhomboid fossa. These are the nuclei of cranial nerves III, VII, X, XII, as well as the ambiguus, solitary, and salivatory nuclei. It conveys impulses from taste and olfactory stimuli as well as motor impulses. B

16 **Spinal tract of trigeminal nerve.** Descending fibers from the trigeminal nerve conveying pain and temperature stimuli. B C, p. 333 A

17 **Amiculum of olive.** Fiber sheath covering the inferior olive. It consists of afferent and efferent fibers from the inferior olivary complex. B, p. 333 A

18 **Spino-olivary tract.** Ascending tract arising from the posterior horns of the spinal column, and crossing to the inferior olive of the contralateral side. From there some of its fibers synapse and project to the cerebellum. It conveys exteroceptive and proprioceptive impulses. C

19 **Olivocerebellar tract.** All ascending fibers from the inferior olive travel in this tract through the inferior cerebellar peduncle to the contralateral side of the cerebellum and end as climbing fibers. B

20 **Inferior cerebellar peduncle.** Various fiber systems connecting the medulla oblongata and cerebellum. It can be divided into the following two parts.

21 *Restiform body.* Posterolateral group of afferent fibers passing to the cerebellum. A

22 *Juxtarestiform body.* Medial fibers connecting the vestibular apparatus with the cerebellum and fastigium. A

23 **Solitary tract.** Bundle of efferent fibers from cranial nerves VII, IX, and X to the nuclei of the solitary tract.

24 **Anterior external arcuate fibers; Ventral external arcuate fibers.** Fibers originating in the arcuate nucleus and traveling laterally around the inferior olive to the inferior cerebellar peduncle. B

25 **Posterior external arcuate fibers; Dorsal external arcuate fibers.** Uncrossed fibers from the lateral part of the arcuate nucleus to the inferior cerebellar peduncle. Above the level of C8 they replace the posterior spinocerebellar tract. The dorsal nucleus is absent here.

17

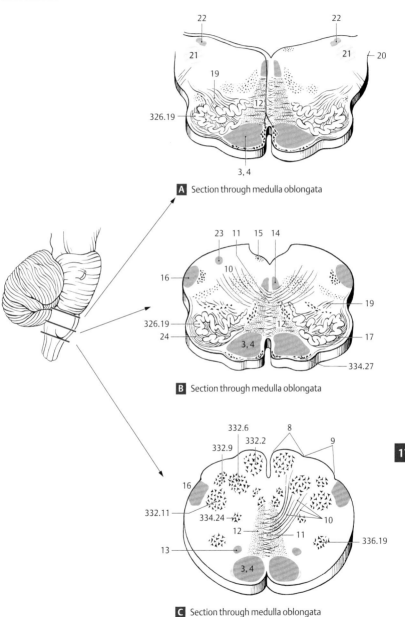

A Section through medulla oblongata

B Section through medulla oblongata

C Section through medulla oblongata

17

1 **Raphe of medulla oblongata.** Seamlike median line at the decussation of medial lemniscus. A

2 **Anterior raphespinal tract.** Portion of the tract in the medial longitudinal fasciculus of the medulla oblongata. A

3 **Anterior reticulospinal tract; Ventral reticulospinal tract.** Descending fibers from the gigantocellular reticular nucleus to the intermediate substance of the spinal cord. B

4 **Anterior spinocerebellar tract; Ventral spinocerebellar tract.** Part of the tract in the medulla oblongata. A B

5 **Hypothalamospinal fibers.** Not yet identified in humans.

6 **Interstitiospinal tract.** Part of the tract within the medial longitudinal fasciculus of the medulla oblongata. A

7 **Lateral raphespinal tract.** Not yet identified in humans.

8 **Lateral bulboreticulospinal tract.** Portion of the tract in the medulla oblongata. A

9 *Medullary reticulospinal fibers.* Fibers from the bulboreticulospinal tract that cross in the medulla oblongata.

10 **Lateral vestibulospinal tract.** Portion of the tract in the medulla oblongata. B

11 **Posterior spinocerebellar tract; Dorsal spinocerebellar tract.** Portion of the tract in the medulla oblongata. B

12 **Cuneocerebellar fibers.** Bundle of fibers passing from the accessory cuneate nucleus (Monakow's tract) through the restiform body to the cerebellum. They transmit information concerning muscle tone and limb position for the upper limb. A

13 **Rubrobulbar tract.** Fibers leaving the rubrospinal tract and traveling to the reticular formation. Their existence is not certain in humans.

14 **Rubro-olivary tract.** Tract arising from the red nucleus and passing uncrossed via the central tegmental tract to the inferior olive and continuing to the cerebellum. Its existence is not certain in humans.

15 **Rubrospinal tract.** Part of the tract in the medulla oblongata. A B

16 **Spinal lemniscus; Anterolateral tracts; Anterolateral system.** Term for the common lemniscus formed by the following eight groups of fibers which mainly convey pain and temperature perception as well as gross tactile sensation and pressure. A B

17 *Spinothalamic fibers.* Common continuation of the anterior and lateral spinothalamic tracts to cranial.

18 *Spinoreticular fibers.* Fibers ascending in the spinothalamic tract and leaving it at the spinal lemniscus.

19 *Spinomesencephalic fibers.* Not all of these fibers have been identified with certainty in humans. Fibers closely accompanying the anterior spinothalamic tract. They terminate in the mesencephalon and are involved in processing pain stimuli.

20 *Spinotectal fibers.* Fibers transmitting pain sensation to the superior colliculus. Involuntary contraction of the pupil in response to pain.

21 *Spinoperiaqueductal fibers.* Fibers passing to the periaqueductal gray substance.

22 *Spinohypothalamic fibers.* Ascending fibers from the intermediolateral nucleus to the hypothalamus that run in the posterior longitudinal fasciculus.

23 *Spinobulbar fibers.* Ascending fibers that pass in the lateral funiculus to a group of cells near the gracile nucleus. They convey information concerning position in space. Their existence is not certain in humans.

24 *Spino-olivary fibers.* Ascending fibers from the posterior horns of the cervical spinal cord to the contralateral side of the inferior olive. B

25 **Spinovestibular tract.** Part of the tract in the medulla oblongata.

26 **Tectobulbar tract.** Efferent fibers from the superior colliculus to brainstem nuclei, mostly passing to the reticular formation, nucleus of abducens nerve, and pontine nuclei. A

17

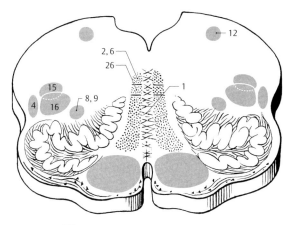

A Section through medulla oblongata

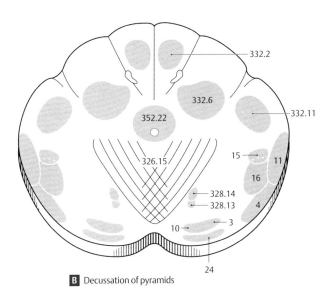

B Decussation of pyramids

17

1 GRAY SUBSTANCE.

2 **Gracile nucleus.** Termination site of tactile and proprioceptive afferents passing in the posterior funiculi from the lower half of the body. It can be divided into various parts differing in terms of cytoarchitecture. A, p. 329 C

3 *Central part*; *Cell nest region*. Central part of the nucleus containing numerous cells and receiving afferents from mechanoreceptors (Meissner corpuscles, Merkel discs; Ruffini corpuscles). A

4 *Rostral part*; *Shell region*. Anterior part containing numerous fibers and receiving afferents mainly from muscle spindles and joints. A

5 *Rostrodorsal subnucleus*; *Cell group Z*. Small group of cells lying anterior to the gracile nucleus that receives muscle spindle afferents from the lower limb and sends projections to the contralateral thalamus.

6 **Cuneate nucleus.** Termination site of tactile and proprioceptive afferent fibers from the upper half of the body running in the posterior funiculus. Its structure and function are similar to those of the gracile nucleus. A B, p. 329 C

7 *Central part*; *Cell nest region*. Comparable to 3 A

8 *Rostral part*; *Shell region*. Comparable to 4 A

9 **Accessory cuneate nucleus.** Origin of the cuneocerebellar fibers. A, p. 329 C

10 **Preaccessory cuneate nucleus; Cell group X.** Cell group for the upper limb that is comparable to the dorsorostral subnucleus. Its existence in humans is not certain.

11 **Spinal nucleus of trigeminal nerve.** Long column of cells in the cervical spinal cord that is bounded rostrally by the principal sensory nucleus, and extends caudally into laminae I–V of the posterior horn of the spinal cord. It constitutes a termination site for protopathic afferents. p. 329 C

12 *Caudal part*. With its laminae I–V, the caudal part of the nucleus resembles a posterior horn of the spinal column in terms of structure. It mainly conveys pain and temperature sensation. It can be subdivided into the following parts. A

13 *Zonal subnucleus*. Comparable to the marginal nucleus of the spinal cord. A

14 *Gelatinous subnucleus*. Comparable to the gelatinous substance of the spinal cord. A

15 *Magnocellular subnucleus*. Comparable to the nucleus proprius of the spinal cord. A

16 *Interpolar part*. Part of the spinal nucleus of the trigeminal nerve adjacent to the caudal part and distinguishable from it in terms of cytoarchitecture. Termination site for tactile afferents from the entire trigeminal nerve as well as cranial nerves VII, IX, X and cervical nerves. B

17 *Oral subnucleus*. Oral part of the spinal nucleus of trigeminal nerve that extends into the tegmentum of pons. Its cytoarchitecture is identical to the interpolar part, and they are closely related in terms of function.

18 **Retrotrigeminal nucleus.** Small cell group lying posterior to the spinal nucleus of trigeminal nerve.

19 **Retrofacial nucleus.** Small cell group lying posterior to the facial nucleus and anterior to the nucleus ambiguus.

20 **Inferior olivary complex.** Nuclear complex of the inferior olive. A B

21 *Principal olivary nucleus*. Principal nucleus of the inferior olive. It is shaped like a thick-walled, folded pouch that is open medially and is connected with the spinal cord and cerebellum.

22 *Dorsal lamella*. Posterior part of the nucleus. B

23 *Ventral lamella*. Anterior part of the nucleus. B

24 *Lateral lamella*. Lateral part of the nucleus. B

25 *Hilum of inferior olivary nucleus*. Medially directed opening of the principal olivary nucleus.

26 *Posterior accessory olivary nucleus*; *Dorsal accessory olivary nucleus*. Accessory nucleus located between the inferior olive and the reticular formation. B

27 *Medial accessory olivary nucleus*. Accessory nucleus located anterior to the hilum of inferior olivary nucleus. A B

28 **Nucleus of hypoglossal nerve.** Paramedian nucleus situated in the floor of the inferior portion of the rhomboid fossa. A B

29 **Posterior paramedian nucleus; Dorsal paramedian nucleus.** Group of nuclei lying medial to the nucleus of hypoglossal nerve and extending nearly to the nucleus of abducens nerve. B

30 **Posterior nucleus of vagus nerve; Dorsal nucleus of vagus nerve.** Nucleus lying on the floor of rhomboid fossa lateral to the nucleus of hypoglossal nerve. It is the origin of the visceromotor fibers of the vagus nerve. A B

17

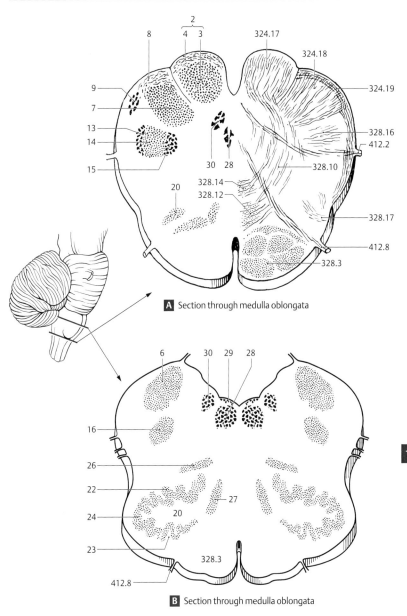

A Section through medulla oblongata

B Section through medulla oblongata

1 **Nuclei of solitary tract; Solitary nuclei.** Column of cells extending from the decussation of pyramids to the middle of the rhomboid fossa. As a functional unit, the nuclear complex receives viscerosensory afferents whose endings are arranged somatotopically. Taste fibers from cranial nerves VII, IX, and X terminate in the anterior portion. As an independent integration center it is connected e.g. with the reticular formation, amygdala, and insular cortex. The current division of nuclei as follows is based mainly on different levels of acetylcholinesterase activity. The various functions of the individual nuclei in humans is unknown. A B

2 *Parasolitary nucleus.* Nucleus lying at the lateral border of the complex. It does not have any enzyme activity. B

3 *Commissural nucleus.* Together with the paracommissural solitary nucleus, it forms the caudal end of the cell column at the decussation of pyramids. It has a low level of enzyme activity. See 8

4 *Gelatinous solitary nucleus.* Nucleus resembling the gelatinous substance of a posterior horn of the spinal cord. It has a high level of enzyme activity. B

5 *Intermediate solitary nucleus.* It contributes to formation of the rostral end of the nuclear complex and has a low level of enzyme activity. B

6 *Interstitial solitary nucleus.* Nucleus situated directly adjacent to the solitary tract. It has a very high level of enzyme activity.

7 *Medial solitary nucleus.* Largest nucleus at the level of the obex. It has a low level of enzyme activity. B

8 *Paracommissural solitary nucleus.* Nucleus with a high level of enzyme activity. See 3 B

9 *Posterior solitary nucleus; Dorsal solitary nucleus.* Nucleus with a high level of enzyme activity, which is also homogeneous.

10 *Posterolateral solitary nucleus; Dorsolateral solitary nucleus.* Nucleus that contributes to the formation of the lateral boundary of the nuclear complex. It contains areas of varying enzyme activity. B

11 *Anterior solitary nucleus; Ventral solitary nucleus.* Nucleus with a moderate level of enzyme activity. B

12 *Anterolateral solitary nucleus; Ventrolateral solitary nucleus.* Nucleus with a moderate level of enzyme activity. B

13 **Vestibular nuclei.** Four nuclei forming a complex lying on the lateral part of the floor of fourth ventricle and extending into the caudal portion of the pons. They receive afferent fibers from the vestibular apparatus and are connected with the spinal column, medulla oblongata, cerebellum, and nuclei of the ocular muscles. They mediate involuntary control of posture and head position, including eye position at rest and during movement. A

14 *Inferior vestibular nucleus.* Group of cells lying inferolateral to the middle nucleus that forms a terminal nucleus mainly for descending afferents from the maculae of saccule and utricle. Its efferents travel in the medial longitudinal fasciculus to the spinal cord. A

15 *Magnocellular part of inferior vestibular nucleus. Cell group F.* Part of the inferior vestibular nucleus consisting of large cells.

16 *Medial vestibular nucleus (Schwalbe's nucleus).* Terminal nucleus located lateral to the sulcus limitans that receives afferents from the ampullary crests and the maculae of saccule and utricle. Its efferents travel bilaterally in the medial longitudinal fasciculus to nuclei of the extraocular muscles, Cajal's interstitial nucleus, and into the spinal cord. A

17 **Marginal nucleus of restiform body; Cell group Y.** Group of cells on the inferior cerebellar peduncle that receives afferent fibers from the vestibular apparatus.

18 **Cochlear nuclei.** Nuclei of the auditory pathway situated in the floor of the lateral recess near the inferior cerebellar peduncle. They constitute the terminal nuclei of the fibers of the cochlear nerve. A

19 *Posterior cochlear nucleus; Dorsal cochlear nucleus.* Its efferent projections form the posterior acoustic striae, running beneath the floor of the lateral recess of rhomboid fossa to the midline, then diving deeper and continuing into the trapezoid body. A

20 *Anterior cochlear nucleus; Ventral cochlear nucleus.* Nucleus that can be subdivided into two parts. A

21 *Anterior part.* Part with crossing fibers that mostly form the trapezoid body.

22 *Posterior part.*

23 **Commissural nucleus of vagus nerve.** Cluster of neurons above the central canal at the level of the decussation of medial lemniscus. Termination site of fibers from the solitary tract.

24 **Nucleus ambiguus.** Nucleus of origin lying posterior to the inferior olive. It gives rise to the motor fibers of CN IX and X as well as the cranial portion of CN XI. It receives afferent projections mainly from the solitary nucleus and reticular formation. A, p. 329 C

25 **Retro-ambiguus nucleus.** Column of cells at the anterolateral end of the nucleus ambiguus. It extends caudally into the upper portion of the cervical spinal cord. It is presumably involved in regulation of respiration and circulation, though its precise function in humans is not certain.

26 **Inferior salivatory nucleus.** Nucleus of origin giving rise to parasympathetic (secretory) fibers of the glossopharyngeal nerve. A

27 **Arcuate nucleus.** Group of cells lying anterior to the pyramidal surface. It gives rise to the anterior and posterior external arcuate fibers of the medulla and the medullary striae of fourth ventricle. p. 329 B

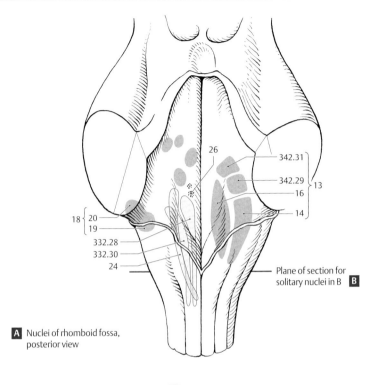

A Nuclei of rhomboid fossa, posterior view

Plane of section for solitary nuclei in B **B**

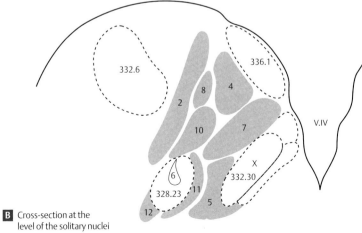

B Cross-section at the level of the solitary nuclei

1 **Area postrema.** Triangular region caudal to the trigone of vagus nerve that contains a circumventricular organ. It atrophies in the adult. p. 335 B

2 **Endolemniscal nucleus.** Small cell group containing cholinesterase that is located in the medial lemniscus at the level of the inferior olive. Its function is unknown.

3 **Medial pericuneate nucleus.** Small cell groups between the accessory cuneate nucleus and solitary tract. Their function is unknown. A

4 **Lateral pericuneate nucleus.** Small cell groups lying lateral to the accessory cuneate nucleus. Their function is unknown. A

5 **Perihypoglossal nuclei.** Nuclear complex consisting of cell groups near the nucleus of the hypoglossal nerve. They are connected with the nuclei of oculomotor nerve, vestibular nuclei, and cerebellum.

6 *Subhypoglossal nucleus (Roller's nucleus).* Group of cells lying beneath the nucleus of the hypoglossal nerve. A

7 *Intercalated nucleus (Staderini's nucleus).* Cell group located between the nuclei of the hypoglossal and dorsal vagus nerves. It extends longitudinally from the obex to the anterior end of the nucleus of the hypoglossal nerve. A

8 *Prepositus nucleus.* Nucleus lying in the floor of rhomboid fossa, rostral to the intercalated nucleus. It receives afferent projections from the vestibular nuclei, Cajal's interstitial nucleus, and cerebellum. Its efferents travel to the cerebellum and nuclei of the ocular muscles. It plays an important role in rapid eye movements and gaze holding.

9 *Peritrigeminal nucleus.* Cell groups of unknown function that largely enclose the spinal nucleus of trigeminal nerve and extend caudally to the inferior olive. A

10 *Pontobulbar nucleus.* Nuclei lying anterior to the inferior cerebellar peduncle. They are considered extrapontine nuclei of the pons.

11 **Supraspinal nucleus.** Anterior horn motor cells of the first cervical spinal nerve that project into the medulla oblongata.

12 **Reticular nuclei.** Medial column of nuclei in the reticular formations of the medulla oblongata and pons.

13 **Gigantocellular reticular nucleus.** Nucleus extending from the anterior one-third of the medulla oblongata to the posterior half of the pons and as deep as the inferior olive or inferior pole of the motor nucleus of trigeminal nerve. A B

14 *Pars alpha.* Portion of the gigantocellular reticular nucleus located in the caudal portion of the pons. It extends over the magnus raphe nucleus.

15 **Anterior gigantocellular reticular nucleus; Ventral gigantocellular reticular nucleus.** Cell area above the posterior accessory olivary nucleus with low levels of acetylcholine. A

16 **Lateral paragigantocellular reticular nucleus.** Nucleus lying anterolateral and directly adjacent to the gigantocellular reticular nucleus. A

17 **Interfascicular nucleus of hypoglossal nerve.** Cell column below the Roller's nucleus. A

18 **Intermediate reticular nucleus.** Group of cells containing catecholamine that are arranged in an anteriorly convex line along the former site of the sulcus limitans where the roots of CN IX and X emerge. A

19 **Lateral reticular nucleus.** Nucleus extending approximately along the lower half of the inferior olive. It receives afferent fibers from the spinal cord. Its efferent fibers travel via the inferior cerebellar peduncle to the cerebellum. A, p. 329 C

20 *Magnocellular part.* Large-cell portion of the nucleus lying adjacent to the inferior olive. A

21 *Parvocellular part.* Portion of the nucleus consisting of small cells. A

22 *Subtrigeminal part.* Narrow segment of cells adjacent to the spinal nucleus of trigeminal nerve. A

23 **Parvocellular reticular nucleus.** Nucleus situated posterior to the intermediate reticular nucleus. A

24 **Posterior paragigantocellular reticular nucleus; Dorsal paragigantocellular reticular nucleus.** Region with low levels of acetylcholine above the gigantocellular reticular nucleus. A

25 **Central reticular nucleus.** Cell region in the inferior part of the medulla oblongata, lying anterolateral to the central canal. It consists of two cytoarchitecturally distinct areas, one overlying the other.

26 *Dorsal part.* Posterior portion of the central reticular nucleus.

27 *Ventral part.* Anterior portion of the central reticular nucleus.

28 **Medial reticular nucleus.** Medial collection of cells lying anterior to the intermediate reticular nucleus.

29 **Raphe nuclei.** Median column of nuclei situated lateral to the raphe of medulla oblongata in the reticular formation. B

30 **Obscurus raphe nucleus.** Nucleus lying medial to the medial longitudinal fasciculus and extending caudally to the first cervical segment. B

31 **Pallidal raphe nucleus.** Small cluster of cells situated medial to the pyramids of medulla oblongata.

32 **Magnus raphe nucleus.** Nucleus overlying the medial lemniscus along the floor of rhomboid fossa. It is especially expansive at the level of the olivary pole. B

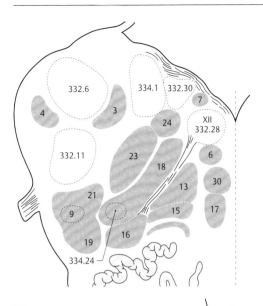

A Schematic representation of distribution of nuclei, level of inferior olive

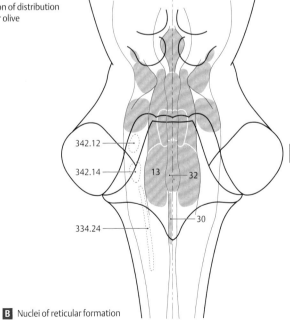

B Nuclei of reticular formation

1 **PONS.** Part of the brain situated between the interpeduncular fossa and the pyramids. It surrounds the anterior part of the fourth ventricle and consists mainly of descending tracts from the cerebrum that travel to nuclei, synapse, cross, and continue to the cerebellum. A

2 **EXTERNAL FEATURES.**

3 **Medullopontine sulcus.** Bounding groove between the medulla oblongata and inferior margin of the pons. Cranial nerve VI emerges at the surface here. A

4 **Basilar sulcus.** Median groove containing the basilar artery. It is formed by the lateral elevation of the fibers of the pyramidal tract. A

5 **Middle cerebellar peduncle.** Part conveying the transverse fibers of the pons, mainly neencephalic tracts, to the cerebellum. A B

6 **Cerebellopontine angle.** Site of emergence of cranial nerves VII and VIII at the surface. Clinically important niche between the pons, medulla oblongata, and cerebellum. A

7 **Frenulum veli.** Band passing between the superior medullary velum and tectal plate. B

8 **Superior cerebellar peduncle.** B

9 **Superior medullary velum.** Layer of white substance stretched between the two cerebellar peduncles. It is fused with the lingula. B

10 **INTERNAL FEATURES.**

11 BASILAR PART OF PONS. Anterior portion mainly formed by fibers from the corticopontocerebellar tract. C

12 WHITE SUBSTANCE.

13 **Longitudinal pontine fibers.** These include the following longitudinal bundles of fibers from projection tracts that terminate in the pontine nuclei or descend to the medulla oblongata or spinal cord.

14 *Corticospinal fibers.* Bundle of fibers in the pyramidal tract. They unite at the inferior margin of the pons and continue to the medulla oblongata. C

15 *Pontine corticonuclear fibers.* Fibers in the pyramidal tract that pass to the motor nuclei of cranial nerves. C

16 *Corticoreticular fibers.* Fiber bundles passing from the cerebral cortex toward the nuclei of the reticular formation.

17 *Corticopontine fibers.* Fibers from the first-order neurons of the corticopontine fibers that pass from the frontal, occipital, parietal, and temporal lobes to the pontine nuclei (second-order neurons).

18 *Tectopontine fibers.* Their existence is not certain in humans.

19 **Transverse pontine fibers.** Crossing pontine fibers and fibers from the pontine nuclei. C

20 *Pontocerebellar fibers.* Group of ascending pontine fibers in the middle cerebellar peduncle. After giving off collaterals to the cerebellar nuclei, they continue to the cortex. C

21 GRAY SUBSTANCE.

22 **Pontine nuclei.** Second-order neurons of the corticopontocerebellar tract. They consist of variously large cell groups scattered between fiber bundles.

23 *Anterior nucleus; Ventral nucleus.* Collection of cells on the ventral side of the pons. C

24 *Lateral nucleus.* Collection of cells on the anterolateral side of the pons. C

25 *Median nucleus.* Collection of cells along the midline. C

26 *Paramedian nucleus.* Collection of cells lateral to the midline. C

27 *Peduncular nucleus; Peripeduncular nucleus.* Cell groups lateral to the red nucleus. C

28 *Posterior nucleus; Dorsal nucleus.* Cell groups in the tegmentum above the medial lemniscus. C

29 *Posterolateral nucleus; Dorsolateral nucleus.* Cell groups lateral to the medial lemniscus. C

30 *Posteromedial nucleus; Dorsomedial nucleus.* Cell groups along the raphe at the level of the medial lemniscus. C

31 *Reticulotegmental nucleus.* Distinguishable nucleus above and in front of the medial lemniscus. C

17

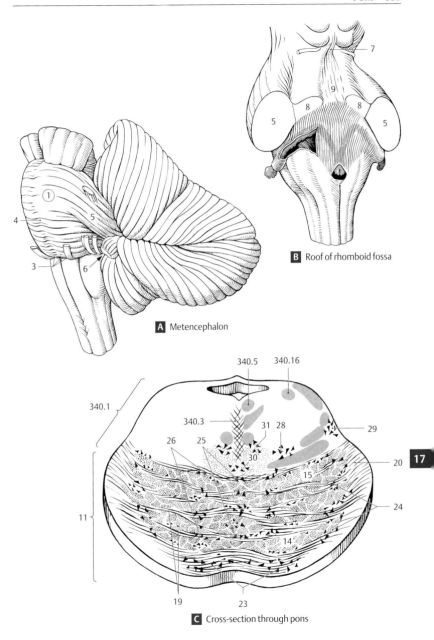

B Roof of rhomboid fossa

A Metencephalon

C Cross-section through pons

17

1 TEGMENTUM OF PONS. Phylogenetically older part of the brainstem situated between the transverse pontine fibers and the fourth ventricle. A

2 WHITE SUBSTANCE.

3 **Raphe of pons.** Middle line of the pons containing fibers from the nucleus of trigeminal nerve. A

4 **Medial longitudinal fasciculus.** Association fibers between, on the one side, the nuclei of the ocular and neck muscles and, on the other, the vestibular apparatus. A

5 **Posterior longitudinal fasciculus; Dorsal longitudinal fasciculus (Fasciculus of Schütz; Bundle of Schütz).** Efferent fibers passing from the hypothalamus to nuclei in the floor of rhomboid fossa. A

6 **Medial lemniscus.** Fibers connecting the nuclei of the posterior longitudinal fasciculus with the thalamus. A

7 **Tectospinal tract.** Fibers connecting the superior colliculus with the propriospinal system of the spinal cord. A

8 **Pretecto-olivary fibers.** Fibers connecting the pretectal nuclei with the inferior olive. Their existence is not certain in humans.

9 **Tecto-olivary fibers.** Fibers connecting the tectum and inferior olive. Their existence is not certain in humans.

10 **Tectoreticular fibers.** Fibers connecting the tectum and reticular formation. Their existence is not certain in humans.

11 **Spinal lemniscus; Anterolateral tracts; Anterolateral system.** Collective term used to describe various groups of fibers. A

12 **Spinal tract of trigeminal nerve.** Descending fibers from the trigeminal nerve for pain and temperature stimuli. B

13 **Trigeminal lemniscus; Trigeminothalamic tract.** Efferents of the principal sensory and spinal nuclei of trigeminal nerve that run, crossed and uncrossed, to the thalamus. A

14 *Anterior trigeminothalamic tract*; *Ventral trigeminothalamic tract.* Crossed fibers from the principal sensory and spinal nuclei of trigeminal nucleus that pass to the thalamus. They mostly convey pain impulses. A

15 *Posterior trigeminothalamic tract*; *Dorsal trigeminothalamic tract.* Uncrossed fibers from the principal sensory nucleus to the thalamus.

16 **Mesencephalic tract of trigeminal nerve.** Fibers for the mesencephalic nucleus of trigeminal nerve that run lateral to the cerebral aqueduct in the floor of fourth ventricle. They convey proprioceptive impulses from the teeth, masticatory muscles, and temporomandibular joints. B

17 **Genu of facial nerve.** Curved facial nerve fibers lying below the facial colliculus and overlying the nucleus of abducens nerve. B

18 **Trapezoid body.** Interwoven, crossing fibers from the two anterior cochlear nuclei. It is part of the auditory pathway. C

19 **Olivocochlear tract.** Fiber bundle from the superior olivary nucleus to the organ of Corti.

20 **Lateral lemniscus.** Ascending continuation of the trapezoid body. It is part of the auditory pathway. C

21 **Medullary striae of fourth ventricle.** Bundle of myelinated nerve fibers that passes from the arcuate nucleus to the cerebellum.

22 **Anterior acoustic stria; Ventral acoustic stria.** Fibers from the posterior cochlear nucleus that cross the floor of rhomboid fossa to the lateral lemniscus of the contralateral side. C

23 **Intermediate acoustic stria.** Fibers from the anterior cochlear nucleus to the inferior olivary complex. C

24 **Posterior acoustic stria; Dorsal acoustic stria.** Fibers from the posterior cochlear nucleus to the lateral lemniscus of the contralateral side. They lie anterior to the anterior acoustic stria. C

25 **Anterior pontoreticulospinal tract; Ventral pontoreticulospinal tract.** Their existence is not certain in humans.

26 **Anterior spinocerebellar tract; Ventral spinocerebellar tract (Gower's tract).** A

27 **Auditory commissure of pons.** Fibers connecting the anterior cochlear nuclei in the trapezoid body.

28 **Central tegmental tract.** Most important descending tract of the extrapyramidal motor system. It extends from the mesencephalon to the inferior olive. In the pons it forms a sheet of fibers lateral to the medial longitudinal fasciculus. It consists of the following groups of fibers. A

29 *Rubro-olivary fibers.* Fibers from the parvocellular part of red nucleus to the inferior olive.

30 *Anulo-olivary fibers.* Fibers traveling from the telencephalon, diencephalon, mesencephalon, and reticular formation to the inferior olive.

31 *Cerebello-olivary fibers.* Mostly crossed fibers from the dentate nucleus that run through the superior cerebellar peduncle to the inferior olive.

17

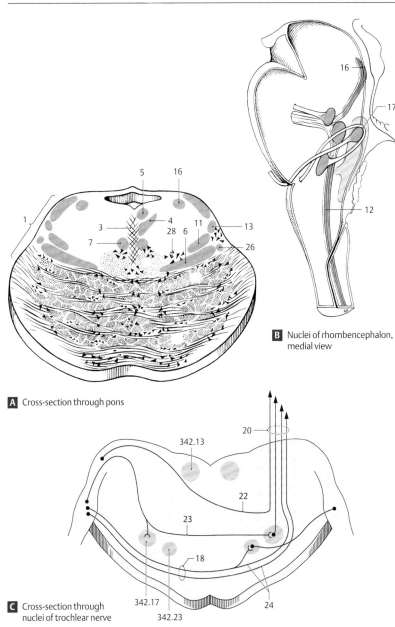

B Nuclei of rhombencephalon, medial view

A Cross-section through pons

C Cross-section through nuclei of trochlear nerve

17

1 **Hypothalamospinal tract.** Its existence is not certain in humans.

2 **Interstitiospinal tract.** Its function in humans is not well understood.

3 **Rubropontine tract.** Portion of the rubrospinal tract in the pons. Its fibers cross in the anterior tegmental decussation (decussation of Forel). A

4 **Rubrospinal tract.** Rudimentary in humans.

5 **Tectobulbar tract.** Portion of the tract in the pons. Its fibers pass to the pontine nuclei and the nucleus of abducens nerve. A

6 **Tectopontine tract.** Fibers from the superior colliculus to the pons, passing along the inferolateral part of the inferior colliculus. A

7 GRAY SUBSTANCE.

8 **Principal sensory nucleus of trigeminal nerve.** Nucleus situated lateral to the motor nucleus that chiefly serves for tactile sensation. It can be divided into two parts. B

9 *Posteromedial nucleus; Dorsomedial nucleus.* Origin of the posterior trigeminothalamic tract.

10 *Anterolateral nucleus; Ventrolateral nucleus.* Origin of the anterior trigeminothalamic tract.

11 **Mesencephalic nucleus of trigeminal nerve.** Nucleus consisting of pseudounipolar neurons extending to beneath the tectal plate. D

12 **Motor nucleus of trigeminal nerve.** Motor nucleus for innervation of the masticatory muscles located near the level of the exit of the nerve. B D

13 **Nucleus of abducens nerve.** Nucleus lying beneath the facial colliculus. B D, p. 341 C

14 **Motor nucleus of facial nerve.** Motor nucleus for innervation of the muscles of facial expression. It is located laterally, beneath the facial nucleus. B D

15 **Superior salivatory nucleus.** Autonomic nucleus providing parasympathetic fibers to the facial nerve. It sends preganglionic fibers to the pterygopalatine and submandibular ganglia. B D

16 **Lacrimal nucleus.** Autonomic cells lying alongside the superior salivatory nucleus that regulate lacrimal secretion. D

17 **Superior olivary nucleus; Superior olivary complex.** Nuclear complex located lateral to the trapezoid body. It receives fibers from the cochlear nuclei and sends fibers forming the olivocochlear tract to the hair cells. It serves as a reflex center and as a relay nucleus of the auditory pathway. C, p. 341 C

18 *Lateral superior olivary nucleus.* Principal lateral nucleus, composed of multipolar cells.

19 *Medial superior olivary nucleus.* Medial nucleus, composed of spindle-shaped cells.

20 *Peri-olivary nuclei.* Cell groups with acetylcholinesterase activity surrounding the inferior olive. It is not clear whether they belong to the superior olivary nucleus in humans.

21 *Medial nuclei.*

22 *Lateral nuclei.*

23 **Nuclei of trapezoid body.** p. 341 C

24 *Anterior nucleus of trapezoid body; Ventral nucleus of trapezoid body.* Small nucleus located on the posterolateral aspect of the trapezoid body. C

25 *Lateral nucleus of trapezoid body.* Nucleus located posterolateral to the anterior nucleus of trapezoid body. C

26 *Medial nucleus of trapezoid body.* Nucleus sometimes located at the exit of the abducens nerve.

27 **Vestibular nuclei of pons.** B D

28 *Medial vestibular nucleus (Schwalbe's nucleus).* Middle vestibular nucleus. B C

29 *Lateral vestibular nucleus (Deiters' nucleus).* Smaller collection of cells near the lateral recess of the rhomboid fossa with projections to the anterior horn of the spinal cord. B C

30 *Parvocellular part; Cell group L.* Small-cell portion of the lateral vestibular nucleus.

31 *Superior vestibular nucleus.* Nucleus situated above the lateral vestibular nucleus that receives afferents from the ampullary crests. It has projections to the medial longitudinal fasciculus and cerebellum. B C

31 **Cochlear nuclei.** Ventral and dorsal terminal nucleus of the cochlear part of the vestibulocochlear nerve. B C

17

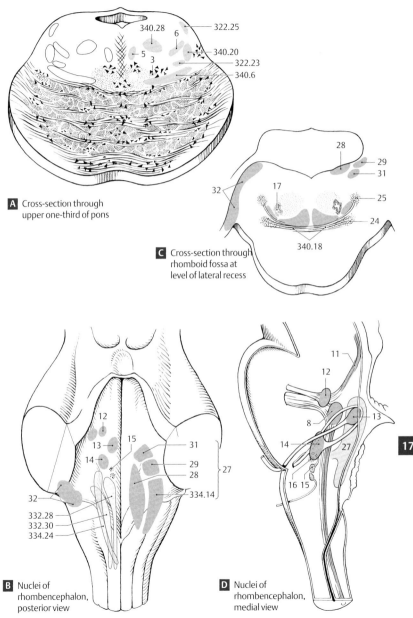

A Cross-section through upper one-third of pons

C Cross-section through rhomboid fossa at level of lateral recess

B Nuclei of rhombencephalon, posterior view

D Nuclei of rhombencephalon, medial view

17

1 **Nuclei of lateral lemniscus.** Groups of cells embedded in the lateral lemniscus.

2 *Posterior nucleus of lateral lemniscus; Dorsal nucleus of lateral lemniscus.* Collection of cells in the posterolateral portion. A

3 *Intermediate nucleus of lateral lemniscus.* Its existence is not certain in humans.

4 *Anterior nucleus of lateral lemniscus; Ventral nucleus of lateral lemniscus.* Collection of cells in the anteromedial portion. A

5 **Anterior tegmental nucleus; Ventral tegmental nucleus.** Nucleus located near the raphe beneath the floor of fourth ventricle. A

6 **Caerulean nucleus.** Elongated column of bluish-black cells situated posterolateral to the anterior tegmental nucleus in the lateral wall of fourth ventricle. It is part of the central catecholamine system. A

7 **Subcaerulean nucleus.** Nucleus that may be considered a diffuse, anterior expansion of the caerulean nucleus. A

8 **Interstitial nuclei of medial longitudinal fasciculus.** Smaller groups of cells lying along the medial longitudinal fasciculus.

9 **Parabrachial nuclei.** Nuclear complex in the rostral portion of the pons, located anteromedial and posterolateral to the superior cerebellar peduncle. They serve, among other things, as a site of synaptic transmission between the solitary nucleus, trigeminal nuclei, spinal cord, and thalamus, as well as the hypothalamus and limbic system.

10 *Subparabrachial nucleus (Kölliker–Fuse nucleus).* Its existence is not certain in humans.

11 *Lateral parabrachial nucleus.* Nucleus located posterolateral to the superior cerebellar peduncle. A B

12 *Lateral part; Lateral subnucleus; Medial part; medial subnucleus; posterior part; dorsal part; posterior subnucleus; dorsal subnucleus; anterior part, ventral part; anterior subnucleus; ventral subnucleus.* These have not yet been identified in human beings.

13 *Medial parabrachial nucleus.* Nucleus located anteromedial to the superior cerebellar peduncle. A B

14 *Medial part; Medial subnucleus; lateral part; lateral subnucleus.* These have not yet been identified in humans.

15 **Posterior tegmental nucleus; Dorsal tegmental nucleus (von Gudden's nucleus).** Cell group in the periaqueductal gray substance near the midline at the border between the pons and mesencephalon. A

16 **Supralemniscal nucleus.** Cell group situated lateral to the reticulotegmental nucleus.

17 **Reticular nuclei.** Medial nuclear column in the reticular formations of the pons and medulla oblongata.

18 **Caudal pontine reticular nucleus.** Medial nuclear column situated between the gigantocellular reticular nucleus and oral pontine reticular nucleus. B

19 **Oral pontine reticular nucleus.** Nuclear column located anterior to the caudal pontine reticular nucleus and medial to the parabrachial nuclei in the floor of the anterior portion of the rhomboid fossa. B

20 **Reticulotegmental nucleus (Nucleus of Bechterew).** Column of cells situated between the pontine raphe nucleus to medial and the caudal pontine reticular nucleus to lateral. B

21 **Paralemniscal nucleus.** Cell group lying lateral to the central nucleus of the inferior colliculus.

22 **Paramedian reticular nucleus.** Cell group situated anterior to the nucleus of the hypoglossal nerve at the level of the middle of the inferior olive.

23 **Raphe nuclei.** Median column of nuclei in the reticular formations of the pons and medulla oblongata.

24 **Magnus raphe nucleus.** Column of cells situated medial to the gigantocellular reticular nucleus. B

25 **Pontine raphe nucleus.** Median column of cells located anterior to the magnus raphe nucleus. B

26 **Median raphe nucleus; Superior central nucleus.** Median column of cells located in the anterior portion of the rhomboid fossa and extending into the mesencephalon. B

27 **Posterior raphe nucleus; Dorsal raphe nucleus.** Column of cells extending from the anterior end of the rhomboid fossa to behind the superior colliculi. B

17

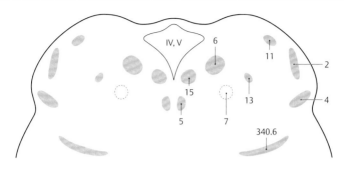

A Pons, section below the decussation of trochlear nerve fibers

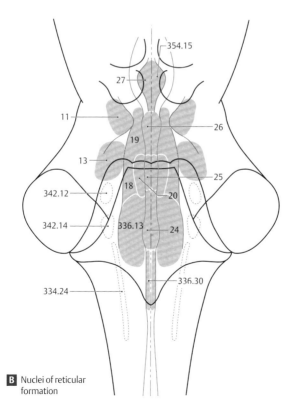

B Nuclei of reticular formation

17

1 **Fourth ventricle.** Dilatation of the embryonic neural tube lumen in the rhombencephalon.

2 **Rhomboid fossa; Floor of fourth ventricle.** A

3 *Median sulcus.* Midline groove running through the rhomboid fossa. A

4 *Medial eminence.* Elongated eminence between the median sulcus and sulcus limitans that is produced by the cranial nerve nuclei. A

5 *Facial colliculus.* Rounded protuberance above the medullary stria of fourth ventricle. It is produced by the internal genu of facial nerve and the nucleus of abducens nerve. A

6 *Locus caeruleus.* Elongated collection of bluish-black cells lying below the lateral wall of the fourth ventricle. A

7 *Medullary stria of fourth ventricle.* Bundles of myelinated nerve fibers extending from the arcuate nuclei to the cerebellum. A

8 *Hypoglossal trigone*; *Trigone of hypoglossal nerve.* Triangular elevation overlying the nucleus of the hypoglossal nerve. It is situated between the median sulcus and the sulcus limitans above the trigone of vagus nerve. A

9 *Vagal trigone*; *Trigone of vagus nerve.* Triangular elevation overlying the dorsal nucleus of the vagus nerve. It lies caudal to the trigone of hypoglossal nerve. A

10 *Vestibular area.* Area overlying the vestibular nuclei lateral to the sulcus limitans at the beginning of the lateral recess. A

11 *Funiculus separans.* Strip of ependyma between the trigone of vagus nerve and the area postrema. A

12 *Gray line*; *Tenia cinerea.* Line along the inferior part of the roof of the rhomboid fossa. A

13 **Roof of fourth ventricle.**

14 *Fastigium.* Transverse summit of the roof of fourth ventricle. A

15 *Choroid plexus.* Paired vascular tufts in the roof of fourth ventricle. Initially oriented sagittally, they bend around near the fastigium toward the lateral aperture. B

16 *Choroid membrane.* Pia mater stretched between the inferior medullary velum and choroid line that bears the choroid plexus. B

17 *Lateral recess.* Lateral outpouching of the fourth ventricle. B

18 *Lateral aperture (Foramen of Luschka).* Opening for the drainage of cerebrospinal fluid at the end of the lateral recess. B

19 *Superior medullary velum.* Layer of white substance stretched between the right and left superior cerebellar peduncles. It is fused with the lingula. B

20 *Frenulum of superior medullary velum.* Bandlike connection between the superior medullary velum and tectal plate. B

21 *Inferior medullary velum.* Layer of white substance in the upper portion of the lower part of the roof of rhomboid fossa that passes from the flocculus peduncle to the nodulus of the cerebellum. B

22 *Median aperture (Foramen of Magendie).* Unpaired opening above the obex for the drainage of cerebrospinal fluid. B

23 *Area postrema.* Triangular field below the trigone of vagus nerve. Its minute structure resembles that of the subfornical organ. A

24 *Obex.* Small bridge at the inferior end of the roof of rhomboid fossa. B

25 **Sulcus limitans.** Lateral groove running lateral to the medial eminence. A

26 **Superior fovea.** Groove running lateral to the facial colliculus. A

27 **Inferior fovea.** Pit at the tip of the trigone of vagus nerve. A

17

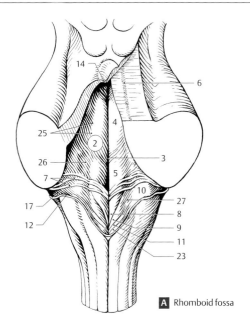

A Rhomboid fossa

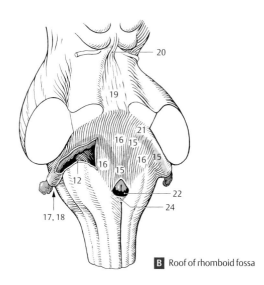

B Roof of rhomboid fossa

1 **MESENCEPHALON; MIDBRAIN.** Portion of the brain situated between the rhombencephalon and prosencephalon. It extends from the superior border of the pons to the anterior boundary of the tectal plate.

2 **EXTERNAL FEATURES.**

3 **Interpeduncular fossa.** Depression between the cerebral crura. B

4 **Posterior perforated substance.** Floor of the interpeduncular fossa with perforations for the passage of vessels. B

5 **Oculomotor sulcus.** Furrow on the medial surface of the cerebral crura where the oculomotor nerve fibers emerge. B

6 **Cerebral peduncle.** Portion of the brain comprising the cerebral crus and the tegmentum, the latter of which extends as far as the cerebral aqueduct. B

7 *Cerebral crus.* Part of the cerebral peduncle resting against the basal part of the tegmentum. It conveys neencephalic tracts to the pons and spinal cord. B

8 *Lateral groove.* Furrow between a cerebral crus and the tegmentum B

9 *Tegmentum of midbrain.* Structural part between the lateral groove of midbrain and a plane through the cerebral aqueduct. B

10 *Trigone of lateral lemniscus.* Triangular field located laterally between the tectal plate, superior cerebellar peduncle, and cerebral crus. A

11 **Superior cerebellar peduncle.** Part conveying fibers mostly from the dentate nucleus to the red nucleus and thalamus. A

12 **Tectal plate; Quadrigeminal plate.** A

13 *Brachium of inferior colliculus.* Connecting arm between the inferior colliculus and medial geniculate body. A

14 *Brachium of superior colliculus.* Connecting arm between the superior colliculus and lateral geniculate body. A

15 *Inferior colliculus.* It is connected to the auditory pathway. A

16 *Superior colliculus.* It is connected to the visual pathway. A

17 **INTERNAL FEATURES.**

18 CEREBRAL PEDUNCLE. See 6

19 **Base of peduncle.** Comparable to the cerebral crus. C

20 **Cerebral crus.** See 7 C

21 **Pyramidal tract.**

22 *Corticospinal fibers.* Nerve fibers traveling in the pyramidal tract into the spinal cord. C

23 *Corticonuclear fibers.* Nerve fibers traveling in the pyramidal tract to the nuclei of cranial nerves. C

24 **Corticopontine fibers.** Nerve fibers traveling to the second-order neurons of the pontine nuclei.

25 *Frontopontine fibers.* Fibers from the frontal lobe lying in the medial part of the cerebral crus. C

26 *Occipitopontine fibers.* Fibers from the occipital lobe.

27 *Parietopontine fibers.* Fibers from the parietal lobe that lie in the lateral part of the cerebral crus. C

28 *Temporopontine fibers.* Fibers from the temporal lobe lying in the lateral part of the cerebral crus. C

29 **Corticoreticular fibers.** Fibers from the cerebrum that pass to nuclei in the reticular formation. See p. 338.16

30 **Substantia nigra.** Black nucleus lying on the cerebral crura. It is characterized by pigmented ganglion cells making it visible to the naked eye. It extends through the entire mesencephalon into the diencephalon. C

31 **Compact part.** Densely pigmented part facing the cerebral peduncle. C

32 **Lateral part.** Part that is present only rostrally at the level of the medial geniculate body and anterior part of the superior colliculus. C

33 **Reticular part.** Part facing the cerebral crura. Its loosely organized cells are scattered irregularly between the fibers of the cerebral crura. C

34 **Retrorubral part.** Part with cells containing iron that extends to the red nucleus.

17

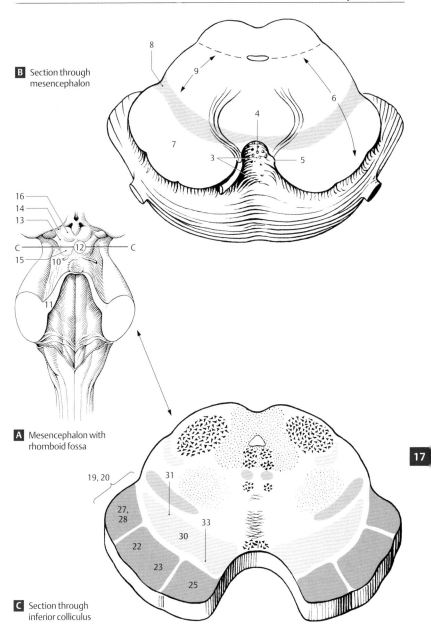

B Section through mesencephalon

A Mesencephalon with rhomboid fossa

C Section through inferior colliculus

17

1 TEGMENTUM OF MIDBRAIN. Continuation of the gray substance of the fourth ventricle that forms the periaqueductal gray substance surrounding the cerebral aqueduct.

2 WHITE SUBSTANCE.

3 **Central tegmental tract.** A B, p. 340.28

4 *Rubro-olivary fibers.* Fibers connecting the red nucleus and inferior olive.

5 *Cerebello-olivary fibers.* Fibers connecting the dentate nucleus and inferior olive.

6 **Mesencephalic corticonuclear fibers.** Fibers passing from the cerebral cortex to the cranial nerve nuclei of the mesencephalon. A

7 **Lateral lemniscus.** Auditory pathway to the inferior colliculus. B

8 **Lateral tectobulbar tract.** Uncrossed fibers from the superior colliculus to nuclei in the reticular formation. A

9 **Medial lemniscus.** A B

10 **Trigeminal lemniscus.** Sensory nerve fibers for innervation of the face. A B

11 **Medial longitudinal fasciculus.** A B

12 **Mesencephalic tract of trigeminal nerve.** Portion of the tract in the mesencephalon. A

13 **Posterior longitudinal fasciculus; Dorsal longitudinal fasciculus.** A

14 **Rubronuclear tract.** See Note.

15 **Rubrospinal tract (Monakow's tract).** Rudimentary structure in humans. A B

16 **Spinal lemniscus; Anterolateral tracts; Anterolateral system.** Mesencephalic part of the lemniscus lying directly adjacent to the medial lemniscus. B, p. 330.16

17 **Superior cerebellar peduncle.**

18 *Decussation of superior cerebellar peduncles.* Crossing of the peduncles below the inferior colliculus and ventral to the medial longitudinal fasciculus. B

19 **Tectobulbar tract.** Nerve fiber tract that passes via the posterior tegmental decussation to the opposite side and then runs anterior to the medial longitudinal fasciculus to the nuclei of the pons and ocular muscles. A

20 **Tectopontine tract.** Nerve fiber tract traveling from the superior colliculus to the pons and lying on the inferolateral part of the inferior colliculus. B

21 **Tectospinal tract.** Nerve fiber tract that initially follows the same course as the tectobulbar tract, but then descends in the anterior funiculus of the spinal cord. A B

22 **Pretecto-olivary fibers.** Fibers connecting a group of nuclei situated anterior to the superior colliculus with the inferior olivary complex. Their existence is not certain in humans.

23 **Tecto-olivary fibers.** Their existence is not certain in humans.

24 **Tegmental decussations.** Crossing of tracts in the mesencephalon.

25 *Posterior tegmental decussation; Dorsal tegmental decussation (Meynert's decussation).* Decussation of the tectospinal and tectobulbar tracts. Fibers from the superior colliculus. A

25 *Anterior tegmental decussation; Ventral tegmental decussation (Decussation of Forel).* Decussation of the rubrospinal tract. Fibers from the magnocellular part of the red nucleus. A

27 **Corticomesencephalic fibers.** Fibers from the cerebral cortex to mesencephalic structures, e.g., substantia nigra, tegmentum, tectum. B

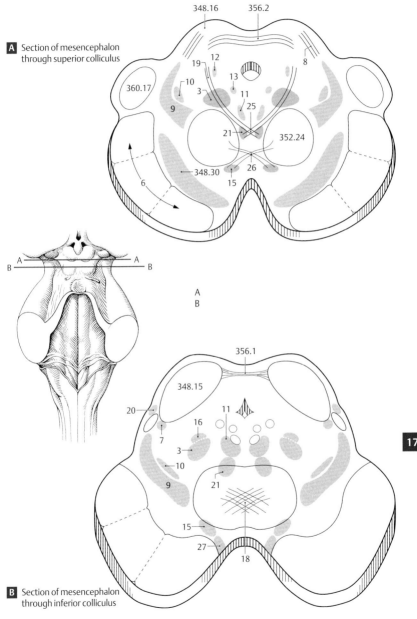

A Section of mesencephalon through superior colliculus

B Section of mesencephalon through inferior colliculus

17

1 GRAY SUBSTANCE.

2 **Nucleus of oculomotor nerve.** Nucleus situated at the level of the superior colliculus anterior to the cerebral aqueduct. A

3 **Accessory nuclei of oculomotor nerve.** Mainly parasympathetic nuclei lying directly medial to the nucleus of the oculomotor nerve. A

4 *Visceral nuclei; Autonomic nuclei.* Parasympathetic nuclei of the oculomotor nerve that supply the ciliary muscle and sphincter pupillae.

5 *Anterior medial nucleus; Ventral medial nucleus.*

6 *Posterior nucleus; Dorsal nucleus.*

7 **Interstitial nucleus (Cajal's interstitial nucleus).** Nucleus situated lateral to the nucleus of oculomotor nerve and separated from it by the medial longitudinal fasciculus. It receives projections from the globus pallidus, vestibular nuclei, and superior colliculus. A

8 **Central precommissural nucleus.** Cell group situated behind the posterior commissure.

9 **Nucleus of posterior commissure (Nucleus of Darkschewitsch).** Cell groups in the posterior commissures.

10 *Ventral subdivision.* Cells lying anteriorly.

11 *Interstitial subdivision.* Dispersed cells.

12 *Dorsal subdivision.* Cells lying posteriorly.

13 **Interpeduncular nucleus.** Cell group overlying the interpeduncular fossa. B

14 **Accessory nuclei of optic tract.** Accessory visual system containing optic fibers that project to three nuclei.

15 *Posterior nucleus; Dorsal nucleus.* Nucleus situated anterior to the rostral portion of the superior colliculus.

16 *Lateral nucleus.* Nucleus situated anteromedial to the medial geniculate body.

17 *Medial nucleus.* Nucleus situated in the mediobasal portion of the mesencephalon, near the substantia nigra.

18 **Lateroposterior tegmental nucleus; Laterodorsal tegmental nucleus.** Group of cells lying anterior to the mesencephalic nucleus of the trigeminal nerve. A

19 **Mesencephalic nucleus of trigeminal nerve.** Sensory nucleus of the trigeminal nerve that extends as far as below the tectal plate. A

20 **Nucleus of trochlear nerve.** Nucleus situated in the periaqueductal gray substance above the medial longitudinal fasciculus. B

21 **Parabigeminal nucleus.** Scattered cells lying lateral to the lateral lemniscus at the level of the inferior colliculus.

22 **Periaqueductal gray substance; Central gray substance.** Gray substance surrounding the cerebral aqueduct. B, p. 331 B

23 **Peripeduncular nucleus.** Cell group lying lateral to the substantia nigra. A

24 **Red nucleus.** Principal nucleus of the central tegmental tract. The iron-containing nucleus is situated between the periaqueductal gray substance and substantia nigra, extending from the superior colliculus into the diencephalon. It is composed of two or possibly more components. A

25 *Magnocellular part.* Portion containing large cells. It is rudimentary in humans.

26 *Parvocellular part.* Small-cell portion that constitutes the chief component of the nucleus.

27 *Posteromedial part; Dorsomedial part.* Part that is sometimes considered a separate nucleus. In terms of cellular composition, it belongs to the parvocellular part.

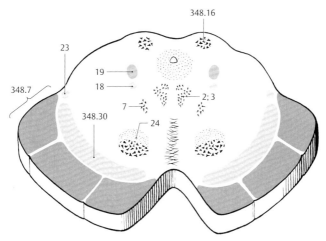

A Section of mesencephalon through superior colliculus

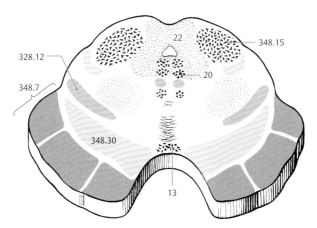

B Section of mesencephalon through inferior colliculus

1 **Sagulum nucleus.** Nucleus situated at the level of the inferior colliculus lateral to the lateral lemniscus. A

2 **Subbrachial nucleus.** Cell group situated at the level of the nucleus of oculomotor nerve lateral to the medial lemniscus.

3 **Anterior tegmental nuclei; Ventral tegmental nuclei.** Collective term for the following three nuclei.

4 *Interfascicular nucleus.* Small group of cells situated in the medial longitudinal fasciculus at the level of the nucleus of trochlear nerve.

5 *Parabrachial pigmented nucleus.* Nucleus situated between the superior cerebellar peduncle and paranigral nucleus. A

6 *Paranigral nucleus.* Nucleus situated posterolateral to the interpeduncular nucleus. A

7 **Reticular nuclei.** Nuclei of the reticular formation.

8 **Cuneiform nucleus.** Cell group lying inferolateral to the superior colliculus. A

9 **Subcuneiform nucleus.** Cell group located anterior to the cuneiform nucleus. A

10 **Pedunculopontine tegmental nucleus.** Two nuclei situated between the medial lemniscus, medial longitudinal fasciculus, and superior cerebellar peduncle.

11 *Compact part; Compact subnucleus.* Portion of the nucleus containing numerous cells situated lateral to the medial longitudinal fasciculus. A

12 *Dissipated part; Dissipated subnucleus.* Portion of the nucleus with sparse cells situated medial to the medial lemniscus. A

13 **Parapeduncular nucleus.** Small group of cells above the interpeduncular fossa anterior to the substantia nigra. A

14 **Raphe nuclei of mesencephalon.**

15 **Posterior raphe nucleus; Dorsal raphe nucleus.** Nucleus extending from the rostral part of the rhomboid fossa to the superior colliculus. p. 345 B

16 [[**Linear nucleus**]]. Dorsoventral medial nuclear column situated near the decussation of superior cerebellar peduncles.

17 **Inferior linear nucleus.** Lower portion of the nuclear column. A

18 **Intermediate linear nucleus.** Middle portion of the nuclear column. A

19 **Superior linear nucleus.** Upper portion of the nuclear column. A

20 **Aqueduct of midbrain; Cerebral aqueduct (Aqueduct of Sylvius).** Narrow canal in the mesencephalon between the third and fourth ventricles. C

21 **Opening of aqueduct of midbrain; Opening of cerebral aqueduct.** Funnel-shaped opening of the cerebral aqueduct into the third ventricle below the posterior commissure of the diencephalon. C

22 **Tectum of midbrain.** Part of the mesencephalon lying on the tegmentum of midbrain. C

23 **Tectal plate; Quadrigeminal plate.** C

24 **Inferior colliculus.** Its cytoarchitectural composition varies. B

25 **Nuclei of inferior colliculus.** Nuclei that serve as relay nuclei and as an integration center for acoustic reflexes.

26 *Central nucleus.* Synaptic site in the auditory pathway formed by the lateral lemniscus. A

27 *External nucleus.* Nucleus presumably involved in the acoustic reflex center. A

28 *Pericentral nucleus.* Nucleus receiving afferents from the auditory cortex. A

29 **Superior colliculus.** Layered structure that functions as an integration site for reflexive saccades and pupillary reflexes. B

30 *Zonal layer; Layer I.* Most superficial layer composed mainly of glial fibers.

31 *Superficial gray layer; Layer II.* Layer containing abundant glial fibers.

32 *Optic layer; Layer III.* Layer containing sparse spindle-shaped and triangular neurons.

33 *Intermediate gray layer; Layer IV.* Layer resembling layer III, but with abundant cells.

34 *Intermediate white layer; Layer V.* Layer resembling layer IV, but with larger cells.

35 *Deep gray layer; Layer VI.* Layer characterized by scattered, plump, multipolar neurons with marked levels of Nissl's substance.

36 *Deep white layer; Layer VII.* Layer containing abundant cells composed of multiform small and medium-sized cells.

17

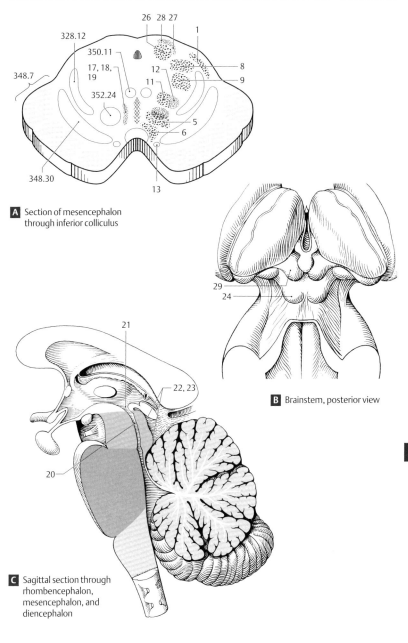

A Section of mesencephalon through inferior colliculus

B Brainstem, posterior view

C Sagittal section through rhombencephalon, mesencephalon, and diencephalon

1 **Commissure of inferior colliculus.** Fiber tract connecting the two inferior colliculi. It also carries nerve fibers from the lateral lemniscus to the opposite side. p. 351 B

2 **Commissure of superior colliculus.** Fiber tract connecting the two superior colliculi. p. 351 A

3 **Decussation of trochlear nerve fibers.** Crossing of the trochlear nerve fibers in the white substance.

4 **CEREBELLUM.** Part of the brain situated above the rhomboid fossa.

5 **EXTERNAL FEATURES.**

6 BODY OF CEREBELLUM. Entire cerebellum excluding the flocculonodular lobe.

7 **Anterior lobe of cerebellum.** Portion located anterior to the primary fissure. B D

8 **Lingula (I).** Unpaired part of the vermis belonging to the archicerebellum that is fused with the superior medullary velum. C D

9 **Precentral fissure; Post-lingual fissure.** Furrow between the lingula and central lobule. A

10 **Central lobule (II and III).** Lobule that is continuous with the wing of the central lobule. It consists of an anterior and a posterior part. A C D

11 *Anterior part*; *Ventral part (II)*. A

12 *Posterior part*; *Dorsal part (III)*. A

13 **Wing of central lobule.** Lateral projection of the central lobule connecting it to the cerebellar hemispheres. B C D

14 *Inferior part*; *Ventral part (H II)*.

15 *Superior part*; *Dorsal part (H III)*.

16 **Preculminate fissure; Post-central fissure.** Cleft in front of the culmen. A D

17 **Culmen (IV and V).** Summit of the vermis of cerebellum. A B C D

18 *Anterior part*; *Ventral part (IV)*. A

19 **Intraculminate fissure.** Cleft dividing the culmen. A

20 *Posterior part*; *Dorsal part (V)*. Posterior part of the culmen. A

21 **Anterior quadrangular lobule (H IV and H V).** Part that is continuous laterally with the declive. C D

22 *Anterior part*; *Ventral part (H IV)*. B

23 *Posterior part*; *Dorsal part (H V)*.

24 **Primary fissure; Preclival fissure.** Depression between the anterior quadrangular and simple lobules. A B D

25 **Posterior lobe of cerebellum.** Structural part of the cerebellum situated between the primary and posterolateral fissures.

26 **Simple lobule (H VI and VI).** Part of the cerebellum situated between the anterior quadrangular lobule and superior semilunar lobule. It contains a portion of the vermis. B C D

27 *Declive (VI)*. Part of the vermis sloping downward and posteriorly from the culmen. A B D

28 *Posterior quadrangular lobule (H VI)*. Lobular part of the simple lobule. B D

29 **Posterior superior fissure; Post-clival fissure.** Depression posterior to the declive. A D

30 **Folium of vermis (VII A).** Narrow, leaflike structure connecting the left and right superior semilunar lobules. B D

31 **Semilunar lobules; Ansiform lobule (H VII A).** Lobules situated anterior and posterior to the horizontal fissure.

32 *Superior semilunar lobule*; *First crus of ansiform lobule (H VII A)*. Lobule situated anterior to the horizontal fissure. B C D

33 **Horizontal fissure; Intercrural fissure.** Deep cleft between the superior and inferior semilunar lobules. A B C D

34 *Inferior semilunar lobule*; *Second crus of ansiform lobule (H VII A)*. Lobule situated posterior to the horizontal fissure. B C D

35 **Lunogracile fissure; Ansoparamedian fissure.** Cleft posterior to H VII A. D

36 **Tuber (VII B).** Median connection between the right and left inferior semilunar lobules. A B C D

37 **Gracile lobule; Paramedian lobule (H VII B).** Lobule situated anterior to the prebiventral fissure. D

38 **Prebiventral fissure; Prepyramidal fissure.** Cleft between the tuber and pyramis. A D

39 **Pyramis (VIII).** Lobule situated posterior to the prepyramidal fissure. C D

40 **Biventral lobule (H VIII).** Lobule situated between the gracile lobule and tonsil of cerebellum. C

41 *Lateral part*; *Pars copularis (H VIII A)*. Anterior part of the lobule. A D

42 **Intrabiventral fissure; Anterior inferior fissure.** Cleft subdividing the lobule laterally. A D

43 *Medial part*; *Dorsal parafloccularis (H VIII B)*. Posterior part of the lobule. A D

44 **Secondary fissure; Post-pyramidal fissure.** Cleft between the biventral lobule and pyramis as well as the tonsil and uvula. A C D

45 **Uvula (IX).** Part of the vermis situated between the tonsils of cerebellum. A C D

46 **Tonsil of cerebellum; Ventral paraflocculus (H IX).** Small, bean-shaped part of the cerebellar hemisphere. C D

47 **Posterolateral fissure.** Furrow above the nodule and flocculus. A C D

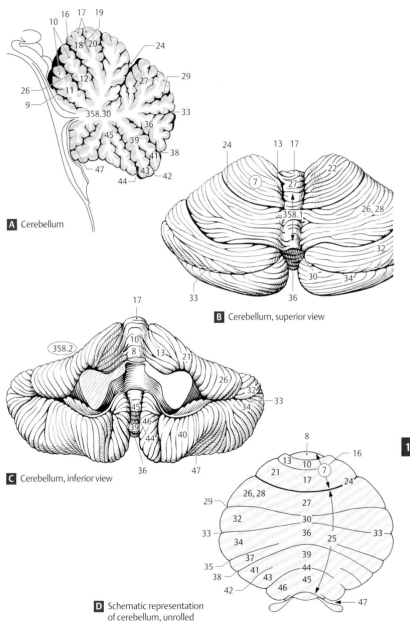

A Cerebellum

B Cerebellum, superior view

C Cerebellum, inferior view

D Schematic representation of cerebellum, unrolled

17

1 **Vermis of cerebellum (I–X).** Middle portion of the embryonic cerebellar plate. p. 357 B

2 **Hemisphere of cerebellum (H II–H X).** p. 357 C

3 **Flocculonodular lobe.** Lobe situated caudal to the posterolateral fissure.

4 **Nodule (X).** Medial protuberance of the vermis. It is connected with the flocculus via the peduncles of flocculus. D

5 **Peduncle of flocculus.** Connecting stalk, part of which is continuous with the inferior medullary velum. D

6 **Flocculus (H X).** Paw-shaped part of the cerebellum located between the inferior cerebellar peduncle and biventral lobule. D

7 **Vestibulocerebellum.** Portion of the cerebellum that is considered part of the vestibular nuclei.

8 **Spinocerebellum.** Portion of the cerebellum receiving projections directly from the spinal cord.

9 **Pontocerebellum.** Part of the cerebellum receiving projections directly from the nuclei of the basilar part of the pons.

10 **Archicerebellum.** Phylogenetically oldest part of the cerebellum comprising the lingula and flocculonodular lobe. A

11 **Paleocerebellum.** Older part of the cerebellum comprising the central lobule, culmen, pyramis, uvula, wing of the central lobule, and anterior quadrangular lobule. A

12 **Neocerebellum.** Most recent part of the cerebellum in terms of evolution. It comprises the declive, folium of the tuber vermis, simple lobule, inferior semilunar lobule, gracile lobule, and tonsil. A

13 **INTERNAL FEATURES.**

14 **Arbor vitae.** "Tree of life." Branchlike appearance of cerebellar white substance in cross-section. C

15 **Cerebellar cortex.** It is about 1 mm thick and consists mainly of nerve cells. B C

16 **Granular layer.** Granular layer at the border to the white substance that is characterized by densely arranged, multipolar neurons with little plasma. B

17 **Purkinje cell layer.** B

18 **Molecular layer.** Cortical layer that contains fewer nerve cells and is rich in dendrites and axons. B

19 **Cerebellar nuclei.**

20 **Dentate nucleus; Nucleus lateralis cerebelli.** Largest cerebellar nucleus. It resembles a folded pouch and is situated in the white substance of cerebellum. C

21 *Hilum of dentate nucleus.* Opening of the dentate nucleus that gives exit to the majority of fibers forming the superior cerebellar peduncle. C

22 **Anterior interpositus nucleus; Emboliform nucleus.** Cerebellar nucleus situated directly in front of the hilum of the dentate nucleus. C

23 **Posterior interpositus nucleus; Globose nucleus.** Collection of cells lying medial to the dentate nucleus. C

24 **Fastigial nucleus; Nucleus medialis cerebelli.** Medially situated nucleus. C

25 **Cerebellar peduncles.** Part of the cerebellum containing nerve fibers passing to and from the cerebellum.

26 **Inferior cerebellar peduncle.** Portion containing the restiform body. D E

27 **Middle cerebellar peduncle.** Portion not clearly distinguishable from the superior cerebellar peduncle. D E

28 **Superior cerebellar peduncle.** Portion not clearly distinguishable from the middle cerebellar peduncle. D E

29 **White substance of cerebellum.** C

30 **Cerebellar commissure.** Fiber bundle connecting right and left cerebellar hemispheres. C

31 **Uncinate fasciculus of cerebellum.** Efferent fibers originating in the fastigium nucleus and passing to the vestibular nuclei, nuclei of the reticular formations of the pons and medulla oblongata, and ascending to the diencephalon. Their existence is not certain in humans.

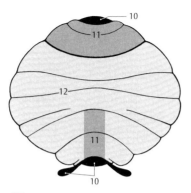

A Schematic representation of cerebellum, unrolled

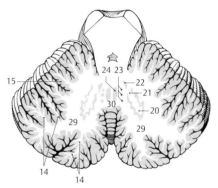

C Transverse section through cerebellum

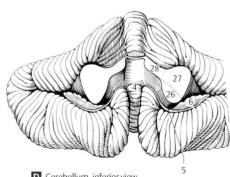

D Cerebellum, inferior view

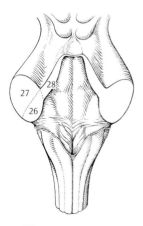

E Cerebellar peduncles

B Layers of cerebellar cortex

17

1 **DIENCEPHALON.** Portion of the brain extending from the interventricular foramen to an imaginary boundary at the anterior border of the superior colliculus. It surrounds most of the third ventricle.

2 **EXTERNAL FEATURES.**

3 EPITHALAMUS. Part comprising the habenulae and pineal gland in the dorsal part of the diencephalon.

4 **Habenula.** Synaptic site between the pineal gland, brainstem, and olfactory centers. A B

5 *Habenular sulcus.* Shallow groove between the habenular trigone and pulvinar. A

6 *Habenular trigone.* Widening of the habenula at its junction with the thalamus. Location of the two nuclei. A B

7 **Pineal gland.** A B C

8 THALAMUS; DORSAL THALAMUS. Part extending from the interventricular foramen to the tectal plate. Medially it borders on the third ventricle, laterally on the internal capsule and basal ganglia. It is formed by a collection of nuclei derived during ontogenetic development from the dorsal thalamus.

9 **Anterior thalamic tubercle.** Small protuberance on the anterior end of the thalamus. Attachment site of the stria medullaris of the thalamus. A

10 **Interthalamic adhesion; Massa intermedia.** Inconstant fusion (70–85%) of the right and left parts of the thalamus. B

11 **Pulvinar.** Posterior, freely projecting portion of the thalamus. A

12 **Tenia thalami.** Upper margin of the stria medullaris of thalamus. Attachment site of the choroid plexus of third ventricle. A

13 **Stria medullaris of thalamus.** Bundle of white fibers running from the anterior thalamic tubercle to the habenula between the dorsal and medial surfaces of the thalamus. B

14 SUBTHALAMUS; VENTRAL THALAMUS. Part arising during ontogenetic development from portions of the tegmentum, basal ganglia, and hypothalamus that is considered part of the extrapyramidal motor system. It lies basal to the hypothalamic sulcus.

15 METATHALAMUS. Geniculate bodies formed by the thalamus. They lie inferolateral to the pulvinar. A C

16 **Lateral geniculate body.** Part of the visual pathway that is connected with the superior colliculus and visual cortex. A C

17 **Medial geniculate body.** Part of the auditory pathway that is connected with the inferior colliculus. A C

18 HYPOTHALAMUS. Basal portion and floor of the diencephalon. B

19 **Mammillary body.** Paired, rounded elevations on the floor of the diencephalon that are connected with the thalamus and mesencephalon. B

20 **Neurohypophysis.** Posterior lobe of pituitary gland formed by an eversion of the floor of the diencephalon. B

21 *Infundibulum.* Pituitary stalk. B

22 *Pars nervosa.* Bundle of unmyelinated fibers forming the neurohypophysis.

23 **Optic chiasm; Optic chiasma.** Decussation of medial optic nerve fibers between the optic tract and optic nerve. B C

24 **Optic tract.** Portion of the visual pathway between the optic chiasm and lateral geniculate body that is visible on the surface of the basal part of the brain. C

25 *Lateral root.* Its fibers pass to the lateral geniculate body. C

26 *Medial root.* Its fibers pass beneath the lateral geniculate body to the superior colliculus. C

27 **Preoptic area.** Area posterior to the lamina terminalis. B

28 **Tuber cinereum.** Condensation of gray substance in the posterior wall of the infundibulum. B

29 *Median eminence.* Median elevation in the tuber cinereum. B

17

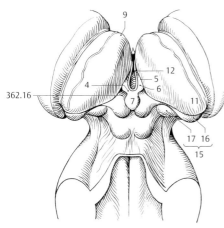

A Brainstem, posterior view

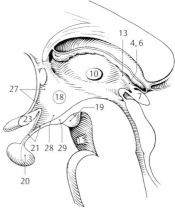

B Brainstem, sagittal section

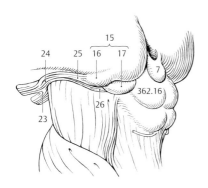

C End of optic tract

1 **Third ventricle.** Diencephalic part of the cerebral ventricular system. It extends from the lamina terminalis to the cerebral aqueduct. A

2 **Interventricular foramen.** Opening between the lateral and third ventricles behind the genu of the fornix. A

3 **Subfornical organ.** Organ in the roof of the third ventricle near the interventricular foramen. A

4 **Suprapineal recess.** Indentation between the roof of the third ventricle and epiphysis. A

5 **Habenular commissure.** Fibers from the habenula that pass over the middle line, crossing cranial to the pineal recess. A

6 **Pineal recess.** Outpocketing of the third ventricle that extends partly into the epiphysis. A

7 **Posterior commissure.** Commissure situated between the pineal recess and the opening of cerebral aqueduct. Crossing site of fibers from the surrounding area. A

8 **Infundibular recess.** Recess of the third ventricle that leads into the infundibulum. A

9 **Supra-optic recess.** Recess of the third ventricle above the optic chiasm. A, p. 365 D

10 **Hypothalamic sulcus.** Furrow extending from the interventricular foramen to the entrance to the cerebral aqueduct. It divides the dorsal and ventral portions of the thalamus. A

11 **INTERNAL FEATURES.**

12 EPITHALAMUS.

13 **Habenulo-interpeduncular tract; Fasciculus retroflexus.** Nerve tract connecting the habenulae and interpeduncular nucleus.

14 **Lateral habenular nucleus.** Lateral nucleus lying in the habenular trigone.

15 **Medial habenular nucleus.** Medial nucleus lying in the habenular trigone.

16 **Pretectal area.** Area extending from in front of the upper border of the superior colliculus to the posterior commissure. Synaptic site for ocular motility and control of visual reflexes. p. 361 A C

17 **Pretectal nuclei.** Subdivisions of nuclei in the pretectal area. They have not yet been identified in humans.

18 **Subcommissural organ.** Area of ependymal cells lying anterior to the tectum of midbrain at the beginning of the cerebral aqueduct. A

19 THALAMUS. Ovoid collection of nuclei in the lateral wall of the third ventricle. It borders laterally on the basal ganglia and internal capsule. Target region of most sensory tracts. It has connections to the cerebral cortex, cerebellum, globus pallidus, striatum, and hypothalamus. B C D

20 **Gray substance of thalamus.**

21 **Anterior nuclei of thalamus.** Three nuclei lying in the sagittal plane in the tip of the thalamus between the internal and external medullary laminae. They receive afferents mainly from the mammillary body and have connections to the cingulate gyrus and limbic system. B

22 *Anterodorsal nucleus.* Narrow anterosuperior sheet of nuclei. C

23 *Anteromedial nucleus.* Small cell group lying below the anteroventral nucleus. C, p. 365 B

24 *Anteroventral nucleus.* Largest and furthest dorsal of the anterior nuclei of thalamus. C, p. 365 B

25 **Dorsal nuclei of thalamus.** Nuclei lying directly adjacent to the anterior nuclei, likewise between the two medullary laminae. They receive afferent projections from the superior colliculus and pretectal area and have reciprocal connections with the parietal, occipital, and temporal cortex. B

26 *Lateral dorsal nucleus.* Nucleus situated anterosuperiorly and directly adjacent to the anterior nuclei. B, p. 365 C D

27 *Lateral posterior nucleus.* Nucleus lying between the lateral dorsal nucleus and pulvinar. B C

28 *Pulvinar nuclei.* Freely-projecting posterior part of the thalamus. B

29 *Anterior pulvinar nucleus.* Group of nuclei that is difficult to distinguish and has largely unknown connections. D

30 *Inferior pulvinar nucleus.* Nucleus located furthest basally that extends rostrally beneath the ventrobasal nuclear complex of thalamus and medially as far as the intralaminar nuclei. Synaptic station for visual pathways. D

31 *Lateral pulvinar nucleus.* Nucleus situated medial to the external medullary lamina and above the lateral geniculate body. Synaptic station for visual pathways. D

32 *Medial pulvinar nucleus.* Nucleus lying caudal and directly adjacent to the medial nuclei of thalamus. It has connections to the prefrontal, parietal, and cingulate cortices and receives afferent projections from the superior colliculus. D

17

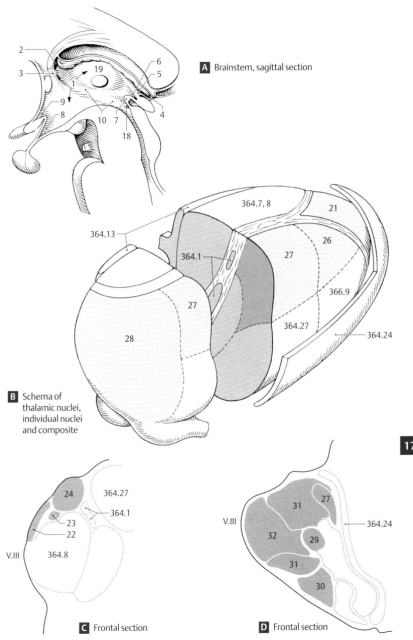

A Brainstem, sagittal section

364.7, 8
364.13
364.1
366.9
364.27
364.24

B Schema of thalamic nuclei, individual nuclei and composite

17

V.III
364.27
364.1
V.III
364.24

C Frontal section

D Frontal section

1 **Intralaminar nuclei of thalamus.** Two consecutive groups of nuclei situated in the internal medullary lamina, extending from the anterior pole of the thalamus to the posterior commissure. They send projections to the cortex and striatum. A B C D

2 *Central medial nucleus.* Nucleus lying in the lower medial end of the internal medullary lamina. It sends projections mainly to the orbitofrontal and prefrontal cortex. A

3 *Central lateral nucleus.* Nucleus lying mostly dorsal to the centromedian nucleus. It sends projections mainly to the parietal and temporal cortex. A

4 *Paracentral nucleus.* Nucleus lying lateral to the centromedian cortex. It sends projections mainly to occipital and prefrontal regions. A

5 *Centromedian nucleus.* Largest of the intralaminar nuclei. It sends projections mainly to motor regions and the striatum. A B C

6 *Parafascicular nucleus.* Nucleus lying medial to the centromedian nucleus. It sends projections to motor regions and the striatum. C

7 **Medial nuclei of thalamus.** Group of nuclei consisting mainly of the dorsomedial nucleus. It receives afferents from other thalamic regions and subcortical structures as well as the amygdaloid body, basal ganglia, and reticular formation of the mesencephalon. A

8 *Medial dorsal nucleus; Dorsomedial nucleus.* Nucleus that is especially large in humans. It is bounded laterally, ventrally, and rostrally by the internal medullary lamina and medially by the median nuclei. It sends projections mainly to the prefrontal cortex. It can be subdivided according to cytoarchitecture and enzyme histochemical composition. A C D

9 *Lateral nucleus; Parvocellular nucleus.* Lateral portion consisting of small cells.

10 *Medial nucleus; Magnocellular nucleus.* Medial portion consisting of large cells.

11 *Paralaminar part; Pars laminaris.* Multiform ventral portion.

12 *Medial ventral nucleus.* Cell group situated anterior to the central medial nucleus that has a high level of acetylcholinesterase activity.

13 **Median nuclei of thalamus.** Perinuclear collection of nuclei lying beneath the ventricular ependyma. It extends from the interventricular foramen to the posterior commissure. A

14 *Paratenial nucleus.* Nucleus lying below the anterodorsal nucleus and above the paraventricular nucleus. B

15 *Paraventricular nuclei of thalamus.* Group lying below the paratenial nucleus, and in front of, above, and behind the interthalamic adhesion. B

16 *Anterior paraventricular nucleus.* Group of nuclei lying anterior to the interthalamic adhesion.

17 *Posterior paraventricular nucleus.* Group of nuclei lying posterior to the interthalamic adhesion.

18 *Nucleus reuniens.* Nucleus lying ventral to the interthalamic adhesion.

19 *Rhomboid nucleus.* Nucleus lying beneath the ependyma of the third ventricle. Its counterparts can partly form the interthalamic adhesion.

20 **Posterior nuclear complex of thalamus.** Nuclear complex lying beneath the dorsomedial nucleus and anterior pulvinar nucleus as well as dorsal to the dorsal nucleus of medial geniculate body. A

21 *Nucleus limitans.* Anteromedial nucleus. D

22 *Posterior nucleus.* Nucleus situated beneath the anterior pulvinar nucleus. D

23 *Suprageniculate nucleus.* Nucleus situated anteroinferior to the posterior nucleus. D

24 **Reticular nucleus of thalamus.** Loosely organized layer of cells. "Reticular" layer on the lateral surface of the thalamus between the external medullary layer and internal capsule. A B C D

25 **Ventral nuclei of thalamus.** Nuclei occupying the caudal half of the diencephalon above the zona incerta and medial to the reticular nucleus.

26 *Ventrobasal complex.* Collective term for the following two nuclei.

27 *Ventral posterolateral nucleus.* Lateral portion of the nucleus that receives the medial lemniscus and spinothalamic tract and sends projections to the postcentral gyrus. A C D

28 *Ventral posteromedial nucleus.* Nucleus lying between the ventral posterolateral nucleus and the centromedian nucleus. It receives fibers from the trigeminal lemniscus. A C

29 Parvocellular part. Portion of the nucleus containing small cells.

17

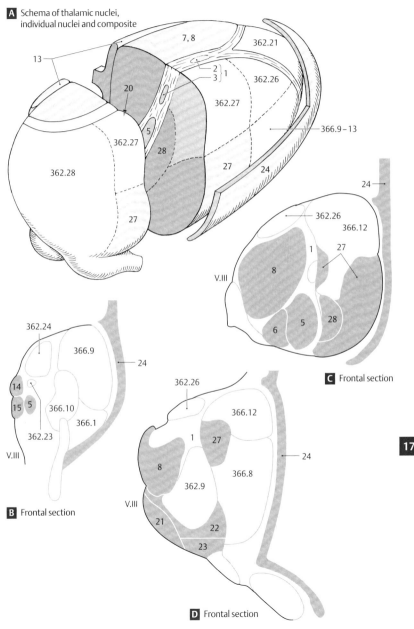

A Schema of thalamic nuclei, individual nuclei and composite

B Frontal section

C Frontal section

D Frontal section

1   *Ventral medial complex.* Nuclear complex lying beneath the ventral lateral complex. p. 365 B

2   *Basal ventral medial nucleus.* Inferior portion of the complex that receives taste fibers.

3   *Principal ventral medial nucleus.* Main portion of the nucleus.

4   *Submedial nucleus.* Rostral portion of the nuclear complex.

5   *Ventral posterior inferior nucleus.* Subnucleus of the ventral group. It has connections to the vestibular nuclei.

6   *Ventral lateral complex.* Ventrolateral nuclear complex situated between the reticular nucleus of thalamus and the dorsomedial nucleus. A

7   *Anterior ventrolateral nucleus.* Anterior and lateral portion of the nucleus. It receives afferent fibers from the globus pallidus and sends projections to the premotor cortex. B

8   *Posterior ventrolateral nucleus.* Posterior and medial portion of the nucleus. It receives afferents from the cerebellum and has reciprocal connections with the motor cortex. B p. 365 D

9   *Ventral anterior nucleus.* Anterior nuclear complex. A p. 365 B

10 *Magnocellular division.* Portion containing large cells.

11 *Principal division.* Main part of the nucleus.

12 *Ventral intermediate nucleus.* Part of the ventral lateral complex. p. 365 C D

13 *Ventral posterior internal nucleus.* Subnucleus of the ventral nuclei of thalamus.

14 *Ventral posterior parvocellular nucleus.* Collection of cells that in humans is located in the ventrobasal complex.

15 **White substance of thalamus.**

16 **External medullary lamina.** Layers of white substance between the reticular nucleus of thalamus and the ventral lateral complex. B

17 **Internal medullary lamina.** Layers of white substance surrounding the anterior nuclei in a Y-shape, separating the medial and lateral portions. B

18 **Acoustic radiation.** Part of the auditory pathway passing from the medial geniculate body to the transverse temporal gyri. It runs through the occipital part of the posterior limb of internal capsule. A

19 **Lateral lemniscus.** Auditory pathway passing into the medial geniculate body. A

20 **Medial lemniscus.** Continuation of fibers of the posterior funiculus from the spinal cord and brainstem to the ventroposterolateral nucleus. A

21 **Spinal lemniscus.** Sensory fibers (mainly pain fibers) passing from the trunk and limbs to the ventroposterolateral nucleus. A

22 **Trigeminal lemniscus.** Fibers passing from the sensory nuclei of trigeminal nerve to the ventroposteromedial nucleus. A

23 **Optic radiation (Gratiolet's radiation).** Portion of the visual pathway leaving the lateral geniculate body. It passes through the occipital portion of the posterior limb of internal capsule around the posterior horn of the lateral ventricle to the visual cortex. A

24 **Intrathalamic fibers.** Fibers connecting individual thalamic nuclei.

25 **Periventricular fibers.** Fibers running beneath the ependyma of the third ventricle between the median nuclei and hypothalamus and then into the posterior longitudinal fasciculus.

26 **Anterior thalamic radiation of thalamus.** Anterior radiation with fibers running through the anterior limb of internal capsule to the frontal lobe. C

27 **Central thalamic radiation.** Central radiation with fibers running through the posterior limb of internal capsule to the precentral and postcentral gyri as well as adjacent cortical regions. C

28 **Posterior thalamic radiation.** Posterior radiation with fibers passing through the occipital region of the posterior limb of internal capsule to the occipital lobe. C

29 **Inferior thalamic radiation.** Inferior radiation with fibers passing through the posterior limb of internal capsule to the temporal lobe and insula. C

17

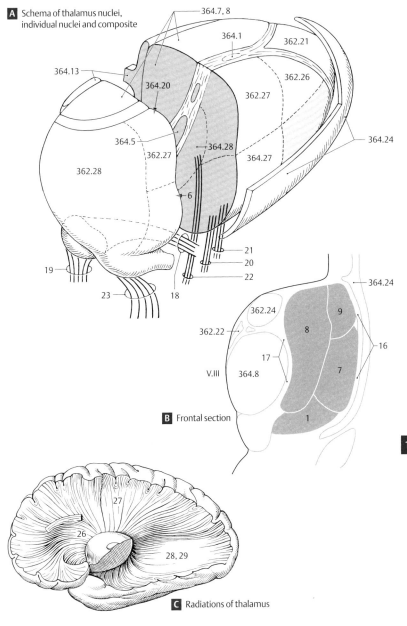

A Schema of thalamus nuclei, individual nuclei and composite

364.7, 8
364.1
362.21
364.13
364.20
362.26
362.27
362.27
364.5
364.28
364.27
364.24
362.28
362.27
364.27
6
21
20
22
19
18
23

B Frontal section

364.24
362.24
9
8
362.22
16
17
7
V.III
364.8
1

17

27
26
28, 29

C Radiations of thalamus

1 **Ansa lenticularis.** Fiber bundle passing from the lentiform nucleus around the anterior margin of the internal capsule to the ventral nuclei of thalamus. A

2 **Lenticular fasciculus.** Fiber bundle passing from the lentiform nucleus through the internal capsule, forming field H2 of Forel, and continuing to the ventral nuclei of thalamus. A

3 **Thalamic fasciculus.** Fasciculus formed by the ansa lenticularis and lenticular fasciculus which forms field H1 of Forel and enters the thalamus. A

4 **Ansa peduncularis.** Fibers from the thalamus and claustrum between the lentiform nucleus and amygdaloid body. A

5 **Subthalamic fasciculus.** Bundle of fibers passing from the globus pallidus to the subthalamic nucleus. A

6 **Brachium of inferior colliculus.** Externally visible connection between the inferior colliculus and medial geniculate body. B

7 **Brachium of superior colliculus.** Externally visible connection between the superior colliculus and lateral geniculate body. Connecting site of the visual pathway and extrapyramidal system. B

8 SUBTHALAMUS. It lies basal to the hypothalamic sulcus and lateral to the hypothalamus. Synaptic station of the extrapyramidal motor system.

9 **Subthalamic nucleus (Nucleus of Luys).** Nucleus lying between the inferior end of the internal capsule and the zona incerta. It has reciprocal connections with the globus pallidus. C

10 **Nuclei of perizonal fields (Nuclei of fields of Forel) (H, H1, H2).** Fibers with interposing nerve cells in the corresponding fields of Forel. C

11 *Nucleus of medial field (H).* Field of Forel situated medial to the zona incerta and anterior to the red nucleus. C

12 *Nucleus of dorsal field (H1).* Field situated between the thalamus and zona incerta. C

13 *Nucleus of ventral field (H2).* Field situated between the zona incerta and subthalamic nucleus. C

14 **Zona incerta.** Fiber bundle interspersed with nerve cells that runs caudal and medial to the reticular nucleus of thalamus. It is presumably a synaptic station in the extrapyramidal motor system. C

15 METATHALAMUS. Nuclear complex attached to the thalamus beneath the pulvinar.

16 **Dorsal lateral geniculate nucleus.** Dorsal nucleus of the lateral geniculate body. It lies on top of the optic tract, from which it receives crossed and uncrossed optic nerve fibers. It is composed of six layers. B

17 *Koniocellular layer.* Wedge-shaped area present in all layers that receives fibers from the macula. D

18 *Magnocellular layers.* Laminae 1 and 2 containing large cells. D

19 *Parvocellular layers.* Laminae 3 through 6 containing small cells. D

20 **Ventral lateral geniculate nucleus; Pregeniculate nucleus.** It lies rostral, dorsal, and medial to the dorsal nucleus. Its function is not well understood. D

21 **Intergeniculate leaf.** Dividing layer between the two geniculate bodies. It contains material from the reticular nucleus of thalamus and pulvinar. B

22 **Medial geniculate nuclei.** Nuclear complex situated directly adjacent to the pulvinar and dorsomedial to the dorsal lateral geniculate nucleus. Synaptic station for all fibers of the auditory pathway and auditory cortex. B

23 *Ventral principal nucleus.* Nucleus composed of small cells. It receives subcortical afferents from the inferior colliculus through the brachium of inferior colliculus. It sends projections to the posterior portion of the auditory cortex.

24 *Dorsal nucleus.* Nucleus that is comparable to the ventral principal nucleus, sending projections to the anterior portion of the auditory cortex.

25 *Medial magnocellular nucleus.* Part consisting of large cells that receives subcortical afferents conveying epicritic and protopathic sensibility as well as fibers from the superior and inferior colliculi. Cortical afferents come from the postcentral gyrus and parietal cortex. It sends projections to the temporal cortex.

17

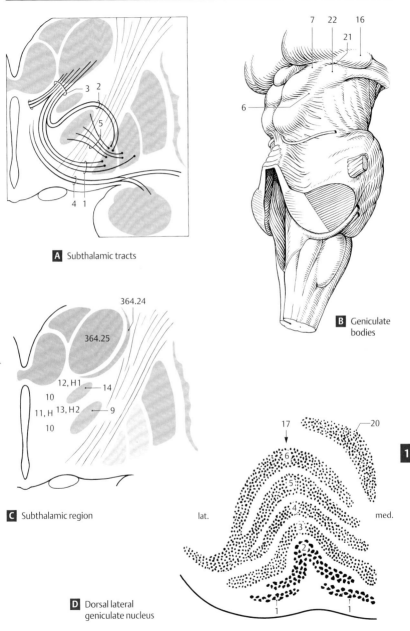

A Subthalamic tracts

B Geniculate bodies

C Subthalamic region

364.24

364.25

12, H1 — 14

10

11, H   13, H2 — 9

10

D Dorsal lateral geniculate nucleus

17

20

lat.   med.

1   HYPOTHALAMUS. Basal portion of the diencephalon. It consists of the floor and, from the hypothalamic sulcus onward, the basal portions of the walls of the third ventricle. It extends from the lamina terminalis to just posterior to the mammillary body and is visible on the base of the brain. It is composed of individual areas that can be distinguished histologically to a greater or lesser extent. It functions as an autonomous control center sending hormonal and nerve efferents.

2   **Anterior hypothalamic area; Anterior hypothalamic region.**

3   *Anterior hypothalamic nucleus.* Nucleus lying posterior to the medial preoptic nucleus. It functions as a relay site between regions of the cerebral cortex, mesencephalon, and nuclei of hypothalamus. A

4   *Anterior periventricular nucleus.* Nuclei situated in the anterior region of the periventricular zone.

5   *Interstitial nuclei of anterior hypothalamus.* Small, scattered groups of cells.

6   *Lateral preoptic nucleus.* Cell group lying near the lateral zone of the hypothalamus. A

7   *Medial preoptic nucleus.* Nucleus lying on the lamina terminalis below the anterior commissure. It has reciprocal connections with the amygdala, septum, and hypothalamic nuclei. A C

8   *Median preoptic nucleus.* Nucleus lying medial to the medial preoptic nucleus that has connections to the subfornical organ and lamina terminalis. C

9   *Periventricular preoptic nucleus.* Rostral continuation of the periventricular zone. C

10   *Paraventricular nucleus.* Patch of cells lying medial to the anterior hypothalamic nucleus at the level of the column of fornix. Its neurosecretory material (e.g., vasopressin, oxytocin) is transported to the posterior lobe of pituitary gland, and its neuropeptidergic cells connect to those of the supra-optic nucleus. A C

11   *Suprachiasmatic nucleus.* Nucleus lying in the periventricular zone on the optic chiasm medial to the medial preoptic nucleus. It receives afferents from the optic system and is probably involved in synchronization of central neuroendocrine rhythms. C

12   *Supra-optic nucleus.* Three-part nucleus containing neurosecretory material (e.g., vasopressin, oxytocin) that is transported by the hypothalamohypophysial tract to the neurohypophysis.

13   *Dorsolateral part.* Larger, magnocellular portion lying dorsolateral to the optic tract. A

14   *Dorsomedial part.* Portion lying on the optic tract. A

15   *Ventromedial part.* Part lying on the medial side of the optic tract. Its projections extend into the tuber cinereum. A

16   **Dorsal hypothalamic area; Dorsal hypothalamic region.** Region of the hypothalamus closest to the vertex of the skull.

17   *Dorsomedial nucleus.* Nucleus lying above the ventromedial nucleus and projecting to the dorsal hypothalamic area.

18   *Endopeduncular nucleus.* Nucleus lying above the optic tract. In humans it is presumably part of the globus pallidus.

19   *Nucleus of ansa lenticularis.* Group of cells located in the ansa lenticularis.

20   **Intermediate hypothalamic area; Intermediate hypothalamic region.** Region located between the anterior and dorsal hypothalamic areas.

21   *Dorsal nucleus.* Group of nuclei situated above the dorsomedial nucleus.

22   *Dorsomedial nucleus.* Nucleus lying closer to the skull vertex than the ventromedial nucleus. It is involved in controlling regulatory hormones for the anterior lobe of pituitary gland. It influences the activity of motor neurons of the spinal cord via the reticular formation. A B C

23   *Arcuate nucleus; Infundibular nucleus.* Nucleus lying nearly in the tip of the funnel of the infundibulum. Among other things, it is the nucleus of origin of the hypothalamoadenohypophysial system. A B C

24   *Periventricular nucleus.* Nuclei of the periventricular zone situated in the intermediate hypothalamic area. They produce regulatory hormones.

25   *Posterior periventricular nucleus.* Cell group lying beneath the ependyma in the posterior portion of the third ventricle. C

26   *Retrochiasmatic area; Retrochiasmatic region.* Region located posterior to the optic chiasm.

27   *Lateral tuberal nuclei.* Groups of nuclei situated in the posterior wall of the infundibulum. A

28   *Ventromedial nucleus of hypothalamus.* Nucleus lying above the entrance to the infundibulum below the dorsomedial nucleus. It is involved in controlling regulatory hormones for the anterior lobe of pituitary gland. A B

17

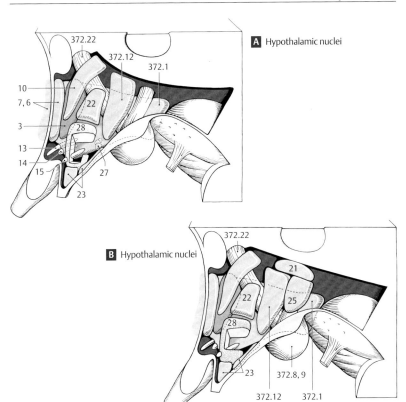

A Hypothalamic nuclei

B Hypothalamic nuclei

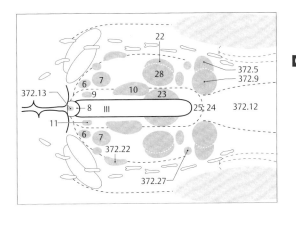

C Hypothalamic nuclei, horizontal section, schematic representation

17

1 **Lateral hypothalamic area.** Region separated from the intermediate hypothalamic area by the fornix and mammillothalamic fasciculus. A

2 *Preoptic area.* Region containing the preoptic nuclei. A

3 *Lateral tuberal nuclei.* Nuclei projecting into the lateral hypothalamic area from the intermediate hypothalamic area. A

4 *Perifornical nucleus.* Strip of nuclei around the fornix. A

5 *Tuberomammillary nucleus.* Group of nuclei situated posterosuperior to the lateral tuberal nuclei. A B

6 **Posterior hypothalamic area; Posterior hypothalamic region.**

7 *Dorsal premammillary nucleus.* Cell groups lying anterior to the true mamillary body. They have not yet been identified in humans. A

8 *Lateral nucleus of mammillary body.* Cell group lying lateral to the medial nucleus. A C

9 *Medial nucleus of mammillary body.* Nucleus forming the main portion of the mammillary body and producing a bulge in it. It is part of the limbic system. A B C

10 *Supramammillary nucleus.* Cell groups situated above the medial nucleus. Their existence is not certain in humans.

11 *Ventral premammillary nucleus.* Dorsorostral group of cells. They have not yet been identified in humans.

12 **Posterior nucleus of hypothalamus.** Its field is continuous caudally with the dorsomedial nucleus. C

13 **Vascular organ of lamina terminalis.** It is rudimentary in humans. Area of capillary loops that produce an elevation in the lamina terminalis of the third ventricle. B

14 **Zones of hypothalamus.** Division of the gray substance of the hypothalamus into three half-shell-shaped layers, arranged from the third ventricle to lateral.

15 *Periventricular zone.* Narrow zone of nuclei bordering on the ventricle. B

16 *Medial zone.* Zone following the periventricular zone and continuous posteriorly with the periaqueductal gray substance. B

17 *Lateral zone.* Area separated from the medial zone by the fornix and mammillothalamic fasciculus. It is bounded laterally by the internal capsule. B

18 **White substance of hypothalamus.**

19 **Posterior longitudinal fasciculus; Dorsal longitudinal fasciculus (Fasciculus of Schütz; Bundle of Schütz).** Caudal continuation of a large portion of the periventricular fibers. It connects the hypothalamus with brainstem nuclei. C

20 **Dorsal supra-optic commissure (Ganser's commissure; Meynert's commissure).** Decussation of fibers from the pons and mesencephalon directly above the optic chiasm.

21 **Fibers of stria terminalis.** Fibers from the amygdaloid body that pass with the stria terminalis to the ventromedial and preoptic nuclei of the hypothalamus. C

22 **Fornix.** Fiber pathway from the hippocampal formation that travels mainly to the mammillary body, but also to the hypothalamus and medial nuclei of the thalamus. A B C

23 **Hypothalamohypophysial tract.** Fiber bundle in the infundibulum of pituitary gland that passes to the capillaries of the posterior lobe of pituitary gland. It consists of the following two parts. C

24 *Paraventricular fibers.* Fibers from the paraventricular nucleus. C

25 *Supra-optic fibers.* Fibers from the supra-optic nucleus. C

26 **Mammillotegmental fasciculus (von Gudden's tract).** Fiber bundle that can be dissected, running between the mammillary body and tegmental nuclei of the mesencephalon. It shares a common origin with the mammillothalamic fasciculus. C

27 **Mammillothalamic fasciculus.** After arising together with the mammillotegmental fasciculus, it passes to the anterior nuclei of the thalamus. A B C

28 **Medial forebrain bundle.** Fibers connecting the hypothalamic nuclei with the olfactory centers and reticular formation of the mesencephalon. C

29 **Paraventriculohypophysial tract.** See 24

30 **Periventricular fibers.** Layer of fibers with interposing neurons lying beneath the ependyma of the third ventricle. It connects the thalamus with the hypothalamus and continues posteriorly in the longitudinal fasciculus. C

31 **Supra-opticohypophysial tract.** See 25

32 **Ventral supra-optic commissure (von Gudden's commissure).** Decussation of fibers from the pons and mesencephalon that partly lies in the optic chiasm.

33 **Retinohypothalamic tract.** Fibers of the optic tract passing to the supra-optic nucleus.

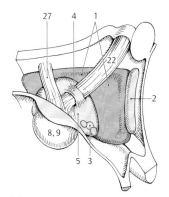

A Hypothalamic nuclei

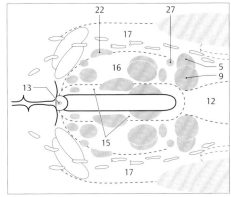

B Hypothalamic nuclei and zones,
horizontal section, schematic representation

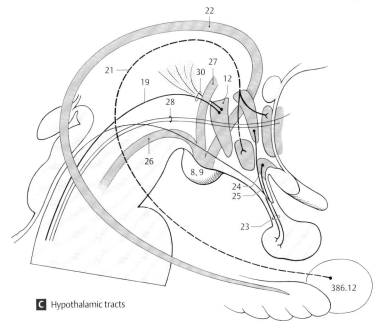

C Hypothalamic tracts

386.12

17

1 **TELENCEPHALON; CEREBRUM.** Endbrain derived from the prosencephalon. It consists of paired portions (hemispheres, cortex, basal ganglia, and primary olfactory regions) as well as unpaired portions (lamina terminalis, corpus callosum, and anterior commissure).

2 CEREBERAL HEMISPHERE.

3 SUPEROLATERAL FACE OF CEREBRAL HEMISPHERE.

4 **Interlobar sulci.** Furrows dividing the cerebral lobes from one another.

5 *Central sulcus.* Groove between the precentral and postcentral gyri. It forms the posterior boundary of the frontal lobe. A B

6 *Lateral sulcus (Sylvian fissure).* Groove running between the frontal and parietal lobes (above) and the temporal lobes (below). A B

7 *Posterior ramus.* Portion of the lateral sulcus that ends at the supramarginal gyrus. A B

8 *Ascending ramus.* Short, ascending portion of the lateral sulcus in the frontal lobe. A B

9 *Anterior ramus.* Short, anteriorly directed portion of the lateral sulcus. A B

10 *Parieto-occipital sulcus.* Terminal portion of the sulcus on the medial surface. A B

11 *Preoccipital notch.* Notch in the inferolateral margin that forms the border between the occipital and temporal lobes. It corresponds to the site on the bony cranium at which the superior border of the petrous part of temporal bone transitions into the lateral wall of the cranium. A B

12 **Frontal lobe.** Portion extending from the frontal pole to the central sulcus. B

13 **Frontal pole.** Anterior end of the frontal lobe. B

14 **Frontal operculum.** Part of the frontal lobe covering the insula. C

15 **Inferior frontal gyrus.** B

16 *Orbital part.* Part of the inferior frontal gyrus below the anterior ramus of the lateral sulcus. B

17 *Triangular part.* Part of the inferior frontal gyrus between the ascending and anterior rami of the lateral sulcus. Central region of Broca's motor speech area. B

18 *Opercular part.* Opercular part of the inferior frontal gyrus lying behind the ascending ramus and covering the insula. Its anterior portion is part of Broca's motor speech area. B

19 **Inferior frontal sulcus.** Groove running between the inferior and middle gyri. A B

20 **Middle frontal gyrus.** B

21 **Precentral gyrus.** Motor area of the frontal lobe lying anterior to the central sulcus. B

22 **Precentral sulcus.** Groove running anterior to the precentral gyrus. A B

23 **Superior frontal gyrus.** A B

24 **Superior frontal sulcus.** Groove below the superior frontal gyrus. B

25 **Parietal lobe.** Lobe bounded anteriorly by the central sulcus and posteriorly by the parieto-occipital sulcus. B

26 **Angular gyrus.** Convolution that curves around the posterior end of the superior temporal sulcus. B

27 **Inferior parietal lobule.** Portion of the parietal lobe situated anteromedial to the intraparietal sulcus. B

28 *Parietal operculum.* Portion of the inferior parietal lobule above the posterior ramus of the lateral sulcus. It covers the insula. C

29 **Intraparietal sulcus.** Inconstant groove between the inferior and superior parietal lobules. A B

30 **Postcentral gyrus.** Chiefly sensory region between the central sulcus and postcentral sulcus. B

31 **Postcentral sulcus.** Posterior boundary of the postcentral gyrus. A B

32 **Superior parietal lobule.** Portion of the parietal lobe situated dorsolateral to the intraparietal sulcus. B

33 **Supramarginal gyrus.** Convolution that curves around the posterior end of the posterior ramus of the lateral sulcus. B

17

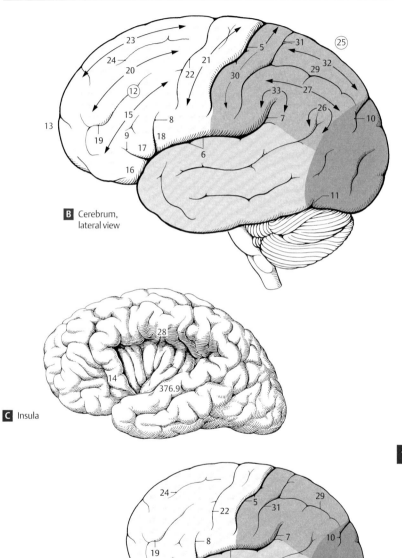

B Cerebrum, lateral view

C Insula

A Interlobar and intralobar sulci

1 **Occipital lobe.** Lobe that is partially bounded by the transverse occipital sulcus, parieto-occipital sulcus, and preoccipital notch. A

2 **Occipital pole.** Posterior end of the occipital lobe. A

3 **Lunate sulcus.** Inconstant groove that forms the anterior boundary of the visual cortex. A

4 **Preoccipital notch.** Indentation on the inferolateral margin. A

5 **Transverse occipital sulcus.** Continuation of the intraparietal sulcus on the occipital lobe. A

6 **Temporal lobe.** Lobe bounded superiorly by the lateral sulcus. A

7 **Temporal pole.** Anterior end of the temporal lobe. A

8 **Superior temporal gyrus.** A C

9 *Temporal operculum.* Portion of the superior temporal gyrus covering the insula. A

10 **Transverse temporal gyri (Heschl's transverse convolutions).** Transverse convolutions (2–4) lying in the floor of the posterior ramus of the lateral sulcus. Area of auditory perception. C

11 *Anterior transverse temporal gyrus.*

12 *Posterior transverse temporal gyrus.*

13 **Temporal plane.** Surface of the temporal lobe after partial removal of the parietal lobe. It corresponds to the floor of the lateral sulcus.

14 **Transverse temporal sulcus.** Transverse grooves between the transverse temporal gyri. C

15 **Superior temporal sulcus.** Groove between the middle and superior temporal gyri. A

16 **Middle temporal gyrus.** A C

17 **Inferior temporal sulcus.** Groove between the middle and inferior temporal gyri. A

18 **Inferior temporal gyrus.** A

19 **Insula; Insular lobe.** Portion of the cerebral cortex situated in the lateral cerebral fossa that is originally uncovered but is overlapped during ontogenesis. B

20 **Insular gyri.**

21 *Long gyrus of insula.* Long, inferior insular gyrus. B

22 *Short gyri of insula.* Short, superior insular gyrus. B

23 **Central sulcus of insula.** Groove between the short and long gyri of the insula. B

24 **Circular sulcus of insula.** Groove bounding the insula. It is interrupted at the limen insulae. B

25 **Limen insulae; Insular threshold.** End of the insula at its junction with the anterior perforated substance. It is covered by the middle cerebral artery. B

26 MEDIAL AND INFERIOR SURFACES OF CEREBERAL HEMISPHERE.

27 **Interlobar sulci.** Grooves dividing the cerebral lobes.

28 *Sulcus of corpus callosum.* Groove between the corpus callosum and cingulate gyrus. D

29 *Cingulate sulcus.* Anterosuperior groove between the cingulate gyrus and middle frontal gyrus. D

30 *Marginal branch; Marginal sulcus.* Ascending terminal branch of the cingulate gyrus. D

31 *Subparietal sulcus.* Terminal portion constituting a prolongation of the cingulate sulcus. D

32 *Parieto-occipital sulcus.* Deep furrow anterior to the cuneus that divides the occipital and parietal lobes. D

33 *Collateral sulcus.* Groove between the parahippocampal and medial occipitotemporal gyri. D

34 *Central sulcus.* Continuation of the groove from the lateral side to medial. A D

17

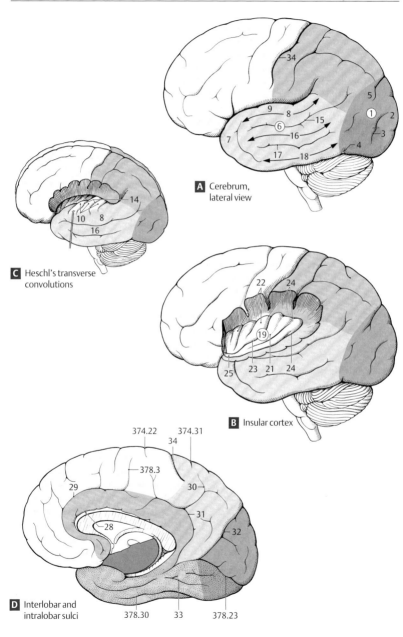

A Cerebrum, lateral view

C Heschl's transverse convolutions

B Insular cortex

D Interlobar and intralobar sulci

17

1 **Frontal lobe.** Lobe extending from the frontal pole to the central sulcus.

2 **Medial frontal gyrus.** Frontal lobe convolution above the cingulate sulcus. A

3 **Paracentral sulcus.** Ascending branch of the cingulate sulcus. It reaches the cortical margin near the precentral sulcus. A

4 **Paracentral lobule.** Hook-shaped connection between the precentral and postcentral gyri. A

5 *Anterior paracentral gyrus.* Part of the paracentral lobule belonging to the frontal lobe. A

6 **Subcallosal area; Subcallosal gyrus.** Region below the genu of corpus callosum. A C

7 *Paraterminal gyrus.* Convolution situated inferior to the rostrum of corpus callosum and anterior to the lamina terminalis. C

8 **Paraolfactory area.** Region lying anterior to the rostrum of corpus callosum and lamina terminalis. A

9 *Paraolfactory gyri.* Variable number of convolutions in the paraolfactory area. C

10 *Paraolfactory sulci.* Grooves between the paraolfactory gyri. C

11 **Orbital gyri.** Convolutions situated lateral to the straight gyrus. B

12 **Orbital sulci.** Grooves between the orbital gyri. B

13 **Straight gyrus.** Straight gyrus above the medial margin of the orbit. B

14 **Olfactory sulcus.** Groove on the inferior surface of the frontal lobe that contains the olfactory tract. B

15 **Lateral olfactory gyrus.** Cellular continuation of the corresponding olfactory striae. B

16 **Medial olfactory gyrus.** Cellular continuation of the corresponding olfactory striae. B

17 **Parietal lobe.** Lobe bounded by the central sulcus, and, posteriorly, by the parieto-occipital sulcus.

18 **Paracentral lobule.** Hook-shaped connection between the precentral and postcentral gyri. A

19 *Posterior paracentral gyrus.* Part of the paracentral lobule belonging to the parietal lobe. A

20 **Precuneus.** Region between the parieto-occipital sulcus, subparietal sulcus, and marginal sulcus. A

21 **Occipital lobe.** See p. 376.1

22 **Cuneus.** Region between the parieto-occipital sulcus and calcarine sulcus. A

23 **Calcarine sulcus.** Deep groove beneath the cuneus in the region of primary visual perception. A

24 **Lingual gyrus.** Continuation of the parahippocampal gyrus to the occipital lobe. B

25 **Lateral occipitotemporal gyrus.** Convolution bordering laterally on the occipitotemporal sulcus. It transitions at the inferolateral margin into the inferior temporal gyrus. A B

26 **Medial occipitotemporal gyrus.** Basal convolution between the collateral sulcus and occipitotemporal sulcus. A B

27 **Occipitotemporal sulcus.** Groove on the inferior surface of the cerebrum between the lateral and medial occipitotemporal gyri. A

28 **Temporal lobe.** Its lateral surface is bounded superiorly by the lateral sulcus. The parahippocampal gyrus and uncus can be considered the uppermost median portions.

29 **Medial occipitotemporal gyrus.** Continuation of the occipital portion in the temporal lobe. A B

30 **Occipitotemporal sulcus.** Continuation of the occipital portion in the temporal lobe. B

31 **Lateral occipitotemporal gyrus.** Continuation of the occipital portion in the temporal lobe. A B

32 **Inferior temporal gyrus.** B

17

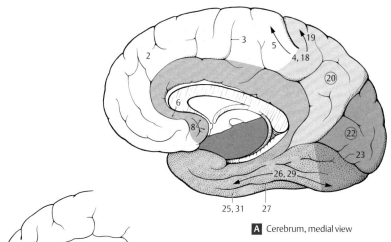

A Cerebrum, medial view

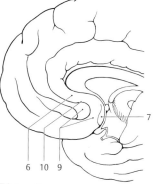

C Paraolfactory area

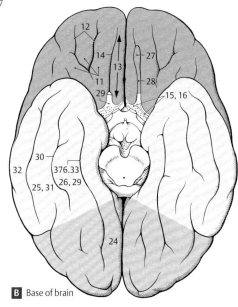

B Base of brain

17

1 **Limbic lobe.** Functional unit formed by structural parts of other lobes.

2 **Cingulate gyrus.** Convolution running parallel and above the corpus callosum. It belongs to the limbic cortex. A B

3 *Isthmus of cingulate gyrus.* Narrowed portion at the transition of the cingulate gyrus into the parahippocampal gyrus posterior and inferior to the splenium of corpus callosum. B

4 **Fasciolar gyrus.** Posterior continuation of the dentate gyrus passing over the splenium of corpus callosum. B

5 **Parahippocampal gyrus.** Convolution situated below the hippocampal sulcus. B

6 *Uncus.* Anterior hook-shaped end of the parahippocampal gyrus. B

7 **Hippocampal sulcus.** Groove between the parahippocampal and dentate gyri. Its anterior end meets with the uncus. B

8 **Dentate gyrus.** Curved convolution of gray substance that has a toothed appearance due to numerous indentations. It forms the inferior continuation of the fasciolar gyrus, extends to the medial surface of the uncus, and lies between the hippocampus and parahippocampal gyrus. B

9 **Fimbriodentate sulcus.** Groove between the dentate gyrus and fimbria of hippocampus. B

10 **Fimbria of hippocampus.** Fibrous band that leaves the hippocampus and extends as the fornix to the mammillary body. B

11 **Rhinal sulcus.** Variable continuation of the collateral sulcus running lateral to the uncus. B

12 **Corpus callosum.** Transverse nerve fibers connecting the two cerebral hemispheres at the base of the longitudinal cerebral fissure. C D

13 **Rostrum.** Anterior end of the corpus callosum that tapers off inferiorly at the lamina terminalis. A C

14 **Genu.** Knee of the corpus callosum situated anterosuperior to the rostrum. A C

15 **Trunk; Body.** Portion between the splenium and genu of corpus callosum. A C

16 **Splenium.** Bulging, exposed posterior end of corpus callosum. A B C

17 **Indusium griseum.** Thin layer of gray substance on the corpus callosum. C

18 **Lateral longitudinal stria.** Paired, longitudinal band of nerve fibers on the corpus callosum that is covered laterally by the cingulate gyrus. It receives efferent fibers from the hippocampus. C

19 **Medial longitudinal stria.** Medial band of longitudinal nerve fibers on the corpus callosum. It receives efferent fibers from the hippocampus. C D

20 **Radiation of corpus callosum.** Fibers radiating from the corpus callosum to the cerebral cortex. D E

21 *Minor forceps; Frontal forceps.* Portion of the radiation of the corpus callosum whose fibers run in a U-shape though the genu. It connects the two frontal lobes with each other. E

22 *Major forceps; Occipital forceps.* Portion of the radiation of the corpus callosum whose fibers run in a U-shape through the splenium, connecting the posterior portions of the occipital lobes with each other. E

23 *Tapetum.* Layer of curving fibers arising from the corpus callosum that extend laterally and inferiorly. They form the lateral wall of the inferior and posterior horns of the lateral ventricle, as well as the roof of the lateral ventricle near the posterior horn. D

24 **Lamina terminalis.** Thin wall forming the anterior boundary of the third ventricle. A C

25 **Anterior commissure.** Transverse nerve fibers between the anterior parts of the right and left cerebral hemispheres. It lies posterior to the lamina terminalis. A

26 *Anterior part.* Anterior portion connecting contralateral anterior olfactory nuclei.

27 *Posterior part.* Posterior portion connecting the inferior and middle temporal gyri.

28 **Fornix.** Bundle of fibers arching in opposite directions to connect the mammillary body and hippocampus. C

29 **Column.** Anterior portion of the fornix that is partly located in the lateral wall of the third ventricle. C

30 *Precommissural fibers.* Fibers lying rostral to the anterior commissure. They pass to the septum pellucidum and anterior hypothalamus, but not to the mammillary body.

31 *Postcommissural fibers.* Fibers lying caudal to the anterior commissure. They pass mainly to the mammillary body.

32 **Body.** Middle, unpaired portion lying below the corpus callosum that is formed by the union of the two crura of the fornix. C

33 **Crus.** Posterior crus of the fornix that is derived from the fimbria of hippocampus. It encircles the pulvinar and joins with the crus from the opposite side to form the body of fornix. C

34 **Commissure.** Triangular sheet of fibers connecting the crura of fornix below the posterior portion of the corpus callosum. It contains crossing fibers from the fimbriae of hippocampus on both sides. C

35 **Tenia.** Thin, lateral margin of the fornix and attachment site for the choroid plexus of the lateral ventricle. C

17

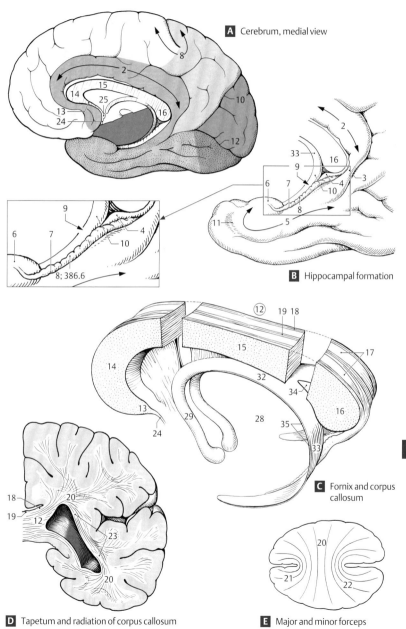

A Cerebrum, medial view

B Hippocampal formation

C Fornix and corpus callosum

D Tapetum and radiation of corpus callosum

E Major and minor forceps

1 **Septum pellucidum.** Thin dual layer of fibers stretched between the corpus callosum and fornix with an irregular slitlike space between them. It divides the anterior horns of the lateral ventricle from each other. B F

2 **Cave.** Enclosed cavity of variable size between the two laminae. B F

3 **Lamina.** Paired layer forming the septum pellucidum. It forms the lateral wall of the cave of septum pellucidum. B F

4 **Precommissural septal nucleus.** Area at the free, medial surface of the frontal lobe situated anterior to the lamina terminalis.

5 **Septal nuclei and related structures.** Findings have not been entirely confirmed in humans. The nuclei are currently divided into three groups according to their position in the septum pellucidum.

6 **Dorsal septal nucleus.** Nuclei lying almost directly beneath the corpus callosum lateral to its midline. F

7 **Lateral septal nucleus.** Nuclei arranged from superior to inferior beneath the dorsal septal nuclei. F

8 **Medial septal nucleus.** Nuclei lying medial to the dorsal and lateral septal nuclei. F

9 **Septofimbrial nucleus.** Small group of cells situated between the dorsal septal nuclei and corpus callosum. F

10 **Subfornical organ.** Organ situated between the right and left portions of the fornix near the interventricular foramen. D

11 **Triangular nucleus.** Small group of cells lying anterior to the subfornical organ.

12 **Lateral ventricle.** Paired ventricles that communicate with the third ventricle via the interventricular foramen.

13 **Frontal horn; Anterior horn.** Portion extending anteriorly from the interventricular foramen. It is bounded medially by the septum pellucidum, laterally by the head of caudate nucleus, superiorly by the body of corpus callosum, and anteriorly and inferiorly by the genu and rostrum of corpus callosum, respectively. A

14 **Interventricular foramen.** Opening that connects the lateral ventricle and third ventricle. It is situated posterior and inferior to the genu of fornix. D

15 **Central part; Body.** Middle portion of the lateral ventricle lying above the thalamus and below the corpus callosum. It contains part of the choroid plexus. A

16 **Stria terminalis.** Longitudinal band of efferent fibers from the amygdaloid body. It is accompanied by the superior thalamostriate vein in the angle between the thalamus and caudate nucleus. C

17 **Lamina affixa.** Floor of the lateral ventricle between the stria terminalis and choroid line. C

18 **Choroid line.** Line of attachment for the choroid plexus of lateral ventricle to the thalamus. The line of separation is visible upon removal of the choroid plexus. C

19 **Choroidal fissure.** Cleft between the thalamus and fornix though which the choroid plexus projects into the lateral ventricle. In the inferior horn it lies between the fimbria of hippocampus and the stria terminalis. C

20 **Choroid plexus.** Well-vascularized, villous garland extending from the interventricular foramen into the inferior horn. It is absent in the posterior horn. C

21 **Collateral trigone.** Widened beginning of the collateral eminence at the border of the posterior horn. E

22 **Atrium.** Expansion of the lateral ventricle at the junction of the posterior and inferior horns. A

23 **Collateral eminence.** Elevation in the lateral arch of the inferior horn produced by the collateral sulcus. E

24 **Choroid enlargement.** Thickened portion of the choroid plexus in the atrium. C

25 **Bulb of occipital horn.** Eminence on the medial side of the posterior horn produced by fibers from the splenium of corpus callosum. E

26 **Calcarine spur.** Elevation on the medial side of the posterior horn produced by the calcarine sulcus. E

27 **Occipital horn; Posterior horn.** It extends into the occipital lobe. A

28 **Temporal horn; Inferior horn.** It extends with the hippocampus laterally and contains the choroid plexus. A

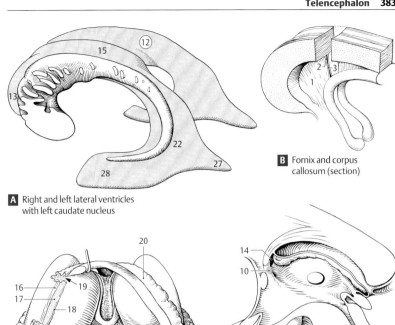

A Right and left lateral ventricles with left caudate nucleus

B Fornix and corpus callosum (section)

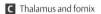

C Thalamus and fornix

D Interventricular foramen

E Left hippocampus

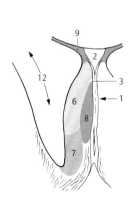

F Right septal area, frontal section, schematic illustration

17

1 **Cerebral cortex.** It is 1.5–4.5 mm thick and consists of six layers in most places.

2 **Archicortex.** Phylogenetically older portion of the cerebral cortex. It consists of three layers formed by the hippocampus and dentate gyrus. The limbic system is mainly located here.

3 **Paleocortex.** Oldest portion of the cerebral cortex containing the areas of the brain that are primarily connected with olfactory sensation. The [[rhinencephalon]] is regressed in human beings. The main origin of this part of the cortex is the piriform lobe.

4 **Neocortex.** Six-layered part comprising the greater portion of the cerebral cortex.

5 **Allocortex.** Part that can be divided in terms of cytoarchitecture and myeloarchitecture into the predominantly triple-layered archicortex and paleocortex.

6 **Mesocortex.** Cytoarchitectural transition between the allocortex and isocortex.

7 **Isocortex.** Part corresponding to the neocortex.

8 **Layers of isocortex.**

9 *Molecular layer (Layer I).* Layer containing scant spindle-shaped neurons and a network of nerve fibers. A

10 *External granular layer (Layer II).* Layer containing numerous small granular cells and a network of nerve fibers. A

11 *External pyramidal layer (Layer III).* Layer containing medium-sized pyramidal cells which, however, do not form longer tracts. A

12 *Internal granular layer (Layer IV).* Layer composed mainly of densely packed small granular cells. It receives stimuli mainly from thalamocortical fibers. A

13 *Internal pyramidal layer (Layer V).* Layer containing large pyramidal cells. It gives rise to the corticospinal tract in the corresponding region of areas 4 and 6. A

14 *Multiform layer (Layer VI).* Layer consisting of numerous, usually small, multiform cells. It transitions into the white substance without a clear boundary. A

15 *Stria of molecular layer.* Tangential fibrous network in layer I. A

16 *Stria of external granular layer.* Superradial network in layer II. A

17 *Stria of internal granular layer.* Baillarger's external stripe (band) found in layer IV. It is produced by ramifying afferent fibers. A

18 *Occipital stripe; Occipital line (Stria of Gennari; Line of Gennari).* Bandlike zone that has scant cells and contains giant stellate neurons.

19 *Stria of internal pyramidal layer.* Baillarger's internal stripe (band) of layer V. It is formed by axon collaterals of pyramidal cells. A

20 *Tangential fibers.* Next layer of fibers, which runs parallel to the surface. A

21 **Hippocampus.** Crescent-shaped, elongated elevation on the floor of the inferior horn of lateral ventricle. It forms the main part of the archicortex.

22 **Parasubiculum.** Part of the subiculum situated directly anterior to the parahippocampal gyrus. C

23 **Pes.** Paw-shaped anterior end of the hippocampus. B

24 **Hippocampal digitations.** Claw-like projections of the pes hippocampi. B

25 **Presubiculum.** Transitional region to the subiculum. C

26 **Subiculum.** Transition between the parahippocampal gyrus and Ammon's horn. C

27 **Hippocampus proper; Ammon's horn.** C

28 *Region I; CA1.* Region situated adjacent to the subiculum. It is particularly well-developed in humans. It is composed of two layers of small pyramidal cells. C

29 *Region II; CA2.* Region adjacent to CA1 that is also composed of two layers of pyramidal cells, the deep layer of which is loosely organized. C

30 *Region III; CA3.* Pyramidal cells arranged in a uniform layer. C

31 *Region IV; CA4.* Region that is not clearly layered and in which the pyramidal cells are irregularly organized. C

32 **Fimbria.** Band of fibers arising from the alveus that lies on the superomedial aspect of the hippocampus. It is continuous with the fornix via the crus of fornix. B C

33 **Alveus.** Layer of fibers on Ammon's horn near the ventricle. It is formed by axons of pyramidal cells. B C

17

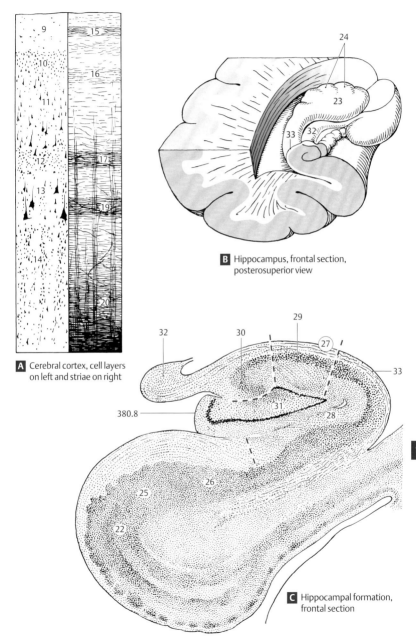

A Cerebral cortex, cell layers on left and striae on right

B Hippocampus, frontal section, posterosuperior view

C Hippocampal formation, frontal section

17

1 **Layers of hippocampus; Layers of Ammon's horn.**

2 *Lacunar-molecular layer.* Layer of apical dendrites of pyramidal cells. A

3 *Oriens layer.* Layer of basal dendrites of pyramidal cells. A

4 *Pyramidal layer.* Layer of pyramidal cell bodies and basket cells. A

5 *Radiate layer.* Layer of collaterals of apical dendrites A

6 **Dentate gyrus.** Convolution between the hippocampal sulcus and fimbriodentate sulcus. It is continuous rostrally with the uncus and caudally with the fasciolar gyrus. Fibers from the neocortex travel through it to Ammon's horn. p. 381 B

7 **Layers of dentate gyrus.**

8 *Molecular layer.* Superficial layer containing a small number of neurons. Ramifying dendrites of granular cells of the granular layer.

9 *Granular layer.* Narrow strip containing densely packed granular cells and little cytoplasm.

10 *Multiform layer.* Layer consisting mainly of collections of neurons of granular cells.

11 BASAL FOREBRAIN. Collective topographical term for basal structures.

12 **Amygdaloid body; Amygdaloid complex.** Group of nuclei connected with the cerebral cortex and lying in the dorsomedial pole of the temporal lobe anterior to the inferior horn of lateral ventricle. It belongs partly to the olfactory tract, partly has autonomic nervous system functions, and partly influences emotional states. C D

13 **Amygdaloclaustral area.** Region between the nuclear complex and claustrum. D

14 **Amygdalohippocampal area.** Region between the nuclear complex and parahippocampal gyrus. D

15 **Amygdalopiriform transition area.** Region between the nuclear complex and temporal lobe. D

16 **Anterior amygdaloid area.** Region situated anterior to the central nucleus and directed toward the anterior perforated substance. Site of entry of the lateral olfactory stria and origin of the (Broca's) diagonal band. C

17 **Basolateral amygdaloid nucleus.** Basal nucleus consisting of large cells. C

18 **Basomedial amygdaloid nucleus.** Basal nucleus consisting of small cells. C

19 **Central amygdaloid nucleus.** C

20 **Cortical amygdaloid nucleus.** Superficially located nucleus. C

21 **Interstitial amygdaloid nucleus.** Variable nucleus between the cortical and lateral amygdaloid nuclei. It can fuse with both.

22 **Lateral amygdaloid nucleus.** C

23 **Medial amygdaloid nucleus.** C

24 **Nucleus of lateral olfactory tract.** Group of cells in the lateral olfactory stria.

25 **Periamygdaloid cortex.** Convolution anterior to the uncus belonging to the paleocortex. B

26 **Anterior olfactory nucleus.** Scattered groups of neurons along the olfactory tract. Their axons project to the tract. B

27 **Basal substance.** It includes the following three areas.

28 *Basal nucleus (Meynert's nucleus).* Part of the innominate substance. D

29 *Bed nucleus of stria terminalis.* Narrow nucleus situated alongside the stria terminalis. It lies just lateral to the septal area.

30 *Sublenticular extended amygdala.* Portion including the central and medial amygdaloid nuclei. D

17

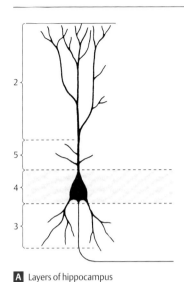

A Layers of hippocampus

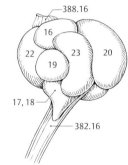

B Cranial base, section

C Amygdaloid body, view from right

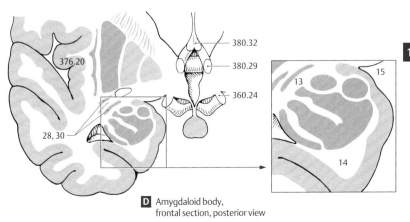

D Amygdaloid body,
frontal section, posterior view

17

1 **Claustrum.** Layer of gray substance between the lentiform nucleus and insular cortex. B

2 **Diagonal band (Broca's diagonal band).** Band of myelinated fibers that usually forms the posterior boundary of the anterior perforated substance. It extends from the amygdaloid body to the paraterminal gyrus. A

3 *Horizontal limb.* Limb on the base of the brain. A B

4 *Vertical limb.* Ascending limb to the paraterminal gyrus. A B

5 *Nucleus of diagonal band.* Group of cells lying caudal to the globus pallidus.

6 **Innominate substance.** Island of gray substance between the lentiform nucleus and amygdaloid body. B

7 **Fasciculus peduncularis.** Collection of fibers connecting the claustrum and thalamus. It contains fibers from the amygdaloid body. p. 391 D

8 **Olfactory islets.** Persistent remnants of an embryonic epithelial area.

9 **Olfactory bulb.** Bulblike expansion at the beginning of the olfactory tract. It lies on top of the cribriform plate of the ethmoid and is part of the allocortex. It serves as a relay station of the olfactory tract. A

10 *Olfactory peduncle.* Rudimentary cortical structure at the end of the olfactory tract.

11 *Olfactory tract.* Narrow band of fibers traveling from the olfactory bulb posteriorly in the olfactory sulcus. A

12 *Olfactory trigone.* Triangular expansion of the olfactory peduncle. A

13 *Olfactory tubercle.* Elevation of the anterior part of the anterior perforated substance. It consists of portions of the striatum and pallidum.

14 **Olfactory striae.** Division of the olfactory tract at the trigone into two bands of fibers.

15 *Medial stria.* Band of fibers extending medially around the trigone to the paraterminal gyrus. A B

16 *Lateral stria.* Band of fibers lying anterior to the trigone and extending laterally to the insula, then posteriorly to the periamygdaloid cortex. A B

17 **Anterior perforated substance.** Perforated area between the olfactory striae produced by the passage of cerebral vessels. It transitions into the gray substance of the tuber cinereum and paraterminal gyrus. A

18 **Ventral pallidum.** Structure formed by portions of the innominate substance, olfactory tubercle, and globus pallidus.

19 **Ventral striatum.** Structure mainly consisting of the accumbens nucleus and part of the olfactory tubercle.

20 *Nucleus accumbens.* Area of cells in the ventral striatum connecting the caudate nucleus and putamen. B

21 *Lateral part; Core region.*

22 *Medial part; Shell region.*

23 **Peduncular loop.** Medio-anterior connection between the amygdaloid body and lateral hypothalamus.

24 **Septal area.** Part of the septum pellucidum containing the septal nuclei. B

17

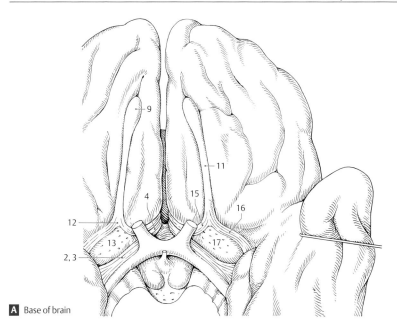

A Base of brain

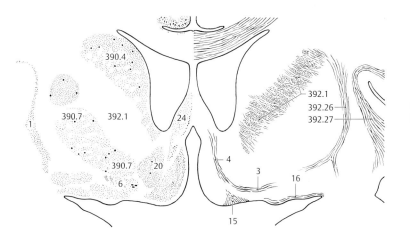

B Nuclei and tracts of septal area,
frontal section

1 BASAL NUCLEI AND RELATED STRUCTURES.

2 **Caudate nucleus.** Elongated nucleus arising from the ganglionic eminence of the telencephalon and curving around the thalamus. B

3 **Head of caudate nucleus.** Anterior portion of the nucleus. It forms that lateral wall of the anterior horn of lateral ventricle. B

4 **Body of caudate nucleus.** Middle portion of the caudate nucleus lying on the thalamus. A B

5 **Tail of caudate nucleus.** Portion of the nucleus that tapers off posteroinferiorly. A B C

6 **Lentiform nucleus; Lenticular nucleus.** Nucleus arising from the telencephalon and diencephalon.

7 **Putamen.** Lateral telencephalic part of the lentiform nucleus. A B C

8 **Lateral medullary lamina; External medullary lamina.** Layer of white substance between the globus pallidus and putamen. A

9 **Globus pallidus lateral segment; Globus pallidus external segment.** Diencephalic portion of the globus pallidus situated between the lateral and medial medullary laminae. A

10 **Medial medullary lamina; Internal medullary lamina.** Layer of white substance between the lateral and medial segments of the globus pallidus. A

11 **Globus pallidus medial segment; Globus pallidus internal segment.** Portion of the globus pallidus situated medial to the medial medullary lamina. In humans it can be subdivided into the following parts. A

12 *Lateral part.* Part located lateral to the accessory medullary lamina.

13 *Accessory medullary lamina.* Layer of white substance that can subdivide the medial segment of the globus pallidus.

14 *Medial part.* Part situated medial to the accessory medullary lamina.

15 **Corpus striatum.** Structure that is currently viewed as consisting of the putamen, caudate nucleus, pallidum, and fasciculi.

16 **Striatum; Neostriatum.** Originally telencephalic mass of cells that is forced apart by the internal capsule during development. The arising cell groups composing the putamen and caudate nucleus remain connected: corpus striatum. It constitutes a central relay station of the extrapyramidal motor system. B C

17 *Dorsal striatum.* Greater portion of the striatum that is nearly identical to it.

18 *Ventral striatum.* Portion basically consisting of the accumbens nucleus, a cellular bridge between the putamen and caudate nucleus, and a part of the olfactory tubercle. C

19 **Pallidum; Paleostriatum.** Structure arising in the diencephalon and forced by the internal capsule away from its original site, with the greater portion of the site giving rise to the subthalamus. C

20 *Dorsal pallidum.* Part including the main part of the globus pallidus and substantia nigra.

21 *Ventral pallidum.* Small ventral part of the globus pallidus. Part of the innominate substance and olfactory tubercle. C

22 **Ansa lenticularis.** Fibers connecting the pallidum and thalamus. They exit from the ventral side of the pallidum. D

23 **Lenticular fasciculus.** Fibers connecting the pallidum and thalamus. They exit from the dorsal side of the pallidum. D

24 **Subthalamic fasciculus.** Fibers connecting the pallidum and subthalamic nucleus. D

25 **Thalamic fasciculus.** Union of the ansa lenticularis and lenticular fasciculus. D

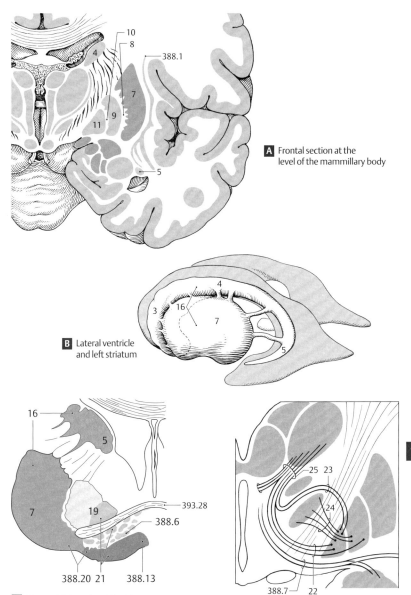

A Frontal section at the level of the mammillary body

B Lateral ventricle and left striatum

C Corpus striatum, frontal section

D Subthalamic tracts

1 **Internal capsule.** Band of nerve fibers lying medial to the lentiform nucleus and medial to the thalamus and caudate nucleus. B

2 **Caudolenticular gray bridges; Transcapsular gray bridges.** Cellular bridges between the putamen and caudate nucleus. A B

3 *Anterior limb of internal capsule.* Portion of the anterior capsule situated between the lentiform nucleus and head of caudate nucleus. A B

4 *Anterior thalamic radiation.* Reciprocal connection between the thalamus as well as frontal lobe and cingulate gyrus. C

5 *Frontopontine fibers.* Fibers from the frontal lobe to the pontine nuclei. C

6 **Genu of internal capsule.** Part situated between the anterior and posterior limbs of internal capsule. It contributes to formation of the lateral wall of the ventricular system A B C

7 *Corticonuclear fibers.* Fibers passing to the motor and sensory cranial nerve nuclei. C

8 **Posterior limb of internal capsule.** Portion situated between the lentiform nucleus as well as thalamus and body of caudate nucleus. A B C

9 *Central thalamic radiation.* Superior thalamic radiation with fibers radiating from the thalamus to the precentral and postcentral gyri as well as adjacent cortical regions. C

10 *Corticoreticular fibers.* Fibers passing from regions around the central sulcus to the reticular formation. C

11 *Corticorubral fibers.* Fibers passing from the frontal lobe to the red nucleus. C

12 *Corticospinal fibers.* Spinal cord portion of the pyramidal tract that is somatotopically organized. Fibers from the most caudal portion of the body lie furthest lateral. C

13 *Corticothalamic fibers.* Portion of the thalamic radiation passing to the thalamus. C

14 *Parietopontine fibers.* Fibers from the parietal lobe to the pontine nuclei.

15 *Thalamoparietal fibers.* Thalamic radiation to the parietal cortex. C

16 *Retrolentiform limb; Retrolenticular limb.* Portion of the internal capsule situated toward the occiput from the lentiform nucleus. B C

17 *Occipitopontine fibers.* Fibers passing from the occipital lobe to the pontine nuclei. C

18 *Occipitotectal fibers.* Fibers connecting the occipital lobe with the tectum.

19 *Optic radiation; Geniculocalcarine fibers.* Optic radiation from the lateral geniculate body to the striate cortex of the occipital lobe. A B C

20 *Posterior thalamic radiation.* C

21 *Sublentiform limb; Sublenticular limb.* Part of the internal capsule beneath the posterior part of the lentiform nucleus. B C

22 *Acoustic radiation; Geniculotemporal fibers.* Portion of acoustic pathway from the medial geniculate body to the transverse temporal gyri (Heschl's transverse convolutions). A B C

23 *Corticotectal fibers.* Fibers connecting the cerebral cortex with the tectum. C

24 *Temporopontine fibers.* Fibers passing from the temporal lobe to the pontine nuclei. C

25 **Corona radiata.** Fanlike arrangement of ascending and descending fibers of the internal capsule. B

26 **External capsule.** White substance between the claustrum and lentiform nucleus. A C

27 **Extreme capsule.** White substance between the insular cortex and claustrum. A C

28 **Anterior commissure.** Commissure located anterior to the fornical column. It is readily visible in the anterior wall of the third ventricle. D

29 *Anterior part.* Part belonging to the phylogenetic [[rhinencephalon]]. It extends into the olfactory peduncle. D

30 *Posterior part.* Part connecting the two temporal lobes. D

17

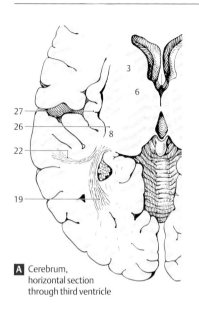

A Cerebrum, horizontal section through third ventricle

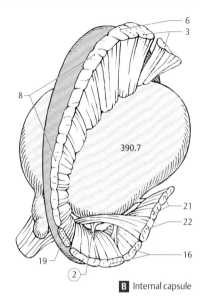

B Internal capsule

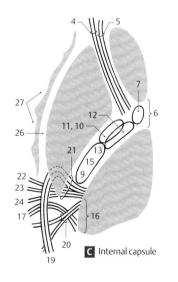

C Internal capsule

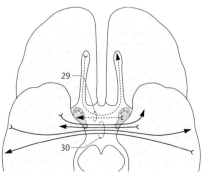

D Anterior commissure

17

1 **Association fibers of telencephalon.** Fibers connecting cortical regions.

2 **Arcuate fibers.** Curving fibers that connect adjacent convolutions. C

3 **Cingulum.** Fiber bundle in the white substance of the cingulate gyrus. It follows the gyrus around the corpus callosum, then continues past the splenium anteriorly to the uncus. B

4 **Inferior longitudinal fasciculus.** Fiber bundle stretching between the occipital and temporal lobes. A B

5 **Superior longitudinal fasciculus; Arcuate fasciculus.** Association fibers traveling between the occipital and frontal lobes with branches to the parietal and temporal lobes. It lies laterodorsal to the putamen and is the largest bundle of association fibers. A

6 **Long association fibers.** Fibers connecting various cerebral lobes.

7 **Short association fibers.** Fibers connecting areas within a single lobe, e.g., immediately adjacent cortical regions, U-fibers.

8 **Uncinate fasciculus.** Fibers connecting the inferior surface of the frontal lobe with the anterior portion of the temporal lobe. A

9 **Inferior occipitofrontal fasciculus.** Fibers connecting the occipital and frontal lobes via the extreme capsule.

10 **Superior occipitofrontal fasciculus; Subcallosal fasciculus.** Fibers connecting the frontal lobes with the temporal and occipital lobes. It lies laterodorsal to the caudate nucleus. A

11 **Vertical occipital fasciculi.** Vertical association fibers in the anterior portion of the occipital lobe. A

12 *Lateral fibers.* Lateral fibers connecting the posterior temporal lobe with the posterior parietal lobe via the occipital lobe.

13 *Caudal fibers.* Fibers connecting the temporal and occipital lobes.

14 **Transverse occipital fasciculi.** Fibers connecting the medial and lateral wall of one hemisphere.

15 *Cuneus fibers.* Fibers connecting the superior margin of the calcarine sulcus with the superolateral cortex of the occipital lobe. B

16 *Lingual fibers.* Fibers connecting the inferior margin of the calcarine sulcus with the inferolateral portion of the occipital lobe. B

17 **Commissural fibers of telencephalon.** Association fibers connecting the cerebral hemispheres.

18 **Corpus callosum fibers.** Broad connection of the white substance of both hemispheres. B

19 **Hippocampal commissure.** Fibers that connect contralateral hippocampi via the crura of the fornix and run beneath the posterior portion of the corpus callosum.

20 **Anterior commissure.** Anterior transverse connection between the two hemispheres. It lies just posterior to the lamina terminalis and is visible in the anterior portion of the third ventricle. B

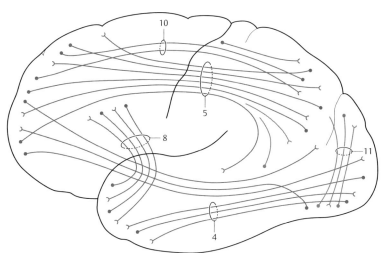

A Association tracts

C Arcuate fibers

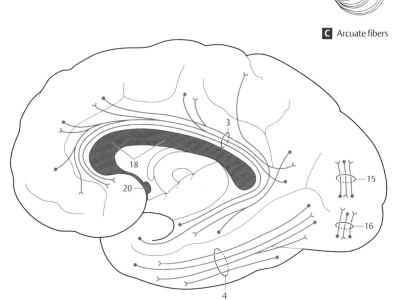

B Association and arcuate fibers

1 CHEMICALLY-DEFINED CELL GROUPS. There is as yet no consensus on their presence and precise location in the human body.

2 **Aminergic cells.**

3 **Noradrenergic cells in medulla; Norepinephric cells in medulla (A1, A2).** Groups lying between the decussation of pyramids and the margin of the pons. A

4 **Noradrenergic cells in nucleus of lateral lemniscus; Norepinephric cells in nucleus of lateral lemniscus (A7).** Cells located anterolateral to the locus caeruleus. A

5 **Noradrenergic cells in locus caeruleus; Norepinephric cells in locus caeruleus (A6).** Cells in the central portion of the locus caeruleus. Noradrenergic principal nucleus. Its ascending and descending fibers are widely dispersed throughout the brain. A

6 **Noradrenergic cells in caudolateral pons; Norepinephric cells in caudolateral pons (A5).** Cells located near the nucleus of the facial nerve and superior olivary nucleus. A

7 **Aminergic cells in reticular formation; Retrobulbar nucleus (A8).** Cells located in the reticular formation of the mesencephalon. A

8 *Dopaminergic cells.* Cells containing dopamine that, together with their counterparts from A9, form the mesostriatal or nigrostriatal dopaminergic system.

9 *Noradrenergic cells*; *Norepinephric cells.* Cells containing norepinephrine (noradrenaline).

10 **Aminergic cells in compact part of substantia nigra (A9).** Cells located in the mesencephalon in the compact part of the substantia nigra. A

11 *Dopaminergic cells.* Cells containing dopamine that, together with their counterparts form A8, form the mesostriatal or nigrostriatal dopaminergic system.

12 *Noradrenergic cells*; *Norepinephric cells.* Cells containing norepinephrine (noradrenaline).

13 **Aminergic cells in ventral tegmental area (A10).** Cells located in the tegmentum of the midbrain. A

14 *Dopaminergic cells.* Cells containing dopamine and forming the mesolimbocortical or mesolimbic dopaminergic system.

15 *Noradrenergic cells*; *Norepinephric cells.* Cells containing norepinephrine (noradrenaline).

16 **Dopaminergic cells in posterior hypothalamus (A11).** Cells located in the diencephalon posterior to the hypothalamus. A

17 **Dopaminergic cells in arcuate nucleus (A12).** Cells in the arcuate nucleus of the diencephalon. They form the tuberoinfundibular system. A

18 **Dopaminergic cells in zona incerta (A13).** Cells in the subthalamus. A

19 **Dopaminergic cells in medial zone and anterior area of hypothalamus (A14).** Cells in the hypothalamus. A

20 **Dopaminergic cells in olfactory bulb (A15).** Cells located in the olfactory bulb of the telencephalon. A

21 **Serotoninergic cells in pallidal raphe nucleus (B1).** Cells located in the medulla oblongata, dorsal to the pyramidal tract. B

22 **Serotoninergic cells in obscurus raphe nucleus (B2).** B

23 **Serotoninergic cells in magnus raphe nucleus (B3).** Cells of the magnus raphe nucleus situated near the reticular formation of the medulla. B

24 **Serotoninergic cells adjacent to medial vestibular nucleus and prepositus nucleus (B4).** Cell group located at the level of the medial vestibular nucleus of the medulla.

25 **Serotoninergic cells in pontine raphe nucleus (B5).** Cells in the rostral part of the pons.

26 **Serotoninergic cells in median raphe nucleus (B6).** Cells in the rostral part of the pons. B

27 **Serotoninergic cells in dorsal raphe nucleus (B7).** B

28 **Adrenergic cells in area postrema and anterior reticular nucleus; Epinephric cells in area postrema and anterior reticular nucleus (C1, C2).** Cells in the dorsal and ventrolateral medulla. A

29 **Cholinergic cells.** Cells containing acetylcholine.

30 **Cholinergic cells of medial septal nuclei (Ch1).** Cells in the basal portion of the telencephalon in the medial septal nuclei. Together with Ch3 they form projections to the hippocampal formation.

31 **Cholinergic cells of globus pallidus, accumbens nucleus and diagonal gyrus (Ch2).** Cells in the telencephalon.

32 **Cholinergic cells of globus pallidus, accumbens nucleus and diagonal band (Ch3).** Cells in the nuclear complex of the diagonal band. They form projections with Ch1 to the hippocampal formation.

33 **Cholinergic cells of substantia innominata, basal nucleus, amygdaloid body and olfactory tubercle (Ch4).** Telencephalic cells that innervate the neocortex.

34 **Cholinergic cells of dorsal tegmental area (Ch5, Ch6, Ch8).** Cells forming the ascending reticular activation system.

35 **Cholinergic cells of epithalamus (Ch7).** Cells in the medial habenular nucleus.

17

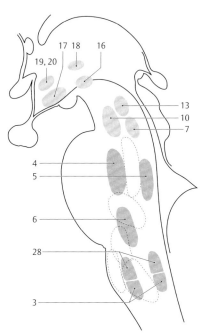

A Scheme of sagittal section with chemically-defined cell groups

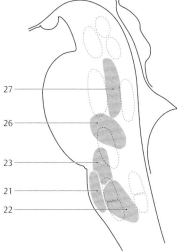

B Scheme of sagittal section with chemically-defined cell groups

17

1 ***PERIPHERAL NERVOUS SYSTEM.*** That part of the nervous system that composes of all peripheral nerve pathways. The surface of the brain and spinal cord forms the boundary between it and the central nervous system.

2 ***CRANIAL NERVES.*** With the exception of CN IV, these 12 pairs of nerves emerge at the base of the brain, exiting the cranium through the skull base. Distribution area: head, neck, and also the thoracic and abdominal cavities via the vagus nerve.

3 TERMINAL NERVE (0). Nerve only detectable in human beings during development stages. It is a tiny and probably autonomic nerve of unknown function situated along the olfactory nerve between the olfactory part and anterior perforated substance. B

4 **Terminal ganglion.** Group of ganglion cells interspersed along the terminal nerve.

5 OLFACTORY NERVE (I). Collection of olfactory nerve fibers. These enter the olfactory bulb through the cribriform plate of the ethmoid bone. Synaptic site. A

6 **Olfactory nerves.** Around 20 small fiber bundles of unmyelinated axons originating from olfactory cells. A

7 OPTIC NERVE (II). Nerve emerging medial to the posterior pole of the eyeball and extending to the optic chiasma. C D

8 OCULOMOTOR NERVE (III). Nerve containing motor and parasympathetic fibers that exits the oculomotor sulcus and passes through the superior orbital fissure into the orbit. C D

9 **Superior branch.** Upper branch innervating the superior rectus muscles and levator palpebrae superioris. C

10 **Inferior branch.** Lower branch supplying the medial rectus, inferior rectus, and inferior oblique muscles. C

11 **Branch to ciliary ganglion; Parasympathetic root of ciliary ganglion; Oculomotor root of ciliary ganglion.** Oculomotor branch containing preganglionic parasympathetic fibers for the ciliary ganglion. C

12 TROCHLEAR NERVE (IV). Nerve exiting on the dorsal side, caudal to the tectal plate. It supplies the superior oblique muscle. C

13 TRIGEMINAL NERVE (V). Nerve innervating the first pharyngeal arch. The fifth cranial nerve, comprised of two groups of fibers exiting laterally from the pons, innervates the muscles of mastication and supplies sensory information for facial sensation. C D

14 **Sensory root.** Sensory part of the nerve that emerges caudally from the pons and extends to the trigeminal ganglion. D

15 *Trigeminal ganglion (gasserian ganglion).* Crescent-shaped equivalent of a spinal ganglion of the trigeminal nerve lying in an outpouching in the subarachnoid space (trigeminal cavity) above the foramen lacerum on the medial, anterior surface of the petrous temporal bone. D

16 **Motor root.** Root emerging from the trigeminal nerve toward the skull vertex and then passing under the trigeminal ganglion, innervating the muscles of mastication. D

17 **Ophthalmic nerve; Ophthalmic division (Va; V1).** First division of the trigeminal nerve, which passes through the superior orbital fissure. D

18 **Tentorial nerve.** Recurrent branch supplying the tentorium cerebelli and falx cerebri. D

19 **Lacrimal nerve.** Nerve passing laterally through the superior orbital fissure to supply the lacrimal gland, conjunctiva, and lateral portion of the upper eyelid. D

20 *Communicating branch with zygomatic nerve.* Connection to the zygomatic nerve via autonomic fibers from the pterygopalatine ganglion to the lacrimal gland. D

21 **Frontal nerve.** Nerve passing through the superior orbital fissure, lies on the levator palpebrae superioris muscle, and continues to the forehead. D

22 *Supra-orbital nerve.* Thickest branch of the frontal nerve which supplies the conjunctiva, upper eyelid, frontal sinus, and the skin of the forehead. D

23 *Lateral branch.* Branch passing laterally through the supraorbital notch. D

24 *Medial branch.* Branch passing medially through the frontal notch. D

25 *Supratrochlear nerve.* Thin, medial branch. It divides at the medial angle of the eye into ascending and descending branches. D

18

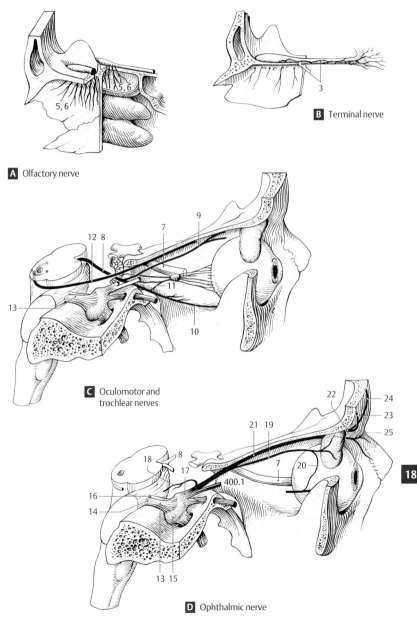

A Olfactory nerve

B Terminal nerve

C Oculomotor and trochlear nerves

D Ophthalmic nerve

18

1   **Nasociliary nerve.** Furthest medial branch of the ophthalmic nerve. It initially lies beneath the superior rectus and then between the superior oblique and medial rectus muscles. A

2   *Communicating branch with ciliary ganglion; Sensory root of ciliary ganglion; Nasociliary root of ciliary ganglion.* Sensory fibers passing through the ciliary ganglion from the eye to the nasociliary nerve. A

3   *Long ciliary nerves.* Two, long, thin branches that carry sympathetic fibers to the dilator pupillae and afferent fibers from the iris, ciliary body, and cornea. A

4   *Posterior ethmoidal nerve.* Nerve emerging at the posterior end of the orbit through the posterior ethmoidal foramen to supply the mucosa of the sphenoidal sinus and posterior ethmoidal cells. A

5   *Anterior meningeal branch.* Branch supplying the anterior part of the anterior cranial fossa.

6   *Anterior ethmoidal nerve.* Nerve emerging through the anterior ethmoidal foramen into the cranial cavity. It travels outside of the dura mater before passing through the cribriform plate of the ethmoid into the nose A B C

7   *Internal nasal branches.* Branches supplying the nasal mucosa anterior to the nasal conchae and anterior nasal septum. B

8   Lateral nasal branches. Branches supplying the lateral wall of the nose. B

9   Medial nasal branches. Branches supplying the nasal septum. C

10   *External nasal nerve.* Branch supplying the skin of the tip of the nose and ala. It passes through the ethmoidal groove of the nasal bone. B

11   *Infratrochlear nerve.* Nerve passing beneath the muscle sling of the superior oblique to the inner angle of the eye. It supplies the lacrimal sac, lacrimal caruncle, and surrounding skin. A

12   *Palpebral branches.* Branches supplying the medial portion of the upper and lower eyelids. A

13   **Maxillary nerve; Maxillary division (Vb; V2).** Second division of the trigeminal nerve. It passes though the foramen rotundum to the pterygopalatine fossa and continues through the orbital fissure into the orbit. A C

14   **Meningeal branch.** Branch given off anterior to the foramen rotundum that passes to the dura mater in the frontal region of the middle meningeal artery. A

15   **Ganglionic branches to pterygopalatine ganglion; Sensory root of pterygopalatine ganglion.** Usually two branches from the pterygopalatine ganglion with parasympathetic fibers supplying the lacrimal glands and small glands of the nose and palate. They also carry sensory fibers from the periosteum of the orbit. A

16   **Orbital branches.** Two or three thin branches that pass through the inferior orbital fissure to the orbit before continuing through the bone to the posterior ethmoidal cells and sphenoidal sinus. B C

17   **Posterior superior lateral nasal branches.** Up to 10 thin branches that pass through the sphenopalatine foramen to the superior and middle nasal conchae and posterior ethmoidal cells. B

18   **Posterior superior medial nasal branches.** Two or three branches that pass through the sphenopalatine foramen to the superior portion of the nasal septum. C

19   **Nasopalatine nerve.** Nerve passing between the periosteum and mucosa of the nasal septum, then through the incisive canal to the anterior portion of the palatine mucosa and gingiva of the upper incisor teeth. C

20   **Pharyngeal nerve.** Thin branch supplying the pharyngeal mucosa. B

21   **Greater palatine nerve.** Nerve traveling in the greater palatine canal and emerging from the greater palatine foramen to supply the mucosa of the hard palate and palatine glands. B

22   *Posterior inferior nasal nerves.* Branches supplying the middle and inferior portions of the nasal passage as well as inferior nasal concha. B

23   **Lesser palatine nerves.** Nerves running in the narrow lesser palatine canals. They emerge through the lesser palatine foramina to supply the soft palate. B

24   *Tonsillar branches.* Branches supplying the palatine tonsils.

25   **Zygomatic nerve.** Nerve that divides in the pterygopalatine fossa. It passes through the inferior orbital fissure to the lateral wall of the orbital cavity and anastomoses with the lacrimal nerve. A

26   *Zygomaticotemporal branch.* Branch passing through the zygomaticotemporal foramen to the skin of the temple. A

27   *Zygomaticofacial branch.* Branch passing through the zygomaticofacial foramen above the zygoma. A

18

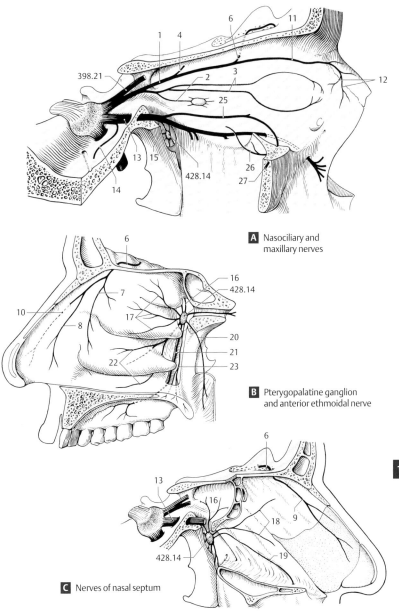

A Nasociliary and maxillary nerves

B Pterygopalatine ganglion and anterior ethmoidal nerve

C Nerves of nasal septum

18

1 **Superior alveolar nerves.** Trunk that gives off the following three branches.

2 *Posterior superior alveolar branches.* Two or three branches that pass through the alveolar foramina to the maxilla. They supply the maxillary sinus, molar teeth, and adjacent buccal gingiva. C

3 *Middle superior alveolar branch.* Branch that enters the maxilla through the infra-orbital groove and runs in the lateral wall of the maxillary sinus to the superior dental plexus, from which it supplies the premolar teeth. C

4 *Anterior superior alveolar branches.* Branches running in a separate canal to the superior dental plexus and from there to the canine, incisor, premolar, and first molar teeth. C

5 *Superior dental plexus.* Network of nerves formed by the superior alveolar branches that lies in the maxilla above the roots of the teeth. C

6 Superior dental branches. Branches supplying individual roots of the teeth. C

7 Superior gingival branches. Branches supplying the gingiva. C

8 **Infra-orbital nerve.** Terminal branch passing through the inferior orbital fissure, infra-orbital groove, infra-orbital canal, and infra-orbital foramen that supplies the skin of the lower lid, nose, upper lip, and cheek. C

9 *Inferior palpebral branches.* Branches given off after traversing the infra-orbital foramen to supply the lower lid. C

10 *External nasal branches.* Branches to the lateral aspect of the ala of the nose. C

11 *Internal nasal branches.* Branches supplying the skin of the nasal vestibule. C

12 *Superior labial branches.* Branches supplying the skin and mucosa of the upper lip. C

13 **Mandibular nerve; Mandibular division (Vc; V3).** Third division of the trigeminal nerve that passes through the foramen ovale into the infratemporal fossa. It contains sensory fibers and motor fibers for the muscles of mastication. A

14 **Meningeal branch; Nervus spinosus.** Nerve passing through the foramen spinosum, accompanying the two branches of the middle meningeal artery. It supplies the dura mater, part of the sphenoidal sinus, and the mastoid cells. A

15 **Nerve to medial pterygoid.** Motor branch supplying the medial pterygoid. Small branches pass to the tensor veli palatini and tensor tympani. A

16 **Branches to otic ganglion; Sensory root of otic ganglion.** Sensory branch communicating with the meningeal branch. It branches off of the nerve to the medial pterygoid. B

17 **Nerve to tensor veli palatini.** Branch supplying the tensor veli palatini. It sometimes arises from the nerve to the medial pterygoid. B

18 **Nerve to tensor tympani.** Branch supplying the tensor tympani that sometimes also supplies the medial pterygoid. B

19 **Masseteric nerve.** Motor branch passing above the lateral pterygoid through the mandibular notch to the masseter. A

20 **Deep temporal nerves.** Motor branches passing from inferior to the temporal muscle. A

21 **Nerve to lateral pterygoid.** Motor branch supplying the lateral pterygoid. It commonly arises together with the buccal nerve. A

22 **Buccal nerve.** Sensory branch supplying the skin and mucosa of the cheek and buccal gingiva near the first molar tooth. A

23 **Auriculotemporal nerve.** Nerve usually encircling the middle meningeal artery. It sends a small branch to the temporomandibular joint and then ascends between the ear and superficial temporal artery to the skin of the temple. A

24 *Nerve to external acoustic meatus.* Usually two small branches that supply the skin of the external acoustic meatus. A

25 *Branches to tympanic membrane.* Tiny branches supplying the tympanic membrane. A

26 *Parotid branches.* Small branches supplying the parotid gland. A

27 *Communicating branches with facial nerve.* Branches communicating with the facial nerve. They convey parasympathetic fibers from the otic ganglion via the facial nerve to the parotid gland. A

28 *Anterior auricular nerves.* Branches supplying the anterior surface of the auricle. A

29 *Superficial temporal branches.* Branches supplying the skin of the temple in front of and above the ear. A

18

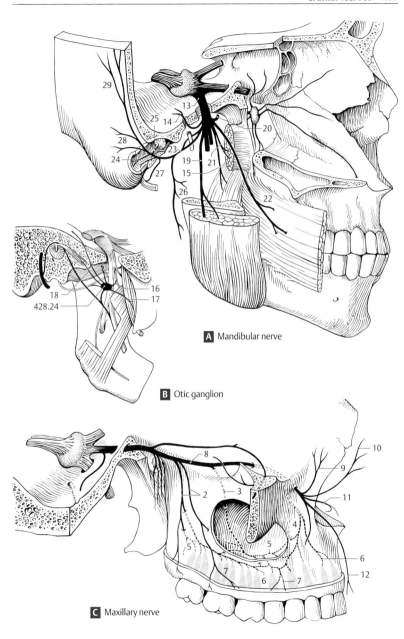

A Mandibular nerve

B Otic ganglion

C Maxillary nerve

18

1 **Lingual nerve.** Branch of the mandibular nerve curving anteriorly between the lateral and medial pterygoid into the floor of the mouth where it lies next to the wisdom tooth immediately beneath the mucosa. A B C

2 *Branches to isthmus of fauces.* Branches supplying the isthmus of the fauces and tonsils. A

3 *Communicating branches with hypoglossal nerve.* Branch communicating with the hypoglossal nerve on the hyoglossus. A

4 *Chorda tympani.* Bundle of parasympathetic fibers to the submandibular ganglion and sensory fibers from the taste buds of the anterior two-thirds of the tongue. As a recurrent nerve it traverses the tympanic cavity, running between the malleus and incus, then continues through the petrotympanic fissure (glaserian fissure) or sphenopetrosal fissure to join the lingual nerve. A

5 *Sublingual nerve.* Branch passing lateral to the sublingual gland into the mucosa of the floor of the mouth and into the gingiva of the anterior mandibular teeth. A

6 *Lingual branches.* Numerous branches to the anterior two-thirds of the mucosa of the tongue containing sensory fibers and taste fibers. A

7 *Ganglionic branches to submandibular ganglion*; *Sensory root of submandibular ganglion.* A

8 *Ganglionic branches to sublingual ganglion*; *Sensory root of sublingual ganglion.* Inconstant branches to the sublingual ganglion, which is also inconstant.

9 **Inferior alveolar nerve.** Thickest branch of the mandibular nerve containing sensory and motor fibers. It enters the mandibular canal through the mandibular foramen approximately 1 cm posterior to the lingual nerve. A B C

10 *Nerve to mylohyoid.* Motor nerve traversing the mylohyoid sulcus and then passing beneath the mylohyoid. It supplies the mylohyoid and anterior belly of the digastric. A B C

11 *Inferior dental plexus.* Nerve plexus lying in the mandibular canal. B

12 *Inferior dental branches.* Branches supplying the teeth of the mandible. B

13 *Inferior gingival branches.* Branches supplying the buccal gingiva of the mandibular teeth (with the exception of the first molar tooth). B

14 **Mental nerve.** Sensory branch emerging through the mental foramen below the second premolar tooth. B

15 *Mental branches.* Branches supplying the chin. B

16 *Labial branches.* Branches supplying the lower lip. B

17 *Gingival branches.* Branches supplying the gingiva of the incisor teeth. B

18 ABDUCENT NERVE; ABDUCENS NERVE (VI). Cranial nerve emerging from the brain at the angle between the pons and medulla oblongata. It penetrates the dura mater at a point half as high as the clivus, continues laterally in the cavernous sinus, and then passes through the superior orbital fissure into the orbit where it supplies the lateral rectus. D

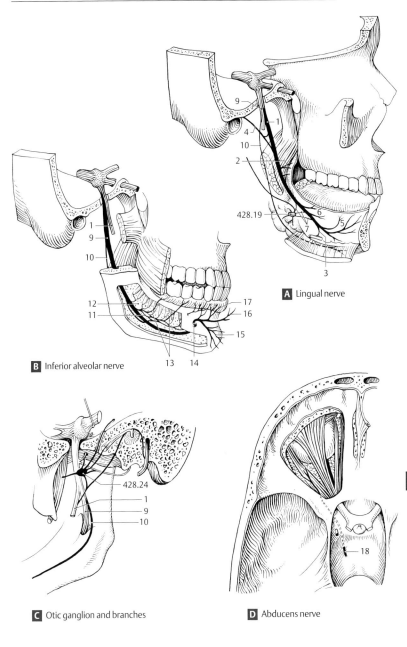

9

4
10

2

428.19

6
7
5

3

A Lingual nerve

1
9
10

12
11

17
16

15

13 14

B Inferior alveolar nerve

428.24

1
9
10

C Otic ganglion and branches

18

D Abducens nerve

18

1   FACIAL NERVE (VII). Nerve arising from the second pharyngeal arch. It emerges from the brain at the pontocerebellar angle between the pons and inferior olive and passes with the vestibulocochlear nerve to the petrous part of the temporal bone, which it exits via the stylomastoid foramen. It supplies the muscles of facial expression. A B C D

2   **Geniculum of facial nerve.** Genu of the facial nerve located just beneath the anterior wall of the petrous part of temporal bone where the facial nerve changes direction from anterolateral to posterolateral. A

3   **Nerve to stapedius.** Branch supplying the stapedius. A

4   **Posterior auricular nerve.** Branch given off below the stylomastoid foramen. It passes superiorly between the mastoid process and external acoustic meatus and supplies the posterior muscles of the ear and occipital belly of occipitofrontalis. B

5   *Occipital branch.* Branch supplying the occipital belly of occipitofrontalis. B

6   *Auricular branch.* Branch to the muscles of the auricle. B

7   **Digastric branch.** Branch supplying the posterior belly of digastric. A B

8   **Stylohyoid branch.** Branch supplying the stylohyoid that sometimes arises together with the lingual branch. A

9   **Communicating branch with glossopharyngeal nerve.** A

10   **Parotid plexus.** Facial nerve plexus in the connective-tissue space between the two portions of the parotid gland. B

11   **Temporal branches.** Branches ascending over the zygomatic arch to supply the muscles of facial expression above the palpebral fissure and ear. B

12   **Zygomatic branches.** Branches supplying the lateral portion of the orbicularis oculi and mimetic muscles between the lid and oral fissure. B

13   **Buccal branches.** Branches supplying the buccinator and mimetic muscles around the mouth. B

14   **[[Lingual branch]].** Inconstant sensory branch supplying the tongue.

15   **Marginal mandibular branch.** Branch traveling above the mandibular margin and supplying the muscles of facial expression below the oral fissure. B

16   **Cervical branch.** Motor branch supplying the platysma. It anastomoses with the transverse cervical nerve. B

17   **Intermediate nerve.** Nonmotor portion of the facial nerve. It emerges from the brainstem between the facial and vestibulocochlear nerves and conveys autonomic and taste fibers. After various anastomoses, it merges with the facial nerve in the petrous part of the temporal bone. D

18   **Geniculate ganglion.** Equivalent of a spinal ganglion located at the geniculum of the facial nerve in the petrous part of the temporal bone. It contains pseudounipolar ganglion cells that form the chorda tympani. A

19   **Chorda tympani; Parasympathetic root of submandibular ganglion.** Parasympathetic fibers of the chorda tympani that travel to the submandibular ganglion. C

20   **Greater petrosal nerve; Parasympathetic root of pterygopalatine ganglion.** Nerve leaving CN VII at the geniculate ganglion as a bundle of parasympathetic fibers. It reaches the anterior surface of the petrous pyramid, passes through the foramen lacerum, and travels with the deep petrosal nerve in the pterygoid canal to the pterygopalatine ganglion. A C

21   **Sympathetic root; Deep petrosal nerve.** Sympathetic fibers from the internal carotid plexus. They unite with the greater petrosal nerve to form the nerve of the pterygoid canal. C

22   **Nerve of pterygoid canal.** Nerve lying in the pterygoid canal situated in the root of the pterygoid process. It contains parasympathetic and sympathetic fibers and passes to the pterygopalatine ganglion. C

23   **Sympathetic root of submandibular ganglion.** Sympathetic fibers from the internal carotid plexus. They pass to the submandibular ganglion via the facial artery and do not synapse. C

24   **Communicating branch with tympanic plexus.** A

25   **Communicating branch with vagus nerve.** Communicating branch located immediately beneath the stylomastoid foramen.

18

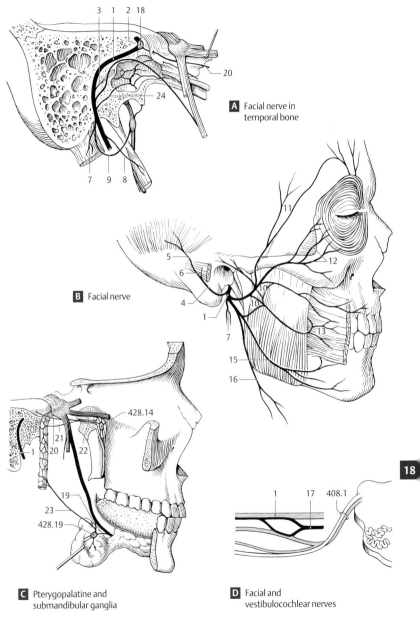

A Facial nerve in temporal bone

B Facial nerve

C Pterygopalatine and submandibular ganglia

D Facial and vestibulocochlear nerves

18

1 VESTIBULOCOCHLEAR NERVE (VIII). Nerve conveying sensory fibers through the internal acoustic meatus. It exits the internal acoustic opening beneath the facial nerve and enters the rhombencephalon at the pontocerebellar angle. A

2 **Vestibular nerve.** Collection of fibers of the vestibular apparatus that travel to the vestibular nuclei. Upper portion of the vestibulocochlear nerve. A

3 **Vestibular ganglion.** Vestibular nerve ganglion lying in the floor of the internal acoustic meatus. It is composed of bipolar nerve cells. A

4 *Cochlear communicating branch.* Branch communicating with the cochlear nerve.

5 *Superior part of vestibular ganglion.* A

6 *Utriculo-ampullary nerve.* Fibers from the macula of the utricle and ampullary crest of the anterior and lateral semicircular canal. A

7 *Utricular nerve.* Fibers from the macula of the utricle. A

8 *Anterior ampullary nerve.* Fibers from the ampullary crest of the anterior semicircular canal. A

9 *Lateral ampullary nerve.* Fibers from the ampullary crest of the lateral semicircular canal. A

10 **Inferior part of vestibular ganglion.** A

11 *Posterior ampullary nerve.* Fibers from the ampullary crest of the posterior semicircular canal. A

12 *Saccular nerve.* Fibers from the macula of saccule. A

13 **Cochlear nerve.** Collection of fibers passing from the cochlea to the cochlear ganglion. A

14 **Cochlear ganglion; Spiral ganglion.** Spiral strip of ganglion cells along the base of the osseous spiral lamina of the axis of the cochlea. A

15 GLOSSOPHARYNGEAL NERVE (IX). Nerve arising from the third pharyngeal arch. It emerges from the medulla oblongata via the retro-olivary groove, passes through the jugular foramen, and descends obliquely behind the stylopharyngeus. It supplies motor fibers innervating the constrictor muscles of the pharynx and stylopharyngeus; sensory fibers innervating the pharyngeal mucosa, tonsils, and posterior one-third of the tongue (taste fibers); and parasympathetic fibers via the tympanic nerve and lesser petrosal nerve to the otic ganglion. B

16 **Superior ganglion.** Upper, small sensory ganglion situated either in or above the jugular foramen. B C

17 **Inferior ganglion.** Lower, larger, sensory ganglion below the jugular foramen. B C

18 **Tympanic nerve.** First branch that leaves the interior ganglion and enters the tympanic cavity through the tympanic canaliculus between the jugular foramen and carotid canal. C

19 *Tympanic enlargement; Tympanic ganglion.* Irregularly scattered ganglion cells interposed in the course of the tympanic nerve. C

20 *Tympanic plexus.* Nerve plexus lying in the mucosa above the promontory of the tympanic cavity. It is formed by the tympanic nerve, the internal carotid plexus, and the communicating branch with tympanic plexus of the facial nerve. C

21 *Tubal branch.* Branch supplying the auditory tube. C

22 *Caroticotympanic nerves.* Sympathetic portion of the tympanic plexus arising from the internal carotid plexus. C

23 **Communicating branch with auricular branch of vagus nerve.** Tiny branch from the inferior ganglion to the auricular branch of vagus nerve. B

24 **Pharyngeal branches.** Three or four branches passing to the pharyngeal plexus. B

25 **Stylopharyngeal branch.** Branch supplying the stylopharyngeus. B

26 **Carotid branch.** Branch supplying the carotid sinus and carotid body. It communicates with the sympathetic trunk and vagus nerve. B

27 **Tonsillar branches.** Branches supplying the mucosa of the palatine tonsil and surrounding region. B

28 **Lingual branches.** Taste fibers for the posterior one-third of the tongue including the vallate papillae, which are also supplied by the lingual nerve via the chorda tympani. B

29 **Lesser petrosal nerve; Parasympathetic root of otic ganglion.** Nerve containing parasympathetic fibers from the glossopharyngeal nerve. It arises from the tympanic plexus, penetrates the anterior wall of the petrous part of temporal bone, and emerges from the middle cranial fossa through the sphenopetrosal fissure. Its fibers synapse in the otic ganglion. C D

30 **Communicating branch with meningeal branch.** Branch communicating with the meningeal branch of mandibular nerve. D

31 **Communicating branch with auriculotemporal nerve.** Branch containing postganglionic parasympathetic fibers that supply the parotid gland. D

32 **Communicating branch with chorda tympani.** Sensory branch that communicates with the chorda tympani. D

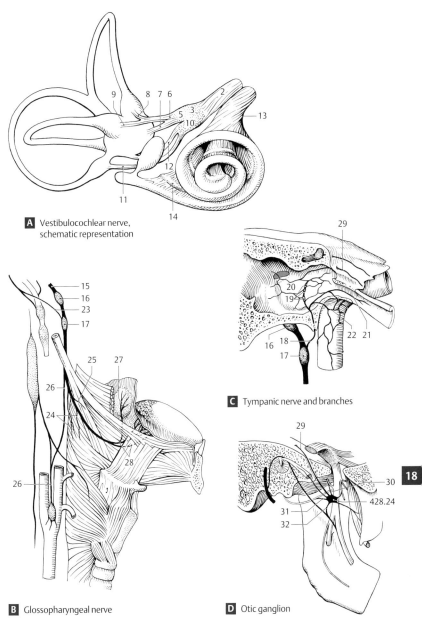

A Vestibulocochlear nerve, schematic representation

B Glossopharyngeal nerve

C Tympanic nerve and branches

D Otic ganglion

18

1 VAGUS NERVE (X). Nerve arising from the fourth and fifth pharyngeal arches. It emerges from the medulla oblongata together with CN IX in the posterolateral sulcus and passes through the jugular foramen. Its distribution area extends into the thoracic and abdominal cavities. A

2 **Superior ganglion.** Small, upper sensory ganglion situated in the jugular foramen. A

3 **Meningeal branch.** Recurrent branch from the superior ganglion to the dura mater of the posterior cranial fossa near the transverse and occipital sinuses. A

4 **Auricular branch.** Branch passing from the superior ganglion into the mastoid canaliculus and through the tympanomastoid fissure to the posterior surface of the auricle and beneath the external acoustic meatus. A

5 **Inferior ganglion.** Lower, larger, spindle-shaped ganglion. A

6 **Communicating branch with glossopharyngeal nerve.** A

7 **Pharyngeal branch.** Branches radiating into the pharyngeal plexus. A

8 *Pharyngeal plexus.* Nerve plexus lying beneath the middle constrictor muscle of the pharynx. It is formed by the glossopharyngeal and vagus nerves as well as the cervical portion of the sympathetic trunk. A

9 **Superior laryngeal nerve.** Nerve arising form the inferior ganglion and descending medial to the internal carotid artery to supply the larynx. A

10 *External branch.* Part giving off branches to the internal constrictor muscle of the pharynx. It travels covered by the infrahyoid muscles to the cricothyroid muscle. A

11 *Internal branch.* Branch piercing the thyrohyoid membrane together with the superior laryngeal artery. It extends to beneath the mucosa of the piriform recess and supplies the mucosa of the epiglottic valleculae, epiglottis, and larynx to near the rima glottidis. A

12 *Communicating branch with recurrent laryngeal nerve.* A

13 **Superior cervical cardiac branches.** Branches to the deep part of the cardiac nerve plexus. They are given off to by the right and left vagus, sometimes at a very high level. A

14 **Inferior cervical cardiac branches.** Branches passing on the right to the deep portion of the cardiac plexus and on the left accompanying the vagus nerve to the superficial part of the cardiac plexus. A

15 **Recurrent laryngeal nerve.** Branch of the vagus nerve that extends on the right around the subclavian artery and on the left around the aortic arch. It runs in the groove between the trachea and esophagus to the larynx. Its terminal portion penetrates the inferior pharyngeal constrictor and supplies the mucosa to about the rima glottis as well as all laryngeal muscles with the exception of the cricothyroid. It communicates with the internal branch of superior laryngeal nerve. A

16 *Tracheal branches.* Branches to the trachea. A

17 *Esophageal branches.* Branches to the esophagus. A

18 *Pharyngeal branches.* Branches to the inferior pharyngeal constrictor.

19 **Thoracic cardiac branches.** Cardiac branches to the thoracic inlet. A

20 **Bronchial branches.** Branches given off below the recurrent laryngeal nerve to the hilum of lung. A

21 **Pulmonary plexus.** Plexus lying anterior and posterior to the hilum of lung that supplies the bronchia, vessels, and visceral pleura. A

22 **Esophageal plexus.** Nerve plexus surrounding the esophagus. It is formed by the two vagus nerves superiorly and also by the left recurrent laryngeal nerve. A

23 **Anterior vagal trunk.** Smaller, anterior nerve plexus arising from the esophageal plexus with fibers from both vagus nerves. A

24 *Anterior gastric branches.* Branches supplying the anterior surface of the stomach. A

25 *Anterior nerve of lesser curvature.* Branch running along the anterior aspect of the lesser curvature of the stomach.

26 *Hepatic branches.* Branches to the porta hepatis. A

27 *Pyloric branch.* Branch to the pylorus.

28 **Posterior vagal trunk.** Larger, posterior nerve plexus arising from the esophageal plexus and formed by the two vagus nerves. A

29 *Posterior gastric branches.* Branches supplying the posterior wall of the stomach. A

30 *Posterior nerve of lesser curvature.* Nerve running along the posterior aspect of the lesser curvature of the stomach.

31 *Celiac branches.* Branches to the celiac plexus. A

32 **Renal branches.** Branches to the renal plexus. A

33 [[Inferior laryngeal nerve]]. Terminal branch of the recurrent laryngeal nerve.

18

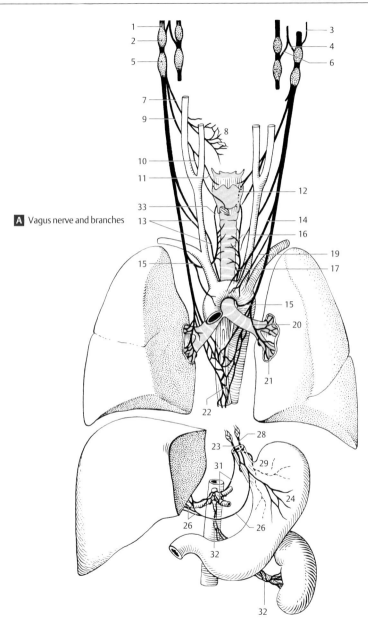

A Vagus nerve and branches

18

1   ACCESSORY NERVE (XI). Nerve arising with two roots forming a single trunk that emerges through the jugular foramen along with CN IX and CN X, before dividing into two branches again. A

2   **Cranial root; Vagal part.** Fibers from the nucleus ambiguus that leave the accessory nerve in the jugular foramen to join the vagus nerve. A

3   **Spinal root; Spinal part.** Fibers traveling from the bases of the anterior horns of C1–C6 through the subarachnoid space into the cranium, where they unite for a short distance with cranial root fibers. A

4   **Trunk of accessory nerve.** Nerve trunk formed by the union of the two roots. A

5   *Internal branch.* Branch formed by united cranial root fibers that joins the vagus nerve. A

6   *External branch.* United spinal root fibers. They supply the sternocleidomastoid and trapezius. A

7   *Muscular branches.* Branches passing to the sternocleidomastoid and trapezius. A

8   HYPOGLOSSAL NERVE (XII). Motor nerve supplying the tongue. It emerges from the brain between the medulla oblongata and inferior olive with numerous roots. Traveling in the hypoglossal canal, it curves anteriorly between the internal jugular vein and internal carotid artery and continues over the posterior border of the floor of the mouth into the tongue. C

9   **Lingual branches.** Branches arising lateral to the hyoglossus that supply the styloglossus, hyoglossus, genioglossus, and intrinsic muscles of the tongue. C

10 *SPINAL NERVES.* Nerves of the spinal cord. Portion of the nerve between the union of both roots and its bifurcation behind the intervertebral foramen: trunk of spinal nerve. B

11 **CERVICAL NERVES (C1–C8).** The eight spinal nerves of the cervical vertebral column. C

12 POSTERIOR RAMI; DORSAL RAMI. Posterior branches of the spinal nerves with branches supplying the neck muscles as well as the skin of the neck and occiput. B

13 **Medial branch.** Branch supplying the shorter autochthonous muscles located close to the vertebrae. It supplies a hand-wide region along the vertebral column as far as the upper thoracic vertebral column. B

14 **Lateral branch.** Branch supplying the generally longer, autochthonous back muscles lying close to the ribs. It supplies the skin to a lesser extent in the cervical region. B

15 *Posterior cutaneous branch.* Branch innervating the skin, usually after T6.

16 **Suboccipital nerve.** Dorsal branch of the first spinal nerve. It exits between the vertebral artery and posterior arch of atlas and supplies the short muscles of the neck. D

17 **Greater occipital nerve.** Dorsal branch of the second spinal nerve. It emerges between the axis and obliquus capitis inferior, penetrates the trapezius, and supplies the neck muscles and skin of the occiput up to the vertex. D

18 **Third occipital nerve.** Dorsal branch of the third spinal nerve. It supplies the skin of the neck close to the midline. D

19 **Posterior cervical plexus.** Plexus formed by the posterior rami of cervical nerves and their intersegmental communicating branches.

20 ANTERIOR RAMI; VENTRAL RAMI. Anterior branches of the spinal nerve. They form the cervical and brachial plexuses. B

21 CERVICAL PLEXUS. Nerve plexus formed by the anterior rami of the first four spinal nerves. It supplies the skin and muscles of the neck.

22 **Ansa cervicalis.** Nerve loop formed by the first, second, and third cervical spinal nerves. It distributes branches to the infrahyoid muscles. C

23 *Superior root; Superior limb.* Root lying for a short distance on the hypoglossal nerve, then descending along the medial side of the internal jugular vein and passing into the inferior root. C

24 *Inferior root; Inferior limb.* Root descending obliquely deep to the sternocleidomastoid and superficial to the internal jugular vein. It anastomoses with the superior root. C

25 *Thyrohyoid branch.* Branch supplying the thyrohyoid. C

26 *[[Geniohyoid branch]].* Branch supplying the geniohyoid. C

27 **Lesser occipital nerve.** Uppermost cutaneous branch of the cervical plexus. It ascends along the posterior margin of the sternocleidomastoid and branches off as a lateral communicating nerve of the greater occipital nerve at the occiput. D

28 **Great auricular nerve.** Nerve ascending vertically near the middle line of the sternocleidomastoid to the ear. D

29 *Posterior branch.* Branch supplying the skin of the posterior surface of the auricle and the adjacent area. D

30 *Anterior branch.* Branch supplying the skin of the anterior surface of the auricle as far as the angle of the mandible. D

19

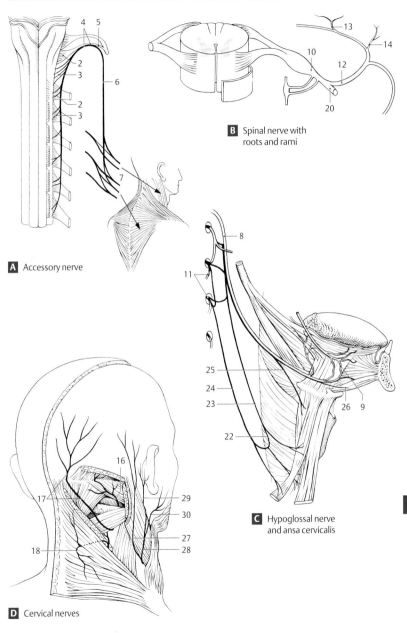

A Accessory nerve

B Spinal nerve with roots and rami

C Hypoglossal nerve and ansa cervicalis

D Cervical nerves

19

1 **Transverse cervical nerve.** Third nerve from the nerve point lying behind the middle of the sternocleidomastoid. It arises from C3 and passes beneath the platysma anteriorly to the skin. It receives motor fibers from the cervical branch of facial nerve that supply the platysma. B

2 *Superior branches.* Ascending branches to the suprahyoid region. B

3 *Inferior branches.* Descending branches to the infrahyoid region. B

4 **Supraclavicular nerves.** Cutaneous branches from C3 and C4 that radiate in a fanlike manner into the shoulder and clavicular regions. B

5 *Medial supraclavicular nerves.* Nerves passing over the medial one-third of the clavicle where they supply the skin of the neck and chest as far as the sternal angle as well as the sternoclavicular joint. B

6 *Intermediate supraclavicular nerves.* Nerves passing beneath the platysma over the middle one-third of the clavicle. They supply the skin to the level of the fourth rib. B

7 *Lateral supraclavicular nerves.* Posterior group of nerves that supplies the skin overlying the acromion, deltoid, and acromioclavicular joint. B

8 **Phrenic nerve.** Nerve arising from C4 with accessory branches from C3 and C5. It lies on the anterior scalene muscle and then passes anterior to the hilum of lung to the diaphragm, with some fibers continuing into the peritoneum. A C

9 **Pericardial branch.** Tiny branch to the anterior surface of the pericardium. A

10 **Phrenico-abdominal branches.** Fibers passing on the right through the caval opening and on the left further anteriorly through the diaphragm at the left margin of the heart to the peritoneum. They supply the peritoneum to as far as the gallbladder and pancreas. A

11 **[Accessory phrenic nerves].** Common accessory roots of the phrenic nerve from C5 and C6 via the subclavian nerve. A C

12 BRACHIAL PLEXUS. Nerve plexus formed by the ventral rami of spinal nerves C5–T1 that supplies the arm and partly also the shoulder girdle. It passes between the anterior and middle scalene muscles to the head of humerus. It can be divided into supraclavicular and infraclavicular parts. C

13 **Roots.**

14 **Trunks.** Three primary trunks of brachial plexus, which are usually formed by one or two ventral spinal nerve rami. They lie superior to the clavicle.

15 *Superior trunk; Upper trunk.* Superior primary trunk of brachial plexus formed by C5 and C6. It usually arises lateral to the scalene space. C

16 *Middle trunk.* Middle primary trunk of brachial plexus formed by C7. C

17 *Inferior trunk; Lower trunk.* Inferior primary trunk of brachial plexus formed by C8 and T1. It lies in the scalene space posterior to the subclavian artery. C

18 **Anterior divisions.** Anterior branches of the three trunks that supply the flexor muscles.

19 **Posterior divisions.** Posterior branches of the three trunks that form the posterior cord and supply the extensor muscles.

20 **Cords.** Branches of the brachial plexus re-allocated to secondary trunks.

21 SUPRACLAVICULAR PART. Portion of the brachial plexus extending as far as the upper margin of the clavicle. Its branches directly supply the shoulder girdle muscles. C

22 **Dorsal scapular nerve.** Nerve arising directly from C5 and piercing the middle scalene muscle. It runs deep to the levator scapulae and the two rhomboids, which it supplies. C

23 **Long thoracic nerve.** Nerve arising from C5–C7, piercing the middle scalene muscle, and then running on the serratus anterior, which it innervates. C

24 **Subclavian nerve.** Thin nerve arising from the superior trunk containing fibers from C4 and C5 that innervates the subclavius. It often distributes a branch to the phrenic nerve. C

25 **Suprascapular nerve.** Nerve formed by C5 and C6 that runs via the brachial plexus to the suprascapular notch and then passes deep to the superior transverse scapular ligament to the supraspinatus and infraspinatus. C

26 **Subscapular nerves.** Two or three branches arising from the brachial plexus, supraclavicular part, or posterior cord. They supply the subscapularis and teres major. p. 419 D

27 **Thoracodorsal nerve.** Longest subscapular nerve arising from C6–C8. It runs along the lateral border of the scapula and supplies the latissimus dorsi. p. 419 D

28 **Medial pectoral nerve.** Fibers from C8 and T1 that supply the pectoralis major and minor. They can arise from the inferior trunk or medial cord. C

29 **Lateral pectoral nerve.** Fibers arising from C5–C7 that supply both pectoral muscles. They can arise from the superior and middle trunk or from the lateral cord. C

30 **Muscular branches.** Variable branches supplying the muscles.

19

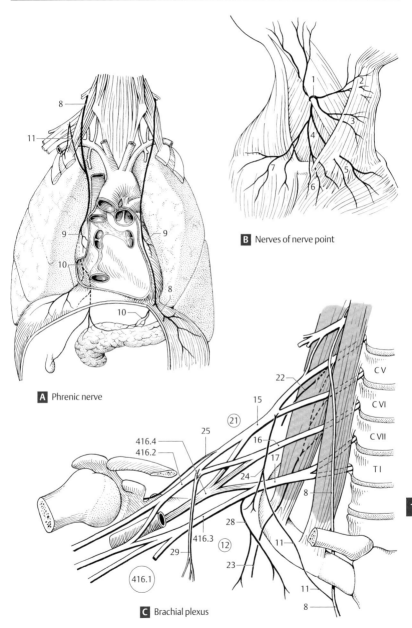

A Phrenic nerve

B Nerves of nerve point

C Brachial plexus

1 INFRACLAVICULAR PART. Inferior portion of the brachial plexus extending from the superior border of the clavicle to the division of the cords into individual nerves. p. 415 C

2 **Lateral cord.** Fascicle formed by the anterior branches of the superior and middle trunks (formed by C5–C7) lying lateral to the axillary artery. p. 415 C

3 **Medial cord.** Fascicle formed by the anterior branch of the inferior trunk (formed by C8, T1) lying medial to the axillary artery. p. 415 C

4 **Posterior cord.** Fascicle formed by the posterior branches of all three trunks (C5–C8) lying posterior to the axillary artery. p. 415 C

5 **Musculocutaneous nerve.** Nerve arising from the lateral cord that pierces the coracobrachialis, which it supplies along with the biceps and brachialis. It ends as the lateral cutaneous nerve of forearm. A

6 **Muscular branches.** Branches to the coracobrachialis, biceps, and brachialis. A

7 **Lateral cutaneous nerve of forearm; Lateral antebrachial cutaneous nerve.** Terminal branch of the musculocutaneous nerve that pierces the brachial fascia at the elbow and supplies the skin of the lateral forearm. A

8 **Medial cutaneous nerve of arm; Medial brachial cutaneous nerve.** Nerve arising from the medial cord and supplying the skin of the medial side of the arm via its communication with the intercostobrachial nerve. A

9 **Medial cutaneous nerve of forearm; Medial antebrachial cutaneous nerve.** Nerve arising from the medial cord, piercing the fascia at about the middle of the arm, and accompanying the basilic vein. It supplies the skin of the medial side of the distal part of the arm and forearm. A

10 **Anterior branch.** Anterior branch of the medial cutaneous nerve of forearm. It supplies the medial flexor aspect of the forearm. A

11 **Posterior branch.** Posterior branch of the medial cutaneous nerve of forearm. It supplies the upper two-thirds of the posterior side of forearm. A B

12 **Median nerve.** Nerve formed by the medial and lateral cords. A

13 **Medial root of median nerve.** Portion of the median nerve arising from the medial cord. A

14 **Lateral root of median nerve.** Portion of the median nerve arising from the lateral cord. A

15 **Anterior interosseous nerve.** Nerve arising at the elbow from the posterior side of the median nerve and running on the interosseous membrane. Distribution area: wrist joint, intercarpal joints, flexor pollicis longus, flexor digitorum profundus (radial portion), and pronator quadratus. A

16 **Muscular branches.** Branches supplying the pronator teres, flexor carpi radialis, palmaris longus, and flexor digitorum superficialis. A

17 **Palmar branch of median nerve.** Branch arising in the distal one-third of the forearm and supplying the skin of the lateral part of the palm. A

18 **Communicating branch with ulnar nerve.** A

19 **Common palmar digital nerves.** Nerves traveling toward the spaces between the first and fourth fingers and then dividing. A

20 *Proper palmar digital nerves.* Terminal branches of the common palmar digital nerves. They supply the skin of the palmar side of the radial 3½ fingers and the skin of the dorsal side of the 2½ radial distal phalanges. A

21 **Ulnar nerve.** Nerve arising from the medial cord that initially travels in the medial bicipital groove, pierces the medial intermuscular septum of the arm, and, after traversing the groove for the ulnar nerve, penetrates the flexor carpi ulnaris. C

22 **Muscular branches.** Branches to the flexor carpi ulnaris and ulnar portion of the flexor digitorum profundus. C

23 **Dorsal branch of ulnar nerve.** Cutaneous branch passing between the distal and middle one-third of the forearm deep to the flexor carpi ulnaris to the dorsum of hand. B C

24 *Dorsal digital nerves.* Individual branches to the little finger, ring finger, and ulnar side of the middle finger. The distribution area can be constricted by the radial nerve. B

25 **Palmar branch of ulnar nerve.** Nerve arising in the distal one-third of the forearm, piercing the deep fascia, and supplying the skin of the ulnar side of the palm. C

26 **Superficial branch.** Branch lying beneath the palmar aponeurosis that divides into the common palmar digital nerves and sends a thin branch to the palmaris brevis. C

27 *Common palmar digital nerves.* Usually a single branch that travels toward the space between the ring finger and little finger. C

28 *Proper palmar digital nerve.* Principal nerves supplying the little finger and ulnar side of the ring finger. They also supply the dorsal aspect of the middle and distal phalanges of the 1 ulnar fingers. C

29 **Deep branch.** Deep branch of the ulnar nerve. It curves around the hamulus, supplies the hypothenar muscles, the interossei, the two ulnar lumbricals, adductor pollicis, and the deep head of flexor pollicis brevis. C

19

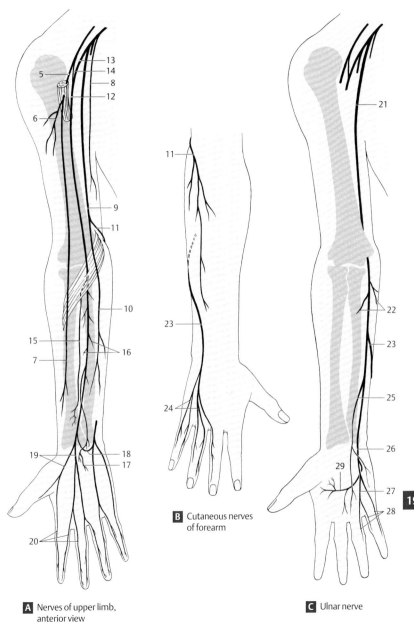

A Nerves of upper limb, anterior view

B Cutaneous nerves of forearm

C Ulnar nerve

19

1 **Radial nerve.** Nerve arising from the posterior cord (usually with fibers from C5–T1) spiraling in the groove for the radial nerve around the posterior side of the humerus, then continuing laterally between the brachialis and brachioradialis as well as the extensor carpi radiales. It divides at the elbow into deep and superficial branches. A B D

2 **Posterior cutaneous nerve of arm; Posterior brachial cutaneous nerve.** Small cutaneous branch on the extensor side of the arm. A

3 **Inferior lateral cutaneous nerve of arm; Inferior lateral brachial cutaneous nerve.** Second cutaneous branch supplying the lateral and dorsal surfaces of the arm below the deltoid. A

4 **Posterior cutaneous nerve of forearm; Posterior antebrachial cutaneous nerve.** Cutaneous branch supplying the area between the lateral and medial cutaneous nerves of forearm. B

5 **Muscular branches.** Motor branches to the triceps, anconeus, brachioradialis, and extensor carpi radialis longus. A

6 **Deep branch.** Deep branch supplying the extensor muscles of the forearm. It penetrates the supinator muscle, and supplies it and all extensor muscles (except the extensor carpi radialis longus) as well as the abductor pollicis longus. A B

7 *Posterior interosseous nerve.* Terminal branch of the deep branch of the radial nerve. It lies in the distal one-third of the forearm beneath the extensor muscles and on top of the interosseous membrane, extending as far as the wrist joint. A

8 **Superficial branch.** Superficial cutaneous branch that runs along the brachioradialis with the radial artery, and then crosses under its accompanying muscle to reach the dorsum of hand and the fingers. A B

9 *Communicating branch with ulnar nerve.* Branch communicating with the dorsal branch of the ulnar nerve on the dorsum of hand. A

10 *Dorsal digital branches.* Terminal branches of the superficial branch of the radial nerve on the ulnar and radial extensor sides of the lateral 2½, and sometimes 3½ fingers. A

11 **Axillary nerve.** Nerve arising from the posterior cord (C5, C6). Accompanied by the posterior circumflex humeral artery, it passes through the lateral (quadrangular) space to the teres minor and deltoid. D

12 **Muscular branches.** Fibers to the teres minor and deltoid. D

13 **Superior lateral cutaneous nerve of arm; Superior lateral brachial cutaneous nerve.** Branch supplying the skin overlying the deltoid. D

14 **THORACIC NERVES (T1–T12).** The twelve thoracic spinal nerves that emerge below T1–T12, respectively. C

15 POSTERIOR RAMI; DORSAL RAMI. Dorsal branches passing through the autochthonous muscles of the back. After supplying these muscles, they divide into a lateral and a medial cutaneous branch. C

16 **Medial branch.** Branches from T1–T6 that supply the skin lateral to the spinous processes. T7–T12 usually do not have any cutaneous branches. C

17 **Lateral branch.** Motor supply of mainly the longissimus thoracic and iliocostalis. T1–T6 only sometimes give off cutaneous branches. T7–T12 have well-developed cutaneous branches. C

18 **Posterior cutaneous branch; Posterior cutaneous nerve.** Descending branches from the lateral branch passing to the skin of the back as far as the level of the iliac crest.

19 INTERCOSTAL NERVES; ANTERIOR RAMI; VENTRAL RAMI. Nerves accompanying vessels to the intercostal spaces. C

20 **Muscular branches.**

21 **Collateral branch.** Branches of the main nerve lying anterior and caudal in the intercostal space, sometimes also present as an accessory cutaneous branches.

22 **Lateral pectoral cutaneous branch.** Branches in the midaxillary line between the slips of the serratus anterior that pass to the lateral thoracic wall. C

23 *Lateral mammary branches.* Nerves leaving the cutaneous branches to the mammary region. C

24 **Lateral abdominal cutaneous branch.** Branches coursing in the midaxillary line between the slips of the serratus anterior to the lateral abdominal wall.

25 **Intercostobrachial nerves.** Fibers from T2 and T3 of the lateral cutaneous branch. The fiber bundle passes through the axilla to the medial cutaneous nerve of arm. C

26 **Anterior pectoral cutaneous branch.** Cutaneous branches emerging anteromedially. C

27 *Medial mammary branches.* Branches of the anterior pectoral cutaneous branch that pass to the mammary region. A

28 **Anterior abdominal cutaneous branch.** Cutaneous branches that course to the anterior abdominal wall.

29 **Subcostal nerve.** Ventral branch of the twelfth thoracic spinal nerve that lies below the twelfth rib.

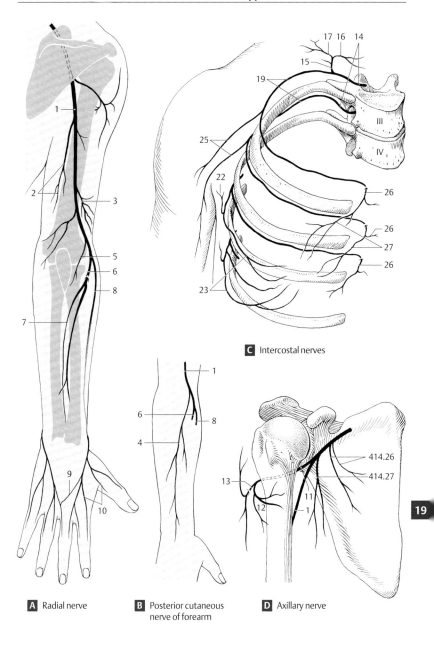

A Radial nerve

B Posterior cutaneous nerve of forearm

C Intercostal nerves

D Axillary nerve

19

1 **LUMBAR NERVES (L1–L5).** The five lumbar spinal nerves that emerge below the respective lumbar vertebrae.

2 POSTERIOR RAMI; DORSAL RAMI. Dorsal branches supplying the autochthonous muscles of the back and overlying skin. C

3 **Medial branch.** Thin, medial branches. C

4 **Lateral branch.** Mostly sensory, lateral branches. C

5 **Posterior cutaneous branch; Posterior cutaneous nerve.** Larger, descending lateral branches.

6 **Superior clunial nerves.** Nerves formed by the posterior rami of L1–L3 that supply the skin as far as the greater trochanter. B

7 **Posterior plexus.** Interconnected posterior rami.

8 ANTERIOR RAMI; VENTRAL RAMI. Anterior branches forming the lumbar plexus. C

9 **SACRAL NERVES AND COCCYGEAL NERVE (S1–S5, Co).** The five sacral spinal nerves and the one coccygeal spinal nerve.

10 POSTERIOR RAMI; DORSAL RAMI. Posterior branches emerging through the posterior sacral foramina. A B

11 **Medial branch.** Branches passing to the multifidus and the skin overlying the sacrum and coccyx. A B

12 **Lateral branch.** Sensory branches emerging from S1–S3 that supply the skin overlying the coccyx. A B

13 **Posterior cutaneous branch; Posterior cutaneous nerve.** Thicker branches of the lateral branches.

14 **Medial clunial nerves.** Sensory nerves formed by the lateral branches of S1–S3. They penetrate the gluteus maximus and innervate the skin of the medial, superior portion of the buttocks. B

15 ANTERIOR RAMI; VENTRAL RAMI. Anterior branches of the sacral nerves that form the sacral plexus. C

16 LUMBOSACRAL PLEXUS. Communication between the lumbar and sacral plexuses via the lumbosacral trunk. C

17 LUMBAR PLEXUS. Plexus formed by the anterior rami of L1–L3 and portions of T12 and L4. Its nerves lie mainly along the inferior abdominal wall and anterior surface of the leg.

18 **Iliohypogastric nerve; Iliopubic nerve.** Nerve containing sensory and motor fibers from L1 and T12 that supplies the abdominal muscles. It traverses the psoas major and continues between the transverse abdominal and internal oblique muscles, which it pierces medial to the anterior superior iliac spine. C

19 **Lateral cutaneous branch.** Branch that can extend as far as the lateral gluteal region. C

20 **Anterior cutaneous branch.** Branch that often penetrates the aponeurosis of the external oblique just above the superficial inguinal ring where it supplies the skin. C

21 **Ilio-inguinal nerve.** It usually arises from L1 and emerges at the lateral border of the psoas. It travels between the kidney and quadratus lumborum, then between the transverse abdominal and internal oblique muscles, continuing through the inguinal canal. C

22 **Anterior labial nerves.** Sensory branches supplying the labia majora, mons pubis, and adjacent skin of the thigh. C

23 **Anterior scrotal nerves.** Sensory branches supplying the anterior scrotal skin, adjacent skin of the thigh and the symphysis. C

24 **Genitofemoral nerve.** Nerve arising from L1 and L2 that pierces and lies on top of the psoas major. C

25 **Genital branch.** Branch running through the inguinal canal that supplies the cremaster, scrotal skin (labium majus), and adjacent skin of the thigh. C

26 **Femoral branch.** Branch passing through the vascular space and continuing through the saphenous opening to supply the overlying skin. C

27 **Lateral cutaneous nerve of thigh; Lateral femoral cutaneous nerve.** It arises from L2 and L3 and emerges at the lateral border of the psoas. It travels beneath the iliac fascia through the lateral part of the muscular space and either deep or superficial to the sartorius, continuing to the skin of the lateral aspect of the thigh. C

28 **Obturator nerve.** It arises from L2–L4 and travels beneath the psoas, posterior to the internal iliac artery, lateral to the ureter, continuing through the obturator canal to the adductors and the skin of the medial aspect of the thigh. C

29 **Anterior branch.** Branch lying on the adductor brevis and obturator externus, beneath the adductor longus and pectineus. It supplies these muscles as well as the gracilis. C

30 *Cutaneous branch.* Variable terminal branch that emerges between the adductor longus and gracilis and supplies the skin of the distal two-thirds of the thigh. C

31 *Muscular branches.* Branches that supply the adductor muscles of the thigh with the exception of the adductor magnus.

19

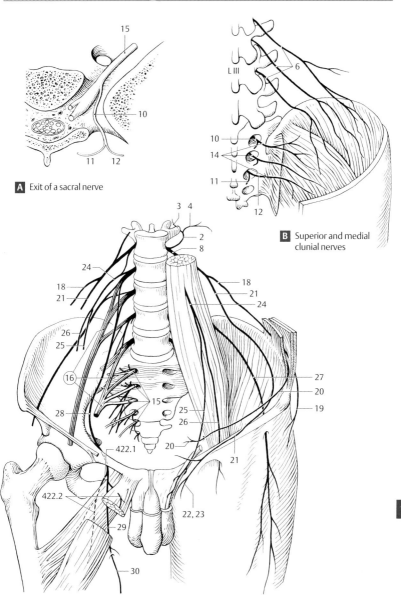

A Exit of a sacral nerve

B Superior and medial clunial nerves

C Lumbar plexus

19

1 **Posterior branch.** Branch piercing the obturator externus and supplying it as well as the adductor magnus and brevis. It sends a sensory branch to the knee joint. p. 421 C

2 *Muscular branches.* Branches supplying the muscles mentioned above. p. 421 C

3 *Articular branch.* Sensory branch that extends into the posterior wall of the knee joint.

4 **Accessory obturator nerve.** Occasional accessory nerve arising from L3 and L4 that supplies the pectineus and hip joint.

5 **Femoral nerve.** Thickest branch of the lumbar plexus, which arises from L2–L4. It emerges at the lateral border of the psoas and travels in the muscular space between it and the iliacus. It divides below the inguinal ligament. A

6 **Muscular branches.** Branches to the sartorius, pectineus, and quadriceps femoris. A

7 **Anterior cutaneous branches.** Cutaneous nerves supplying the distal three-fourths of the anterior side of the thigh as far as the patella. A

8 **Saphenous nerve.** Longest, purely sensory branch of the femoral nerve. It begins in the femoral triangle, passes beneath the "vastoadductor membrane," which it pierces, continues between the sartorius and gracilis to beneath the skin, and then travels with the great saphenous vein as far as the medial side of the foot. A, p. 425 B

9 *Infrapatellar branch.* Branch that penetrates the sartorius and reaches the skin below the patella. A

10 *Medial cutaneous nerve of leg; Medial crural cutaneous nerve.* Branches of the saphenous nerve that extend to the skin of the leg and foot. p. 425 B

11 **Lumbosacral trunk.** Communication with the lumbar plexus formed by L5 and part of L4. A

12 SACRAL PLEXUS. Plexus formed by L5–S3 and part of L4 and S4. It lies on the anterior aspect of the piriformis deep to the fascia and sends nerves to the posterior aspect of the leg. A

13 **Nerve to obturator internus.** Nerve arising from L5–S2, passing through the greater sciatic foramen into the ischioanal fossa from where it travels into the obturator internus.

14 **Nerve to piriformis.** Nerve arising from S1–S2 that passes to the anterior side of the piriformis.

15 **Nerve to quadratus femoris.** Nerve arising from L4–S1 that passes through the greater sciatic foramen and continues along a very deep course to the quadratus femoris and hip joint.

16 **Superior gluteal nerve.** Nerve arising from L4–S1 that passes through the greater sciatic foramen cranial to the piriformis and then between the gluteus medius and minimus to the tensor muscle of fascia lata, which it supplies as well as the above-mentioned muscles. B

17 **Inferior gluteal nerve.** Nerve arising from L5–S2 that travels through the infrapiriform foramen and supplies the gluteus maximus. B

18 **Posterior cutaneous nerve of thigh; Posterior femoral cutaneous nerve.** Nerve arising from S1–S3 that travels through the greater sciatic foramen distal to the piriformis and supplies the skin on the posterior side of the thigh as well as the proximal part of the leg. B

19 *Inferior clunial nerves.* Cutaneous branches ascending along the inferior margin of the gluteus maximus.

20 *Perineal branches.* Branches that ramify at the inferior border of the gluteus maximus and then continue below the ischial tuberosity medially to the scrotum (labia), sending an ascending branch as far as the coccyx. B

21 **Perforating cutaneous nerve.** Branch of the posterior femoral cutaneous nerve that supplies the anal skin. B

22 **Pudendal nerve.** Nerve arising from the second, third, and fourth sacral spinal nerves. It travels through the greater sciatic foramen distal to the piriformis into the ischioanal fossa. C

23 **Inferior anal nerves; Inferior rectal nerves.** Fibers arising from the third and fourth sacral spinal nerves that supply the external anal sphincter and anal skin. C

24 **Perineal nerves.** Collective term for the following two perineal nerves.

25 *Posterior scrotal/labial nerves.* Branches traveling from posterior to the scrotum (labia majora). C

26 *Muscular branches.* Branches supplying the perineal muscles.

27 *Dorsal nerve of penis.* Paired nerve lying on the dorsum of penis that also sends branches to its inferior aspect. C

28 *Dorsal nerve of clitoris.* Small nerve that corresponds to the dorsal nerve of the penis. C

29 **Coccygeal nerve.** Last spinal nerve. It emerges between the coccyx and sacrum and communicates with the fourth and fifth sacral spinal nerves. C

30 **Coccygeal plexus.** Nerve plexus formed by S5, part of S4, and the coccygeal nerve. It supplies the skin overlying the coccyx. C

31 **Anococcygeal nerve.** Several thin nerves from the coccygeal plexus that penetrate the anococcygeal ligament and supply the overlying skin. C

19

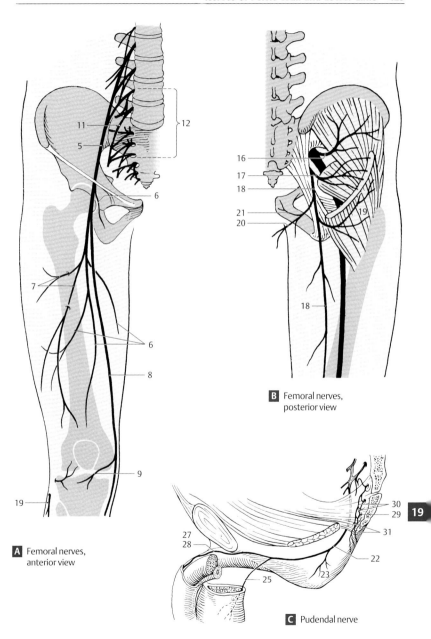

A Femoral nerves,
anterior view

B Femoral nerves,
posterior view

C Pudendal nerve

19

1 SCIATIC NERVE. Thickest nerve in the body, arising from the pelvis through the greater sciatic foramen distal to the piriformis and descends lateral to the ischial tuberosity, than travels deep to the gluteus maximus and long head of biceps femoris. A

2 **Common fibular nerve; Common peroneal nerve.** Branch of the sciatic nerve arising from L4–S2. It accompanies the tendon of the biceps femoris to posterior to the head of fibula and then crosses obliquely forward between the skin and the fibula. A B

3 **Lateral sural cutaneous nerve.** Nerve given off in the popliteal fossa that supplies the skin of the lateral side of the leg as well as the upper two-thirds of its posterior side. A B

4 **Sural communicating branch.** Branch that travels deep to the fascia over the lateral head of gastrocnemius. It joins the medial sural cutaneous nerve to form the sural nerve. C

5 **Superficial fibular nerve; Superficial peroneal nerve.** Terminal branch of the common fibular nerve. It descends between the peroneus muscles and extensor digitorum longus. A B

6 *Muscular branches.* Branches to the peroneus longus and brevis.

7 *Medial dorsal cutaneous nerve.* Branch traveling over the extensor retinaculum and supplying the skin of the dorsum of foot, the medial side of the great toe, and the adjacent halves of the second and third toes. C

8 *Intermediate dorsal cutaneous nerve.* Lateral cutaneous branch of the superficial fibular nerve lying in the middle portion of the dorsum of foot. B

9 *Dorsal digital nerves of foot.* Branches supplying the toes with the exception of the distal phalanges. B

10 **Deep fibular nerve; Deep peroneal nerve.** Nerve passing deep to the peroneus longus and then lateral to the tibialis anterior to the dorsum of foot. A B

11 *Muscular branches.* Branches to the tibialis anterior, extensor hallucis longus and brevis, and extensor digitorum longus and brevis.

12 *Dorsal digital nerves of foot.* Sensory branches to the adjacent sides of the great toe and second toes. B

19 13 **Tibial nerve.** Second terminal branch of the sciatic nerve arising from L4–S3. It travels through the popliteal fossa, passes deep to the tendinous arch of the soleus, and accompanies the posterior tibial artery around the medial malleolus to the sole of the foot. A

14 **Muscular branches.** Branches to the gastrocnemius, plantaris, soleus, and deep flexors of the leg. A

15 **Interosseous nerve of leg; Crural interosseous nerve.** Nerve accompanying the anterior tibial artery that contains fibers for the tibia and tibiofibular joint. A

16 **Medial sural cutaneous nerve.** Nerve given off by the tibial nerve in the popliteal fossa that descends subfascially lateral to the small saphenous vein and joins the sural communicating branch to form the sural nerve. A C

17 **Sural nerve.** Continuation of the medial sural cutaneous nerve after it joins the sural communicating branch. C

18 *Lateral dorsal cutaneous nerve.* Branch to the lateral portion of the dorsum of foot. It anastomoses with the intermediate dorsal cutaneous nerve. C

19 *Lateral calcaneal branches.* Lateral branches to the heel. C

20 **Medial calcaneal branches.** Medial branches to the heel that arise directly from the tibial nerve. C

21 **Medial plantar nerve.** Thicker terminal branch of the tibial nerve. It travels beneath the flexor retinaculum and abductor hallucis to the sole of foot. It supplies the skin, abductor hallucis and flexor digitorum brevis. A

22 **Common plantar digital nerves.** Nerves to the interdigital spaces 1–4 of toes. They divide into the proper plantar digital nerves. A

23 *Proper plantar digital nerves.* Cutaneous nerves to the fibular and tibial flexor aspects of the medial 3½ toes. They supply the distal phalanges, including their dorsal aspects. A

24 **Lateral plantar nerve.** Terminal branch of the tibial nerve. It passes below the flexor digitorum brevis alongside the lateral plantar artery to the base of the fifth metatarsal. A

25 *Superficial branch.* Mainly sensory, superficial branch. A

26 *Common plantar digital nerves.* Two branches, one of which passes to the little toe and gives off a branch to the flexor digiti minimi brevis; the other to the space between the fifth and fourth toes. A

27 *Proper plantar digital nerves.* Nerves that supply the fibular and tibial sides of the little toe as well as the fibular side of the fourth toe. A

28 *Deep branch.* It accompanies the deep plantar arch to the interossei, adductor hallucis, and three lateral lumbricals. A

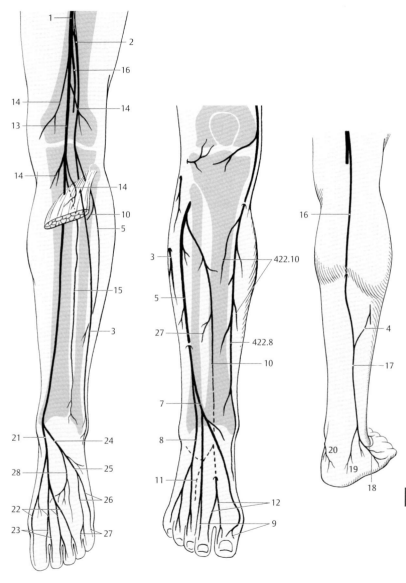

A Nerves of leg and foot, posterior view

B Nerves of leg, anterior view

C Cutaneous nerves of leg, posterior view

19

1 *AUTONOMIC DIVISION; AUTONOMIC PART OF PERIPHERAL NERVOUS SYSTEM.*

2 SYMPATHETIC PART.

3 **Sympathetic trunk.** Chain of ganglia that are connected by nerve fibers and lie on the left and right sides of the vertebral column, extending from the base of the cranium to the coccyx. B

4 **Ganglion of sympathetic trunk.** Collection of mostly multipolar ganglion cells. Preganglionic myelinated fibers synapse in the ganglion and leave as postganglionic unmyelinated fibers. B

5 **Interganglionic branches.** White and gray fibers interconnecting the ganglia of the sympathetic trunk. B

6 **Rami communicantes.** Communicating branches of the sympathetic trunk to and from the spinal nerves.

7 *Gray ramus communicans.* Unmyelinated postganglionic fibers returning to the spinal nerve. A

8 *White ramus communicans.* Preganglionic myelinated fibers to the ganglion of the sympathetic trunk. B

9 **Intermediate ganglia.** Collections of displaced ganglion cells, e.g., in the rami communicantes. B

10 **Superior cervical ganglion.** Uppermost ganglion of the sympathetic trunk, measuring about 2.5 cm in length. It lies directly beneath the cranial base between the longus capitis and posterior belly of digastric. A

11 *Jugular nerve.* Branch to the inferior ganglion of glossopharyngeal nerve and superior ganglion of vagus nerve. A

12 **Internal carotid nerve.** Nerve whose postganglionic fibers form the internal carotid plexus in the carotid canal, from which point its fibers travel to the head. A

13 *Pineal nerve.* Branch to the pineal gland.

14 **External carotid nerves.** Nerves forming the plexus surrounding the common carotid artery and external carotid artery. A

15 **Laryngopharyngeal branches.** Postganglionic fibers to the pharyngeal plexus. C

16 **Superior cervical cardiac nerve.** Fibers to the cardiac plexus at the aortic arch. C

17 **Middle cervical ganglion.** Often very small cervical ganglion of the sympathetic trunk at the level of C6 that lies either anterior or posterior to the inferior thyroid artery. C D

18 **Vertebral ganglion.** Ganglion at the level of the transverse foramen of C6. C

19 **Middle cervical cardiac nerve.** Branch from the middle cervical ganglion to the deep portion of the cardiac plexus. C

20 **[Inferior cervical ganglion].** Ganglion that usually does not exist independently; it is often connected with the first thoracic ganglion.

21 **Cervicothoracic ganglion; Stellate ganglion.** Fusion of the inferior cervical ganglion with the first and sometimes also second thoracic ganglion in about 75%. C D

22 **Ansa subclavia.** Loop formed by fibers from the sympathetic trunk anterior and posterior to the subclavian artery. C

23 **Inferior cervical cardiac nerve.** Branch to the deep portion of the cardiac plexus. C

24 **Vertebral nerve.** Nerve running posterior to the vertebral artery that forms the vertebral plexus. C

25 **Thoracic ganglia.** Eleven or twelve thickened portions of the thoracic sympathetic trunk. C D

26 **Thoracic cardiac branches.** Fibers passing from the second, third, and fourth (fifth) thoracic ganglia to the cardiac plexus. They contain efferent and afferent components. C D

27 **Thoracic pulmonary branches.** Efferent fibers from the second, third, and fourth thoracic ganglia to the pulmonary plexus at the hilum of lung.

28 **Esophageal branches.** Efferent fibers from the second through fifth thoracic ganglia.

29 **Greater splanchnic nerve.** Nerve running from the fifth through ninth (tenth) ganglia of the sympathetic trunk to the celiac ganglia. It contains preganglionic and postganglionic fibers and conveys pain perception from upper abdominal organs. D

30 **Thoracic splanchnic ganglion.** Accessory ganglion at the level of T9 that is interposed in the course of the greater splanchnic nerve. D

31 **Lesser splanchnic nerve.** Nerve arising from the ninth, tenth, and eleventh ganglia of the sympathetic trunk that behaves similarly to the greater splanchnic nerve. D

32 **Renal branch.** Occasional branch of the lesser splanchnic nerve to the renal plexus. D

33 **Least splanchnic nerve; Lowest splanchnic nerve.** Variable branch from the twelfth thoracic ganglion to the renal plexus. D

20

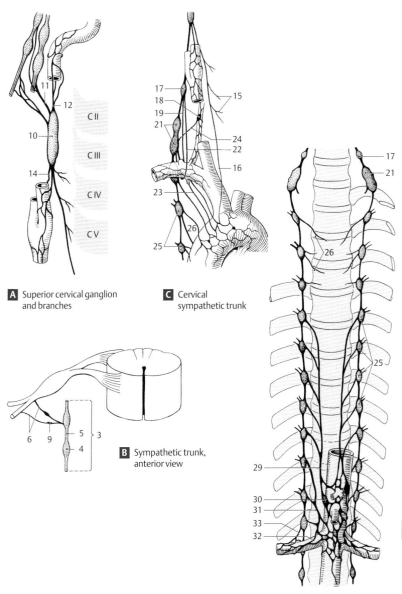

A Superior cervical ganglion and branches

C Cervical sympathetic trunk

B Sympathetic trunk, anterior view

D Splanchnic nerves

20

1 **Lumbar ganglia.** Often four sympathetic ganglia of the lumbar vertebral column. C

2 **Lumbar splanchnic nerves.** Usually four nerves arising from the lumbar sympathetic trunk forming a plexus on the fifth lumbar vertebra. C

3 **Sacral ganglia.** Four ganglia near the lower end of the vertebral column lying medial to the anterior sacral foramina. C

4 **Sacral splanchnic nerves.** Two or three thin nerves arising from the second, third, and fourth sacral ganglia. C

5 **Ganglion impar.** Last, unpaired ganglion of the sympathetic trunk lying anterior to the coccyx. C

6 **Sympathetic paraganglia.**

7 **PARASYMPATHETIC PART.**

8 **Cranial part.**

9 **Ciliary ganglion.** Ganglion situated on the posterolateral aspect of the optic nerve that contains cells for the postganglionic parasympathetic fibers to the ocular muscles. They constrict the pupils and contract the ciliary muscle for near vision. A B

10 *Parasympathetic root; Oculomotor root; Branch of oculomotor nerve to ciliary ganglion.* Preganglionic parasympathetic fibers from CN III. A

11 *Sympathetic root.* Postganglionic sympathetic fibers from the internal carotid plexus. A

12 *Sensory root; Nasociliary root; Communicating branch of nasociliary nerve with ciliary ganglion.* Sensory fibers that leave the eye via the short ciliary nerves and continue through the ganglion to the nasociliary nerve A

13 *Short ciliary nerves.* Up to 20 short nerves that pierce the sclera around CN II. They contain postganglionic parasympathetic fibers from the ciliary ganglion as well as postganglionic sympathetic fibers of the sympathetic root that carry information to the eye. They contain sensory fibers of the nasociliary root that carry impulses away from the eye. A

14 **Pterygopalatine ganglion.** Ganglion measuring 4–5 mm that lies lateral to the sphenopalatine foramen in the pterygopalatine fossa. It contains cells for the postganglionic parasympathetic fibers to the lacrimal gland and the small nasal and palatine glands. A B

15 *Nerve of pterygoid canal.* Nerve lying in the pterygoid canal at the root of the pterygoid process. It is composed of the greater and deep petrosal nerves.

16 *Parasympathetic root; Greater petrosal nerve.* Portion of the intermediate nerve that leaves CN VII in the geniculate ganglion with preganglionic parasympathetic fibers. It synapses in the pterygopalatine ganglion. A

17 *Sympathetic root; Deep petrosal nerve.* Postganglionic sympathetic fibers from the internal carotid plexus that travel through the ganglion. A

18 *Sensory root; Ganglionic branches of maxillary nerve.* Sensory fibers from the maxillary nerve that travel through the ganglion. A

19 **Submandibular ganglion.** Ganglion that varies in shape and lies along the lingual nerve, usually above the submandibular gland. It contains cells for the postganglionic parasympathetic fibers to the submandibular and sublingual glands. A B

20 *Parasympathetic root; Chorda tympani.* It conveys preganglionic parasympathetic fibers from the intermediate nerve, which leave CN VII before the stylomastoid foramen. They synapse in the ganglion. A

21 *Sympathetic root.* Postganglionic sympathetic fibers from the vascular plexus of the facial nerve that pass through the ganglion.

22 *Sensory root; Ganglionic branches of mandibular nerve.* Sensory fibers of the lingual nerve that pass through the ganglion.

23 **Sublingual ganglion.** Inconstant ganglion with similar components as the submandibular ganglion.

24 **Otic ganglion.** Flattened ganglion that varies in shape. It lies directly beneath the foramen ovale medial to the mandibular nerve and contains cells of postganglionic parasympathetic fibers to the parotid gland. A B

25 *Parasympathetic root; Lesser petrosal nerve.* Preganglionic parasympathetic fibers from the tympanic nerve that travel to the otic ganglion where they synapse. A

26 *Sympathetic root.* Postganglionic fibers above the vascular plexus of the middle meningeal artery that travel through the ganglion.

27 *Sensory root; Ganglionic branches of mandibular nerve.* Sensory fibers of the lingual nerve that travel through the ganglion.

28 **Pelvic part. Sacral part.**

29 **Pelvic ganglia.** Autonomic ganglia in the inferior hypogastric plexus where the preganglionic fibers synapse and leave as postganglionic fibers to the pelvic and genital organs. p. 433 D

30 *Parasympathetic root; Pelvic splanchnic nerves.* Preganglionic parasympathetic fibers from S2–S4. They synapse in the ganglia. C

31 *Sympathetic root.* Postganglionic sympathetic fibers lying along vascular plexuses.

32 *Sensory root.* Sensory fibers from the pelvic region.

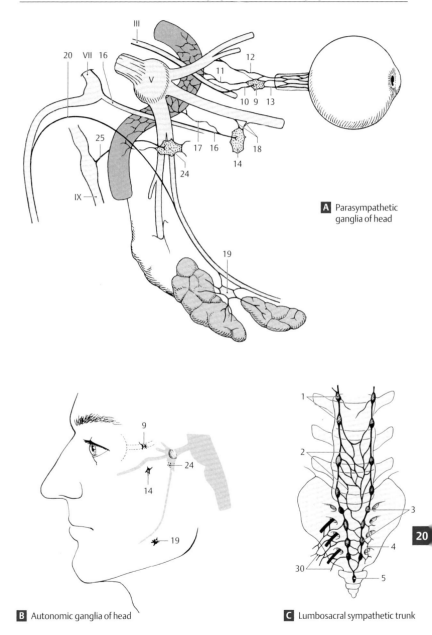

A Parasympathetic ganglia of head

B Autonomic ganglia of head

C Lumbosacral sympathetic trunk

20

1   **PERIPHERAL AUTONOMIC PLEXUSES AND GANGLIA.** Autonomic nerve plexuses interspersed with ganglia, mainly along vessels.

2   **Craniocervical part.**

3   **Common carotid plexus.** Sympathetic nerve plexus accompanying the common carotid artery. B

4   **Internal carotid plexus.** Continuation of the plexus to the internal carotid artery. From here it sends fibers to the cranial ganglia.

5   **Cavernous plexus.** Plexus accompanying the internal carotid artery to the cavernous sinus.

6   **External carotid plexus.** Plexus accompanying the external carotid artery from the common carotid plexus, which it helps form.

7   **Subclavian plexus.** Plexus whose fibers leave the sympathetic trunk at the inferior cervical ganglion and travel along the vessel wall.

8   **Brachial autonomic plexus.** Plexus lying alongside the brachial artery.

9   **Vertebral plexus.** Plexus extending into the vertebral canal via the carotid plexus, after receiving fibers from the vertebral ganglion at its entrance. B

10 **Thoracic part.**

11 **Thoracic aortic plexus.** Autonomic nerve plexus around the aorta with fibers from the first five thoracic ganglia and the splanchnic nerve. It also contains afferent fibers of the vagus nerve. B

12 **Cardiac plexus.** Autonomic nerve plexus formed by sympathetic and vagus nerve fibers at the base of the heart, especially around the aortic arch and at the root of the pulmonary trunk, as well as along the coronary vessels and between the aorta and tracheal bifurcation. B

13 **Cardiac ganglia.** Small macroscopically visible collections of ganglion cells mainly located to the right of the ligamentum arteriosum. B

14 **Esophageal plexus.** Autonomic nerve plexus around the esophagus.

15 **Pulmonary plexus.** Plexus formed by fibers from the vagus nerve and sympathetic trunk lying anterior and posterior to the hilum of lung. It communicates across the midline with the pulmonary plexus of the opposite side and with the cardiac plexus. B

16 *Pulmonary branches.* Branches from the third and fourth thoracic sympathetic ganglia mainly to the posterior parts of the pulmonary plexus. B

17 **Abdominal part.**

18 **Abdominal aortic plexus.** Nerve plexus lying anterior to and on both sides of the aorta. It extends from the celiac plexus to the aortic bifurcation, receiving fibers from both superior lumbar ganglia, and continues caudally as the superior hypogastric plexus.

19 **Phrenic ganglia.** Small collections of ganglion cells in the nerve plexus accompanying the inferior phrenic artery. A

20 **Celiac plexus.** Nerve plexus around the celiac trunk that communicates with the adjacent plexuses. It receives fibers from the two splanchnic nerves and the vagus nerve. A C

21 *Hepatic plexus.* Continuation of the celiac plexus to the liver that contains fibers from the vagus and phrenic nerves. A C

22 *Splenic plexus.* Plexus formed by branches from the celiac plexus along the splenic artery to the spleen. A C

23 *Gastric plexuses.* Autonomic nerve plexuses supplying the stomach. The anterior and posterior portions are formed by the vagus nerve; the left portion forms the continuation of the celiac plexus along the left gastric artery. C

24 *Pancreatic plexus.* Continuation of the celiac plexus to the pancreatic vessels. C

25 *Suprarenal plexus.* Continuation of the celiac plexus along the suprarenal vessels that contains preganglionic fibers to the medulla of suprarenal gland. A

26 *Celiac ganglia.* Collection of ganglion cells that communicates with the celiac plexus and lies on the right and left of the aorta adjacent to the celiac trunk. A

27 **Aorticorenal ganglia.** Collection of ganglion cells at the departure of the renal artery that receive the lesser splanchnic nerve. They are sometimes fused with the celiac ganglia. A

28 **Superior mesenteric plexus.** Nerve plexus accompanying the superior mesenteric artery and its branches. It contains sympathetic fibers from the celiac plexus and parasympathetic fibers from the vagus nerve. A

29 *Superior mesenteric ganglion.* Group of ganglion cells on the right and left of the aorta adjacent to the superior mesenteric artery and its branches. It is often fused with the adjacent ganglia. A

30 **Intermesenteric plexus.** Nerve plexus lying between the superior and inferior mesenteric plexuses. A

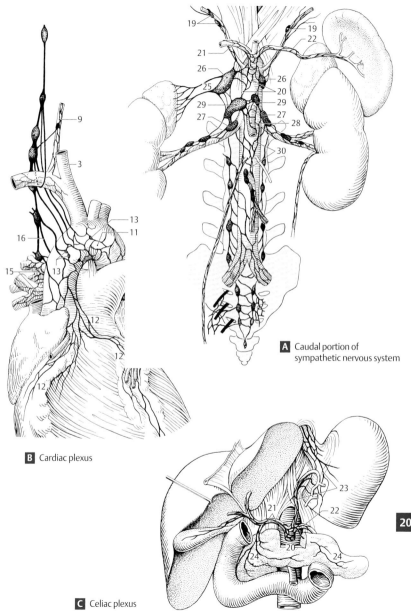

A Caudal portion of sympathetic nervous system

B Cardiac plexus

C Celiac plexus

1 **Renal plexus.** Plexus accompanying the renal artery. It also contains fibers from the vagus nerve. A

2 *Renal ganglia.* Microscopic groups of ganglion cells interspersed in the renal plexus. A

3 **Ureteric plexus.** Nerve plexus lying alongside the ureter that contains fibers from the renal plexus, abdominal aortic plexus, and aorticorenal ganglia. A

4 **Testicular plexus.** Nerve plexus accompanying the testicular artery as far as the testes. It receives fibers from the renal plexus and abdominal aortic plexus. A

5 **Ovarian plexus.** Autonomic nerve plexus lying alongside the ovarian artery. It receives fibers from the abdominal aortic plexus and renal plexus. A

6 **Inferior mesenteric plexus.** Continuation of the abdominal aortic plexus along the inferior mesenteric artery and its branches. B

7 *Inferior mesenteric ganglion.* All ganglion cells situated in the inferior mesenteric plexus. A

8 **Superior rectal plexus.** Continuation of the inferior mesenteric plexus to the superior rectal artery and rectum. It also receives parasympathetic fibers from the inferior hypogastric plexus. B

9 **Enteric plexus.** Collective term for the autonomic nerve plexuses situated in the wall of the intestinal tract.

10 *Subserous plexus.* Tiny autonomic nerve plexus lying directly beneath the serosa. C

11 *Myenteric plexus (Auerbach's plexus).* Plexus containing a large number of ganglion cells situated between the longitudinal and circular muscle layers. It regulates peristalsis. C

12 *Submucous plexus (Meissner's plexus).* Plexus containing a large number of ganglion cells in the submucosa. It regulates the muscularis mucosae and villi. C

13 **Iliac plexus.** Continuation of the abdominal aortic plexus to both iliac arteries. B D

14 **Femoral plexus.** Continuation of the iliac plexus to the femoral artery. D

15 **Pelvic part.**

16 **Superior hypogastric plexus; Presacral nerve.** Plexuslike communication between the abdominal aortic plexus and inferior hypogastric plexus that mostly lies anterior to the fifth lumbar vertebra. It contains branches from the lumbar sympathetic ganglia. B D

17 *Hypogastric nerve.* Right and left branches of the superior hypogastric plexus passing to the pelvic viscera. It communicates with the inferior hypogastric plexus. B D

18 **Inferior hypogastric plexus; Pelvic plexus.** Nerve plexus consisting of sympathetic and parasympathetic fibers. It lies on the right and left sides of the rectum and anterior to it. B

19 *Middle rectal plexus.* Continuation of the inferior hypogastric plexus to the wall of the rectum. D

20 *Inferior rectal plexus.* Autonomic nerve plexuses accompanying the corresponding branches of the internal iliac artery to both sides of the rectum. D

21 *Superior anal nerves.* Branches to the anus. D

22 **Uterovaginal plexus.** Nerve plexus situated in the parametrium that is interspersed with numerous ganglia. It sends branches to the uterus, vagina, uterine tube, and ovary. It communicates with the inferior hypogastric plexus in the recto-uterine fold. B

23 *Vaginal nerves.* Branches from the uterovaginal plexus of the vagina. B

24 **Prostatic plexus.** Branches from the inferior hypogastric plexus to the lateral surfaces of the prostate. D

25 **Deferential plexus; Plexus of ductus deferens.** Branches from the vesical plexus to the seminal vesicle and ductus deferens. D

26 **Vesical plexus.** Plexuses lying on both sides of the urinary bladder containing parasympathetic fibers. They regulate the emptying mechanism of the urinary bladder. D

27 **Cavernous nerves of penis.** Branches from the prostatic plexus to the corpus cavernosum of penis. D

28 **Cavernous nerves of clitoris.** Nerves in the female that correspond to the cavernous nerves of penis. D

20

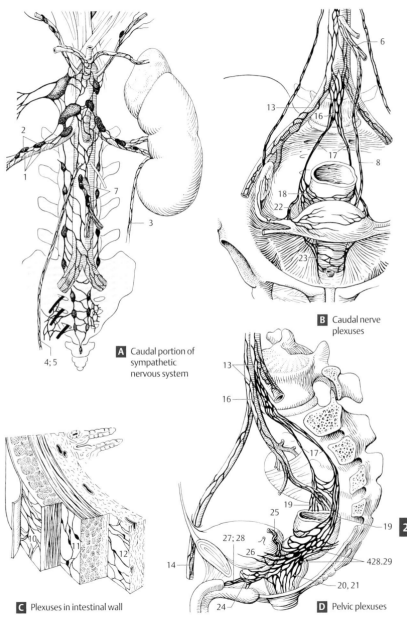

A Caudal portion of sympathetic nervous system

B Caudal nerve plexuses

C Plexuses in intestinal wall

D Pelvic plexuses

20

1 *SENSE ORGANS.* The organs of vision, hearing, olfaction, and taste.

2 *OLFACTORY ORGAN.*

3 **Olfactory part of nasal mucosa; Olfactory area.** Dime-sized area lined with olfactory cells located on the upper part of the nasal septum below the cribriform plate and on the lateral wall of the nose. A

4 **Olfactory glands.** Small, branched tubular glands. The discharge of these cleansing glands presumably binds odorants. A B

5 *EYE AND RELATED STRUCTURES.*

6 **EYEBALL.**

7 **Anterior pole.** It is determined by the corneal vertex. F

8 **Posterior pole.** It lies opposite to the anterior pole and lateral to the exit of the optic nerve. F

9 **Equator.** Greatest circumference encircling the eyeball equidistant between the anterior and posterior poles. F

10 **Meridians.** Imaginary half-circles passing at right angles to the equator between the anterior and posterior poles. F

11 **External axis of eyeball.** Imaginary line connecting the anterior and posterior poles. D

12 **Internal axis of eyeball.** Distance from the posterior surface of the cornea to the inner surface of the retina, measured along an imaginary line that extends through the anterior and posterior poles (external axis of eyeball). D

13 **Optic axis.** Imaginary line passing through the midpoints of the cornea and lens. It meets the retina between the fovea centralis and the optic disc. D

14 **Anterior segment.** Portion of the eye including the cornea and lens.

15 **Posterior segment.** Portion of the eye posterior to the lens and ciliary zonule.

16 FIBROUS LAYER OF EYEBALL. Wall of the eyeball consisting of the cornea and sclera. D

17 **Sclera.** Membrane of the eyeball composed of interwoven collagen fibers. It has a bluish-white appearance and is visible through the conjunctiva. C D E

18 **Sulcus sclerae.** Shallow groove between the cornea and sclera produced by the stronger curvature of the cornea. D E F

19 **Trabecular tissue.** Connective-tissue meshwork in the angle between the cornea and iris.

20 *Corneoscleral part.* Portion of the trabecular meshwork attached to the sclera. E

21 *Uveal part.* Portion of the trabecular meshwork attached to the iris. E

22 *Scleral spur.* Wedge-shaped, anular elevation that opens toward the scleral venous sinus. It encloses the posterior portion of the sinus. E

23 **Scleral venous sinus (Canal of Schlemm).** Circular vessel that borders on the inner aspect of the trabecular tissue. The channel can be either interrupted or double and collects aqueous humor from the anterior chamber of eyeball. E

24 **Episcleral layer.** Delicate, sliding layer of tissue between the outer surface of the sclera and the fascial sheath of eyeball.

25 **Substantia propria.** Main component forming the wall of the eyeball. It is composed of interwoven, collagen connective-tissue fibers and sparse elastic fibers. C E

26 **Suprachoroid lamina.** Layer of loose connective tissue between the sclera and the choroid lying internal to it. Scattered melanocytes give it a yellow appearance. C

27 **Lamina cribrosa of sclera.** Perforated layer of the substantia propria for the passage of optic nerve fibers. C

28 **Cornea.** Transparent, anterior part (1/6) of the eyeball that is anteriorly convex and posteriorly concave. It is 0.9 mm thick in the middle and 1.2 mm thick at the margin. E

29 **Conjunctival ring.** Transition of the conjunctival epithelium into the epithelium of the anterior surface of cornea. E

30 **Corneoscleral junction; Corneal limbus.** Margin of the cornea that is continuous with the sclera. E

31 **Corneal vertex.** Furthest anteriorly projecting point on the anterior surface of the cornea. D

32 **Anterior surface.** Surface of the cornea facing the outside air. E

33 **Posterior surface.** Surface of the cornea facing the anterior chamber. E

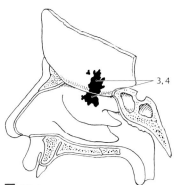

A Olfactory area

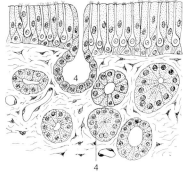

B Olfactory mucosa

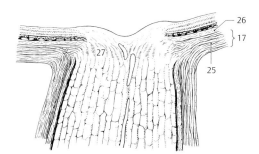

C Exit of optic nerve and tunics of eye

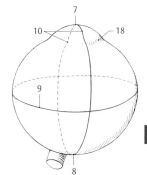

D Eyeball, overview

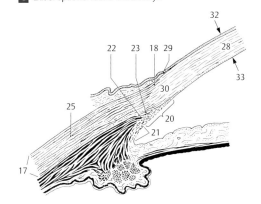

E Iridocorneal angle

F Eyeball, lines of orientation

21

1 **Corneal epithelium.** Approximately five layers of squamous epithelium covering the anterior surface of the cornea. Its surface is very smooth. B D

2 **Anterior limiting lamina (Bowman's membrane).** Basal membrane of the corneal epithelium that is about 10–20 µm thick. It is continuous posteriorly with the substantia propria. B

3 **Substantia propria.** Main, avascular component of the cornea that consists of a lamellar arrangement of connective tissue and a ground substance containing mucopolysaccharides. Corneal transparency is produced by turgescence of the fibers and colloidal fluid distribution. B D

4 **Posterior limiting lamina (Descemet's membrane).** Basal membrane of the posterior corneal epithelium. Along its lateral margin it divides into fibers which radiate into the sclera and iris. Aqueous humor passes through the interstices between fibers into the scleral venous sinus. B D

5 **Endothelium of anterior chamber.** Simple squamous epithelium covering the posterior surface of the cornea. B D

6 VASCULAR LAYER OF EYEBALL. Uveal tract. It consists of the choroid, ciliary body, and iris.

7 **Choroid.** Portion situated between the retina and sclera. A

8 **Suprachoroid lamina.** Poorly vascularized, sliding layer lying directly beneath the sclera that contains pigment cells. Its fibers are partly covered with endothelium. A

9 **Perichoroidal space.** System of spaces in the suprachoroid lamina that partly belongs to the lymphoid system. It contains the ciliary nerves, long and short posterior ciliary arteries, and vorticose veins. A

10 **Vascular lamina.** Layer containing branches of the short posterior ciliary arteries. A

11 **Capillary lamina.** Layer containing a dense capillary network and no pigment cells that extends as for as the ora serrata. It is often separated from the vascular lamina by a special layer of connective tissue. A

12 **Basal lamina (Bruch's membrane).** Homogeneous zone measuring 2–4 mm thick between the capillary lamina and the retinal pigment epithelium. A

13 **Choroid blood vessels.** All blood vessels contained in the uveal tract.

14 **Ciliary body.** Thickened area situated between the ora serrata and root of the iris that contains the ciliary muscle and ciliary processes. C

15 **Corona ciliaris.** Circular zone formed by the ciliary processes. C

16 **Ciliary processes.** Between 70 and 80 radiating folds containing numerous capillaries measuring 0.1–0.2 mm wide, 1 mm high, and 2–3 mm long. Their epithelium produces aqueous humor. C

17 **Ciliary plicae.** Low folds in the corona ciliaris, some of which are also situated between the ciliary processes. C

18 **Orbiculus ciliaris.** Circular zone between the corona ciliaris and ora serrata that is covered with ciliary plicae. C

19 **Ciliary muscle.** Smooth muscle of the ciliary body. It draws the choroid anteriorly, thereby relaxing the zonular fibers, allowing the lens to take its own, more strongly convex form for near vision. D

20 *Meridional fibers (Brücke's muscle).* Larger group of fibers running meridionally that mostly arise from the scleral spur and pass along the choroid to the sclera. D

21 *Longitudinal fibers.* Fibers arising from the corneoscleral part that follow the path of the meridional fibers for the rest of their course. D

22 *Radial fibers.* Middle, radial portion of the ciliary muscle with fibers crossing from medial to lateral. D

23 *Circular fibers (Müller's muscles).* Anular inner muscle layer. D

24 **Basal lamina.** Continuation of the basal lamina of the choroid on which the epithelium sits. D

21

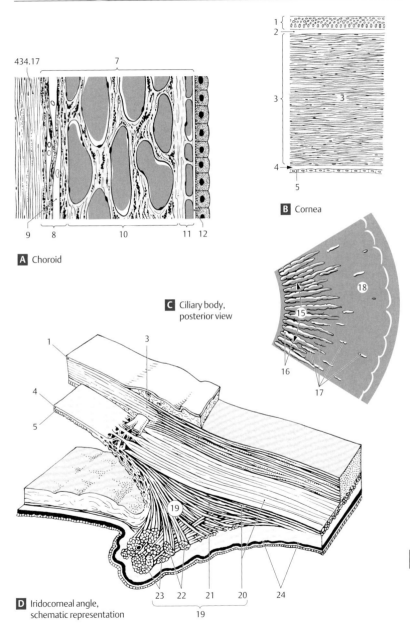

A Choroid

B Cornea

C Ciliary body, posterior view

D Iridocorneal angle, schematic representation

1 **Iris.** Round disc with a central opening (pupil) situated in the frontal plane that varies in color in different individuals. It forms the posterior end of the anterior chamber and becomes continuous at its margin with the ciliary body. It has a diameter of 10–12 mm. A

2 **Pupillary margin.** Inner border of the iris encircling the pupil. A B

3 **Ciliary margin.** Outer border of the iris that is attached to the ciliary body and at the iridocorneal angle. B

5 **Anterior surface.** Anterior surface of the iris facing the anterior chamber. B

5 **Posterior surface.** Posterior surface of the iris facing the posterior chamber. A B

6 **Outer border of iris.** Ciliary portion of the iris. Outer, wider zone that is distinguishable from the inner border of the iris by its coarser structure. A

7 **Inner border of iris.** Pupillary portion of the iris. Narrower zone that is distinguishable from the outer border of iris by its more delicate structure. A

8 **Folds of iris.** Folds passing around the border of the anterior surface of iris. They produce the slightly scalloped appearance of the border of the iris. A

9 **Pupil.** Opening in the iris surrounded by the pupillary margin. Its diameter can change in response to light entering the eye and the distance to an object being viewed. A

10 *Sphincter pupillae.* Meshwork of spiraling muscle fibers. In the dilated pupil its long axes run nearly parallel to the pupillary margin. It is innervated by parasympathetic fibers from the oculomotor nerve. B

11 *Dilator pupillae.* Thin layer of smooth muscle whose cells are mainly oriented radially. It is innervated by sympathetic nerve fibers via the carotid plexus.

12 **Stroma of iris.** Vascular framework of the iris interspersed with pigmented connective-tissue cells. Its anterior and posterior portions are denser, with fine fibers in between. A B

13 **Pigmented epithelium.** Double-layered pigmented epithelium on the posterior aspect of the iris. The surface facing the posterior chamber is so heavily pigmented that no nuclei are visible. A

14 **Spaces of iridocorneal angle (Spaces of Fontana).** Spaces between the fibers of the trabecular tissue through which the aqueous humor drains into the scleral venous sinus. A

15 **Major circulus arteriosus of iris.** Vascular circle with radiating branches formed by anastomoses between the long and short posterior ciliary arteries. A

16 **Minor circulus arteriosus of iris.** Vascular circle near the pupillary margin that is formed by anastomoses between the radiating branches of the major circulus arteriosus of the iris. A

17 **[Pupillary membrane].** Anterior portion of the embryonic vascular sheath surrounding the lens that lies behind the pupil. It is fused with the pupillary margin, from which it also receives blood vessels.

18 INNER LAYER OF EYEBALL. Layer comprising the retina and pigmented epithelium.

19 **Retina.** Inner lining of the eyeball whose greater portion (optic part) is light sensitive. It is derived from the two layers of the optic cup. B

20 **Nonvisual retina.** Part of the retina that is not sensitive to light.

21 *Ciliary part of retina.* Part situated on the posterior surface ciliary body. It is composed of simple, cuboidal, pigmented epithelium. B

22 *Iridial part of retina.* Part situated on the posterior surface of the iris. It is composed of a double layer of pigmented, cuboidal epithelium. B

23 **Ora serrata.** Serrated border between the light-sensitive and light-insensitive portions of the retina. B C

24 **Optic part of retina.** Portion of the retina capable of transforming light impulses into nerve impulses. It borders posteriorly with the ora serrata. B

25 *Pigmented layer.* Pigmented epithelium derived from the outer layer of the optic cup. B

26 *Neural layer.* True retina lying immediately internal to the pigmented layer. It contains the layers listed on the following page. B

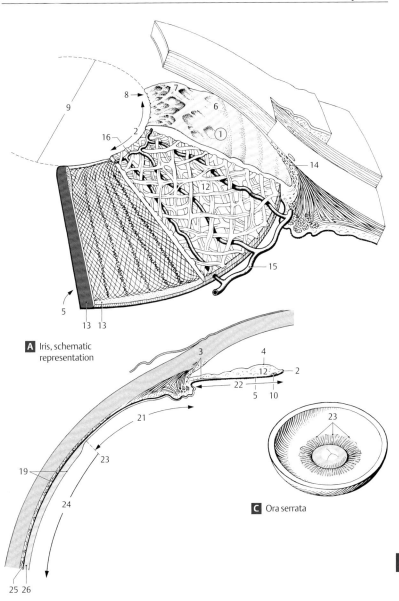

A Iris, schematic representation

B Parts of retina

C Ora serrata

1 *Layer of inner and outer segments.* Layer of rods and cones. A

2 *Outer limiting layer.* A

3 *Outer nuclear layer.* A

4 *Outer plexiform layer.* A

5 *Inner nuclear layer.* A

6 *Inner plexiform layer.* A

7 *Ganglionic layer.* A

8 *Layer of nerve fibers.* A

9 *Inner limiting layer.* A

10 **Optic disc.** Beginning of the optic nerve in the fundus of the eye about 3 or 4 mm medial to the macula with a diameter of about 1.6 mm. B

11 *Depression of optic disc; Physiological cup.* Depression in the middle of the optic disc containing the trunks of the central retinal artery and vein. B

12 **Macula.** Pigmented, transversely oval region on the posterior pole of the eyeball that is yellow in color and measures 2–4 mm in diameter. B

13 *Fovea centralis.* Pit in the macula that is produced by a reduction of upper retinal layers. Its diameter, measured from the beginning of decreasing retinal thickness to the opposite side, is 1–2 mm. A B

14 *Foveola.* Thinnest site in the fovea centralis where the retina consists of virtually only cone cells. It measures 0.2–0.4 mm in diameter and contains 2500 cone cells.

15 **Optic nerve.** Fiber bundle beginning in the retina and passing to the optic chiasm. In terms of histology and development, it is an eversion of the brain and thus surrounded by a dural sheath as far as the posterior side of the eyeball. Its axons are not covered with a sheath of Schwann cells. Those axons covered with myelin have a sheath produced by oligodendrocytes. C D

16 **Intracranial part.** Portion between the optic canal and chiasm. C

17 **Part in canal.** Segment lying in the optic canal. It is partly connected with the canal wall. C

18 **Orbital part.** Rather tortuous portion of about 3 cm in length running in the orbit. C

19 **Intra-ocular part.** Part situated in the eyeball.

20 *Postlaminar part.* Part situated posterior to the lamina cribrosa of sclera and thus alongside the site where the outer sheath (dural sheath) of optic nerve becomes continuous with the sclera. D

21 *Intralaminar part.* Part lying in the lamina cribrosa of the sclera. D

22 *Prelaminar part.* Portion between the lamina cribrosa of the sclera and the optic nerve fiber layer of the retina. D

23 **Outer sheath.** Dural sheath surrounding the optic nerve as far as the eyeball. D

24 **Inner sheath.** Pial and arachnoidal covering accompanying the optic nerve as far as the eyeball. A

25 *Subarachnoid space; Leptomeningeal space.* Subarachnoid space around the optic nerve and the capillary layer between arachnoid and dura mater. D

26 **Retinal blood vessels.** Branches of the central retinal artery and vein situated on the inner surface of the retina.

27 **Central retinal artery, intraocular part.** Part supplying the eyeball.

28 **Central retinal vein, intraocular part.** Part draining the eyeball.

29 **Vascular circle of optic nerve.** Small vascular circle piercing the sclera around the optic nerve.

30 *Superior temporal retinal arteriole/venule.* Superolateral branches. B

31 *Inferior temporal retinal arteriole/venule.* Inferolateral branches. B

32 *Superior nasal retinal arteriole/venule.* Superomedial branches. B

33 *Inferior nasal retinal arteriole/venule.* Inferomedial branches. B

34 *Superior macular arteriole/venule.* Branches of the superior part of the macula. B

35 *Inferior macular arteriole/venule.* Branches of the inferior part of the macula. B

36 *Middle macular arteriole/venule.* Small branches for the medial part of the retina lying directly adjacent to the optic disc. B

21

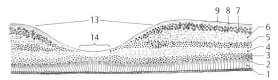

A Fovea centralis

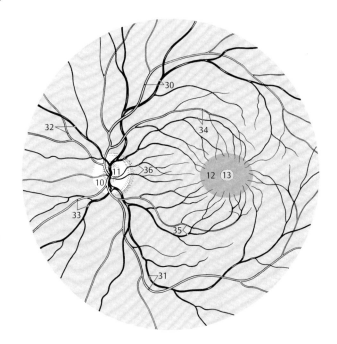

B Fundus of eye

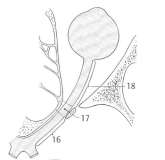

C Segments of optic nerve

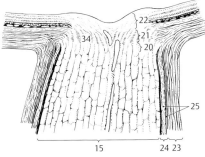

D Exit of optic nerve and sheaths

21

1 LENS. Lens suspended by the ciliary zonule between the pupil and vitreous body. It measures 9–10 mm in diameter and is about 4 mm thick. B C D

2 **Lens substance.** Substance forming the lens that lies beneath the lens epithelium and consists of the lens nucleus and cortex. It has a refractive index of 1.44–1.55. C

3 **Cortex of lens.** Outer zone of the lens that is softer due to higher water content. It transitions into the nucleus of the lens without a distinct boundary between them. C

4 **Nucleus of lens.** Part that is less well hydrated and thus harder, especially in older age. C

5 **Lens fibers.** Lens fibers corresponding to the lens epithelium. They form the acellular lens substance and are 2.5–12 µm thick and up to 10 mm long. C

6 **Lens epithelium.** Epithelium of the lens that extends to the equator of the lens. It is derived during embryonic development from the anterior wall epithelium of the lens vesicle. C

7 **Capsule of lens.** Crystal-clear membrane up to 15 µm thick covering the lens and its epithelium. It is thicker at the anterior pole than at the posterior pole. It gives attachment to zonular fibers. C

8 **Anterior pole.** D

9 **Posterior pole.** D

10 **Anterior surface.** Anterior, less convex surface of the lens that has a radius of 8.3–10 mm. C

11 **Posterior surface.** Posterior, more strongly convex surface of the lens that has a radius of about 6.5 mm. C

12 **Axis.** Imaginary line connecting the anterior and posterior poles. D

13 **Equator.** Perimeter of the lens. D

14 **Radii.** Suture lines formed by individual lens fibers that are present in the young and resemble a three-pointed star. D

15 **Ciliary zonule.** Suspensory apparatus of zonular fibers and spaces encircling the equator. It is composed of system of radiating fibers of varying lengths and the folds between them. C

16 *Zonular fibers.* Suspensory fibers attached at the equator and adjacent anterior and posterior surfaces of the lens. They are fixed distally to the basal lamina of the ciliary body and the ciliary part of retina. C

17 *Zonular spaces.* Interstices between the zonular fibers with aqueous humor flowing through them. C

18 CHAMBERS OF EYEBALL. Intra-ocular space.

19 **Aqueous humor.** Fluid produced by the ciliary processes. It flows through the interstices of the ciliary zonule to the anterior surface of the lens and from there between the iris and lens and through the pupil into the anterior chamber. Total amount: 0.2–0.3 cm^3. It is transparent, consisting of up to 98 % water, 1.4 % sodium chloride, and trace amounts of protein and glucose. Its refractive index is 1.336.

20 **Anterior chamber.** Space extending from the anterior surface of the iris to the posterior side of the cornea and communicating though the pupil with the posterior chamber. A

21 *Iridocorneal angle.* Angle between the iris and cornea. It contains the trabecular tissue, which allows drainage of aqueous humor through its interstices into the scleral venous sinus. A

22 **Posterior chamber.** Space extending from the iris and ciliary body to the anterior surface of the vitreous body. A

23 **Postremal chamber; Vitreous chamber.** Space occupied by the vitreous body. B

24 **Retrozonular space.** Crevice behind the zonular fibers. C

25 **Vitreous body.** It consists of about 98 % water and contains trace amounts of protein and sodium chloride as well as a mixture of tiny fibers that become denser toward the surface and form a limiting membrane. Its gelatinous consistency is due to its high hyaluronic acid content. A

26 **[Hyaloid artery].** Branch of the ophthalmic artery present only during embryonic stages, supplying the vascular membrane of the lens. Its trunk persists as the central retinal artery near the optic nerve. B

27 **Hyaloid canal.** Canal spiraling in corkscrew fashion that dips inferiorly during its course. Its walls are formed by a condensation of fibers. It is a vestige of the embryonic hyaloid artery, extending from the optic disc to the posterior surface of the lens. A

28 **Hyaloid fossa.** Depression on the anterior side of the vitreous body for the lens. A

29 **Vitreous membrane.** Condensation of fibers at the surface of the vitreous body. A

30 **Vitreous stroma.** Fine meshwork of fibers in the vitreous body that is condensed at the surface meeting the vitreous membrane.

31 **Vitreous humor.** Fluid of the vitreous body between the fibers of the vitreous stroma. It contains mucopolysaccharides.

21

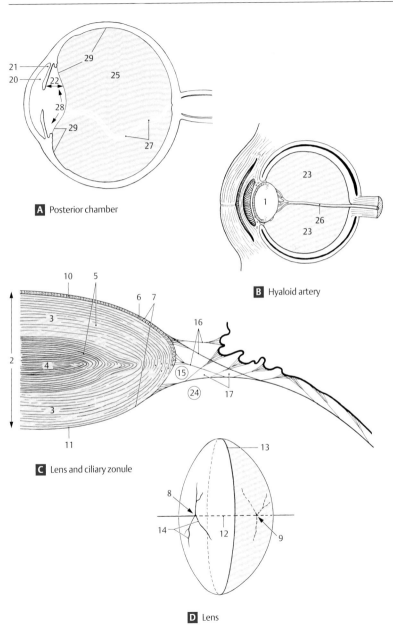

A Posterior chamber

B Hyaloid artery

C Lens and ciliary zonule

D Lens

1   ACCESSORY VISUAL STRUCTURES.

2   **Periorbita.** Delicate periosteal covering of the orbit that is firmly attached to the bone at the entry and exit sites of the orbit. It is continuous anteriorly with the adjacent periosteum and posteriorly with the dura mater. A

3   **Orbital septum.** Sheet of connective tissue that is partly reinforced by tendons. It extends from the orbital margin beneath the orbicularis oculi to the outer margins of the tarsi and closes off the orbital cavity anteriorly. A

4   **Fascial sheath of eyeball (Tenon's capsule).** Connective-tissue sheath between the eyeball and orbital fat. It is attached posteriorly at the optic nerve to the sclera. It ends anteriorly below the conjunctiva. It is separated from the sclera mostly by the episcleral space. A C

5   *Suspensory ligament of eyeball.* Expansion of the check ligaments of the lateral and medius rectus muscles beneath the eyeball. C

6   **Episcleral space.** Gliding space between the eyeball and fascial sheath of the eyeball that is crossed by long, delicate connective-tissue fibers. A

7   **Retrobulbar fat; Orbital fat body.** Fat body filling the spaces around the extra-ocular muscles, eyeball, and optic nerve. It is bounded anteriorly by the orbital septum. A E

8   **Muscular fascia.** Sheaths of the Tenon's capsule that are reflected on the tendons and bellies of the six extra-ocular muscles. A

9   **Extra-ocular muscles; Extrinsic muscles of eyeball.**

10   **Orbitalis; Orbital muscle.** Thin layer of smooth muscle bridging the inferior orbital fissure. D

11   **Superior rectus.** o: Common tendinous ring. i: Along an oblique line passing anterior to the equator, 7–8 mm behind the corneal margin. Action: Elevation and intorsion of superior pole. I: Oculomotor nerve. B D E

12   **Inferior rectus.** o: Common tendinous ring. i: Along an oblique line about 6 mm from the corneal margin. Action: Depression of the eye and extorsion of the superior pole. I: Oculomotor nerve. B D E

13   **Medial rectus.** o: Common tendinous ring. i: About 5.5 mm from the corneal margin. Action: Adduction of the corneal pole. I: Oculomotor nerve. B C D

14   *[[Check ligament of medial rectus muscle]].* Sheet of fascia extending to the lacrimal bone. C

15   **Lateral rectus.** o: Common tendinous ring and lesser wing of sphenoid. i: 5.5 mm behind the corneal margin. Action: Abduction of the corneal pole. I: Abducent nerve. B C D E

16   *Check ligament of lateral rectus muscle.* Sheet of fascia extending to the zygomatic bone. C

17   **Common tendinous ring; Common anular tendon.** Tendinous ring giving origin to the rectus muscles. It surrounds the optic canal and medial part of the superior orbital fissure. D

18   **Superior oblique.** o: Medial to the common tendinous ring on the body of sphenoid. i: After a hook shaped course, obliquely behind the equator. Its tendon passes through the trochlea. Action: Abduction, intorsion, and depression of the eye. I: Trochlear nerve. D

19   *Trochlea.* Short, curved fibrocartilage tubes that serve as a pulley for the tendon of the superior oblique. They are fixed to the medial wall of the orbital cavity. B

20   *Tendinous sheath of superior oblique.* Tubes resembling tendinous sheaths that assist in guiding the tendon of the superior oblique in the trochlea. B

21   **Inferior oblique.** o: Lateral alongside the nasolacrimal canal. i: Behind the equator. Action: Gaze elevation, abduction, and extorsion. I: Oculomotor nerve. E

22   **Levator palpebrae superioris.** o: Upper portion of optic canal and dural sheath of optic nerve. Its insertion tendon widens anteriorly and divides into a superior and an inferior layer. I: Oculomotor nerve. A B D E

23   *Superficial layer.* Layer passing between the tarsus and orbicularis oculi into the connective tissue of the upper lid lying just beneath the skin. It is so wide that it reaches the orbital wall, especially the lateral wall. A

24   *Deep layer.* Layer attached at the upper margin and anterior surface of the tarsus. A

21

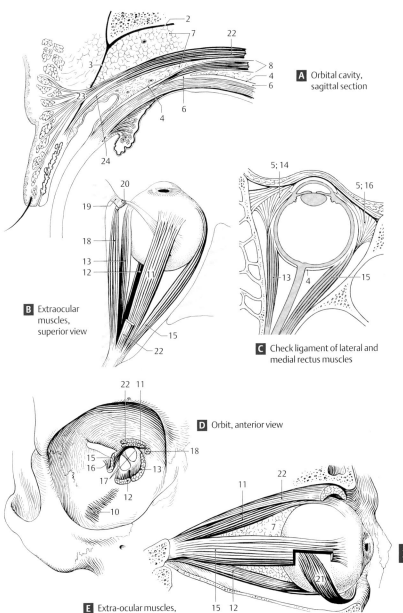

A Orbital cavity, sagittal section

B Extraocular muscles, superior view

C Check ligament of lateral and medial rectus muscles

D Orbit, anterior view

E Extra-ocular muscles, lateral view

21

1 **Eyebrow.** Eyebrow with its thicker, brushlike hair. A

2 **Eyelids.**

3 **Superior eyelid; Upper eyelid.** Larger, upper eyelid. A

4 **Inferior eyelid; Lower eyelid.** Smaller, lower eyelid. A

5 **Anterior surface of eyelid.** Anterior surface that is covered by the outer layer of skin. E

6 **Palpebronasal fold; Medial canthic fold.** Continuation of the covering fold of the upper eyelid to the lateral wall of the nose, overlapping the medial angle of eye. C

7 **Posterior surface of eyelid.** Surface lined with conjunctival epithelium which contains scattered goblet cells. E

8 **Palpebral fissure.** Opening between the margins of the upper and lower eyelids. A

9 **Lateral palpebral commissure.** Junction of the upper and lower eyelids at the lateral angle of eye. A

10 **Medial palpebral commissure.** Junction of the upper and lower eyelids at the medial angle of eye. A

11 **Lateral angle of eye.** Sharp lateral angle of the eye that simultaneously forms the lateral end of the palpebral fissure. A

12 **Medial angle of eye.** Medial end of the palpebral fissure that has a convex, rounded shape for the lacrimal lake. A

13 **Anterior palpebral margin.** Margin of the eyelids facing the outer skin of the eyelid. E

14 **Posterior palpebral margin.** Inner margin of the eyelids facing the conjunctiva. E

15 **Eyelash.** Eyelashes arranged in 3–4 rows near the anterior palpebral margin. E F

16 **Superior tarsus.** Semilunar fibrous plate that is curved like a bowl and forms the upper eyelid. It measures about 10 mm vertically and consists of tough, connective tissue of interwoven collagen fibers. It contains the tarsal glands. B E

17 **Inferior tarsus.** Semilunar fibrous plate forming the lower eyelid that measures about 5 mm vertically. It consists of tough, connective tissue of interwoven collagen fibers and contains the tarsal glands. B E

18 **Medial palpebral ligament.** Connective-tissue band connecting the medial palpebral commissure and medial wall of the orbit, lying immediately anterior to the fossa for the lacrimal sac. B D

19 **[[Lateral palpebral raphe]].** Thin band on the lateral palpebral ligament that is reinforced by the orbicularis oculi. D

20 **Lateral palpebral ligament.** Attachment of the lateral palpebral commissure at the lateral wall of the orbit, anterior to the orbital septum. B

21 **Tarsal glands (meibomian glands).** Elongated string of holocrine glands in the superior and inferior tarsi with openings near the posterior palpebral margin. They produce a sebaceous discharge that lubricates the margins of the eyelids. E

22 **Ciliary glands (Moll's glands).** Apocrine glands situated at the margin of the eyelid. They open either into the hair follicles of the eyelashes or on the margin of the eyelid. E

23 **Sebaceous glands (Glands of Zeis).** Small sebaceous glands with openings into the hair follicles of the eyelashes. E

24 **Superior tarsal muscle.** Smooth muscle between the musculotendinous junction of the levator palpebrae and superior tarsus. E

25 **Inferior tarsal muscle.** Smooth muscle between the inferior conjunctival fornix and the inferior tarsus. E

26 **Conjunctiva.** Membrane covering the inner surface of the eyelids where it is composed of stratified (dual-layered or multilayered) columnar epithelium with goblet cells and a loosely organized, well-vascularized lamina propria containing numerous cells. It reflects at the conjunctival fornix onto the eyeball, covering it with stratified squamous epithelium as far as the corneal margin. E

27 **Plica semilunaris.** Fold at the medial angle of eye that connects the superior and inferior conjunctival fornices. F

28 **Lacrimal caruncle.** Mucosal protuberance at the medial angle of eye with stratified squamous or columnar epithelium. F

21

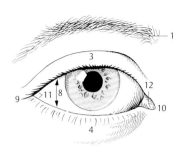

A Palpebral fissure

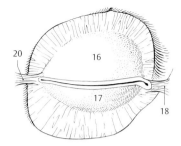

B Tarsi and ligaments

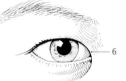

C Medial canthic fold

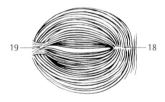

D Orbicularis oculi, posterior view

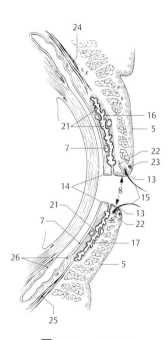

E Eyelids, sagittal section

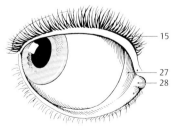

F Medial angle of eye

21

1 **Bulbar conjunctiva.** Portion of the conjunctiva covering the eyeball. It consists of stratified, nonkeratinized squamous epithelium with only a small number of goblet cells and a lamina propria of loosely organized structures, containing few cells and permeated by elastic fibers. A

2 **Palpebral conjunctiva.** Conjunctiva lining the posterior surface of the eyelids. It consists of stratified (dual-layered or multilayered) columnar epithelium with goblet cells and a well-vascularized lamina propria with loosely organized structures. A

3 **Superior conjunctival fornix.** Reflection of bulbar conjunctiva onto the palpebral conjunctiva located high up behind the superior eyelid. A

4 **Inferior conjunctival fornix.** Reflection of bulbar conjunctiva onto the palpebral conjunctiva behind the inferior eyelid. A

5 **Conjunctival sac.** Crevice between the palpebral conjunctiva and bulbar conjunctiva. It ends at the superior and inferior conjunctival fornices. A

6 **Conjunctival glands.** Follicle-like aggregations of lymphocytes at the medial angle of eye.

7 **Lacrimal apparatus.** Structure serving to maintain the moistness of the cornea and conjunctiva. B

8 **Lacrimal gland.** Gland located above the lateral angle of eye. It is divided by the tendon of the levator palpebrae into an upper and lower portion. Its excretory ducts open laterally in the superior conjunctival fornix. B

9 *Orbital part.* Larger portion of the lacrimal gland situated above the tendon of the levator palpebrae. B

10 *Palpebral part.* Smaller portion of the lacrimal gland situated below the tendon of the levator palpebrae. B

11 *Excretory ducts.* Between 6 and 14 excretory ducts of the lacrimal gland that open into the superior conjunctival fornix. B

12 **[Accessory lacrimal glands].** Additional smaller, scattered lacrimal glands that are mostly situated near the superior conjunctival fornix. A

13 **Lacrimal pathway.** Groove between the closed margins of the eyelids and the eyeball.

14 **Lacus lacrimalis; Lacrimal lake.** Space in the medial angle of eye around the lacrimal caruncle. B C

15 **Lacrimal papilla.** Single small, medial, conical elevation on each eye at the inner margin of the upper and lower eyelids on top of which the lacrimal punctum sits. C

16 **Lacrimal punctum.** Punctate beginning of the lacrimal drainage system situated on the lacrimal papilla. C

17 **Lacrimal canaliculus.** One duct present on each eye that measures up to 1 cm in length and extends from the lacrimal punctum to the lacrimal sac. C

18 *Ampulla of lacrimal canaliculus.* Slight dilatation at the bend in the lacrimal duct. C

19 **Lacrimal sac.** Sac measuring about 1.5 cm long and 0.5 cm wide lying in the lacrimal fossa. Its inferior portion is directly continuous with the nasolacrimal duct. C

20 *Fornix of lacrimal sac.* Domelike space in the upper part of the lacrimal sac. C

21 **Nasolacrimal duct.** Duct arising directly from the lacrimal sac. Measuring 1.2–2.4 cm in length, it travels through the nasolacrimal canal and opens into the inferior nasal meatus. Its flattened lumen has a mucosal lining covered with stratified (dual-layered or multilayered) columnar epithelium that in places is ciliated. C

22 *Lacrimal fold.* Mucosal fold at the opening of the nasolacrimal duct located 3–3.5 cm posterior to the piriform aperture in the inferior nasal meatus. C

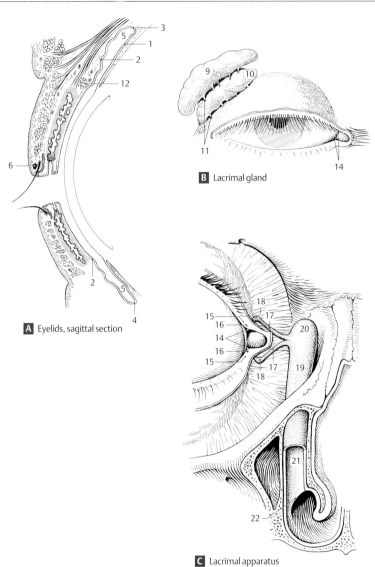

A Eyelids, sagittal section

B Lacrimal gland

C Lacrimal apparatus

1 *EAR.*

2 **EXTERNAL EAR.** Outer portion of the ear consisting of the auricle, external acoustic meatus, and tympanic membrane.

3 **Auricle; Pinna.** A B

4 **Lobule of auricle; Lobe of ear.** Noncartilaginous, inferior end of the auricle. A B

5 **Auricular cartilage.** Supporting framework of the auricle that is composed of elastic cartilage. C

6 **Helix.** Outer, curved margin of the auricle. A B C

7 *Crus of helix.* Beginning of the helix at the concha of auricle. A B C

8 *Spine of helix.* Small protuberance projecting anteriorly from the crus of helix. C

9 *Tail of helix.* Posteroinferior end of the helix that is separated by a notch from the antitragus. C

10 **Antihelix.** Curved elevation in front of the tail of helix. A B C

11 *Triangular fossa.* Anterosuperior depression that is bordered by both crura of antihelix. A C

12 *Crura of antihelix.* Two limbs formed by the superior bifurcation of the antihelix. They bound the triangular fossa. A C

13 **Scapha.** Groove between the helix and antihelix. A C

14 **Concha of auricle.** Hollow of the auricle that is bordered by the antihelix, antitragus, and tragus. A

15 *Cymba conchae.* Upper, slitlike portion of the concha located between the crus of helix and crus of antihelix. A

16 *Cavity of concha.* Main part of the concha situated below the crus of helix and behind the tragus. A

17 **Antitragus.** Small elevation that forms a continuation of the antihelix. It is separated from the tragus by the intertragic incisure. A C

18 **Tragus.** Flat prominence in front the external acoustic pore. A

19 **Anterior notch (of ear).** Furrow between the tragus (supratragic tubercle) and crus of helix. A

20 **Intertragic incisure; Intertragic notch.** Notch between the tragus and antitragus. A C

21 **[Auricular tubercle]. (Darwin's tubercle).** Occasional elevation on the superior posterior aspect of the inner margin of the auricle. A

22 **[Apex of auricle; Tip of ear].** Occasional protrusion of the outer margin of the auricle that is directed outward and to posterosuperior. B

23 **Posterior auricular groove.** Faint notch between the antitragus and antihelix. A

24 **[Supratragic tubercle].** Occasional, small tubercle on the superior end of the tragus. A

25 **Isthmus of cartilaginous auricle.** Narrow junction where the cartilage of the external acoustic meatus and tragal lamina meet the auricular cartilage. D

26 **Terminal notch of auricle.** Deep notch dividing the tragal lamina from the auricular cartilage. D

27 **Fissura antitragohelicina.** Deep furrow dividing the inferior portions of the antitragus and helix near its inferior end and the antihelix and helix near its superior end. D

28 **[[Sulcus anthelicis transversus]].** Furrow visible from posteromedial that is situated between the eminentia fossae triangularis and eminentia conchae. D

29 **Groove of crus of helix.** Faint groove on the posterior surface of the auricular cartilage. It corresponds to the crus of helix on the anterior surface. D

30 **Fossa antihelica; Antihelical fossa.** Groove on the posterior surface of the auricular cartilage that corresponds to the antihelix on the anterior surface. D

31 **Eminentia conchae.** Elevation on the posterior surface of the auricular cartilage corresponding to the cavity of the concha. D

32 **Eminentia scaphae.** Curved elevation on the posterior surface of the auricular cartilage corresponding to the scapha on the anterior surface. D

33 **Eminentia fossae triangularis.** Elevation on the posterior surface of the auricular cartilage corresponding to the triangular fossa. D

21

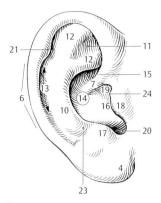

A Auricle

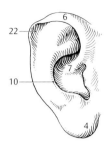

B Auricle and eminences

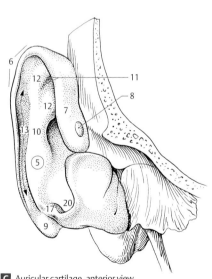

C Auricular cartilage, anterior view

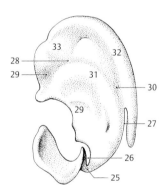

D Auricular cartilage, medial view

21

1 **Ligaments of auricle.** Bands attaching the auricular cartilage to the temporal bone.

2 **Anterior ligament of auricle.** Band of fibers extending from the root of the zygomatic arch to the spine of the helix. A

3 **Superior ligament of auricle.** Band passing from the upper margin of the bony external meatus to the spine of helix. A

4 **Posterior ligament of auricle.** Band of connective tissue passing from the eminentia concha to the mastoid process. B

5 **Auricular muscles.**

6 **Helicis major.** Muscle ascending from the spine of helix to the helix. A

7 **Helicis minor.** Muscle lying on the crus of helix. A

8 **Tragicus.** Vertically-oriented muscle lying on the tragal lamina. A

9 **[Muscle of terminal notch].** Inconstant portion of the tragicus that extends to the terminal notch of the auricle.

10 **Pyramidal muscle of auricle.** Muscle fibers that occasionally split off from the tragicus and extend to the spine of helix. A

11 **Antitragicus.** Muscle fibers on the antitragus, some of which pass to the tail of helix. A

12 **Transverse muscle of auricle.** Muscle lying on the posterior surface of the auricular cartilage. It stretches between the eminentia scaphae and eminentia conchae. B

13 **Oblique muscle of auricle.** Muscle fibers passing between the eminentia conchae and eminentia fossae triangularis. B

14 **External acoustic meatus.** Canal that is shaped like a flattened "S" and consists of cartilaginous and bony segments. It is about 2.4 cm long with a diameter of about 6 mm. D

15 **External acoustic pore; External acoustic aperture.** Opening of the acoustic meatus to external. D

16 **Tympanic notch.** Notch between the greater and lesser tympanic spines. In the newborn it is formed by the unclosed upper ends of the tympanic ring.

17 **Cartilaginous external acoustic meatus.** Lateral, cartilaginous one-third of the external acoustic meatus. C

18 *Cartilage of acoustic meatus.* Cartilage connected with that of the auricle. It forms a furrow that opens superiorly and posteriorly. C

19 *Notch in cartilage of acoustic meatus.* Usually two anteriorly directed gaps in the cartilage of acoustic meatus that are bridged by connective tissue. C

20 **Tragal lamina.** Lateral part of the cartilage of acoustic meatus. It lies in front of the external acoustic pore. C

21 **Tympanic membrane.** Membrane stretched diagonally at the end of the external acoustic meatus. It has a diameter of 9–11 mm. E F

22 **Pars flaccida (Shrapnell's membrane).** Smaller, flaccid part of the tympanic membrane above the anterior and posterior malleolar folds. E F

23 **Pars tensa.** Much larger portion of the tympanic membrane that is stretched within the tympanic ring. E F

24 **Anterior malleolar fold.** Fold on the inner surface of the tympanic membrane that extends anteriorly with a concave inferior border from the base of the handle of malleus. F

25 **Posterior malleolar fold.** Fold on the inner surface of the tympanic membrane that curves posteriorly with a concave inferior border from the root of the handle of malleus. F

26 **Malleolar prominence.** Small elevation on the outer surface of the tympanic membrane produced by the lateral process of the malleus. E

27 **Malleolar stria.** Lighter strip on the outer surface of the tympanic membrane that is produced by the handle of malleus attached there, visible through the membrane. E

28 **Umbo of tympanic membrane.** Portion of the membrane lying at the tip of the handle of malleus that draws the tympanic membrane inward. E

29 **Fibrocartilaginous ring.** Ring of tissue anchoring the tympanic membrane in the tympanic sulcus. G

21

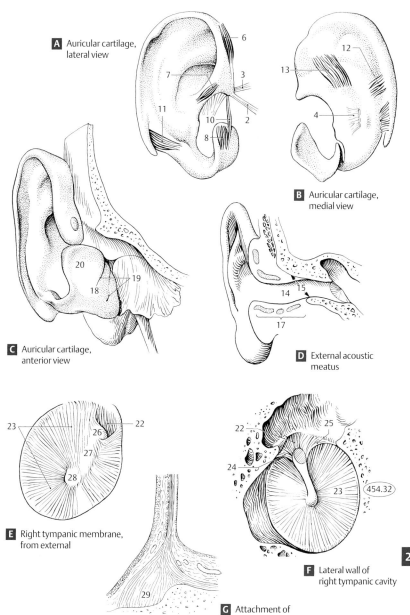

A Auricular cartilage, lateral view

B Auricular cartilage, medial view

C Auricular cartilage, anterior view

D External acoustic meatus

E Right tympanic membrane, from external

F Lateral wall of right tympanic cavity

G Attachment of tympanic membrane

454.32

21

1 **MIDDLE EAR.** Portion of the ear comprising the tympanic cavity, auditory tube, and mastoid cells.

2 TYMPANIC CAVITY. Oblique crevice situated medial to the tympanic membrane. It contains the auditory ossicles and communicates posterosuperiorly with the pneumatized mastoid cells and anterosuperiorly with the nasopharynx via the auditory tube.

3 **Tegmental wall; Tegmental roof.** Thin roof of the tympanic cavity that lies lateral to the arcuate eminence of the petrous part of temporal bone. A

4 *Epitympanic recess.* Dome of the tympanic cavity above the upper border of the tympanic membrane that arches upward and laterally. A

5 *Cupular part.* Superior portion of the epitympanic recess. A

6 **Jugular wall; Floor.** Inferior wall of the tympanic cavity facing the jugular fossa. A

7 *Styloid prominence.* Elevation in the floor of the tympanic cavity caused by the styloid process. A

8 **Labyrinthine wall; Medial wall.** Medial wall of the tympanic cavity.

9 *Oval window.* Opening that is closed off by the base of the stapes. A

10 *Fossa of oval window.* Small depression in the medial wall of the tympanic cavity between the malleus and incus. A

11 *Promontory.* Elevation produced by the basal turn of the cochlea. A

12 *Groove of promontory.* Branched groove on the promontory that is produced by the tympanic plexus. A

13 *Subiculum of promontory.* Thin, bony ridge behind the promontory and round window. A

14 *Sinus tympani.* Deep depression behind the promontory and round window. B

15 *Round window.* Round opening at the end of the scala tympani that is closed off by the secondary tympanic membrane. B

16 *Fossa of round window.* Depression leading to the round window. B

17 *Crest of round window.* Bony ridge along the round window that gives attachment to the secondary tympanic membrane. B

18 *Processus cochleariformis.* Spoon-shaped bony process above the promontory at the end of the canal for the tensor tympani. Together with a connective-tissue sling it serves as a pulley for the tensor tympani. B

19 *Secondary tympanic membrane.* Membranous septum stretched in the round window between the scala tympani and tympanic cavity.

20 **Mastoid wall; Posterior wall.** Wall of the tympanic cavity facing the mastoid process.

21 *Aditus to mastoid antrum.* Entrance from the tympanic cavity into the mastoid antrum. B

22 *Prominence of lateral semicircular canal.* Elevation above the prominence of the facial canal that is produced by the lateral semicircular canal. B

23 *Prominence of facial canal.* Elevation produced by the facial canal between the oval window and the prominence of the lateral semicircular canal. B

24 *Pyramidal eminence.* Conical, bony prominence at the level of the oval window with a perforated summit. It contains the stapedius and gives its tendon exit through the opening at its tip. B

25 *Fossa of incus.* Small depression in the aditus to mastoid antrum that contains the posterior ligament of incus. B

26 *Posterior sinus.* Small pit between the fossa of incus and the pyramidal eminence. B

27 *Tympanic aperture of canaliculus for chorda tympani.* Opening into the tympanic cavity lying at the posterior margin of the tympanic membrane at the level of the pyramidal eminence. B

28 **Mastoid antrum.** Space continuous with the tympanic cavity to posterosuperior. The mastoid cells extend from here downward. B

29 *Mastoid cells.* Pneumatized cells that, like the tympanic cavity, are lined with squamous or cuboidal epithelium. B

30 *Tympanic cells.* Small, cell-like pits in the floor of the tympanic cavity. B

31 **Carotid wall.** Anterior wall that is formed partly by the carotid canal and partly by the opening of the auditory tube. B

32 **Membranous wall; Lateral wall.** Lateral wall of the tympanic cavity that is mostly formed by the tympanic membrane. p. 453 F

21

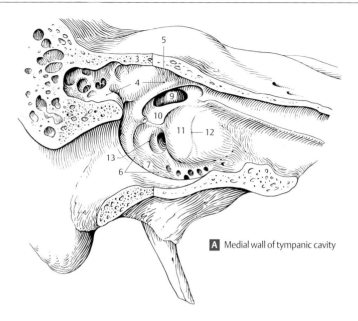

A Medial wall of tympanic cavity

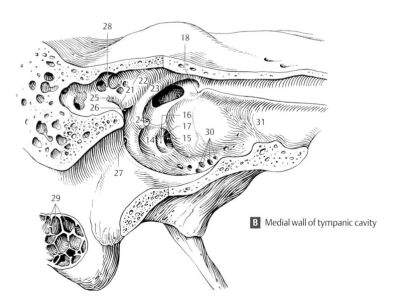

B Medial wall of tympanic cavity

21

1 AUDITORY OSSICLES. Malleus, incus, and stapes. They form a type of lever system that transmits sound from the tympanic membrane to the internal ear.

2 **Stapes.** Stirrup-shaped ossicle, the base of which is integrated into the oval window. A B

3 **Head of stapes.** Portion of the stapes situated opposite its base that articulates via the lenticular process with the long limb of incus. A B

4 **Anterior limb.** Nearly straight, anterior limb of stapes. A B

5 **Posterior limb.** Curved, posterior limb of stapes. A B

6 **Base of stapes; Footplate.** Part inserted in the oval window. A B

7 **Incus.** Ossicle interposed between the stapes and the head of the malleus. A D

8 **Body of incus.** Portion that articulates via a saddle-shaped articular surface with the malleus. A

9 **Long limb.** Limb descending nearly vertically behind the handle of malleus with the lenticular process at its end. A

10 *Lenticular process.* Tiny bony process at the end of the long limb of incus. It articulates with the stapes. A

11 **Short limb.** Limb pointing horizontally backward and attached by a ligament to the fossa of incus. A

12 **Malleus.** Ossicle interposed between the tympanic membrane and incus. A C

13 **Handle of malleus.** Manubrium of malleus that is fused along its lateral surface with the tympanic membrane as far as the lateral process. A

14 **Head of malleus.** Portion bearing a convex facet for articulation with the body of incus. A

15 **Neck of malleus.** Segment connecting the head and handle of malleus. A

16 **Lateral process.** Short, lateral process at the end of the handle of malleus. It produces the malleolar prominence in the tympanic membrane. A

17 **Anterior process.** Longer, very thin process. In the newborn it extends into the petrotympanic fissure. It regresses in the adult. A

18 ARTICULATIONS OF AUDITORY OSSICLES. These are not true joints, but rather syndesmoses.

19 **Incudomallear joint.** Articulation between the malleus and incus. It occasionally has an articular cavity. A

20 **Incudostapedial joint.** Articulation between the stapes and the lenticular process of the long limb of incus. A

21 **Tympanostapedial syndesmosis.** Connective tissue inserted at the base of the stapes in the oval window. Its anterior part is wider than its posterior part. B

22 **Ligaments of auditory ossicles.**

23 **Anterior ligament of malleus.** Band arising from the anterior process of the malleus, lying in the anterior malleolar fold, and passing into the petrotympanic fissure. D

24 **Superior ligament of malleus.** Band passing from the head of malleus to the roof of the epitympanic recess. C D

25 **Lateral ligament of malleus.** Band connecting the neck of malleus with the upper margin of the tympanic notch. C

26 **Superior ligament of incus.** Band running nearly parallel to the superior ligament of malleus, connecting the body of incus with the roof of the epitympanic recess. C D

27 **Posterior ligament of incus.** Band passing from the short limb of incus to the lateral wall of the tympanic cavity. C D

28 **Stapedial membrane.** Thin membrane between the limbs of the stapes and its base. B

29 **Anular ligament of stapes.** Band connecting the base of stapes and the margins of the oval window. Its anterior portion is wider than its posterior portion. B

21

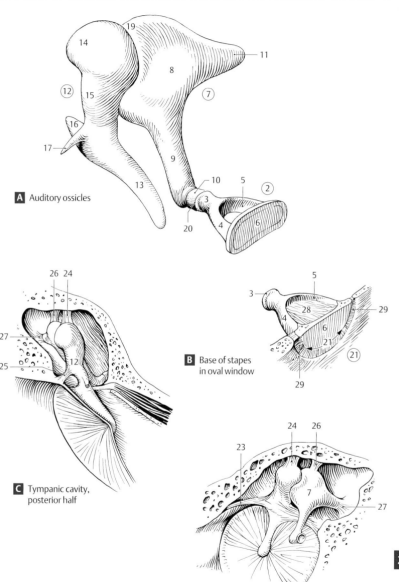

A Auditory ossicles

B Base of stapes in oval window

C Tympanic cavity, posterior half

D Lateral wall of tympanic cavity

21

1 MUSCLES OF AUDITORY OSSICLES. The following two muscles attached to the auditory ossicles.

2 **Tensor tympani.** Muscle lying in the canal for the tensor tympani above the auditory tube. Its tendon runs laterally at nearly a right angle around the processus cochleariformis and attaches to the base of the handle of malleus. I: Mandibular nerve. A

3 **Stapedius.** Muscle arising in a bony canal in the posterior wall of the tympanic cavity. It emerges at the tip of the pyramidal eminentia and attaches to the head of stapes. It tilts the base of stapes, dampening its vibrations. I: Nerve to stapedius, given off by the facial nerve. B

4 **Mucosa of tympanic cavity.** Thin mucosal lining of the tympanic cavity. It consists of simple squamous or cuboidal epithelium and a delicate, well-vascularized lamina propria.

5 **Posterior fold of malleus.** Fold extending from the base of the handle of malleus as far as the posterosuperior portion of the tympanic ring. It contains the posterior portion of the chorda tympani. D

6 **Anterior fold of malleus.** Fold extending from the base of the handle of malleus as far as the anterosuperior portion of the tympanic ring. It contains the anterior portion of the chorda tympani, the anterior process of malleus, and the anterior ligament of malleus. D

7 **Fold of chorda tympani.** Fold produced by the chorda tympani on the neck of the malleus between the anterior and posterior folds of malleus. D

8 **Recesses of tympanic membrane.** Mucosal pouches in the tympanic cavity.

9 *Anterior recess.* Mucosal pouch between the anterior fold of malleus and the tympanic membrane. D

10 *Superior recess (Pouch of Prussak).* Mucosal pouch bordered laterally by the pars flaccida of the tympanic membrane and medially by the head and neck of malleus as well as the body of incus. D

11 *Posterior recess.* Mucosal pouch between the posterior fold of malleus and the tympanic membrane. D

12 **Fold of incus.** Mucosal fold extending from the roof of the epitympanic recess to the head of incus or from the short limb of incus to the posterior wall of the tympanic cavity. D

13 **Fold of stapedius.** Mucosal fold passing from the posterior wall of the tympanic cavity to the stapes. It encloses the stapedius and stapes. B

14 PHARYNGOTYMPANIC TUBE; AUDITORY TUBE. Nearly 4 cm long, partly cartilaginous, partly bony passageway connecting the middle ear and nasopharynx that serves to ventilate the tympanic cavity. A C

15 **Tympanic opening.** Opening of the auditory tube in the anterior wall of the tympanic cavity. It usually lies slightly above the floor of the tympanic cavity. A

16 **Bony part (of auditory tube).** Lateral, posterior, superior bony part of auditory tube, comprising about one-third of its entire length. It lies beneath the canal for the tensor tympani and emerges between the carotid canal and foramen spinosum. A

17 **Isthmus of auditory tube.** Narrow part of the auditory tube between the cartilaginous and bony parts. A

18 **Tubal air cells.** Small depressions in the wall of the bony part of auditory tube. A

19 **Cartilaginous part (of auditory tube).** Anteromedial, cartilaginous part of auditory tube measuring about 2.5 cm in length. A

20 **Cartilage of tube.** Auditory tube cartilage that appears hook-shaped in cross-section. It decreases in height posterolaterally and is composed of elastic cartilage only in the angle between its two laminae. A

21 *Medial lamina.* Wider, medial sheet of cartilage. C

22 *Lateral lamina.* Low sheet of cartilage directed anterolaterally. C

23 *Membranous lamina.* Membranous part in the wall of the cartilaginous part of auditory tube. A C

24 **Mucosa; Mucous membrane.** Auditory tube mucosa consisting of simple, ciliated epithelium. C

25 *Tubal glands.* Mucoid glands situated mostly in the cartilaginous part of auditory tube. C

26 **Pharyngeal opening.** Funnel-shaped or slitlike opening of the auditory tube above the levator eminence at the level of the inferior nasal meatus 1 cm in front of the posterior wall of the pharynx. A

21

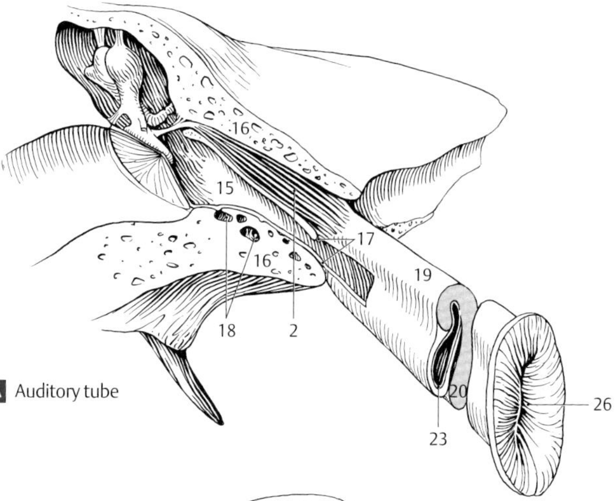

A Auditory tube

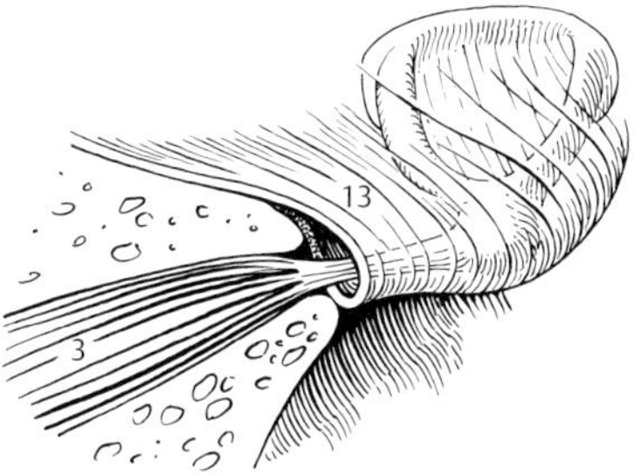

B Stapedius

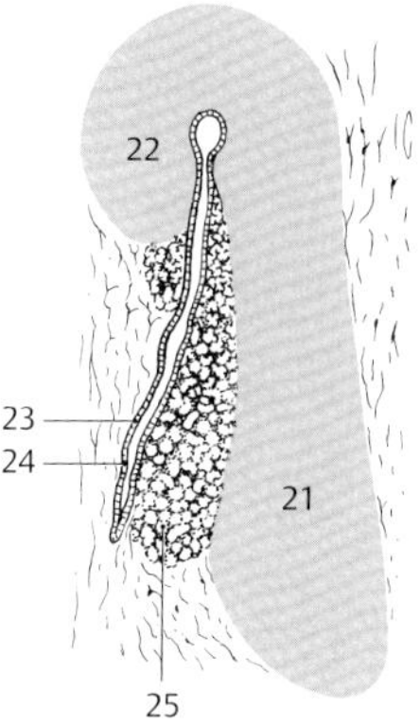

C Auditory tube, cross-section

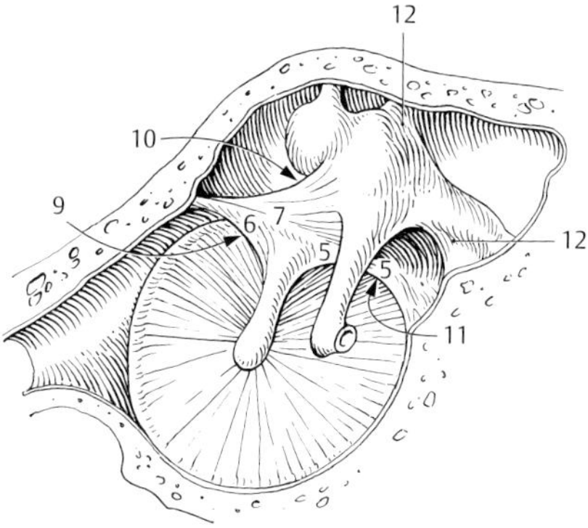

D Lateral wall of tympanic cavity

1 **INTERNAL EAR.** Portion of the vestibulo-cochlear organ housed in the petrous part of temporal bone.

2 **Vestibulocochlear organ.** Sensory system located in the temporal bone for perception of sound, head position, and positional changes.

3 BONY LABYRINTH. Bony capsule containing the membranous labyrinth. B

4 **Vestibule.** Portion of the bony labyrinth containing the utricle and saccule. B

5 **Elliptical recess; Utricular recess.** Elongated depression in the medial wall of the vestibule. It lodges the portion of the utricle between the posterior bony ampulla and common bony limb. B

6 *Internal opening of vestibular canaliculus.* Beginning of the canaliculus in the elliptical recess.

7 **Vestibular crest.** Ridge between the spherical recess and elliptical recess. B

8 *Pyramid of vestibule.* Upper, broader portion of the vestibular crest. B

9 **Spherical recess; Saccular recess.** Round niche in the medial wall of the vestibule that lodges the saccule. B

10 **Cochlear recess.** Depression situated beneath and anterior to the spherical recess. It lodges the inferior end of the cochlear duct. A

11 **Maculae cribrosae.** Perforated areas in the bone giving passage to fibers from the vestibulocochlear nerve.

12 *Macula cribrosa superior.* Perforated area in the bone giving passage to fibers from the utriculoampullary nerve. A

13 *Macula cribrosa media.* Perforated area in the bone near the base of cochlea giving passage to fibers from the saccular nerve. A

14 *Macula cribrosa inferior.* Perforated area in the wall of the posterior bony ampulla giving passage to fibers from the posterior ampullary nerve. A

15 **Semicircular (bony) canals.** Semicircular spaces surrounded by a bony wall that can be dissected. They contain the perilymphatic and endolymphatic spaces. A

16 **Anterior semicircular canal.** Anterior (superior) semicircular canal. It shares a common limb with the posterior semicircular canal and is situated vertically, nearly perpendicular to the axis of the petrous part of temporal bone. C

17 *Anterior bony ampulla.* Anterior ampulla lying directly adjacent to the lateral bony ampulla. C

18 **Posterior semicircular canal.** Canal situated furthest to inferior. It is situated nearly parallel to the axis of the petrous part of temporal bone. C

19 *Posterior bony ampulla.* Posterior ampulla lying beneath the level of the lateral semicircular canal. C

20 **Common bony limb.** Posterior limb formed by the union of the limbs of the anterior (superior) and posterior semicircular canals. C

21 *Ampullary bony limbs.* Limbs of the semicircular canals that are correspondingly widened for reception of the ampullae of the membranous labyrinth. C

22 **Lateral semicircular canal.** It lies horizontally and can produce a prominence in the medial wall of the tympanic cavity. C

23 *Lateral bony ampulla.* Ampulla lying anteriorly, directly adjacent to the anterior bony ampulla. C

24 *Simple bony limb.* Posterior limb of the lateral semicircular canal that opens alone into the wall of the vestibule. C

25 **Cochlea.** Part of the internal ear that in humans consists of $2^{1}/_{2}$–$2^{3}/_{4}$ turns with a base measuring 8–9 mm in width and a total height of 4 5mm. C

26 **Cochlear cupula.** Part directed anteriorly, inferiorly, and laterally in the cranium. C

21

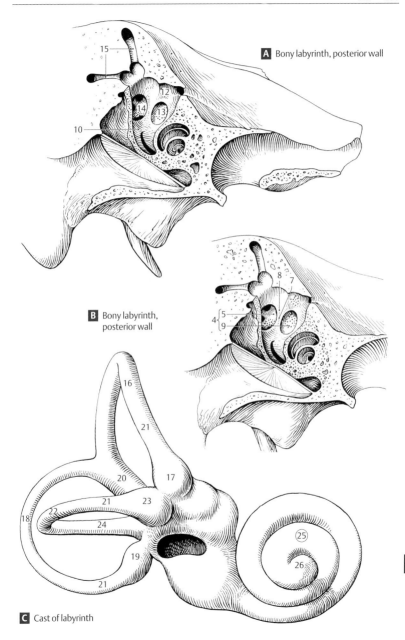

A Bony labyrinth, posterior wall

B Bony labyrinth, posterior wall

C Cast of labyrinth

21

1 **Base of cochlea.** Its surface faces toward the internal acoustic meatus. A

2 **Spiral canal of cochlea.** Three canals subdivided by, on the one side, the osseous spiral lamina and basal lamina, and on the other the vestibular wall of the cochlear duct. A

3 *Osseous spiral lamina.* One of the spiral, dual-layered bony ledges projecting from the modiolus into the spiral canal of cochlea. It does not completely divide the scala vestibuli and scala tympani until it is augmented by the cochlear duct. B

4 *Vestibular lamella.* Osseous lamina situated medial to and beneath the scala vestibuli. B

5 *Tympanic lamella.* Osseous lamina lying medial to and above the scala tympani. B

6 **Foramina nervosa.** Openings for the passage of nerve fibers from the organ of Corti to the spiral ganglion. p. 467 B

7 *Hamulus of spiral lamina.* Free, hook-shaped upper end of the osseous spiral lamina at the cochlear cupula. B

8 *Secondary spiral lamina.* Bony ridge situated in the lower half of the basal turn of the cochlea. It projects from the lateral wall of the spiral canal of cochlea opposite to the osseous spiral lamina. The inferior portion of the basal lamina is stretched between the two. B

9 *Internal opening of cochlear canaliculus.* Opening for the cochlear canaliculus in the scala tympani.

10 **Cochlear septum.** Bony roof or floor in the spiral canal of cochlea. A B

11 **Modiolus.** Conical part of the cochlea that is hollowed out to lodge the cochlear nerve. It forms the medial wall of the spiral canal of cochlea. A

12 *Base of modiolus.* Beginning of the modiolus at the base. A

13 *Lamina of modiolus.* Upright end of the osseous spiral lamina. A

14 *Spiral canal of modiolus.* Tiny canal in the wall of the modiolus near the base of the osseous spiral lamina. It contains the spiral ganglion of cochlea. A

15 *Longitudinal canals of modiolus.* Centrally located bony canals that lodge the fibers of the cochlear nerve arising from the spiral ganglion of the cochlea. A

16 **Scala vestibuli.** Passageway filled with perilymph that ascends as far as the cochlear cupula above the osseous spiral lamina and cochlear duct. A

17 **Helicotrema.** Opening at the cochlear cupula connecting the scala vestibuli and scala tympani. It arises because the osseous spiral lamina and cochlear duct end before the cochlear cupula. A B

18 **Scala tympani.** Passageway filled with perilymph below the osseous spiral lamina and basal lamina. A

19 **Internal acoustic meatus.** Passageway beginning at the posterior wall of the petrous part of temporal bone. It measures up to 1 cm in length and contains the vestibulocochlear nerve, facial nerve, and labyrinthine artery and vein. C

20 **Internal acoustic opening.** Entrance of the internal acoustic meatus at the posterior wall of the petrous part of temporal bone above the jugular foramen. C

21 **Fundus of internal acoustic meatus.** Floor of the internal acoustic meatus that is divided into several areas. C

22 *Transverse crest.* Transverse ridge dividing the fundus of internal acoustic meatus into upper and lower portions. C

23 *Facial area.* Area beginning with the facial canal. C

24 *Vertical crest.* Bony ridge between the facial area and the superior vestibular area. C

25 *Superior vestibular area.* Area situated lateral to the facial canal that gives passage to fibers from the utriculoampullary nerve. C

26 *Inferior vestibular area.* Area situated lateral to the tractus spiralis foraminosus that gives passage to fibers from the saccular nerve. C

27 *Foramen singulare.* Small opening behind the inferior vestibular area that transmits the posterior ampullary nerve. C

28 *Cochlear area.* Spacious area below the transverse crest that contains the tractus spiralis foraminosus. C

29 *Tractus spiralis foraminosus.* Perforated area corresponding to the spiral canal of cochlea. It gives passage to fibers from the spiral ganglion to the cochlear nerve. C

30 **Perilymphatic space.** Spaces containing perilymph that are partly traversed by connective-tissue fibers. They also include the scala vestibuli and scala tympani. p. 465 B

31 **Perilymph.** Fluid in the space between the membranous and bony labyrinth.

32 **Vestibular aqueduct.** Passageway connecting the endolymphatic space with the endolymphatic sac.

33 **Cochlear aqueduct.** Passageway connecting the perilymphatic space with the subarachnoid space. pp. 467 A, 469 A

21

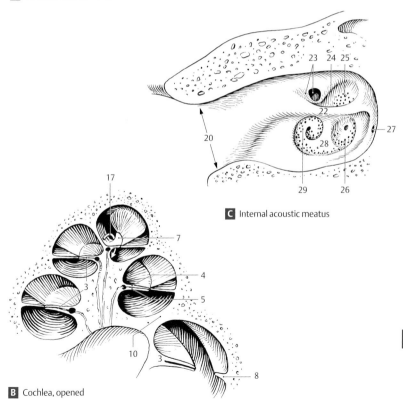

A Cochlea, longitudinal section

C Internal acoustic meatus

B Cochlea, opened

21

1 MEMBRANOUS LABYRINTH. Complicated system of tiny canals and dilatations lined with sensory epithelia that is suspended by connective-tissue bands in the bony labyrinth. A B

2 **Endolymphatic space.** Space in the membranous labyrinth.

3 *Endolymph.* Fluid in the membranous labyrinth.

4 VESTIBULAR LABYRINTH. Contents of the labyrinth including the semicircular canals, but excluding the cochlea.

5 **Utricle.** Small pouch serving as the base for the three semicircular canals. It measures 2.5–3.5 mm in diameter. A B

6 **Utricular recess.** Space in the utricle.

7 **Saccule.** Round vesicle measuring 2–3 mm that contains a sensory area. A B

8 **Semicircular ducts.** Three semicircular canals that form three semicircles within the bony semicircular canals, arranged perpendicularly, one above the other. Each duct corresponds to about 2/3 of a circle.

9 **Anterior semicircular duct.** Anterior (superior), vertical semicircular duct that stands nearly perpendicular to the axis of the petrous part of temporal bone. B

10 *Anterior membranous ampulla.* Anterior dilatation of the anterior (superior) semicircular duct situated near the lateral membranous ampulla. B

11 **Posterior semicircular duct.** Posterior semicircular duct that is situated in a vertical plane that runs nearly parallel to the long axis of the petrous part of temporal bone. B

12 *Posterior membranous ampulla.* Dilatation of the posterior semicircular duct that situated at some distance from the other two ampullae. B

13 **Common membranous limb.** Common opening of the anterior and posterior semicircular ducts into the utricle. B

14 *Ampullary membranous limbs.* Portions of the semicircular duct situated between the ampullae and utricle. B

15 **Lateral semicircular duct.** Horizontal duct that is situated furthest to lateral. It can produce a prominence in the medial wall of the tympanic cavity. B

16 *Lateral membranous ampulla.* Ampulla situated directly adjacent to the anterior membranous ampulla. B

17 *Simple membranous limb.* Posterior limb of the lateral semicircular duct that opens alone into the utricle. B

18 **Utriculosaccular duct.** Y-shaped connection joining the endolymphatic duct with the utricle and saccule. B

19 **Utricular duct.** Connection between the utricle and utriculosaccular duct. B

20 **Saccular duct.** Connection between the saccule and utriculosaccular duct. B

21 **Endolymphatic duct.** Thin endolymphatic duct arising from the saccule. It passes through the bony vestibular aqueduct and ends at the endolymphatic sac. B

22 **Endolymphatic sac.** Blind-ending pouch at the end of the endolymphatic duct, situated on the posterior wall of the petrous part of temporal bone between two layers of dura mater. B

23 **Ductus reuniens.** Thin tube connecting the saccule and cochlear duct. A B

24 **Maculae.** Sensory areas for perception of head position in space. A B

25 *Macula of utricle.* Horizontal sensory area on the floor of the utricle measuring 2.3–3 mm. A B

26 *Macula of saccule.* Vertical, curved sensory area on the medial wall of the saccule that is about 1.5 mm wide. A

27 *Otolithic membrane.* Membrane consisting of a gelatinous ground substance embedded with statoconia that forms a layer covering the maculae. It is permeated by brushlike processes of sensory cells. D E

28 *Otolith.* Up to 15 μm large calcareous particles that are embedded in a gelatinous substance along with the sensory hair cells. D E

29 *Striola.* Striplike depression (macula of utricle) or elevation (macula of saccule) of the statolithic membrane caused by a decrease or increase of statoconia. These strips contain an increased number of Type 1 hair cells. D E

30 **Ampullary crest.** Crescent-shaped ridge projecting into the ampullary space. It is covered with sensory epithelium and is comprised of nerve fibers and connective tissue. C

31 *Ampullary groove.* Groove below the ampullary crest that transmits a branch of the ampullary nerve to the ampullary crest. C

32 *Ampullary cupula.* Gelatinous body overhanging the epithelium of the ampullary crest and extending to its roof. The sensory hair cells are immersed in it. C

33 [[Neuroepithelium]]. Simple, columnar, sensory epithelium of the maculae that consists of supporting cells and sensory cells. The 20–25 **µ**m long brushlike processes of the sensory cells project into the statoconic membrane. D E

21

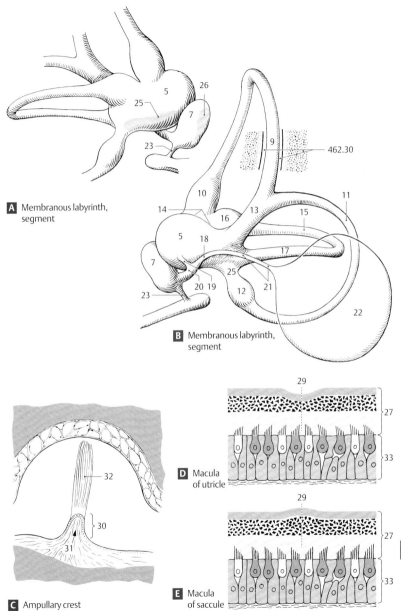

A Membranous labyrinth, segment

B Membranous labyrinth, segment

C Ampullary crest

D Macula of utricle

E Macula of saccule

1 COCHLEAR LABYRINTH. Contents of the bony cochlea.

2 **Scala media.**

3 **Cochlear duct.** Endolymphatic duct that in humans has $2^1/_2$–$2^3/_4$ turns and extends to the cochlear cupula. It is triangular in cross-section and contains sensory epithelium for sound perception. A C D

4 **Vestibular surface of cochlear duct; Vestibular membrane.** Upper wall of the cochlear duct. It is about 3 μm thick. C D

5 **External surface of cochlear duct.** Lateral wall of the cochlear duct. C D

6 *Stria vascularis.* Broad, highly vascularized strip with specially structured epithelial cells overlying the spiral prominence. It presumably secretes endolymph. D

7 *Spiral prominence.* Ridge running over the outer spiral sulcus. It consists of connective tissue and a blood vessel. C D

8 *Vas prominens.* Blood vessel running in the spiral prominence. C D

9 *Spiral ligament.* Layer of connective tissue on the bony wall of the cochlear duct. C

10 **Tympanic surface; Spiral membrane.** Inferior wall of the cochlear duct above the scala tympani. C

11 *Basal crest*; *Spiral crest.* Medial continuation of fibers from the spiral ligament. Attachment site of the basal lamina. C D

12 *Basal lamina.* Layer of connective tissue between the cochlear duct and scala tympani. It is stretched between the tympanic lamellae of the osseous spiral lamina and the spiral crest and bears the organ of Corti. C D

13 *Vas spirale.* Small blood vessel running in the tympanic layer of the basal lamina beneath the tunnel. D

14 **Spiral limbus.** Thickening and conversion of the terminal portion on the superior layer of the osseous spiral lamina. Its outer surface is grooved by the inner spiral sulcus. C

15 *Tympanic lip.* Upper, shorter extension of the limbus. Attachment site for the tectorial membrane. C

16 *Vestibular lip.* Lower, longer extension of the limbus. It lies on the basal lamina. B C

17 *Acoustic teeth.* Ridge of projecting rows of cells on the surface of the vestibular lip. Area giving attachment to the tectorial membrane. B

18 **Tectorial membrane.** Fibrous membrane that is thin at its attachment site on the vestibular lip. It overlies the organ of Corti and ends with a free margin outside the outer row of hair cells. B C

19 **Vestibular cecum.** Blind end of the cochlear duct in the cochlear cupula. A

20 **Cupular cecum.** Blind end of the cochlear duct facing the vestibule. A

21 **Spiral organ (Organ of Corti).** Sensory region lying on the basal lamina that converts sound waves into nerve impulses. B

22 *Reticular membrane.* Membranous covering of the organ of Corti. It consists of the heads of Corti's rods and Deiters' cells with the processes of the hair cells projecting in the spaces between them. B

23 *Inner spiral sulcus.* Groove between the vestibular lip and tympanic lip. B C

24 *Outer spiral sulcus.* Furrow on the outer wall of the cochlear duct between the spiral prominence and the organ of Corti. C

25 **Spiral ganglion.** Collection of bipolar ganglion cells in the spiral canal of the modiolus. Their peripheral nerve fibers arise from the hair cells and the central fibers form the cochlear nerve.

21

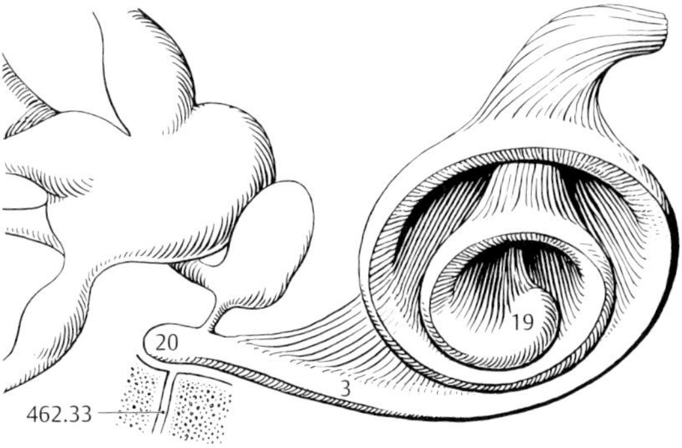

A Membranous labyrinth, segment

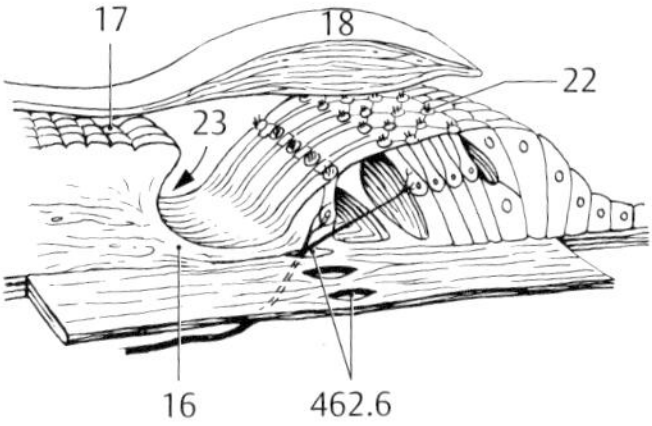

B Organ of Corti

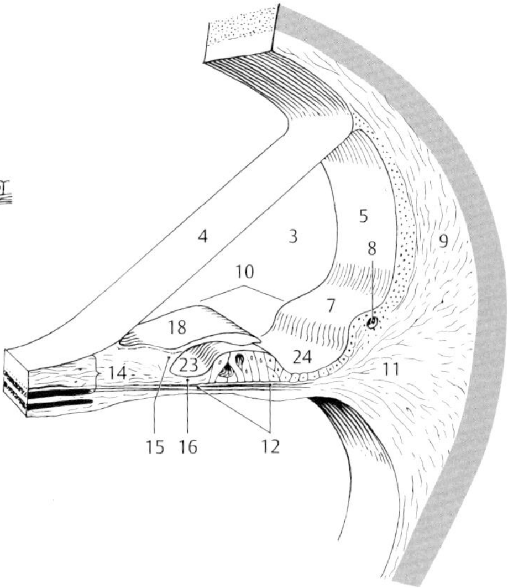

C Cochlear duct

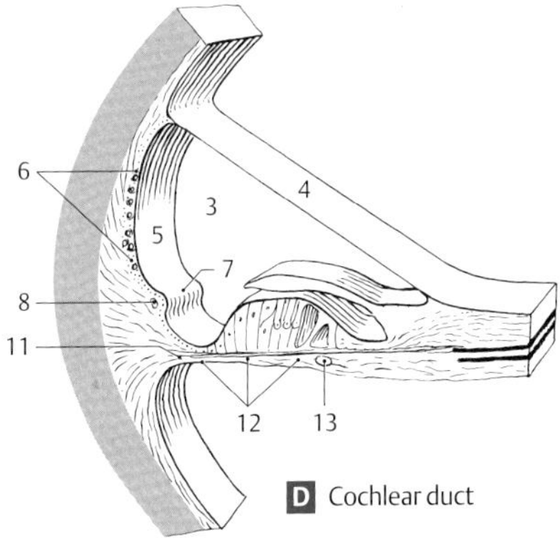

D Cochlear duct

21

1 Vessels of internal ear.

2 **Labyrinthine artery.** Principal artery that is usually a branch of the anterior inferior cerebellar artery. It accompanies the eighth cranial nerve through the internal acoustic meatus into the petrous part of temporal bone where it ramifies and supplies the internal ear. A

3 *Anterior vestibular artery.* Artery supplying the vestibule, macula of utricle, part of the macula of saccule, as well as the utricle, ampullae, and parts of the anterior and lateral semicircular canals. A

4 *Common cochlear artery.* Ramifying branch of the labyrinthine artery supplying the cochlea. A

5 *Vestibulocochlear artery.* Artery dividing into two branches at the base of the osseous spiral lamina. A

6 Posterior vestibular branch. Branch supplying parts of the vestibule, saccule, and utricle, as well as the macula of saccule, parts of the posterior semicircular canal, and the common bony limb of all semicircular canals. A

7 Cochlear branch. Branch passing along the base of the osseous spiral lamina and anastomosing in the middle one-third of the basal turn of the cochlea with the proper cochlear artery. A

8 *Proper cochlear artery.* Artery giving off branches to the scala tympani and scala media. Its course parallels the spiral ganglion. A

9 *Spiral modiolar artery.* Branches supplying the scala vestibuli. A

10 **Vein of vestibular aqueduct.** Companion vein of the endolymphatic duct. It drains the semicircular ducts and opens into the inferior petrosal sinus. A

11 *Veins of semicircular ducts.* Veins draining the individual semicircular ducts.

12 **Vein of cochlear aqueduct.** Companion vein of the perilymphatic duct. Principal vein draining the cochlea. A

13 *Common modiolar vein.* Union of the vein of the scala vestibuli and the vein of the scala tympani at the inferior end of the basal turn of the cochlea. A

14 *Vein of scala vestibuli.* Vein that mostly drains the scala vestibuli. A

15 *Vein of scala tympani.* Vein draining the scala tympani and the wall of the cochlear duct. A

16 *Vestibulocochlear vein.* Vein arising from the union of the following three veins. A

17 *Anterior vestibular vein.* Vein draining the utricle, and anterior and lateral ampullae. A

18 *Posterior vestibular vein.* Vein draining the saccule and posterior ampulla. A

19 *Vein of cochlear window.* Vein draining the secondary tympanic membrane and surrounding area. A

20 **Labyrinthine veins.** Veins opening into the inferior venous sinus that drain the dura mater and nerves of the internal acoustic meatus. A

21 *GUSTATORY ORGAN.* Organ comprising the taste buds.

22 **Taste bud.** It is as tall as the epithelium and consists of supporting cells and taste cells, each of which bears a microvillar process on its surface that acts as a chemoreceptor. Distribution of taste buds: accumulations in the epithelium of the vallate and foliate papillae, but also occurring as individual taste buds elsewhere than on the tongue. B

23 **Taste pore.** Gaps in the epithelium overlying the apex of the taste buds into which the microvillar processes project. B

21

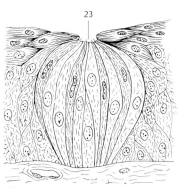

A Labyrinthine vessels

B Taste buds

1 THE INTEGUMENT. Outer skin consisting of three layers: epidermis, dermis, and subcutaneous tissue. On the adult body it covers an area of about 1.8 m^2.

2 SKIN. Collective term for the epidermis and dermis.

3 **Skin sulci.** Variously large furrows in the skin, e.g., the nasolabial sulcus, skin sulci at the joints, small furrows in hairy skin, and grooves between the ridges of hairless skin. A

4 **Dermal ridges; Papillary ridges.** Ridges with underlying connective-tissue papillae on the hairless skin of the palmar side of the hand and plantar side of the foot. A

5 **Skin ligaments.** Connective-tissue bands attaching the skin to the underlying surface. A

6 **Retinaculum caudale.** Connective-tissue remnant of the embryonic notochord between the coccygeal foveola and coccyx. C

7 **Tactile elevations.** Regions of the skin that are better cushioned with fat, e.g., on the phalanges of the fingers and on the balls of the thumb and little finger. B

8 **Tension lines; Cleavage lines.** Lines indicating the course of the collagen fibers in the dermis.

9 **Epidermis.** Outer layer of skin covering the body, ranging in thickness from 30 μm to 4 mm or more. It is stratified and keratinized, and consists of squamous epithelial cells. A

10 **Dermis; Corium.** Layer consisting of tightly woven collagen and elastic fibers that has abundant nerves and vessels but no fatty tissue. A

11 **Papillary layer.** Upper dermal layer that contains numerous cells and fibers. Its connective-tissue papillae interlock with the epidermis. A

12 Papillae. Connective-tissue elevations projecting into the epidermis. They can be arranged in rows (hairless skin) or form branches and vary greatly in terms of form and organization. A E

13 **Reticular layer.** Dermal layer situated directly beneath the papillary layer that contains few cells. It consists of tough, tightly woven bundles of collagen fibers that determine the mechanical characteristics of the skin. A

14 **Hairs.** Collective term of any type of hair.

15 **Downy hair; Primary hair.** Fine, downy hairs that can be distributed over the entire body, especially in neonates. They generally do not contain medullary cells.

16 **Hairs of head.**

17 **Eyebrows.**

18 **Eyelashes.**

19 **Beard.**

20 **Hairs of tragus.**

21 **Hairs of vestibule of nose.**

22 **Axillary hairs.**

23 **Pubic hairs.**

24 **Hair follicle.** Sheath of connective tissue and epithelium enclosing the root of the hair. E

25 **Arrector muscles of hair.** Bundles of smooth muscle that pass from the middle of the hair follicle to the papillary layer of the dermis. They are absent on the eyelashes, eyebrows, hairs of the vestibule of the nose, tragus, and beard. They cause the hair to stand erect (goose bumps) and probably also compress and empty the sebaceous glands. They are innervated by sympathetic nerve fibers arising from the sympathetic trunk. E

26 **Hair streams.** Direction of hair growth.

27 **Hair whorls.** D

28 **Hair crosses.** Sites at which hair streams from two directions meet and then diverge in two new directions perpendicular to their original orientation. D

29 **Skin glands.** Glands arising from the epithelium and in close relationship to the skin.

30 Sweat gland. Usually small eccrine glands, although in specific regions (anus, genitals, axilla) they are present as large apocrine glands. E

31 Sebaceous gland. Holocrine glands that open into the hair follicle. E

32 **Nerve terminals.** Nerve endings that are present as end organs or as free nerve endings. A

33 [Coccygeal foveola]. Depression overlying the coccyx that is produced by the retinaculum caudale.

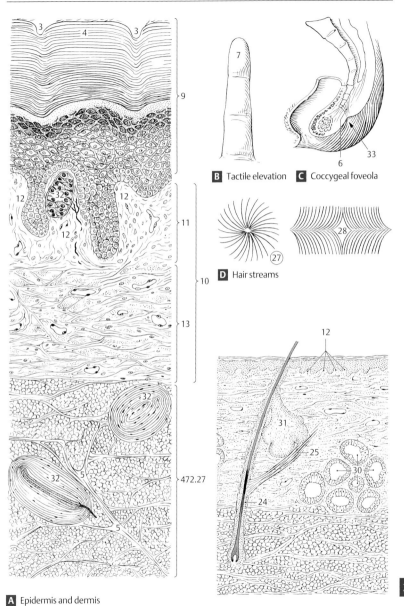

A Epidermis and dermis

B Tactile elevation

C Coccygeal foveola

D Hair streams

E Hair and cutaneous glands

22

1   **Nail.** Fingernail or toenail. A

2   **Nail matrix.** Nail bed epithelium at the root of the nail and lunule. In the lunule region it forms the nail substance. A D

3   **Nail wall.** Fold of skin surrounding the nail on the sides and near the root. A B

4   **Body of nail.** A B D

5   **Lunule.** Whitish, semilunar area at the posterior nail root. Its anterior margin corresponds to the anterior border of the nail-forming tissue. B

6   **Hidden border.** Proximal, posterior border of the nail that is hidden in the nail fold. A

7   **Lateral border.** Lateral margin of the nail lying beneath the nail wall. C

8   **Free border.** Anterior, free margin of the nail. It corresponds to the margin that is cut or worn down. C

9   **Perionyx.** Protruding border of the eponychium. It covers the proximal strip of the lunule. A

10 **Eponychium.** Epithelium lying on the root of the nail that advances slightly at the posterior wall. A

11 **Hyponychium.** Epithelium of the nail bed that lies beneath the nail. Its posterior portion, in the regions of the lunule region and nail root, forms the nail matrix. A

12 **Breast.** Female breast consisting of glandular tissue, connective tissue fibers, and fat. E

13 **Intermammary cleft.** Depression between the left and right breasts.

14 **[Accessory breast].** Additional mammary gland along the embryonic mammary line. F

15 **Nipple.** Structure containing the openings of the lactiferous duct and abundant smooth-muscle tissue. E

16 **Body of breast.** Glandular tissue and surrounding fatty tissue.

17 **Mammary gland.** Glandular tissue of the female breast. E

18 *Axillary process; Axillary tail.* Glandular process directed toward the axilla.

19 *Lobes of mammary gland.* Fifteen to twenty conical lobes of the mammary gland. E

20 *Lobules of mammary gland.* Lobules of each lobe that are divided by connective tissue. E

21 *Lactiferous duct.* Fifteen to twenty ducts draining the lobes of the mammary gland. They have a diameter of 1.7–2.3 mm and open at the nipple. E

22 *Lactiferous sinus.* Spindle-shaped dilatations of the lactiferous ducts with a diameter of 1–2 mm (up to 8 mm during lactation) just before they open at the tip of the nipple. E

23 *Areola.* Round, pigmented area around the nipple with small, scattered bumps produced by the areolar glands. E

24 *Areolar glands.* Ten to fifteen apocrine glands in the areolar region. E

25 *Areolar tubercles.* Irregularly distributed projections in the areola produced by sebaceous glands and small lactiferous glands.

26 *Suspensory ligaments of breast; Suspensory retinaculum of breast.* Connective-tissue bands passing from the skin of the breast to the pectoralis fascia to which they are connected via a thin layer of loose, sliding tissue. E

27 SUBCUTANEOUS TISSUE. G

28 **Fatty layer.** G

29 *Muscle layer.* Local muscle fibers. Cutaneous muscles.

30 *Fibrous layer.* Connective-tissue framework of the fatty layer. G

31 **Membranous layer.** Sheetlike collection of fibers from the fibrous layer beneath the fatty layer, e.g., overlying muscle fascia. G

32 **Loose connective tissue.**

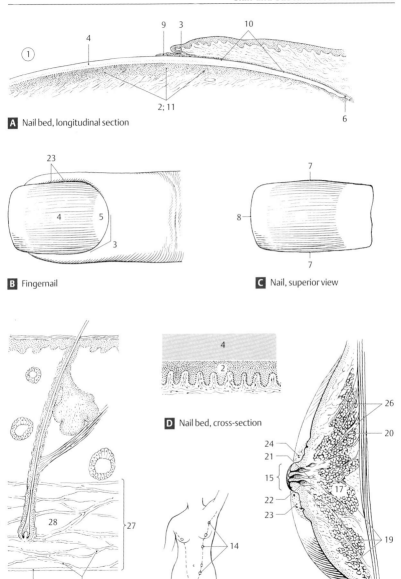

① **A** Nail bed, longitudinal section

B Fingernail

C Nail, superior view

D Nail bed, cross-section

G Subcutaneous tissue

F Mammary line

E Mammary gland

22

Further Reading

Baehr M, Frotscher M. Duus' Topical Diagnosis in Neurology. Anatomy, Physiology, Signs, Symptoms. 4th ed. Stuttgart: Thieme; 2005

Benninghoff A. Anatomie. 15th ed. Munich: Urban & Schwarzenberg; 1994

Benninghoff A,Goerttler K. Lehrbuch der Anatomie des Menschen. 7th ed. Munich: Urban & Schwarzenberg; 1964

Braus H, Elze C. Anatomie des Menschen. 2nd ed. Berlin: Springer; 1960–1965

Bucher O, Wartenberg H. Cytologie, Histologie und mikroskopische Anatomie des Menschen. 12th ed. Bern: Huber; 1997

Carpenter BM. Human Neuroanatomy. 7th ed. Baltimore: Williams & Wilkins; 1976

Clara M. Das Nervensystem des Menschen. 3rd ed. Leipzig: Barth; 1959

Corning HK. Lehrbuch der Topographischen Anatomie, 20th and 21st eds. Munich: Bergmann; 1942

Couinaud . Le foie. Etudes anatomiques et chirurgicales. Paris: Masson; 1957

Crosby EC, Humphrey Tr, Lauer EW. Correlative Anatomy of the Nervous System. New York: Macmillan; 1962

Cunningham DJ. Textbook of Anatomy. 11th ed. London: Oxford University Press; 1972

Dauber W. Anatomische Grundlagen der Funktionsdiagnostik. In: Siebert GK, Atlas der zahnärztlichen Funktionsdiagnostik. 3rd ed. Munich: Hanser Verlag; 1996:20–39

Duvernoy HM. The Superficial Veins of the Human Brain. Heidelberg: Springer; 1975

Duvernoy HM. Human Brainstem Vessels. Berlin: Springer; 1978

Fasel J. The exit of the chorda tympani nerve through the external surface of the base of the skull. Acta Anat. 1986;126:205–207

Frick H, Leonhardt H, Starck D. Human Anatomy. Vol. 1: General Anatomy; Special Anatomy: Limbs, Trunk Wall, Head and Neck. Stuttgart: Thieme; 1991

Fritsch H, Kuehnel W. Color Atlas and Textbook of Human Anatomy. Vol. 2. Internal Organs. 5th ed. Stuttgart: Thieme; in press

Graumann W, Sasse D (eds). Compact Lehrbuch Anatomie. Vol. 2, Bewegungsapparat. Stuttgart: Schattauer; 2003

Gray's Anatomy. 36th ed. Edinburgh: Churchill Livingstone; 1980. 38th ed. 1995

Hafferl A. Lehrbuch der topographischen Anatomie. 2nd ed. Berlin: Springer; 1957

Haines DE. Neuroanatomy. An Atlas of Structures, Sections and Systems. Munich: Urban & Schwarzenberg; 1987

Hamilton WJ. Textbook of Human Anatomy. London: Macmillan; 1958

Heimer L. The Human Brain and Spinal Cord. 2nd ed. New York: Springer; 1995

Henle J. Handbuch der Systematischen Anatomie des Menschen. Braunschweig: Vieweg und Sohn; 1868–1871

Kahle W, Frotscher M. Color Atlas and Textbook of Human Anatomy. Vol. 3. Nervous System and Sensory Organs. 5th ed. Stuttgart: Thieme; 2003

Kaplan HA, Ford DH. The Brain Vascular System. Amsterdam: Elsevier; 1966

Köpf-Maier P (ed). Wolf-Heideggers Atlas der Anatomie des Menschen. 5th ed. Basel: Karger; 2000

Krayenbühl H, Yasargil MG. Zerebrale Angiographie für Klinik und Praxis. 3rd ed. Stuttgart: Thieme; 1979

Kretschmann H-J, Weinrich W. Neurofunctional Systems. Stuttgart: Thieme; 1998

Kubik S. Klinische Anatomie Vol III. 2nd ed. Stuttgart: Thieme; 1969

Lang J. Klinische Anatomie des Kopfes, Neurokranium, Orbita, Kraniozervikaler Übergang. Berlin: Springer; 1981

Lazorthes G. Le systeme nerveux central. 2nd ed. Paris: Masson; 1973

Lierse W. Becken. In: v. Lanz Wachsmuth, Praktische Anatomie Vol II/8a. Berlin: Springer; 1984

Mac Nalty AS. Butterworths Medical Dictionary. London: Butterworths; 1965

Morris J, Parsons J, Schaeffer. Human Anatomy. 12th ed. Philadelphia: Blakiston; 1966

Mühlreiter E. Anatomie des menschlichen Gebisses. 5th ed. Leipzig: Felix; 1928

Mumenthaler M, Schliack H. Peripheral Nerve Lesions. Diagnosis and Therapy. Thieme: Stuttgart; 1991.

Netter FH. The Ciba Collection of Medical Illustrations. New York: Ciba; 1983–1997

Neubert K. Die Basilarmembran des Menschen und ihr Verankerungssystem. Z. Anat. Entwickl.-Gesch. 1949/50; 114:539–588

Nieuwenhuys R, Voogd J, van Huijzen Chr. The Human Central Nervous System. 3rd ed. Berlin: Springer; 1988

Oelrich TM. The striated urogenital sphincter muscle in the female. Anat Rec. 1983;205

Olszewski J, Baxter D. Cytoarchitecture of the Human Brain Stem. Basel: Karger; 1982

Paturet G. Anatomie Humaine. Vols I, II, III. Paris: Masson; 1958

Paxinos G (ed). The Human Nervous System. New York: Academic Press; 1990

Paxinos G, Huang X-F. Atlas of the Human Brain Stem. New York: Academic Press; 1995

Peele TL. The Neuroanatomic Basis for Clinical Neurology. New York: Mc Graw-Hill; 1977

Pernkopf E. Topographische Anatomie des Menschen. Munich: Urban & Schwarzenberg; 1960

Pernkopf E. Atlas der topographischen und abgewandten Anatomie des Menschen. 3rd ed. Munich: Urban & Schwarzenberg; 1994

Platzer W. Atlas der topographischen Anatomie. Stuttgart: Thieme; 1982

Platzer W. Color Atlas of Human Anatomy. Vol. 1. Locomotor System. 5th ed. Stuttgart: Thieme; 2004

Poirier P, Charpy A. D'anatomie humaine. 3rd ed. Paris: Masson; 1920

Rauber A, Kopsch F. Anatomie des Menschen. In 4 vols. Stuttgart: Thieme; 1987–1997

Rauber A, Kopsch F. Lehrbuch und Atlas der Anatomie des Menschen. 19th ed. Stuttgart: Thieme; 1955

Rohen JW. Topographische Anatomie. Stuttgart: Schattauer; 1966, 9th ed. 1992

Schultze O. Atlas und kurzgefaßtes Lehrbuch der topographischen und angewandten Anatomie. 4th ed. Munich: von W. Lubosch, J.F. Lehmanns Verlag; 1935

Schuenke M, Schulte E, Schumacher U. Thieme Atlas of Anatomy: General Anatomy and Musculoskeletal System (consulting editors LM Ross and ED Lamperti). Stuttgart–New York: Thieme; 2006

Schuenke M, Schulte E, Schumacher U. Thieme Atlas of Anatomy: Neck and Internal Organs (consulting editors LM Ross and ED Lamperti). Stuttgart–New York: Thieme; 2006

Schuenke M, Schulte E, Schumacher U. Thieme Atlas of Anatomy: Head and Neuroanatomy (consulting editors LM Ross and ED Lamperti). Stuttgart–New York: Thieme; 2006

Schumacher GH, Schmidt H, Börnig H, Richter W. Anatomie und Biochemie der Zähne. 4th ed. G. Stuttgart: Fischer; 1990

Sicher H. Oral Anatomy. 4th ed. Saint Louis: Mosby; 1965

Sieglbauer F. Lehrbuch der normalen Anatomie des Menschen. 8th ed. Munich: Urban & Schwarzenberg: Munich; 1958

Sobotta J, Becher H. Atlas der Anatomie des Menschen. 16th ed. Munich: Urban & Schwarzenberg; 1962

Sobotta J, Becher H. Atlas der Anatomie des Menschen. In 2 vols. Munich: Urban & Schwarzenberg; 1993

Sobotta J. Atlas der Anatomie des Menschen, Vols 1 und 2. Edited by R Putz and R Pabst. 21th ed. Urban & Fischer; 2000

Spalteholz W, Spanner R. Handatlas der Anatomie des Menschen. 16th ed. Amsterdam: Scheltema & Holkema; 1961

Stephens RB, Stillwell DL. Arteries and Veins of the Human Brain. Thomas Springfield/III; 1969

Steriade M, Jones EG, Mc Cormick DA. Thalamus, Vols. I and II. Oxford: Elsevier; 1997

Tandler J. Lehrbuch der Systematischen Anatomie. Leipzig: Vogel; 1926

Testut L. D'anatomie humaine. 4th ed. Paris; 1900

Tillmann B. Farbatlas der Anatomie, Zahnmedizin–Humanmedizin. Stuttgart: Thieme; 1997

Toldt C, Hochstetter F. Anatomischer Atlas. 23rd ed. Vienna: Urban & Schwarzenberg; 1961; 27th ed. Munich: Urban & Schwarzenberg; 1979

Töndury G. Anatomie der Lungengefäße. Ergebn. ges. Tuberk.- u. Lung.-Forsch. 1958;14:61–100

Töndury G. Angewandte und topographische Anatomie. 3rd ed. Stuttgart: Thieme; 1965; 5th ed. 1981

Truex RC, Carpenter MB. Strong and Elwyn's Human Neuroanatomy. 5th ed. Baltimore: Williams & Wilkins; 1964

van Damme J.-P.J. Behavioral Anatomy of the Abdominal Arteries. Surg Clin North Am. 1993; 73:699–725

Viamonte jr. M, Ruttimann A. Atlas of Lymphography. Stuttgart: Thieme; 1980

Villiger E, Ludwig E. Gehirn und Rückenmark, 11th–13rd ed. Leipzig: Engelmann; 1940

von Hayek H. Die menschliche Lunge. 2nd ed. Berlin–Heidelberg: Springer; 1970

von Lüdinghausen M. The Venous Drainage of the Human Myocardium Advances in anatomy, embryology and cell biology, Vol. 168. Berlin: Springer; 2003

Waldeyer A, Mayet A. Anatomie des Menschen. 16th ed. Berlin: De Gruyter; 1993

Wolf-Heidegger G. Atlas der systematischen Anatomie. Basel: Karger; 1957

W

Y

Z